P9-DHP-274

NUTRITION IN AGING

NUTRITION IN AGING

ELEANOR D. SCHLENKER, *Ph.D., R.D.*

Professor and Head
Department of Human Nutrition, Foods, and Exercise
College of Human Resources and Education
Virginia Polytechnic Institute and State University
Blacksburg, Virginia

THIRD EDITION
illustrated

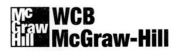

Boston, Massachusetts   Burr Ridge, Illinois   Dubuque, Iowa
Madison, Wisconsin   New York, New York   San Francisco, California   St. Louis, Missouri

WCB/McGraw-Hill

A Division of The **McGraw·Hill** Companies

NUTRITION IN AGING

Copyright © 1998 by The McGraw-Hill Companies, Inc. All rights reserved.
Previous editions © by Mosby—Year Book, Inc. Printed in the United States of America.
Except as permitted under the United States Copyright Act of 1976, no part of this
publication may be reproduced or distributed in any form or by any means, or stored
in a data base or retrieval system, without the prior written permission of the publisher.

 This book is printed on recycled, acid-free paper containing 10% postconsumer waste.

1 2 3 4 5 7 8 9 0 QPD/QPD 9 0 9 8 7

ISBN 0–8151–8504–9

Publisher: *Ed Bartell*
Executive editor: *Vicki Malinee*
Developmental editor: *Jean Babrick*
Senior marketing manager: *Pamela S. Cooper*
Project manager: *Donna Nemmers*
Design freelance coordinator: *Mary Christianson*
Cover designer: *Ben Neff*
Cover illustrator: *Jason Dowd*
Compositor: *Shepherd, Inc.*
Typeface: *10/11 Galliard*
Printer: *Quebecor Printing Dubuque, Inc.*

Library of Congress Cataloging-in-Publication Data

Schlenker, Eleanor D.
    Nutrition in aging/Eleanor D. Schlenker.—3rd ed.
        p.   cm.
    Includes bibliographical references and index.
    ISBN 0–8151–8504–9
    1. Aging—Nutritional aspects. 2. Aged—Nutrition. 3. Nutrition
disorders in old age. I. Title.
    QP86.S35   1997
    613.2′084′6–dc21   97–9477
                                                             CIP

http://www.mhcollege.com

WT
100
S 34 n
1997

Contributors

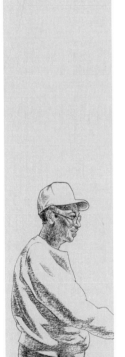

MARIE FANELLI KUCZMARSKI, PH.D., R.D., L.D.

Associate Professor
Department of Nutrition and Dietetics
University of Delaware
Newark, Delaware

ROBERT J. KUCZMARSKI, DR.P.H., R.D., L.D.

Nutritionist
National Center for Health Statistics
Centers for Disease Control and Prevention
United States Department of Health and Human Services
Hyattsville, Maryland

CONNIE E. VICKERY, PH.D., R.D., L.D.

Professor
Department of Nutrition and Dietetics
University of Delaware
Newark, Delaware

MARSHA READ, PH.D., R.D.

Professor
Department of Nutrition
University of Nevada-Reno
Reno, Nevada
(material reprinted from second edition)

366 29955

To my father, Harold Schlenker, who
throughout his 81 years continued to
learn, grow, and be a role model of
successful aging.

Preface

Throughout this decade and into the next century the older population will continue to expand in size and diversity. Individual older people differ greatly from one another in their nutrient requirements and need for nutrition services. The aging individual in good health who exercises regularly and takes few medications may have nutrient requirements that are similar to those of younger adults of the same sex, build, and health status. Conversely, the chronically ill elderly adult who is regularly taking a wide variety of over-the-counter and prescription drugs is likely to have increased needs for particular nutrients as compared to his or her peers who enjoy good health. An active older person living in the community who is able to obtain and prepare adequate meals will also need reliable sources of nutrition information to support self-care, whereas the homebound older adult must depend on nutrition programs and services to deliver appropriate preprepared or shelf-stable foods to meet his or her nutritional needs. The frail institutionalized elderly person is likely to need nutrient-dense, easily swallowed foods that provide substantial levels of nutrients, and may require help with feeding. Each of these individuals presents a unique challenge to the professional responsible for his or her nutritional care. Older people will comprise a significant and growing proportion of the future consumers of health care.

AUDIENCE

This book has been designed to serve as a resource or textbook for upper level undergraduate or graduate nutrition students, or students in other health professions who are preparing to work with older people. It is expected that the reader will have a science background that includes chemistry and physiology as well as a strong foundation in applied and metabolic nutrition, although several chapters could be helpful to a student or practitioner with a limited knowledge of nutrition.

APPROACH

The third edition of Nutrition in Aging has been expanded to include both emerging issues and new research information bearing on the nutrition needs, problems, and delivery of care in aging. It is designed to provide the student or practitioner with the knowledge and skills necessary to assume an active role on the health care team that makes decisions regarding the food and nutrition needs of the older individual and provides helpful advice to the older client or caregiver regarding food selection. An overall theme of this edition is successful aging, and the role of the nutrition or health professional is helping older people reach this goal. Appropriate dietary and exercise patterns are the cornerstone of successful aging and can improve the quality of life of all older individuals regardless of their health status.

COMPREHENSIVE COVERAGE OF TOPICS

The third edition of this book has been updated throughout and continues to provide a broad background in many subject areas that will be useful to the nutrition or health professional working with older people. In this edition some topics have been grouped differently to provide greater depth and integration and to facilitate understanding, and new sections have been added. The professional working in the field of aging needs to recognize the increasing growth and diversity of the older population, know which groups are expanding most rapidly, and understand the underlying causes of these changes. Chapter 1 provides a brief overview of the current and emerging aging population, their social and health characteristics, and the implications of these characteristics for the delivery of health care. Chapter 2 emphasizes current research in aging with a newly added section on the theories of aging and their relationship to physiological aging. Also included is expanded and updated information on the impact of nutrition and lifestyle on physical well-being in light of current health promotion and intervention strategies. Succeeding chapters focus on current understanding and research limitations regarding the changing nutrient requirements of aging adults. Chapter 3 describes the existing Recommended Dietary Allowances for older people and the need for reevaluation of these recommendations. Current standards for dietary intakes of the macronutrients are addressed in terms of both nutritional adequacy and the dietary goals for health. The following chapter provides an overview of the known changes in the physiology and secretions within the gastrointestinal tract that occur with advancing age and influence food intake and digestion and the absorption of nutrients. There is expanded coverage of changes in the oral cavity as influenced by the aging process and chronic disease, and a new section on food sensitivity and food allergy in older people. Chapters 5 through 7 focus on new research describing energy, vitamin, and mineral requirements in the aging adult. Energy needs are related to both changes in body composition and physical activity. Alterations in hormonal patterns that influence changes in body composition throughout the adult years are explored. Vitamin and mineral requirements are interpreted in light of physiologic and metabolic changes that are observed in the older individual. Recent evidence from metabolic studies conducted with community-living older people that suggest alterations in vitamin and mineral requirements in the elderly is described in detail. The reader is also alerted to particular subgroups of older people who are particularly vulnerable to low intakes of important nutrients because of ethnic background, race, and socioeconomic or health status.

The second half of the new edition is devoted to application of the basic principles of nutrition and aging that have been learned. Chapters 8 through 11 describe the myriad of factors that affect food selection and overall nutritional status and nutrition assessment methods in elderly people. Chapter 8 contains in-depth analysis of the influence of race, sex, income level, health, and functional disability on selecting, obtaining, and preparing nourishing food and the serious implications when multiple risk factors affect food intake. The following chapter provides detailed national statistics describing the dietary, anthropometric, and biochemical status of aging populations in the United States. Older groups are compared on the basis of income and poverty status, sex, race, and ethnic background, and differences among white, black, and Hispanic elderly groups are emphasized. New data presented were obtained from the most recent phase of the Continuing Survey of Food Intakes of Individuals conducted by the U.S. Department of Agriculture, and the ongoing Third

National Health and Nutrition Examination Survey being conducted by the U.S. Department of Health and Human Services. Both over-the-counter and prescription medications influence food intake and nutritional status, and professionals working with the elderly need to be aware of these effects. Chapter 10 provides a helpful overview of the various types, classes, and brand names of drugs commonly prescribed for and used by the older population in the management of pain, neurological conditions, and chronic disease. The nutritional implications of each type of drug including the effects on food intake or, conversely, the effects of food on drug utilization, as well as any specific nutrients of concern are described in this chapter. The last chapter in this section focuses on the methods of nutritional assessment appropriate for older people. It begins by providing an overview of assessment and follows with specific methods that can be selected based on the goals for the assessment, the facility or community setting where the assessment will take place, and the level of resources available. A new section focuses on nutrition assessment in congregate meal sites and adult day care settings, and includes new assessment tools adapted for and validated with older people.

The last section of the new edition groups together information on nutrition problems and the nutritional implications of chronic disease in elderly people with practical intervention strategies. Specific and updated nutrition-related topics included in chapter 12 are bone health, anemia, body weight management, protein energy malnutrition, and gastrointestinal problems. A new topic not included in the previous edition is the etiology and management of pressure sores, an issue of increasing concern in long term care facilities. The following chapter addresses chronic diseases and medical problems arising from the physiological changes occurring with advancing age. In order to better integrate these areas of study, the discussion of physiologic changes formerly included in chapter 1 were moved to chapter 13 in the new edition. Interventions to reduce or delay the physiologic and pathologic changes leading to chronic disease are stressed throughout this section. The final chapter provides an overview of new trends in long term care that directly impact the nutritional care of the elderly in community and institutional settings. Included is an analysis of changes in government policy that have made available funds for the delivery of community-based long term care within the continuum of care. Data from the recently completed evaluation of the federally funded Elderly Nutrition Program provide a basis for understanding the importance and limitations of the congregate and home delivered meal programs in the United States. The new nutrition guidelines for long term care facilities established through the OBRA legislation are also discussed.

RECOGNITION OF CONTROVERSY

Despite the increasing emphasis on research in nutrition and aging, many questions remain unanswered. Researchers or clinicians at times report conflicting findings in studies evaluating the nutrient requirements and metabolism of older people, or the relationship of particular nutrients and nonnutrients to the development of chronic and nutrition-related disorders. Alternative points of view along with supporting experimental evidence are presented to encourage the reader to critically evaluate available data and develop appropriate conclusions.

BALANCE OF THEORY AND APPLICATION

Working with older adults demands a clear understanding of nutrition theory and principles along with the skills to translate these principles into dietary advice or nutrition care plans that are both practical and appropriate in a variety of settings. The nutrition and health professional must understand why a problem exists, identify alternative solutions, and involve the older client and caregiver in defining the most realistic plan of action. Meeting the food and nutrition needs of older individuals often requires compromise between what is ideal and what is possible in the situation presented.

FOCUS ON DIVERSITY

Since the preparation of the second edition, increasing information has become available describing the socioeconomic, health, and nutritional characteristics of older individuals from various ethnic backgrounds and races, including African American, Mexican-American, Hispanic, American Indian, and Asian-American groups, and these data are included throughout the new edition. A new section describing the food habits and food selection patterns of several ethnic and racial groups has been added to chapter 8. When available, data are presented that allow comparison of the young-old (ages 65–74) with the oldest-old (ages 85+), who often differ in health status, functional ability, nutrient needs, and the types of nutrition services required.

HEALTH ISSUES
AND LONG-TERM CARE

As older persons are and will continue to be the largest users of health care services, positive nutrition and lifestyle practices and intervention strategies to promote the highest level of health and function possible are a constant theme throughout this text. The final chapter focusing on nutrition services and nutrition education within the continuum of health care builds awareness of the opportunities, challenges, and creative approaches for delivering quality food and nutrition services at all levels of care.

RESOURCES FOR FUTURE USE

To maximize the usefulness of this text for students and practitioners with professional responsibilities, an extensive bibliography is provided with each chapter that includes both current and classical references. Screening tools and dietary assessment materials found in Chapter 11 and in the Appendix can be adapted to various community and clinical situations. The resource lists of nutrition education and program development materials have been updated and audiovisual resources are included.

PEDAGOGICAL AIDS

Several features facilitate the use of the book by educators, students, and practitioners:
- **Learning Objectives** direct the reader's attention to specific subject areas and outcomes to be achieved by studying the chapter.
- **Review Questions** aid in the study and discussion of the material. These questions are designed to reinforce the important content to be retained from the chapter and encourage critical thinking in respect to controversies and challenges.
- **Suggested Learning Activities** provide opportunities for students to apply the theories and principles learned to clinical and professional situations. These activities also encourage students to interact with older people in various facilities and develop communication skills with this client group. Current controversies in the field are defined for further study or evaluation.
- **Case Studies** have been added to the third edition to encourage students to apply their learning to solving practical nutrition problems similar to those encountered in community or clinical settings.
- **Glossary** has been expanded to include new words and terms in each chapter.

ACKNOWLEDGMENTS

I continue to be indebted to the many people who make possible the preparation of each new edition. Both the content and organization of this edition were improved immeasurably by the following reviewers who devoted much time and effort to evaluating the second edition and offering many helpful suggestions: LuAnn Soliah, Baylor University, Ira Wolinsky, University of Houston, Winifred Morse, University of Wisconsin-Eau Claire, Karen Kubena, Texas A and M University, and Christopher Melby, Colorado State University.

I would also like to recognize the continuing contributors to this edition who have shared their expertise on important topics: Marie Fanelli Kuczmarski, Robert Kuczmarski, and

Connie Vickery. Included in this edition is material prepared by Marsha Read, a contributor to the second edition. Elizabeth Thomas, Kathryn Reynolds, and Rita Sigmon developed the pedagogical aids included in each chapter.

It is important that I acknowledge the ongoing help of Jean Babrick, my developmental editor at Mosby—Year Book who put together the new organization of this edition and provided technical support and expertise through this time of transition. Karen Bankston, my copy editor, took struggling sentences and turned them into something we could both be happy with. Others who contributed to this effort included Maryam Majidy, Nyira Lugogo, Kristen Coyne, Jeannine Simon, Joy Breneman, Tracy Wagner, and Alicia Hogbin, who assisted with library research and found new references and new information; Mary Taylor, who turned my ragged copy into readable manuscript and produced many of the new illustrations; the faculty, students, and staff of the Department of Human Nutrition, Foods, and Exercise, who provided continuing encouragement through this long process; and Dean Janet Johnson of the College of Human Resources and Education, who supported this endeavor. Finally, I would like to thank Donna Nemmers, project manager at McGraw-Hill, who has facilitated the transfer of this manuscript from Mosby—Year Book to McGraw-Hill.

Eleanor D. Schlenker
Blacksburg, Virginia

Contents

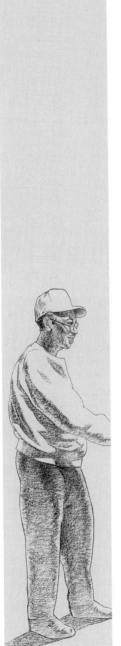

13 NUTRITION, PHYSIOLOGIC FUNCTION, AND CHRONIC DISEASE

14 NUTRITION AND THE CONTINUUM OF CARE FOR OLDER ADULTS

APPENDICES

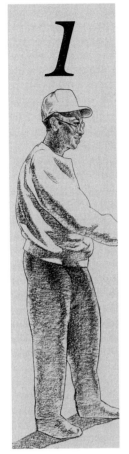

1

Who Are the Aging?

✦✦✦

Objectives

After studying the chapter, the student should be able to:

✔ *Recognize the current and projected size and diversity of the aging population in the United States.*

✔ *Define the demographic and health characteristics of the aging population and the implications for nutrition services, health promotion, and health care.*

✔ *Describe how life expectancy differs depending on age, gender, and race.*

✔ *Understand the aging process and be able to develop ways to help individuals move from usual to successful aging.*

✔ *Identify the activities of daily living that influence the quality of life of older people and their capacity to live independently.*

INTRODUCTION

America is an aging society. One of every eight people is now age 65 or older, and by the year 2030, that ratio will be one in five.[20] These population trends have far-reaching implications for our society, from public concern about rising health care costs to increasing efforts by food manufacturers to develop easy-to-prepare products that will appeal to older consumers. The growing number of older people presents both a challenge and a responsibility for the health professional. For the older population in good health, nutrition and fitness education

that promotes continuing physical well-being is a priority. Older individuals in declining health need specialized nutrition services designed to maintain the highest possible level of independence and functional capacity. The growing elderly population has diverse needs and resources. These people will require health and nutrition services that do not exist today. Our knowledge of the nutritional needs and problems and factors that influence food intake in older people is very limited; furthermore, we do not understand the biologic and physiologic changes that occur as part of the aging process or how these changes influence nutritional status. Our challenge is to begin developing nutrition recommendations and services that will meet the changing nutrient needs of tomorrow's elderly.

POPULATION TRENDS
Definition of Age

In legal matters age is defined on the basis of chronologic age, or the number of years a person has lived. Reaching a particular age usually determines eligibility for benefits or services, although standards are not consistent. One becomes eligible at age 60 to participate in the Nutrition Program for the Elderly and other services mandated under the Older Americans Act, one becomes eligible to receive Medicare and full Social Security benefits at age 65, and laws protecting the older worker against age discrimination become effective at age 55. In the United States age 65, still the typical age of retirement, is viewed as the benchmark of the older population.

When older people were fewer in number, census and health statistics grouped together all individuals over the age of 64. This practice failed to recognize the physical and socioeconomic changes that occur in older people as they continue to age. For example, those age 65 who recently retired are likely to be in good health; those age 85 or older are likely to have some functional disability and need assistance with housekeeping, meal preparation, or transportation. Most women ages 65 to 74 live with a spouse; most women over the age of 84 live alone.[18] So that we might evaluate these differences and recognize when they occur, current census statistics categorize older people into three groups: ages 65 to 74 are the young-old, ages 75 to 84 are the aged, and ages 85 and older are the oldest-old.[18]

Although chronologic age is relatively easy to determine, it is a poor measure of the physical health, mental alertness, or vitality of an older individual. Despite the fact that advancing age increases the likelihood of chronic disease or functional disability, many older people entering their eighth or ninth decade have independent, active lifestyles that include household chores, regular exercise, and visiting with friends. A health professional should never form an opinion about the physical or mental status or functional abilities of an older client solely on the basis of chronologic age.

Growth of the Aging Population

Diversity and growth are two terms that describe the elderly population in the United States.[18] Although generally we refer to the population age 65 and older as the elderly, each age, gender, race, and ethnic group has distinctive characteristics. Individuals within the elderly population differ greatly in their needs, abilities, and resources. Some older people either by choice or because of financial necessity continue to work for pay, whereas others fill their leisure time with travel, hobbies, or volunteer work. Many grandparents spend their time caring for their grandchildren. Rural elderly as compared to urban elderly have reduced access to community centers, social activities, and health and support services such as home delivered meals. However, both urban and rural older people may feel socially isolated or lonely. Deteriorating health status and difficulty in preparing meals limits the nutritional choices of some older people, whereas those in better health who have discretionary income can more easily prepare their own meals or eat in restaurants.

There are more elderly people now than ever before in history. At one time we were a nation of youth. In colonial times half of the population was under the age of 16, and most people did not survive to old age. In 1990 less than one person in four, or only 23% of the population, was under the age of 16, and about half were age 33 or older.[18] During this century older age groups have increased in size far more rapidly than have younger age groups, both in absolute numbers and as a proportion of the total population (fig. 1-1). Since 1900 the general population has tripled but the population of people age 65 and older increased by a factor of 10, from 3.1 million to 31.1 million. By the year 2050, this number could double.[18]

A common assumption is that this increase in number of older people is the result of increased longevity. In fact, an increased average life span is only part of the explanation. Another primary

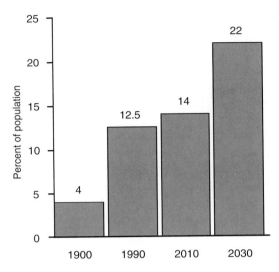

FIG. 1-1   Proportion of Older People in the General Population. People age 65 and older are increasing both in absolute numbers and as a percentage of the total population.

Taeuber, C.: Sixty-five plus in America, Curr. Pop. Reports P23-278, Washington, D.C., 1992, U.S. Bureau of the Census.

cause is the high number of births before 1920 and after World War II. The aging of those born prior to 1920 has resulted in the rising number of people now in their 80s and 90s. Future increases in the elderly population relate to the high number of births immediately following World War II, often referred to as the baby boom. Seventy-five million babies were born between 1946 and 1964, almost 70% more than were born in the 20 years prior.[18] The aging of the baby boom generation will cause the rapid increase in the number of older people that is expected to begin about 2010. Based on projected mortality rates and birth rates, by 2030 the United States will have more than 64 million people over age 64, accounting for 18% of the population.[18] The low birth rate between 1964 and 1980 also reduced the proportion of younger groups in the general population. Because the growth in the elderly population will be fairly slow until 2010, health planners are urging that we use this window of opportunity to prepare for the future.

Composition of the Aging Population

Age. The projected increase in numbers of older people will not be equal across all age groups (fig. 1-2). Currently, most older people are among the young-old (ages 65 to 74). By the year 2000 nearly half of the older population will have reached age 75. The 85 and older group is the fastest growing among all age groups. In 1900 very few people reached age 85, but by 1990, 3 million people were at least age 85. By 2010 this number will double to over 6 million, and by 2030 it will reach more than 8 million. Although people age 85 and older represent only about 1% of the U.S. population, they have begun to have a major impact on available health and social service systems. Centenarians, people age 100 or older, are also increasing in number. The 1990 census identified 36,000 centenarians in the United States.[18]

Race. Older age groups will also increase in ethnicity. Today, the older population is predominantly white. Only 8% of African Americans, 5% of Hispanics, and 6% of American Indians and Asian Americans are age 65 or older, as compared to 13% of whites.[18] This difference relates in part to the higher fertility rates among the African American and Hispanic populations, resulting in greater proportions of children and young people. Another factor contributing to this difference is the lower life expectancy of these ethnic groups as compared to the white population. In the future, however, the proportion of older people in the African American and Hispanic populations will increase, as life expectancy continues to rise in these groups. Ethnic groups now account for 10% of all people age 65 or older and will increase to 17% by the year 2000.[26] By 2050 one of every three people above age 64 will be African American, American Indian, Asian American, or Hispanic.[18]

Sex. The ratio of women to men varies dramatically among different age groups. At younger ages the numbers of women and men are about equal, but at older ages women outnumber men. This disparity becomes even greater as individuals continue to age. Between ages 65 and 69, women outnumber men five to four; by age 85, there are five women for every two men.[18] The relative numbers of men and

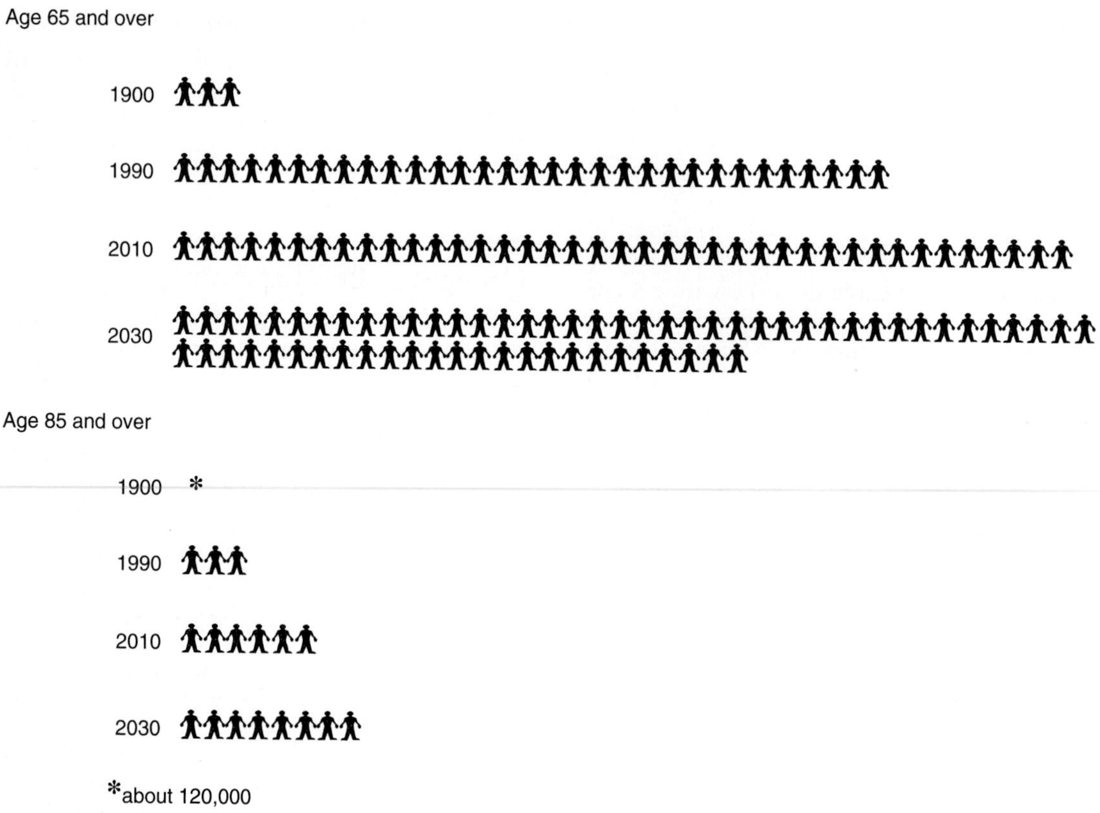

Age 65 and over

1900 𝍓𝍓𝍓

1990 𝍓𝍓𝍓𝍓𝍓𝍓𝍓𝍓𝍓𝍓𝍓𝍓𝍓𝍓𝍓𝍓𝍓𝍓𝍓𝍓𝍓𝍓𝍓𝍓𝍓𝍓𝍓𝍓𝍓𝍓𝍓

2010 𝍓𝍓𝍓𝍓𝍓𝍓𝍓𝍓𝍓𝍓𝍓𝍓𝍓𝍓𝍓𝍓𝍓𝍓𝍓𝍓𝍓𝍓𝍓𝍓𝍓𝍓𝍓𝍓𝍓𝍓𝍓𝍓𝍓𝍓𝍓𝍓𝍓𝍓𝍓

2030 𝍓𝍓

Age 85 and over

1900 *

1990 𝍓𝍓𝍓

2010 𝍓𝍓𝍓𝍓𝍓

2030 𝍓𝍓𝍓𝍓𝍓𝍓𝍓

*about 120,000

FIG. 1-2 Growth of the Older Population (each figure equals 1 million people). The older population has undergone explosive growth in this century and this growth will continue. Between 1990 and 2030, the 65 and over age group will increase over twofold and the 85 and over age group will increase about threefold.

Taeuber, C.: Sixty-five plus in America, Curr. Pop. Reports P23-278, Washington, D.C., 1992, U.S. Bureau of the Census.

women are one of the most striking characteristics of the oldest-old population group. At every age men have a higher mortality than women, and for many years the female advantage in life expectancy continued to widen. Because women live longer, they have a longer period of retirement and are more likely to live alone or with nonrelatives in their later years. These factors also increase the vulnerability of older women to economic insecurity at advanced ages.

Implications of Present Trends

The projected increases in the number and proportion of older people in the population have implications for both the family and our society as a whole. As improved health care and medical technology continue to increase life expectancy, the issues of active life expectancy and quality of life are receiving more attention. More people will live to older ages but may suffer physical or mental disabilities. People in their

60s who are recently retired will have the responsibility of providing economic and emotional support, assistance with household tasks such as shopping or meal preparation, and daily personal care to very old or frail family members. Currently, one-third of older women with some degree of disability receive their primary care from their children, whereas disabled older men usually are cared for by their wives.[26] Unmarried older people or those with no children are more likely to be institutionalized. In the coming years support services for an increasing number of older people with no close family will have to be provided by government or private agencies.

Older people are the most frequent users of health services, including visits to physicians, hospital stays, and prescription drugs. Although people over age 65 represent only 12% of the population, $3 of every $5 in government-funded health care goes toward care of the elderly.[18] As their number increases, older people will require an ever-growing share of both public and private health insurance resources. Health promotion activities focusing on appropriate diet, exercise, and lifestyle patterns should be emphasized among young and middle-aged segments of the population to ensure their continuing good health at older ages.

In future years the aging population will exert an ever-increasing influence in a society which has been youth oriented. With increasing numbers of older consumers wielding buying power, more products, services, and advertising will be targeted toward this market. Nutrition professionals should be teaming with food industry specialists and social service providers to develop unique food products and food and nutrition services that will meet the needs of tomorrow's burgeoning older population.

TRENDS IN MORTALITY AND MORBIDITY

Life expectancy, mortality rates, and the prevalence of chronic diseases have all changed dramatically during this century. Medical advances in the treatment of diseases as well as alterations in lifestyle have contributed to these differences. Such changes as improved diets and use of new medications to control blood pressure have had a positive effect. Because all major causes of death in middle age and beyond are influenced by modifiable risk factors, efforts toward promoting health and reducing disease risk could further increase life expectancy.

Changes in Life Expectancy

Basis for changes in life expectancy. Life expectancy, or the average remaining years of life for a person of a given age, has increased in all age groups since 1900. The most striking increases occurred during the first half of this century as infant mortality declined and antibiotics to control pneumonia, influenza, and other infectious diseases were discovered.[26] Prior to these discoveries many people died at young ages. People now survive to older ages and over time develop chronic diseases. Decreased mortality from heart disease and stroke, achieved by reducing hypertension and adopting appropriate diet, exercise, and lifestyle patterns, has contributed to the increase in life expectancy. Overall life expectancy at birth increased from a mean of 47 years in 1900 to 75.5 years in 1992.[22]

Although gains in life expectancy at birth have been substantial, gains in life expectancy at age 65 and older have been relatively small, especially in men.[25] Since 1900, life expectancy at age 65 has increased by 3.8 years for men and 6.9 years for women. Life expectancy at age 85 has increased by about 1.5 years for men and 2.5 years for women. A 65-year-old in the United States can expect to live another 17 years. Currently, 20% of the U.S. population lives to age 85 or older. If projected trends continue, by 2010 half of the population will survive to at least age 85.[17] This has important implications for both health care institutions and community service agencies, since individuals over age 85 are more likely to have some functional disability or require specialized health care.

Differences in life expectancy between men and women. Gains in life span have not been equal in both sex groups[22] (fig. 1-3). Women have made increasing strides in life expectancy compared to men. In 1900 women could expect

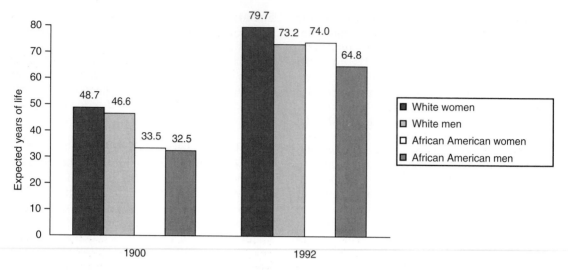

FIG. 1-3   Increases In Life Expectancy Since 1900. Significant increases in life expectancy since 1900 were made possible through medical discoveries to control infectious diseases; more recently improved medical management of chronic diseases and lifestyle changes have reduced cardiovascular risk. Unfortunately gains were not equal for both sexes and all ethnic groups.

United States Department of Health and Human Services: Health, United States, 1993, DHHS Publication No. (PHS) 94-1232, Hyattsville, MD, 1994, National Center for Health Statistics.

to live two years longer than men of similar age; women now live about seven years longer. The gender gap in life expectancy has been decreasing somewhat, as men continue to make gains. The current difference in life expectancy at birth between men and women is 6.9 years, compared to 7.7 years in 1970.

The basis for the increased **life span,** or average number of years of life, of women has received much attention. In experimental animals the increased life span of females is believed to relate to genetic factors. The difference in life span between men and women could be the result of genetic factors or environmental factors or a combination of both. One major influence on the life span in men and women is the pattern of incidence of heart disease; men are more likely to die of heart disease at younger ages. Mortality rates from heart disease between ages 55 and 59 are 402 per 100,000 men and only 152 per 100,000 women.[18] The death rates from heart disease continue to be twice as high

in men than in women until age 75. The biological basis for this difference in deaths from heart disease may involve estrogen, the female sex hormone, which exerts a favorable influence on serum lipoprotein patterns and the distribution of body fat.

Lifestyle behaviors influence mortality patterns in both sexes. Cigarette smoking, for example, has brought about changes in mortality patterns among women. In the first half of this century smoking was uncommon among women, and in the early 1970s it was concluded that two-thirds of the difference in life span between men and women in middle age and beyond could be explained by differences in smoking habits.[1] As the use of cigarettes by women has increased, their incidence of lung cancer has risen to be nearly identical to that of men 30 years ago. Ironically, smoking has declined among men, and this change is reflected in the decreasing rates of lung cancer in men and increasing life expectancy.[23]

Differences in life expectancy among ethnic groups. African American men and women have experienced lower gains in life expectancy both at birth and at age 65 than white men and women[22] (fig. 1-3). Expected years of life at birth are eight years longer for white men as compared to African American men, and almost six years longer for white women as compared to African American women. Although white men at age 65 can expect to live another 15.4 years, their African American counterparts can expect to live only 13.4 years. Life expectancy at age 65 is 19.2 years for white women and 17.2 years for African American women. It is interesting to note, however, that after age 84 advantages in life expectancy shift from white people to African Americans, with African Americans living longer.[18] Several ideas[5] have been put forth to explain this crossover in mortality risk. First, the relationship between age and health status may be stronger in white elderly than in African American elderly. Among African Americans reduced lifelong access to medical care or occupations demanding a high level of physical activity may have a greater influence on general health than age per se. The older African American who survives to an advanced age may have enjoyed better health throughout adulthood. Also, African American elderly appear to be more likely to "recover" or regain function after a debilitating illness.

Mortality rates differed between African American adults and white adults, ages 35 to 77, who participated in the First National Health and Nutrition Examination Survey (NHANES I).[11] About 70% of the higher mortality observed among the African Americans was related to smoking habits, a high prevalence of diabetes, elevated systolic blood pressure (160 mg Hg or higher), high body mass index, and low family income. Otten and colleagues also pointed to racial inequalities in the use of medical procedures to treat coronary heart disease, noting that white adults are more likely to receive specialized treatment or surgical intervention. Inadequate medical supervision and lack of nutrition counseling for appropriate management of obesity, diabetes, and hypertension very likely contribute to the higher death rates observed among African Americans.

TABLE 1-1   Leading Causes of Death in Older People (Deaths per 100,000 in Age Group)

Cause of Death	65–74	75–84	85+
All causes	2,651	5,979	15,231
Diseases of the heart	897	2,292	6,717
Cancer	870	1,339	1,739
Cerebrovascular disease	144	497	1,625
Chronic obstructive pulmonary disease	156	327	447
Pneumonia and influenza	57	235	1,029

Data from United States Department of Health and Human Services: Health, United States, 1993, DHHS Publication No. (PHS) 94-1232, Hyattsville, MD, 1994, National Center for Health Statistics; and, United States Senate Special Committee on Aging: Aging America. Trends and projections (annotated), Serial No. 101-J, Washington, DC, 1990, U.S. Government Printing Office.

Leading Causes of Death

The leading causes of death in the United States are heart disease, cancer, and cerebrovascular disease (stroke). These three conditions are responsible for three of every four deaths in people age 65 or over[26] (table 1-1). Influenza and pneumonia are important causes of death in people over age 85. The number of deaths caused by cancer, especially lung cancer, is rising among elderly people, and in particular among African American men.[18] This is in contrast to the continuing decline in deaths from coronary heart disease in all age and sex groups. Nevertheless, eliminating deaths from cancer would have relatively little effect on life expectancy, increasing the average life span by only two years. Eliminating deaths from heart disease, however, would add an average of five years to life expectancy in the over 65 age group.[26] The increasing vulnerability of the older individual to infection and the life-threatening events associated with advanced chronic disease is evident in the dramatic increase in mortality rates between ages 65 to 74 and ages 85 and over.

In general, deaths associated with chronic diseases have declined significantly in recent years.

Since 1970 death rates from ischemic heart disease and cerebrovascular disease have dropped by more than 40%.[24] This decline has been attributed to the adoption of preventive health practices, including reduced dietary fat, regular physical exercise, avoidance of smoking, and limited use of alcohol. Moreover, an increasing number of older adults are rating their health as good to excellent rather than fair to poor.[22] This would suggest that the older people who are enjoying an increased life span are actually healthier. Nevertheless, the observed decline in mortality rates could have come about through heroic medical interventions that rescued frail or debilitated individuals from death. Such survivors would continue to suffer from serious disease and disability.

According to Verbrugge,[27] prevalence rates for heart disease, hypertension, and arthritis have actually increased in recent years along with the use of health services. This suggests an increasing burden of illness among older people but could reflect an increased awareness of health issues and more honest reporting, not an actual increase in disease prevalence and disability. Encouraging news from the National Long-Term Care Survey[2] indicated that the proportions of elderly people with chronic disability, including people over age 85, actually declined in the past decade. Despite this trend of improved health status, the absolute numbers of older people requiring community services will continue to escalate. Health promotion programs should be available to all age groups to ensure the highest possible level of physical well-being among current and future older adults.

Aging in the World

The projected increase in the proportion of older people in the United States mirrors the population trends in other parts of the world. During the 1990s the number of people over age 64 worldwide will increase from 332 million to 426 million.[18] Surprisingly, the numerical growth in the elderly population is occurring in the developing as well as the developed nations, although at a slower rate (1.5% per year as compared to 3% per year). Over half of the world's population ages 65 and older now live in developing countries and by the year 2020, four-fifths of the world's elderly will live in developing nations. Reduction in the overall birth rate and infant mortality rate, reduced incidence of infectious and parasitic diseases, and improvements in health and education are all contributing to this increase. By 2020, 25% of the population in many European countries and Japan will have reached age 65. China and India, followed by the United States, will have the largest numbers of people age 80 and older.

The country with the highest life expectancy for both sexes is Japan, followed by Sweden and Hong Kong for men and France and Switzerland for women.[10] Life expectancy in Japan is 82.1 years for women and 76.1 years for men. In comparison, the life expectancy of white Americans is 2.4 years shorter for women and 3.1 years shorter for men. Life expectancy for African Americans is 5.9 years shorter for women and 8 years shorter for men. It is important to note that alcohol consumption per person is almost twice as high in the United States as compared to Japan and use of tobacco products is about 30% higher.

Future Trends

Cigarette smoking is the greatest single preventable cause of illness and premature death in the United States, contributing to 19% of all deaths.[9] Smokers have a 70% greater risk of death from all causes than nonsmokers, and it is believed that coronary deaths would decrease by 30% if all Americans stopped smoking. Chronic obstructive pulmonary disease is now the fifth leading cause of death in older age groups. Environmental smoke is responsible for about 3,000 deaths each year from lung cancer among nonsmokers. Although smoking prevalence continues to decline in the adult population, 18% of teenagers ages 16 and 17 smoke.[22]

The report *Healthy People 2000: National Health Promotion and Disease Prevention Objectives*[23] issued in 1991 addressed many health-related factors in addition to smoking that contribute to disease risk and established goals for behavior change. According to that report almost 30% of adults had high blood pressure (above 140/90 mm Hg) and less than one-fourth of these had it under control. Excess weight was a problem for about one quarter of

Americans, and most people were not following sound practices for weight reduction. Fewer than half of adult Americans exercised three or more times per week. Dietary fats, both saturated and unsaturated, accounted for more than 36% of total kilocalories in the American diet. The Healthy People 2000: Midcourse Review report[9] released in 1995 indicated progress toward some but not all of the defined goals. More people are now exercising regularly, but about the same number of people never exercise. Although total dietary fat has decreased from 36% to 34% of total kilocalories, more people are overweight; in fact the prevalence of overweight has increased from 26% to 34% of the population. More adults have stopped smoking but the number of high school seniors who smoke has risen. Increased numbers of people are receiving intervention for their high blood pressure. All of these health factors contribute measurably to the development of chronic disease and should be prime targets for health and nutrition education.

SOCIOECONOMIC CHARACTERISTICS OF THE AGING POPULATION

The increasing ethnic diversity of the older population and differences in life expectancy contribute to differences in living arrangements and income.[18] Most older people (95% percent) live in the community with their spouse, with other family members, with nonrelatives, or alone; only 5% of older people are institutionalized. Living arrangements of those age 65 and older are influenced by sex, marital status, and age. Most older men remain married until they die and continue to live in a family setting. Most older women are widowed and many live alone. Widowed white women tend to maintain individual households, whereas widowed African American and Hispanic women are more likely to live with family members.

Since the 1980s the median income of people over age 64 has more than doubled; however, not all groups have shared in these gains.[18] Older African American and Hispanic households are more likely to have lower incomes after retirement, based on their lower earnings while in the workplace. The young-old, individuals between ages 65 and 74, and married couples have higher incomes than people ages 75 and older and elderly single people. Social Security benefits, which are based on one's income while working, are the principal source of income for most older Americans. Because many older people are limited in their ability to increase their income by working, they become vulnerable to economic uncertainty and more likely to fall below the poverty level. The loss of a husband is critical for a wife who was dependent on his pension and is eligible for very limited Social Security or pension benefits in her own right. Deteriorating health resulting in continuing medical costs that may not be covered by Medicare or private health insurance can deplete the older person's savings, creating financial anxiety. Costly prescription drugs often divert money from the food budget.

The elderly people of tomorrow are expected to have an improved economic status as compared to the current elderly. The educational level and therefore the lifelong income level of older people will be higher in future years, as more will have completed high school and college. In future years more women will have been in the workforce long enough to have established retirement plans and pensions in their own names. Despite expected increases in income, elderly people will continue to face economic uncertainties as life expectancy and potential health care costs continue to rise.

PHYSICAL HEALTH IN THE AGING POPULATION
Changes in Physical Health

The progression of biologic and physiologic events that occur in individuals as they age has been observed for centuries but only in recent years has the study of aging begun to emerge as a science. Researchers who are studying physiologic aging have tried to separate those changes that occur in all people from those changes that are associated with the development of chronic diseases. This is not as easy as we would like it to be. For example, atherosclerotic lesions could be the result of an age-related change in the cells in the wall of the artery or a disease-related change caused by a virus or inappropriate serum lipoprotein levels and diet. Mental and cognitive function is another area for study. Although changes in brain cells and metabolism have been observed with aging, not all older people suffer dementia, leading one biologist[19] to suggest that this be studied as any other disease. The *sequence* of age-related changes is the same in all members of a species or sex group, although the *rate* at which changes occur differs widely from one individual to another.[16] Changes that are believed to occur in all individuals and therefore are considered to be age-related are often referred to as **normal aging.**

The identification of age-related versus disease-related changes is complicated further by the fact that physiologic, psychologic, or cognitive changes occurring over adulthood are influenced by both genetic and environmental factors. In his treatise on how to live to be at least 70 years of age, Oliver Wendell Holmes facetiously recommended that individuals advertise for parents from families whose members survived to age 80 or 90.[16] One very obvious genetic characteristic influencing aging and, consequently, life expectancy is one's sex; in most species, including humans, females live longer. Genetic control of the rate of aging could be exerted through the regulation of protein synthesis. The individual with an increased ability to produce HDL-cholesterol may enjoy increased protection against coronary heart disease. Aging could to some extent be under hormonal control. The lower waist-to-hip ratio, characteristic of women, may play a role in reduction of cardiovascular risk.

Environmental and lifestyle factors can either enhance or reduce the effects of existing biological traits. Individuals with less than optimum serum HDL-cholesterol levels who adopt a diet that limits total fat and saturated fat, avoid alcohol, and exercise regularly may improve their HDL to LDL ratio and mitigate their risk of cardiovascular disease.

In broad terms the definition of aging includes all of the structural and functional changes that occur throughout the life span from embryonic development through maturation

and senescence. The term **gerontology,** which we will use in our study of aging, includes not only the physiologic or behavioral changes observed as people age, but also the factors—biologic, sociologic, or psychologic—that influence these changes. The term **geriatrics,** in contrast to the term gerontology, is a medical specialty dealing with the health problems of older people and the study of diseases associated with the aging process. Unfortunately, research in aging has tended to emphasize age-related losses and the time-dependent changes that increase one's vulnerability to disease, rather than positive approaches to the maintenance of physical and mental well-being. We will take a closer look at available research on aging in chapter 2.

Usual versus Successful Aging

The study of age-related changes, or normal aging, has taken place using healthy populations that were carefully screened to exclude individuals with obvious disease. This work has allowed us to evaluate the physical and psychological differences that exist between adults of different ages. At the same time this emphasis on normal aging has serious limitations for health professionals with responsibility for the future well-being of the aging population.[14] First, the emphasis on normal aging in healthy individuals fails to recognize the heterogeneity among older people who are relatively free of disease. Many physiologic characteristics such as bone mineral mass are related to one's ethnic group. An older individual's performance on tests of mental function can be influenced by level of education. It is important to recognize differences both within and between ethnic and cultural groups. Second, the idea of normal aging implies that such changes carry no risk to well-being. This is not an appropriate assumption as changes in cardiovascular response have implications for the initiation of vigorous exercise by the older individual. Finally, the idea of normal aging implies that such changes are natural and therefore unresponsive to intervention.

To meet this need Rowe and Kahn[14] have introduced the concept of "usual" versus "successful" aging. They believe the portrayal of the aging process as unpreventable or irreversible

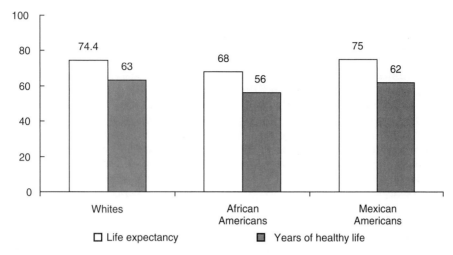

FIG. 1-4   Life Expectancy and Years of Healthy Life. As life expectancy edges upward, it is important to promote healthy lifestyles that will delay the onset of chronic disease and disability. African Americans have the least years of healthy life.

United States Department of Health and Human Services: Healthy people 2000. National health promotion and disease prevention objectives, DHHS Publication No. (PHS) 91-50212, Washington, DC, 1991, U.S. Government Printing Office.

has been exaggerated, and the potential modifying effects of positive lifestyle factors have been underestimated. Based on their definition, usual aging refers to the physiologic or cognitive changes occurring in older people that represent age-related changes that have been exacerbated by adverse environmental and lifestyle factors and the presence of disease. **Successful aging** is demonstrated in individuals in whom age-related changes have not been augmented or accelerated by environmental influences or disease and in fact may have been delayed by the adoption of appropriate intervention strategies.

Successful aging will influence the years of healthy life enjoyed by an aging individual. As described in figure 1-4, white and Hispanic elderly not only enjoy longer life expectancies, but also more years of healthy life than African American elderly.[23] Access to an appropriate diet, adequate and safe housing, and preventive health care can play a role in determining the years of healthy life within particular ethnic groups. Positive lifestyle intervention and health promotion practices can slow the progression of age-related changes or reduce their severity and

decrease the number of years of poor health. Examples of physiologic changes ameliorated by improvement in diet or exercise patterns include body composition, glucose tolerance, and cardiovascular function. The goal of nutrition intervention in both younger and older adults is to implement the transition from usual to successful aging. Positive intervention strategies and their demonstrated effects are emphasized in succeeding chapters.

Physical Health Status

Functional assessment. Changes in physical appearance such as graying of the hair or use of a cane for walking may provide clues as to chronologic age; however, an individual's ability to perform tasks related to personal care or independent living is less easily defined. When assessing acute conditions such as a bone fracture or pneumonia, the medical diagnosis and the ability to function are closely linked. This is not true for chronic diseases. An older individual with compensated cardiac failure or well-controlled diabetes mellitus can function quite well and lead an active, independent life. Thus disease-oriented models are limited in their power to identify those who require help with personal or household tasks. Two indices that have been developed to measure functional status as related to the ability to live independently or the need for care are the Activities of Daily Living and the Instrumental Activities of Daily Living.[25]

The **Activities of Daily Living** (ADLs) relate to personal care:

- Bathing
- Dressing
- Feeding oneself
- Using the toilet
- Transferring between bed and chair

The **Instrumental Activities of Daily Living** (IADLs) assess the ability to perform household and social tasks:

- Meal preparation
- House cleaning
- Handling money
- Shopping
- Using the telephone

Difficulty in walking is not always a predictor of dependence, since individuals may overcome the problem with the use of canes, walkers, or wheelchairs.

The ability to perform both the ADLs and the IADLs influences the quality of life and the capacity to live independently. In a recent national survey[25] nearly 19% of noninstitutionalized people age 65 and older had difficulty with walking or with at least one ADL task; the same was true for 40% of people 85 years of age and older. Walking, going outside, and bathing or showering were the most common problems. Of those reporting difficulty with walking, 18% lived with others and 20% lived alone. More people age 65 and older had difficulty with at least one IADL than at least one ADL (24% versus 19%), and heavy housework, shopping, and preparing meals were mentioned most frequently. Preparing meals and shopping were problems for 26% to 37% of people over age 84.

Functional limitations are related to one's sex and ethnic group as well as one's age.[25] Women are more likely to report difficulty in carrying out daily activities than are men. Many older women with functional limitations related to a health or physical problem live alone; most older men with functional limitations live with their spouse who can assist with daily activities. The proportion of African American and Hispanic elderly requiring assistance with everyday activities are 23% and 19%, respectively, as compared to 15% of white elderly. Helping the older person who has problems with food shopping or meal preparation make appropriate choices from the foods available or making referrals to support services such as home delivered meals is an important task for the health professional.

Health perception. It is often assumed that the health of older people has improved because they are living longer. Conversely, older people are sometimes perceived to be dependent and frail. Neither viewpoint is completely correct.[18] In fact 41% of people ages 65 to 74 rate their health as excellent or very good. In the group age 85 or older, the proportion rating their health as excellent or very good falls to 31%. Eighteen percent of the young-old (ages 65 to 74) rate their health as fair, and 8% rate their health as poor.[25] Surprisingly, ratings of fair or poor do not change appreciably when individuals age 85 and older are evaluated separately. The rating of fair increases by 4% and the rating of poor by 3%. Although chronic problems do increase in number and severity with advancing age, people age 85 and older may hold a different perspective on what constitutes good health. This evaluation was conducted with noninstitutionalized elderly people who do have fewer physical problems than their institutionalized counterparts.

A person's perception of his or her health is also related to income.[25] Only 11% of those with the lowest incomes reported their health to be excellent, and 14% reported their health to be poor. Conversely, 25% of those with the highest incomes considered their health to be excellent, and only 4% considered it to be poor. African American elderly are more likely to rate their health as fair or poor than are white elderly. A comparison of adult health in the United States and developing nations also suggests an influence of income on health. The proportion of people over age 50 reporting poor health in Jamaica, Malaysia, and Bangladesh ranged from 40% to 60% as compared to 20% to

30% in the United States (based on that author's calculations).[12] After corrections for differences in mortality rates and socioeconomic factors, women in the developing nations still fared worse than men in all health measures. The cumulative effect of repeated pregnancies with less than optimum diets and health care may contribute to this gender difference in health.

Despite generally positive attitudes toward their health, depression and mental health problems play a significant role in the perception of health status in older people. Depression may adversely affect the course of an illness.[26] Older people are at particular risk for depression because of physical illness and high use of prescription drugs that can alter mental function. Poor self-rated health can be a significant predictor of hospital stays and nursing home placement among low income elderly. For older participants in NHANES I,[6] however, health behaviors such as smoking and demographic characteristics such as age, race, and marital status were stronger predictors of mortality over a 12-year period than poor self-rated health.

Presence of chronic disease. As people grow older, so does the probability of their having multiple chronic diseases. Chronic conditions are those which last for more than three months and for which there is no immediate cure. Among people age 80 and older, 70% of the women and 53% of the men have two or more chronic conditions.[21] Watkin[28] quoted a survey of congregate meal participants in which 60% had one to six chronic disorders. Common chronic conditions among older people are arthritis (49%), heart disease (31%), hypertension (35%), impaired hearing (31%), orthopedic problems (18%), cataracts (15%), and diabetes (10%).[21] The prevalence of arthritis is especially high among women and African Americans; hypertension is most common among African American women.[18] Heart disease, hypertension, and arthritis all require dietary counseling to assist in controlling dietary fat and sodium and body weight.

Use of health services. In general the use of health services increases with age; although older

Americans make up only one-eighth of the total population, they account for more than one-third of the total health care expenditures.[22] On the average, young adults have contact with a physician about 5 times a year; in contrast, adults ages 65 to 74 contact a physician about 10 times a year, and for those above age 74 the number of contacts increases to 12. Older people are more likely to be hospitalized during the year and, when admitted, will have a longer length of stay. On an annual basis 9% of young adults enter a hospital and stay about five days as compared to 24% of the 65- to 74-year-old group who will stay an average of seven days. Among those over age 75, 30% will be hospitalized during the course of a year.[21] Many of these hospital admissions are for acute episodes relating to a chronic condition such as heart disease or diabetes.

Although these statistics provide an overview of the health care needs of the older population, they do not address the differences that exist between groups.[18] For example, older women have a higher number of physician contacts but are less likely to be hospitalized than older men. African American elderly who are more likely to report fair or poor health also have a higher rate of hospital admissions and longer hospital stays than white elderly. In contrast to what might be expected, older people with low incomes are more likely to be admitted to the hospital than those with high incomes.

A comparison of health services provided to people ages 65 to 79 and age 80 and older by a health maintenance organization (HMO)[7] indicated few differences in services provided, despite the differences in age. The chronic conditions reported by both groups were similar, although the younger group was more likely to have hypertension and the older group was more likely to have congestive heart failure. The number of physician visits was the same for both, but those ages 80 and older were more likely to be admitted to the hospital. Johnson and coworkers suggested that chronic conditions such as cardiac failure or respiratory disease could be more serious in the elderly. On the other hand, physicians may be more likely to hospitalize an older individual who does not have a caregiver to help during episodes of illness.

Perspective on Aging— Biologic or Medical: Implications for Health Care

The association of aging with physical changes and the development of chronic disease has led to the view that aging is a medical problem. This biomedical approach emphasizes illness and disability rather than the overall biologic, social, and behavioral aspects of the aging process.[3] Our society will soon experience a rapid increase in the number of older people, including the oldest-old who are likely to have multiple chronic diseases and require medical services. An important issue now being discussed by health care planners, providers, and consumers is the future impact of the growing aging population on demand for health care services and related costs. Schneider and Guralnik[15] have predicted that the unprecedented growth of the oldest-old could lead to a sixfold increase in health care costs over the next 40 years. Medicare costs now increase from $2,017 per year for people ages 65 to 74 to $3,215 for those ages 85 and older, and these numbers do not include the cost of nursing home care. Nearly half of all nursing home beds are occupied by individuals over age 84. By 2040 the number of people over age 84 needing nursing home care could be two to three times the total number of people age 65 and older who are now receiving nursing home care. Research and education relating to the causes and prevention of chronic disease are of major importance and could reduce these numbers substantially.

Looking at these issues from the positive point of view, half of the individuals who now reside in nursing homes have chronic diseases whose risk factors have been identified and can be modified.[4] It is clear that good nutrition and appropriate levels of exercise can prevent or ameliorate the problems arising from major chronic diseases, including diabetes mellitus, cardiovascular disease, and osteoporosis, and should be the keystone of preventive health care.[8] Recent studies have provided evidence that optimum nutritional status, especially optimum vitamin B-12, vitamin B-6, and folate status, may contribute to continued efficient mental function[13] and an improved quality of life. Fries[4] reminds us that 99 of every 100 people below age 75 are living independently, and 80 of every 100 people above age 85 are still living in the community. We should not lose sight of the complex issues that affect the health status and quality of life of all older people. Appropriate housing, income, and social services as well as a sense of physical and emotional well-being are all important in determining appropriate food intake and other positive lifestyle choices. Successful aging is already a reality for many older people, and healthy lifestyles that preserve fitness, energy, and independence can make it so for the aging population of the future. In succeeding chapters we will discuss the role of nutrition in achieving this goal.

❖ ❖ ❖

CASE STUDY

Mrs. M. is a 69-year-old African American woman who lives alone in a house in a large city. Her only income is from Social Security. She has high blood pressure but sometimes is unable to refill her prescription for medication because she does not have the money. Mrs. M. does not have a car and must depend on public transportation. Her arthritis is worsening and she finds it difficult to walk for more than one city block without resting.

1. What is her life expectancy?

2. How would you assess her ability to live independently?
3. Determine the current amount of money she would be allotted under the U.S. Department of Agriculture (USDA) Thrifty Food Plan. (See: Cost of Food at Home, Fam. Econ. Nutr. Rev. 9(1):60, 1996.)
4. Develop an appropriate three-day menu that provides 70% of the RDAs for all nutrients and stays within this budget allotment.

Summary

America has a diverse and growing elderly population. One of every eight people is now age 65 and older, and by the year 2030, it will be one in five. With most older people currently among the young-old (ages 65–74), that population is also aging. By the year 2000 nearly half of the older population will have reached age 75. The 85 and older group is the fastest growing among all age groups. Although a variety of factors, including age, gender, and race, influence life expectancy, the adoption of preventive health practices, such as reduced dietary fat intake, regular physical activity, avoidance of smoking, and limited alcohol use, has contributed to a decreased number of deaths from chronic disease. These lifestyle changes result in an improvement in both the quantity and quality of life. The exaggerated portrayal of the aging process as unpreventable and irreversible has led to the concept of usual versus successful aging. Usual aging refers to age-associated changes that have been exacerbated by adverse environmental and lifestyle factors and the presence of disease. Successful aging occurs in individuals who in fact may have delayed or diminished age-related changes by the adoption of appropriate intervention strategies. As the population ages, the proportion of health care services and related costs used by these individuals will continue to increase. Currently, older Americans account for more than one-third of the total health care expenditures in the United States. The predicted growth of the oldest-old could lead to a sixfold increase in health care costs over the next 40 years. Appropriate lifestyle choices can help prevent or reduce that increase in health care costs.

REVIEW QUESTIONS

1. What factors will contribute to the projected increase in both the number and proportion of older people in the general population? Will all segments of the 65 and older population increase to the same extent? Explain. What are the social and economic implications of the increase in the older segment of the population?
2. Explain the factors that have contributed to the increased life expectancy in the United States. What additional factors may lead to an even longer life expectancy in the future? What are the differences in life expectancy between men and women? What factors contribute to these differences and how have they changed over the years?
3. What chronic diseases are most common among older people? How has the prevalence of these diseases changed throughout the 20th century?
4. What is the difference between usual and successful aging? What are some intervention strategies that would promote successful aging?
5. What are the Activities of Daily Living (ADLs) and the Instrumental Activities of Daily Living (IADLs)? How are they used?

SUGGESTED LEARNING ACTIVITIES

1. Visit a local library and review current census statistics for your community. Determine the relative proportion of older people in your geographic area and their demographic characteristics. How do they compare to your state and the United States as a whole?
2. Visit a senior center or a congregate meal program and an adult day care center and interview the directors of each program about their participants. Compare the groups on the basis of ADLs, IADLs, and general health.
3. Make a list of community agencies that provide services to older people, and determine what food- and nutrition-related services are available.
4. Prepare a lesson plan for a course designed to educate a group of healthy young-old on diet and lifestyle interventions for prevention of heart disease.

REFERENCES

1. Brown, C.C., and Kessler, L.G.: Projections of lung cancer mortality in the United States: 1985–2025, J. Natl. Cancer Inst. 80(1):43, 1988.
2. Corder, L.S.: Compression of disability: evidence from the national long-term care survey, Nutr. Rev. 54(1, Part II):S9, 1996.
3. Estes, C.L., and Binney, E.A.: The biomedicalization of aging: dangers and dilemmas, Gerontologist 29(5):587, 1989.
4. Fries, J.F.: The sunny side of aging, J.A.M.A. 263(17):2354, 1990.
5. Gibson, R.C.: The age-by-race gap in health and mortality in the older population: a social science research agenda, Gerontologist 34(4):454, 1994.
6. Idler, E.L., and Angel, R.J.: Self-rated health and mortality in the NHANES-I epidemiologic follow-up study, Am. J. Public Health 80:446, 1990.

7. Johnson, R.E., Mullooly, J.P., and Greenlick, M.R.: Morbidity and medical care utilization of old and very old persons, H.S.R. 25:4, 1990.
8. Kretchmer, N.: Nutrition is the keystone of prevention, Am. J. Clin. Nutr. 60:1, 1994.
9. McGinnis, J.M., and Lee, P.R.: Healthy people 2000 at mid decade, J.A.M.A. 273(14):1123, 1995.
10. Miller, D.K., Morley, J.E., and Rubenstein, L.Z.: An overview of international aging and nutrition. In: Morley, J.E., Glick, Z., and Rubenstein, L.Z., editors: Geriatric nutrition: a comprehensive review, New York, 1995, Raven Press.
11. Otten, M.W., and others: The effect of known risk factors on the excess mortality of black adults in the United States, J.A.M.A. 263(6):845, 1990.
12. Rahman, O., and others: Gender differences in adult health: an international comparison, Gerontologist 34(4):463, 1994.
13. Rosenberg, I.H., and Miller, J.W.: Nutritional factors in physical and cognitive functions of elderly people, Am. J. Clin. Nutr. 55:1237S, 1992.
14. Rowe, J.W., and Kahn, R.L.: Human aging: usual and successful, Science 237:143, 1987.
15. Schneider, E.L., and Guralnik, J.M.: The aging of America. Impact on health care costs, J.A.M.A. 263(17):2335, 1990.
16. Shock, N.W.: Biologic concepts of aging, Psych. Res. Rep. 23:1, 1968.
17. Sutherland, J.E., Persky, V.W., and Brody, J.A.: Proportionate mortality trends: 1950 through 1986, J.A.M.A. 264(24):3178, 1990.
18. Taeuber, C.: Sixty-five plus in America, Curr. Pop. Reports P23-278, Washington, DC, 1992, U.S. Bureau of the Census.
19. Timiras, P.S.: Physiological basis of aging and geriatrics, ed. 2, Boca Raton, FL, 1994, CRC Press.
20. U.S. Bureau of the Census: Projections of the population of the United States, by age, sex, and race: 1988 to 2080, Curr. Pop. Reports Series P-25, No 1018, Washington, DC, 1989, U.S. Government Printing Office.
21. U.S. Department of Health and Human Services: Current estimates from the national health interview survey, 1993, Vital and Health Statistics, Series 10, No. 190, DHHS Publication No. (PHS) 95-1518, Hyattsville, MD, 1994, National Center for Health Statistics.
22. U.S. Department of Health and Human Services: Health, United States, 1993, DHHS Publication No. (PHS) 94-1232, Hyattsville, Md, 1994, National Center for Health Statistics.
23. U.S. Department of Health and Human Services: Healthy people 2000. National health promotion and disease prevention objectives, DHHS Publication No. (PHS) 91-50212, Washington, DC, 1991, U.S. Government Printing Office.
24. U.S. Department of Health and Human Services: The surgeon general's report on nutrition and health, DHHS Publication No. (PHS) 88-50210, Washington, DC, 1988, U.S. Government Printing Office.
25. U.S. Department of Health and Human Services: Trends in the health of older Americans: United States, 1994, Vital Health Statistics, Series 3, Analytic and Epidemiological Studies No. 30, DHHS Publication No. (PHS) 95-1414, Hyattsville, MD, 1995, National Center for Health Statistics.
26. U.S. Senate Special Committee on Aging: Aging America. Trends and projections (annotated), Serial No. 101-J, Washington, DC, 1990, U.S. Government Printing Office.
27. Verbrugge, L.M.: Recent, present, and future health of American adults, Annu. Rev. Public Health 10:333, 1989.
28. Watkin, D.M.: The physiology of aging, Am. J. Clin. Nutr. 36:750, 1982.

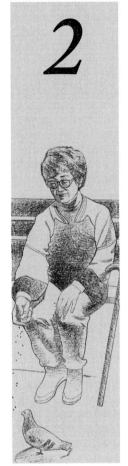

2 How Do We Age?

THE ROLE OF NUTRITION RESEARCH

✦✦

Objectives

After studying the chapter, the student should be able to:

✔ *Appreciate the theories of aging involving genetic control and cellular damage and their relation to human aging.*

✔ *Recognize the contribution of animal studies to our knowledge of nutrition and aging.*

✔ *Recognize the nutritional and lifestyle factors that contribute to mortality risk in younger and older adults.*

✔ *Understand the role of nutrition in decreasing an individual's risk of cardiovascular disease and cancer.*

✔ *Apply the nutrition principles related to diet and lifestyle that promote successful aging.*

INTRODUCTION

Since antiquity people have been searching for magical potions to preserve youth and prolong life. Early explorers came to the New World seeking the "fountain of youth." Hormonal and herbal preparations that promise to retard aging or restore physical health have a widespread market. Today researchers are examining the alterations at the molecular and cellular level that are the root of the changes we observe in aging animals and humans. Many theories about why and how these changes occur appear in the public media and in scientific studies. Both biologists and nutritionists are identifying genetic and environmental factors that accelerate the progression of aging changes and the development of chronic disease. Older people in good health who exemplify successful aging are being studied to isolate those health practices and food habits that have contributed to their lifelong health and well-being. Clinical researchers are looking at possible links between diet early in life—even the nutritional environment during fetal development—and the likelihood of developing obesity, coronary heart disease, or hypertension. This chapter will consider the types of aging studies now in progress and findings that are important toward our goal of successful aging.

HISTORICAL PERSPECTIVE

Historical writings contain many directives for maintaining good health and prolonging life. Cornaro, whose book, *The Art of Living Long*, was published in 1558,[5] became an ardent advocate of a temperate diet after becoming ill with fever, pains in the stomach, and perpetual thirst. Previously given to excessive food and drink, from that time on he ate sparingly of bread, meat, milk, egg yolk, and soup, and at the age of 95 wrote his final treatise on the wisdom of a moderate diet. Cornaro suggested that one needs less food as the body grows older. He limited himself to 12 ounces of food and 14 ounces of wine a day and exhorted young people to avoid overindulgence. We might consider what a current diagnosis of Cornaro's sudden illness might be.

Francis Bacon (1561–1626) was the first author to recommend a scientific approach to the evaluation of diet and longevity.[5] He advocated a frugal diet and encouraged the study of people living in different climates and eating different diets to determine those characteristics that influence the life span. In his opinion, diet was the most important component in prolonging life. Unfortunately, Bacon's recommendation to evaluate the influence of diet and lifestyle on mortality has only recently begun to receive attention. Suggested practices regarding food and health were popular reading in colonial America. Benjamin Franklin's *Poor Richard's Almanac*, published in 1733, advised readers to limit the amount they ate. Franklin urged his followers to "eat to live and not live to eat."[13]

Early medical writings also stressed a prudent diet for the elderly.[5] A physician living in A.D. 1000 urged his older patients to eat only small amounts of food at a time and to avoid foods that could lead to digestive upset, such as spiced and pickled items. A treatise on geriatric medicine that appeared in 1796 advised older people to avoid sugar and confectionery foods, to consume liberal amounts of vegetables, to limit the amount of meat they ate, and to eat only sparingly at night. A paper titled "Food and Hygiene of Old Age," which appeared in the *Journal of the American Medical Association* in 1892, suggested that errors in food selection are less serious in the young, who can recover from such mistakes.[6]

In this century Metchnikoff, a Russian physiologist, proposed the theory of autointoxication, suggesting that death occurred as a result of toxins that were produced in the large intestine by fecal waste and then absorbed into the body.[13] Yogurt and other fermented milk products containing lactic acid-producing bacilli were recommended to destroy the intestinal microbes responsible for the poisonous waste. Although Metchnikoff's theory is no longer considered valid, it provides an example of early research on the association between diet and human aging.

The first study evaluating the relationship between body weight and mortality was reported in 1913,[67] as life insurance companies began to recognize that policyholders with higher body weights in proportion to their heights had shorter lives. Central to the insurance industry's profitability is its ability to predict how long a policyholder might live or, conversely, how soon the life insurance claim must be paid. Life insurance statistics have continued to be a source of both information and controversy about the relationship between nutrition and life span. It is rather interesting to note that throughout history, writers have emphasized limiting one's intake of food both for physical health and spiritual good. Current research is focusing on energy intake and obesity and their influence on molecular and cellular aging.

THEORIES OF AGING

Numerous theories focus on what causes aging. In fact over 300 theories have been developed in this century alone. Aging is a multifactorial process.[68] No one single theory or cause can explain all of the mechanisms involved at the molecular, cellular, organ, and whole body levels. Just as many mechanisms lead to the development of a particular disease such as cancer, so do many factors, both genetic and environmental, cause us to age.[53] Although more people are surviving into old age as a result of improvements in public health, nutrition, and medical care, the maximum life span has remained unchanged. This underscores the importance of one's genetic inheritance in controlling longevity and establishing a biological barrier beyond which life cannot be sustained.

There are several ways to categorize the theories of aging. The **genetic theories** assume that aging occurs as a predetermined sequence of events in the ongoing continuum of growth and development. The **environmental theories** propose that aging events occur at random and damage accumulates until eventually the cell or organism can no longer function. Another way to look at theories of aging is by **level of organization,** moving from the whole organism to the organ system and finally to the cell. Many of these theories overlap; however, it is useful to become familiar with the variety of processes that together form aging.[41]

Organism Level

The **rate of living concept** proposes that the rate of development and maturation is related to longevity. This concept is rooted in the idea that the total amount of energy expended over the life span is constant across all species; thus, animals that have a high metabolic rate have a shorter life span than animals who have a slow metabolic rate. Across animal species, life span is correlated with metabolic rate or age at sexual maturation; nevertheless, research studies do not support this theory.[41]

Organ Level

Theories of aging related to organ system function have focused on the roles of the endocrine system under the control of the hypothalamus and the immune system. These organ systems are considered the pacemakers of the aging process, genetically programmed to decline in function in later life. The programmed senescence of these organ systems is believed to bring about the aging sequence in the whole organism.[53] Immune response does decline with advancing age, and there are

changes in endocrine function as, for example, alterations in secretion of the sex steroid hormones. However, as Rowe[53] pointed out, none of these theories explain the basis of the changes in the pacemaker system itself.

Cellular and Molecular Level

The most popular theories of aging are those based on changes that occur at the level of the cell and its molecular constituents. In 1891 Weismann proposed the **"wear and tear" theory,** which suggested that aging was the result of body cells wearing down from constant use over a lifetime.[68] Since then researchers have looked at age-related changes in cellular DNA and control proteins and lipid membranes. The major theories receiving current attention are 1) the somatic mutation theory, 2) the error catastrophe theory, 3) the free radical theory, 4) the glycation theory, and 5) the genetic code theory.[68]

Somatic mutation theory. This theory suggests that alterations and mutations in DNA structure result in the synthesis of protein molecules that cannot carry out their intended function. This loss of functional proteins over time leads to cell death.[41] Evidence for this theory came from the observation that animals exposed to irradiation died at a younger age than control animals. However, the rate at which changes occur in the genetic code under normal circumstances is too slow to account for general aging.

Error catastrophe theory. This theory suggests that errors in protein synthesis occurring over time contribute to the production of abnormal proteins and impaired cell function. These errors would occur in transcription and translation, the process by which an RNA template is produced from an existing DNA strand and then used to produce a new DNA strand. Existing evidence does not support this theory. For example, amino acid sequences do not differ between younger and older animals, and defective RNA strands do not increase in number. Also, if this theory were correct, aging would occur at a continuous rate from birth.[53]

Free radical theory. Free radicals, oxygen molecules with an unpaired electron, are high energy molecules that attack double bonds. These peroxidation reactions damage membranes, enzymes, and DNA. Animals fed supplements of nutrients that act as antioxidants, such as vitamin E, have a longer life span but also have a lower body weight, which may contribute to the longer life.[53] Animals treated with a monoamine oxidase inhibitor that reduces the oxidation of neurotransmitters had a life span 34% longer than untreated control animals. The inhibition of monoamine oxidase reduces free radical damage to tissues of the central nervous system.

Glycation theory. This theory is based on the changes in existing proteins that occur through a reaction involving glucose and lysine residues (the Maillard or Browning reaction). The glycation of proteins has biological consequences, including a reduction in enzyme activity and alterations in antigen responses. The accumulation of glycated proteins in diabetes has been related in part to the slowed nerve conduction velocity observed in that disease.[41]

Alteration of the genetic code. Genetic factors appear to be important determinants of aging although the mechanisms are still unknown. Life span is remarkably distinct for each species. The effect of genetic factors in human life span is evident in the fact that life expectancy in monozygous twins is more similar than in dizygous twins. Aging does bring about some chemical changes in DNA; however, a more significant finding has been the identification of RNA with cell growth inhibitory activity. Young cells do not have detectable levels of this genetic material. When RNA is injected into young cells, growth ceases.[68]

Current experimental evidence supports the genetic code theory as a basis for cellular aging; however, other theories very likely contribute to overall aging. Changes at the cellular level form the basis of changes occurring in organ systems and the whole body; thus all theories are not mutually exclusive. In spite of recent progress we still lack techniques with the accuracy and sensitivity to quantitatively measure cellular changes. The next important step will be to relate cellular and molecular changes to the functional alterations and diseases observed in older age.[68] In later sections we will discuss the effects of particular environmental factors, including diet, activity level, and use of alcohol, which may influence the rate and degree of aging changes in body cells.

RESEARCH TOWARD SUCCESSFUL AGING: ANIMAL MODELS

In the past many biological gerontologists believed that a single aging process was responsible for the changes that occur in all species after maturity and into senescence. Most contemporary researchers believe that several fundamental processes exist, and many aging interventions have been studied in animal models to try to identify these processes.[37] Nutrition interventions have included feeding of natural and synthetic antioxidants and diet experiments involving energy restriction, overfeeding, diets high in fat or protein, and changes in body weight. An impressive number of studies by many researchers indicate that energy restriction, regardless of dietary fat or protein, influences a process that controls the rate of aging.

Energy Restriction and Length of Life

Studies over the past 60 years using experimental animals have confirmed that **energy restriction** increases the life span. The classic studies of McCay and coworkers[39] in the 1930s revealed that energy intake controls not only the rate of growth but also the rate of development and aging. Those researchers demonstrated that laboratory rats fed diets adequate in protein, vitamins, and minerals but limited in kilocalories could be maintained at their weaning stage and weight for several years. When additional kilocalories were provided, the animals would begin to grow and mature. The life span of these animals was nearly twice as long as the life span of those given the usual amount of food throughout their lives. This work established the principle that energy intake controls fundamental metabolic processes that influence aging changes and provided the foundation for current research to identify the site and mechanism of the metabolic control.

Current studies using energy restriction provide a level of kilocalories that supports growth and maturation.[38] Restricted animals are fed 50% to 60% of the kilocalories eaten by the control animals who have free access to food (**ad**

libitum-fed). It is important to recognize that the energy-restricted diets are formulated to provide adequate levels of protein, vitamins, and minerals; only kilocalories are below the usual level.

The profound effect of energy restriction is evident when comparing the median and maximum length of life in restricted and ad libitum-fed rats.[38] Those given free access to food had a median life span of 701 days, compared to 956 days for the restricted animals; the maximum life span was 941 days for the ad libitum-fed and 1,295 days for the restricted animals, respectively. More than half of the restricted animals were still alive when the last ad libitum-fed animal died. Length of life is an acceptable measure of outcome when evaluating an aging intervention in animal models. In humans, qualitative measures of health and well-being and reduced morbidity are also important measures of outcome.

Physiologic Effects of Energy Restriction

In animals age-related and detrimental changes in physiologic function are prevented, delayed, or reduced in severity by energy restriction. These effects range from delaying and blunting the age-related increase in serum cholesterol to slowing alterations in the proteins in the eye's lens and retarding the decline in the ability to learn a maze (see box).[37]

Energy restriction also slows the development of chronic disease. Laboratory animals develop both heart disease and kidney disease in older age.[38] As described in table 2-1, the incidence and severity of both chronic diseases are lower in restricted animals. Energy restriction influences the cause of death in experimental animals. Kidney disease is the major cause of death among ad libitum-fed animals, whereas the major causes of death among restricted animals are tumors and leukemia. Energy restriction does delay the development of tumors, and tumor growth is not increased at younger ages in restricted animals; older restricted animals show a greater prevalence of tumors because they live longer and have additional time to develop tumors.

❖

AGE-RELATED CHANGES DELAYED BY ENERGY RESTRICTION IN ANIMAL MODELS

Physiologic function
Increase in plasma cholesterol level
Increase in plasma parathyroid hormone level
Decrease in immune function
Decrease in dopamine receptors in the brain
Decrease in hepatic enzymes
Changes in proteins in the eye
Decreased ability to learn a maze
Chronic disease
Renal disease
Cardiac disease
Leukemia
Cataract
Cancers

Adapted from Masoro, E.J.: Dietary restriction and aging, J. Am. Geriatr. Soc. 41:994, 1993.

TABLE 2-1 Energy Intake and Incidence of Age-Related Chronic Disease in Older Rats

	Energy Restricted	Ad Libitum-Fed
Kidney disease		
Absent or minimal	93%	18%
Severe	7%	82%
Heart disease		
Absent or minimal	75%	41%
Severe	25%	59%

Modified from Masoro, E.J., Shimokawa, I., Yu, B.P.: Retardation of the aging processes in rats by food restriction, Ann. NY Acad. Sci. 621:337, 1991.

Energy Restriction and Metabolic Outcome

Although the influence of energy intake on the rate of aging in animal models is well recognized, what is still to be determined is the mechanism by which energy restriction exerts its effect. Many explanations have been presented, but no single theory has withstood careful scrutiny.[37] An enhanced growth rate and more body fat have been suggested as factors that accelerate the aging process. Animals restricted in energy intake grow more slowly and have a lower content of body fat per gram of body weight than unrestricted animals. In restricted animals the level of body fat is positively related to the length of life. In contrast, ad libitum-fed animals have a higher body weight and larger amount of body fat than restricted animals, but these measurements do not always correlate with their length of life. One piece of evidence suggesting that factors other than growth rate and maximum body weight influence life span is that food restriction begun in mature animals, later in life, leads to gains in the life span similar to those achieved when restriction is begun at weaning.[38]

A decrease in the metabolic rate, or slowing of the "rate of living" also has been proposed to explain the observed increase in life span in restricted animals. The metabolic rate per unit of body weight does fall when energy restriction is first begun, but it returns to normal shortly thereafter.[37] Although a reduction in energy expenditure per unit of metabolic mass is not responsible for the delay in aging changes, reduced energy intake does play a role. Masoro[37] considers it likely that energy restriction alters a neural or endocrine regulatory system that changes the way carbohydrate is used. Both plasma glucose and plasma insulin are lower in restricted animals despite a rate of glucose use per kg of body weight that is similar to ad libitum-fed animals. It would appear that either glucose effectiveness or insulin sensitivity or both are enhanced by dietary restriction. Hyperglycemia and hyperinsulinemia enhance the development of chronic disease, and even normal levels may over a lifetime contribute to cellular and molecular aging.

Dietary restriction may influence aging processes by reducing free radical and oxidative damage to body proteins and tissues. Energy-restricted animals have higher glutathione reductase activity which decreases lipid peroxidation and free radical damage.[37]

We have discussed possible mechanisms by which energy restriction may influence primary aging processes. An alternate point of view suggests that energy restriction may enhance an animal's ability to protect itself against the harmful effects of physiologic stress or damage caused by normal aging. Restricted animals have a more rapid recovery from surgery and their hepatocytes produce higher levels of stress-induced proteins after a mild heat stress. The ability to respond to heat stress declines with age in ad libitum-fed animals. The higher plasma glucocorticoid levels observed in restricted animals may play a role in protecting against age-related damage.[37] At this time there is no clear evidence to establish a cause and effect relationship for any particular action.

The use of food restriction as a tool by experimental gerontologists has stirred controversy regarding its use as an intervention in human aging.[37] Optimal feeding is important during the period of growth, but, at the same time, avoiding the accumulation of excessive body fat in childhood holds promise for lifelong health and successful aging. A balance between a moderate energy intake and regular physical activity may promote the positive benefits observed in energy-restricted animals.

NUTRIENT INTAKE AND HUMAN AGING
Scope of the Problem

Limited information is available to evaluate the influence of lifelong dietary habits on health and longevity. Major studies evaluating the impact of diet and lifestyle on the incidence of chronic disease examined key nutrients, such as the intake of saturated fat, but not the diet as a whole. Moreover, we need to evaluate intervention strategies that we can apply after chronic disease becomes apparent that may retard its progression or reduce its severity. Finally, it is important to establish a base of knowledge about how people age. Several types of research studies can provide important pieces of information.[40]

Epidemiologic studies. Epidemiology is the study of the occurrence, distribution, and causes of disease. Epidemiologic studies are used to establish the extent of a nutrition or health problem within a population and learn who is most likely to have the problem.[40] Gender, race, nutrient intake, income, or health practices (e.g., smoking) influence who has a health problem. Elderly African American women with an income below the poverty level are at high risk for a poor diet. High intakes of fruits and vegetables are associated with a lower risk of stroke in middle-aged and elderly men. Epidemiologic studies can suggest associations between diet and disease although they *do not* establish cause and effect.

Cohort studies. A cohort study, which focuses on a group of the same age, race or other commonality, is used to monitor the nutritional or health consequences of a dietary pattern, health practice, or lifestyle. Groups who are free of the disease or health problem when the study begins are observed for a predetermined period of time.[40] Postmenopausal women with moderate calcium intake might be monitored for the occurrence of a hip fracture. Cohort studies can be prospective or retrospective. In a prospective study current records or an interview are used to establish an information base of current practices or risk factors and a plan for follow-up; in a prospective study the health consequence has not yet occurred. In a retrospective study both exposure to any risk factors or preventive behavior and the health outcome have occurred and existing records are used for evaluation.

Cross-sectional studies. A cross-sectional study compares information obtained from two or more groups at the same time;[40] cross-sectional studies may compare a physiologic characteristic such as kidney function in younger and older people or the vitamin intake of adults of different ages.

Longitudinal studies. A longitudinal study follows the same individual over time and provides information on not only the rate of change but also the time when changes occur. The Baltimore Longitudinal Study of Aging (BLSA) has been studying the same men for 30 years and established that energy intake and expenditure actually begin to decline about

❖

RESEARCH NEEDS IN NUTRITION AND AGING

- Effect of diet on the biological mechanisms that control the aging process
- Effect of diet at all stages of the life cycle on development of chronic disease
- Nutrient requirements in elderly people
- Interactions of diet, the aging process, and chronic disease in elderly people
- Psychological, social, and environmental factors that influence food intake in elderly people
- Effective strategies to promote optimum food availability and food intake in elderly people

---

age 35 to 45 and then stabilize until age 75 and after.

Clinical trials. A clinical trial is a research study that has an experimental group and a control group, which have similar characteristics at the beginning of the study.[40] The experimental group receives an intervention such as a nutritional supplement, drug, exercise regimen, or nutrition education program and the control group does not; both groups are evaluated based on set parameters. Clinical trials have evaluated the effect of vitamin B supplements on immune function in elderly people and the efficacy of added protein in healing pressure sores.

All of these methods can contribute to our knowledge of nutrition and lifestyle intervention in modulating the aging process. Longitudinal evaluations, although costly and arduous, are urgently needed to provide important information as to the effect of particular dietary habits and daily lifestyle practices throughout adulthood on the development of chronic disease. We also need to understand how nutrient intake, nutrient requirements, and health practices change in older people as they continue to age. (Some goals for future research are outlined in the box above.)

EARLY NUTRITION, LENGTH OF LIFE, AND CHRONIC DISEASE

Years of research have established that genetic inheritance plays a role in determining the length of life and an individual's resistance to chronic disease. We have learned also through animal studies that energy intake influences the rate at which aging changes occur. Recent research from England[2] and the Netherlands[34] indicates that adverse nutritional experiences before birth and during the first year of life result in lifelong effects observed in middle age and beyond. This concept of nutritional programming is being used to study the relationships between fetal growth and chronic disease in adult life.[17] During fetal life different tissues undergo rapid growth at different times, and an inadequate level of nutrients or oxygen during a period of critical growth will slow cell division in that organ system, causing permanent differences in the distribution of particular cells, in hormonal feedback, or in metabolic activity. Early undernutrition thereby can lead to pathologic changes that bring about endocrine and immune patterns associated with disease. These in utero relationships and consequences have long been recognized in animals; however, only recently have we studied these relationships in humans.

Records available in several counties in England have made it possible to evaluate the health status of middle-aged and older men and women in relation to their size and weight at birth and one year of age.[2] Follow-up on 15,726 individuals revealed that those with a very low birth weight had higher death rates from coronary heart disease. Babies who were small because they failed to grow in utero, not small because of premature birth, were at increased risk as adults. This relationship between low birth weight and heightened disease risk was independent of smoking, obesity, and social class, confirming that it was the growth pattern in utero and not environmental factors or deprivation thereafter that influenced the development of disease. Low birth weight also appears to predispose an individual to hypertension and non-insulin-dependent diabetes, which no doubt contributes to coronary risk. Individuals

with a low birth weight who become obese as adults are at particular risk.

Various mechanisms have been proposed to explain the association between low birth weight and chronic disease in later life. The thin newborn has a lower amount of muscle as well as fat. It has been suggested that in utero existing muscle becomes resistant to insulin so that all available nutrients are directed to the brain, allowing brain cell growth to continue normally.[2] This insulin resistance then continues into adulthood. Babies undernourished in utero also may have fewer beta cells in the pancreas. The fetal pattern of diverting nutrients from other organ tissues to the brain in undernutrition also seems to result in low liver weight with disturbed cholesterol metabolism and blood clotting. The size and weight of the placenta influences the development of chronic disease.[17] Placental size increases as a way to extract more nutrients in an environment of undernutrition; however, as the ratio of placental weight to birth weight rises, so does the likelihood of elevated blood pressure in later life.

Growth patterns after birth involve the development and enlargement of existing cells, and babies with a low birth weight tend to grow slowly. The English men with poor growth were three times more likely to die from coronary heart disease than those with normal weight gain.[2] Babies with low weight gain develop hypertrophy of the left ventricle as adults. This condition is an independent predictor of heart disease.

Nutrition in fetal life also appears to influence the offspring born to mothers nutritionally deprived in utero.[34] During the winter of 1944, Amsterdam, Holland, suffered a severe famine causing a per capita food availability of 1,300 kcal or less. Toward the end of the famine the food supply consisted of bread and potatoes. The famine lasted seven months after which food again became plentiful. Birth weights of infants born to women who in utero were undernourished in the first, second, or third trimester of their mother's pregnancy were compared to control infants with mothers of the same age, physical characteristics, and geographic region. The first offspring of women who in utero were undernourished in the first trimester was heavier

(73 g), and the second offspring was lighter (96 g) than control infants. This effect may be the result of alterations in the mother's ovaries or uterus which are laid down in fetal life.

The observation that undernutrition in utero exerts a strong effect on health and morbidity in middle and older age has important implications for today's mothers. Increasing numbers of infants are being born to women in their teenage years who require nutrients for their own growth and so may have lower levels of nutrients available for the growth of the fetus. The idea that poor nutrition before or immediately after birth can predispose the individual to life-threatening complications in adulthood emphasizes the importance of optimum prenatal care and nutrition for all mothers and food assistance programs to support appropriate infant feeding after birth.

NUTRITION AND PREVENTION OF CHRONIC DISEASE

A major health initiative in recent years has been public education defining the risk factors for chronic disease and strategies for their modification. The initiative *Healthy People 2000: National Health Promotion and Disease Prevention Objectives* has directed attention to research findings that suggest health behaviors to reduce the incidence of heart disease, cancer, and cerebral hemorrhage, the three major causes of death in the older population. Dietary intake, body fat content, exercise patterns, and use of tobacco and alcohol contribute to disease risk in both younger and older adults. Each of these is subject to intervention toward the goal of successful aging. In the following sections we will look at research evidence that suggests appropriate goals.

Occurrence of Cardiovascular Disease

The early 1960s marked the beginning of a significant decline in mortality from coronary heart disease. Changes in food consumption that contributed to this decline, the substitution of vegetable fats for animal fats, and the movement toward foods lower in total fat began in the late 1940s and accelerated from that time on.[58] Food patterns indicating reduced consumption of total fat and saturated fat were evident 10 to 15 years before the downward trend in mortality from coronary heart disease was observed.[58] This interval of 10 to 15 years between the initiation of positive dietary changes and the reduction in the incidence of chronic disease reinforces the need to encourage lifestyle changes among young and middle-aged individuals to ensure their successful aging.

Factors Contributing to Cardiovascular Risk

A common belief is that the risk factors known to predispose middle-aged people to heart disease do not apply to older people. In fact, elevated blood pressure, inappropriate blood lipoprotein patterns, obesity, smoking, and glucose intolerance are also strong predictors of coronary risk in the elderly.[26] When examined on an individual basis, some risk factors decrease in importance. Current evidence suggests that after age 65, stopping smoking does not measurably decrease cardiovascular risk, because the incidence of stroke increases among both smokers and nonsmokers after that age.[50] In contrast, elevated blood pressure and, possibly, an undesirable serum lipid profile remain powerful predictors of cardiovascular risk into the late 70s. Elevated systolic or diastolic blood pressure multiplies the risk of heart disease in all individuals after age 45.[26] Only two factors change in risk between middle and older age: gender and total cholesterol level.[60] Before menopause women have some protection from coronary heart disease, but morbidity and mortality from coronary heart disease for women in their late 60s and 70s are comparable to men of similar age. More women die of heart disease than from all forms of cancer combined. Total cholesterol appears to be less important to overall risk as people age; however, high density lipoprotein (HDL) cholesterol and low density lipoprotein (LDL) cholesterol levels continue to influence cardiovascular risk into advanced age.

Older men and women with several risk factors are especially vulnerable to heart attack or stroke. Results from the Framingham Heart Study indicate that the risk of coronary heart disease is about doubled in older people with

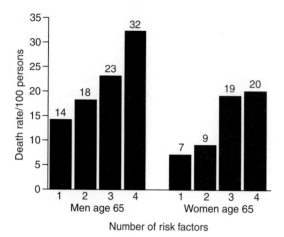

FIG. 2-1 Probability of Death from Coronary Heart Disease According to Number of Risk Factors. The risk of death from coronary heart disease rises progressively in both older men and older women as the number of risk factors increases. Risk factors include obesity, elevated blood pressure, abnormal glucose tolerance, elevated serum lipids, and smoking.

Data from Castelli, W.P., and others: Cardiovascular risk factors in the elderly, Am. J. Cardiol. 63:124, 1989.

three risk factors as compared to those with one risk factor (fig. 2-1).[63] Elevated blood pressure and abnormal glucose tolerance, if associated with obesity, increase the risk of coronary heart disease and stroke in women even before menopause. Conversely, dietary and lifestyle interventions can have an additive effect on risk reduction.[49] Models for coronary risk derived from the Framingham Heart Study suggest that among people ages 30 to 80, a 10% reduction in total serum cholesterol would be expected to result in a 12% reduction in coronary risk among men and a 14% reduction in women with elevated cholesterol levels (240 mg/dl or higher). An individual who lowered his or her blood cholesterol and also stopped smoking would have a 28% to 38% decline in cardiovascular risk.

Serum Lipoprotein Levels and Cardiovascular Risk

The role of **blood lipoprotein levels** in predicting coronary risk in people of all ages remains a topic of intensive research. Three major areas of

inquiry are 1) the influence of total cholesterol versus particular lipoprotein fractions, 2) the ages at which blood lipoprotein levels influence coronary risk, and 3) the genetic versus the environmental (e.g., dietary intake, obesity) influence on blood lipoprotein levels.[60]

Serum total cholesterol has served as a marker for coronary disease risk since the classic studies of Ancel Keys in the 1950s, which associated diet, serum total cholesterol, and the development of coronary heart disease.[72] Serum total cholesterol increases as intake of saturated fat and cholesterol increases and decreases when polyunsaturated fat replaces saturated fat. Serum total cholesterol levels are influenced less by monounsaturated fat. A recent finding from the Framingham Heart Study[12] was that HDL cholesterol is the strongest independent predictor of coronary artery disease and cardiovascular death. Higher levels of HDL cholesterol were associated with a lower incidence of coronary artery disease and coronary death in both midlife and older age. In the Bronx Aging Study[60] HDL cholesterol levels less than or equal to 30 mg/dl were associated with myocardial infarction, cardiovascular disease, and total mortality in older men and older women. HDL cholesterol may decrease cardiovascular risk by returning cholesterol to the liver and promoting its excretion. HDL cholesterol levels may be more important in reducing risk in individuals who already show symptoms of heart disease and in men, as heart disease occurs about 10 to 15 years earlier in men than in women.[12]

Conversely, LDL cholesterol, which carries cholesterol to the tissues and is responsible for the deposition of cholesterol in the arterial wall, is positively associated with coronary risk. In the Framingham Heart Study individuals ages 50 to 80 whose serum LDL cholesterol was one standard deviation above the mean had a risk of coronary heart disease that was 1.9 (men) to 2.5 (women) times higher than other members of their age group.[27]

Although lipoprotein patterns remain strong indicators of coronary risk in midlife and beyond, the role of serum total cholesterol, especially in those over age 75, is less clear. Serum total cholesterol was not associated with myocardial infarction, coronary death, or deaths from all causes in 997 people above age 70 (mean age was about 79).[30] After four years of follow-up, mortality from coronary heart disease was about 5% in men and women with desirable serum total cholesterol (less than 200 mg/dl) and 2.1% to 2.4% in men and women with high-risk total cholesterol (equal to or above 240 mg/dl). There are several reasons why serum total cholesterol may not be a risk factor for coronary heart disease in people after the late 70s. Krumholz and coworkers[30] suggested that the total cholesterol level in very elderly people may not represent their true cholesterol level over their lifetime. Also, individuals who survive to an advanced age despite elevated cholesterol may be resistant to its effects. Finally, other health factors, such as hypertension, smoking, diabetes, aging, or preexisting coronary heart disease, could obscure the effect of elevated total cholesterol.[60] It is also pertinent that very low serum cholesterol signals declining health status in the elderly adult. In the NHANES I Epidemiologic Follow-up Study of 10,295 people ages 35 to 74,[20] a serum total cholesterol below 158 mg/dl was associated with an increased risk of death in men and women ages 70 to 74. Risk of death in that age group was associated also with a low activity level, recent weight loss, and chronic disease.

Clinicians advise that individuals in their late 70s and beyond not be screened or treated for high blood cholesterol.[22] Yet screening and treatment are both appropriate and important for the young-old, and dietary and weight loss interventions can be effective in reducing risk factors in people age 60 and older. (Intervention studies will be discussed in chapter 13.) In young adults, interventions to reduce elevated serum cholesterol levels will promote successful aging. The increased cardiovascular risk in middle age resulting from a high serum cholesterol as a young adult was demonstrated in a prospective study of 1,017 men, with a mean age of 22, who were followed for 27 to 42 years.[29] A serum cholesterol difference of 36 mg/dl separated the lowest quartile of men from the highest quartile when the study began. This difference of 36 mg/dl doubled the risk of coronary heart disease and death at older ages and strongly increased risk of death before age 50.

Dietary Fat and Cardiovascular Risk

In light of the known association between increased dietary fat, especially saturated fat, and serum cholesterol levels, the National Cholesterol Education Program (NCEP) recommends dietary intervention as a first step.[66] NCEP guidelines[66] indicate that dietary fat should provide no more than 30% of total kilocalories. This fat should be divided as follows.

Type of fat	Percentage of total kilocalories
Saturated fatty acids	less than 10%
Polyunsaturated fatty acids	10% or less
Monounsaturated fatty acids	10% to 15%

Recent studies evaluating the abilities of individual fatty acids to raise or lower serum total cholesterol have complicated this issue.[66,72] Although saturated fatty acids generally are expected to raise total cholesterol, stearic acid does not have this effect. **Linoleic acid** (an n-6 fatty acid) decreases LDL cholesterol but decreases HDL cholesterol as well. **Oleic acid,** a monounsaturated fatty acid, is receiving increasing attention because it appears to lower LDL cholesterol to the same degree that polyunsaturated fatty acids do without also lowering HDL cholesterol. The increasing use of table fats that have been produced through chemical hydrogenation has focused attention on the effect of trans fatty acids on serum lipid levels. Trans fatty acids are found in higher amounts in fats subjected to chemical hydrogenation as part of their processing. Trans fatty acids increase serum LDL cholesterol levels and reduce serum HDL cholesterol levels. Trans fatty acid intake was related to an increased incidence of coronary heart disease in a study of middle-aged and older white women.[72]

Polyunsaturated fatty acids found in fish (n-3 fatty acids) decrease serum very-low-density lipoprotein (VLDL) cholesterol and also reduce the aggregation of blood platelets and blood-clotting.[1] Evidence from geographical regions such as Alaska, where fish is consumed in large amounts and the prevalence of coronary heart disease is low, suggested that eating fish might protect against cardiovascular disease.[14] Continuing research, however, has not provided definitive answers. Ascherio and coworkers[1] completed a six-year follow-up of nearly 45,000 male health professionals ages 40 to 75 years. Risk of cardiovascular disease as measured by a heart attack or heart surgery did not differ between the men who ate six or more servings of fish a week and those who ate fish once a month or less. The risk of coronary death did fall by 25% in men who ate any fish as compared to those who ate no fish. It may be that a favorable effect is possible with the consumption of just a few grams of fish oil a day.

Micronutrients and Cardiovascular Disease

In past years primary attention was directed toward dietary fat in the development and worsening of cardiovascular disease. Recent research points to the importance of several micronutrients in maintaining cardiovascular health and emphasizes our need to focus on the overall adequacy of the diet.

A major factor in the development of atherosclerotic lesions in the coronary arteries is the oxidation of LDL cholesterol, which exacerbates its damage-promoting ability. Peroxidation of existing lipids in the aorta promote the progression of vascular damage.[66] Vitamins C and E play a role in reducing lipid peroxidation and may lower cardiovascular risk. Prospective studies[10] of 87,000 female nurses ages 34 to 59 and 40,000 male health professionals ages 40 to 75 indicated that the risk of heart attack or cardiovascular death in the women in the highest quintile of vitamin E intake was reduced by 34% after eight years, and the risk in the men was reduced by 36% after four years as compared to those in the lowest quintile of intake. In the men supplements of vitamin C or multivitamins also reduced risk. One issue to be resolved is the need for vitamin E supplements. Although use of supplements contributed to the reduced risk in the women, it is important to determine if a higher dietary intake (or a more accurate calculation of dietary intake) might serve the same purpose.

A 13-year follow-up study[42] of 1,899 middle-aged men who participated in a trial of lipid-lowering drugs found that men with higher serum carotenoids had a lower risk of a subsequent heart attack. Folate status plays a role in preventing coronary heart disease. Folate is a necessary cofactor in the metabolism of methionine. When folate is not available in adequate amounts, homocysteine, an intermediary metabolite, accumulates in the plasma in excessive amounts. Even moderately high levels of plasma homocysteine were associated with a threefold increase in risk of heart attack and coronary death among nearly 15,000 male physicians.[61] Because high levels of plasma homocysteine can be reduced with increased dietary folate, this would appear to be a modifiable risk factor for heart disease.

Copper may be important to antioxidant function as it acts as a cofactor for the enzyme superoxide dimutase, which prevents lipid peroxidation. High iron stores were associated with myocardial infarction in a group of Finnish men studied for three years.[4] It was proposed that free iron from their iron stores participated in the production of free radicals and increased the oxidation of LDL cholesterol. This relationship between high iron stores as measured by serum ferritin and cardiovascular risk has not been duplicated in other studies. Measurements were not available to ascertain possible hemochromatosis in this population. It is important to note that vitamins E and C, the carotenoids, folate, and copper are all found in fruits and vegetables and can be obtained through diet.

Alcohol Intake and Cardiovascular Risk

A dietary practice that is both popular and controversial is the use of alcohol. Alcohol is believed to raise HDL cholesterol levels, and regular use of wine with meals has been suggested as one of the factors contributing to reduced cardiovascular disease in the Mediterranean region.[32] Conversely, some research points to a detrimental effect of alcohol on health and chronic disease patterns. Epidemiologic evidence suggests that up to two drinks a day can decrease cardiovascular risk by as much as 30%.[32] In over 8,000 men and women studied in the NHANES I Epidemiologic Follow-Up Study,[55] a pattern of less than two drinks a day was associated with a 20% reduction in total mortality in older men and women with preexisting disease as compared to nondrinkers. Preexisting diseases included heart disease, cerebral vascular disease, and cancer. Although up to two drinks a day was associated with a positive health outcome, more than two drinks a day increased risk of death from all causes in both sexes.

The biological mechanisms by which alcohol lowers coronary risk is an area of intensive research. Alcohol intake raises serum HDL cholesterol levels, and this effect is believed to account for 30% to 50% of the reduction in coronary heart disease that is attributed to alcohol. Alcohol also reduces the aggregation of blood platelets, an important component in blood clotting. Men consuming alcohol on a daily basis have higher levels of plasminogen activator than men consuming alcohol weekly, monthly, or never.[52] Plasminogen activator plays a role in breaking down small fibrin clots in the plasma. These effects of alcohol on HDL cholesterol and blood clotting activators likely contributed to the reduction in mortality among the men and women with preexisting heart disease examined in the NHANES I Follow-Up Study[55] described earlier.

The presumed positive effects of alcohol in lowering the risk of heart disease must be weighed against the increased risk of cancer, especially breast cancer in women.[32] Alcohol consumption is inappropriate in pregnancy and in the opinion of the Committee on Diet and Health[11] carries the risk of addiction as well as other types of injury. An expert panel[66] on evaluation and treatment of high blood cholesterol concluded that use of alcohol cannot be recommended for the prevention of coronary heart disease.

Physical Activity and Cardiovascular Risk

Increasing physical activity can improve fitness and health and prevent or ameliorate cardiovascular disease in men and women at middle and older ages. Among 14,786 male Harvard alumni between the ages of 45 and 84,[48] groups who reported walking, stair climbing, or engaging in sports activity had fewer deaths from all causes. Individuals who walked less than 9 miles (15 km) a week, climbed less than 20 flights of stairs a week, or expended fewer than 1,500 kcal a week in physical activity had a 38% higher risk of death. Over time the men who increased their energy expenditure by at least 750 kcal a week decreased their risk of death by 17%; conversely, those who decreased their energy expenditure by at least 750 kcal increased their risk of death by 25%. This was true for both younger and older men. Increased energy expenditure offers some protection against developing chronic diseases that contribute to coronary heart disease. Hypertension and non-insulin-dependent diabetes were less frequent among the men who were more physically active.[47]

Sherman and coworkers[57] evaluated physical activity and mortality in 1,404 women ages 50 to 74 in the Framingham Heart Study. All of the women were free of cardiovascular disease at the time of entry and were monitored for 16 years. At that time the women were ranked in quartiles based on level of physical activity. The two more physically active groups had an overall mortality that was about 30% lower than the two more sedentary groups. It is of interest, however, that there were no significant differences in cardiovascular deaths between groups. The higher mortality in the sedentary women was the result of cancer or other causes.

Older people may benefit more from exercise than younger people, because younger people have a lower risk of death regardless of their level of physical activity. Regular physical activity had health benefits even for women age 75 and over, followed for a period of 10 years.[56] Walking 30 minutes a day lowered the risk of death from all causes in older men and older women. Physical activity can help to raise HDL cholesterol levels, reduce the resting heart rate, lower the waist-to-hip ratio, and improve glucose tolerance. Physical activity throughout life contributes to successful aging.

Body Measurements and Cardiovascular Risk

The influence of body weight on mortality was first examined by life insurance companies nearly 100 years ago.[67] Based on the heights and weights of policyholders who lived the longest, insurance companies derived tables listing appropriate body weights for people of a particular sex and height. Although such tables are still widely used by insurance companies and health professionals (see chapter 11), they have many limitations. The body weights given as standards are presumed to represent an appropriate proportion of lean body tissue and body fat, and deviations from these weights are presumed to be a gain or loss of body fat. However, for a person participating in an exercise program, body weight can remain unchanged despite an increase in fitness if body fat is replaced by lean muscle tissue. Conversely, an older individual may have a low muscle mass and an excessive amount of body fat, yet meet the suggested weight for height. Finally, height and weight tables derived from life insurance statistics are not representative of the general population. Whites and individuals from middle and upper socioeconomic groups are more likely to buy life insurance than are low-income or minority groups. Nevertheless, body weight standards derived from life insurance records are used to evaluate mortality risk.

Body weight and mortality. The most recent compilation of life insurance data is the 1979 Build Study, which traced the mortality of 4.2 million policyholders between 1954 and 1972.[67] In general, the greater the deviation from average weight, the greater the mortality risk (table 2-2). Among both older men and older women, mortality ratios, or the risk of death, increased sharply for those 25% to 35% underweight. These mortality ratios represent a decrease in life expectancy of about 2 years in men and 1.5 years in women. In men optimal mortality ratios (ratios < 100) occur at about average weight whereas in women mortality ratios are most favorable at a body weight 5% to 15% below average. Mortality ratios increase sharply at a body weight that is 35% or more above average, with a decrease in life expectancy of 1 to 1.5 years. These findings suggest that overweight, unless 35% or more above average weight, carries somewhat less risk than severe underweight, particularly in women.

Issues in evaluating body weight and mortality. Although life insurance statistics point to the increased vulnerability of both overweight

TABLE 2-2 *Mortality Risk and Body Weight in Older People*

Classification	Mortality Risk* (Ratio of actual to expected mortality)	
	Men	Women
25%–35% underweight	137	143
15%–25% underweight	120	108
5%–15% underweight	100	91
Average weight	96	99
5%–15% overweight	98	100
25%–35% overweight	103	107
35%–45% overweight	148	128

*Average risk = 100 (Mortality ratios above 100 indicate a higher risk of death; mortality ratios below 100 indicate a lower risk of death.)

Modified from Van Itallie, T.B., and Lew, E.A.: Health implications of overweight in the elderly. In Prinsley, D., and Sandstead, H.H., editors: Nutrition and aging, New York, 1990, Alan R. Liss.

and underweight individuals, underweight rather than overweight appears to be more dangerous at older ages. Manson and coworkers[35] have pointed to several biases within data that contribute to the apparent increased mortality in the underweight and should be kept in mind when evaluating studies of body weight and mortality.

1. Smoking is more prevalent among people with low body weight. In the Framingham Heart Study, only 55% of those in the highest overweight category reported smoking, compared to 80% of those in the lowest weight category.

2. High mortality rates associated with underweight can be caused by an underlying clinical disease such as cancer or respiratory disease that was present when the study began. This bias can be avoided by carefully screening subjects for a prospective study or by disregarding data collected during the first few years of follow-up when weight loss from underlying disease will be most evident.

3. Whether the study was long term or short term will affect the conclusion reached about the impact of body weight on mortality. Short-term evaluations are influenced by underlying disease and often suggest that underweight per se carries a high mortality risk. Obesity, on the other hand, may appear to have less effect when evaluated over the short term, since the mortality rates of the most obese may be similar to those of average-weight individuals. This is because the risk factors associated with obesity, hypertension, glucose intolerance, or hyperlipidemia, develop slowly over several years. The longer the period of overweight, the more likely are these conditions to develop.

These relationships were evident in two recent studies that evaluated the influence of **body mass index (BMI)** on health and mortality in men[33] and women[75] in middle age. The BMI (body weight in kilograms divided by height in meters squared) provides a useful estimate of body fatness and is a better evaluation tool than height and weight tables. Willett and coworkers[75] reviewed the incidence of nonfatal heart attacks and cardiovascular mortality among 11,581 women in the Nurses Health Study. All were between the ages of 30 and 55 when the study began and were followed for 14 years. A higher BMI, even within the normal range, increased the risk of coronary heart disease in these middle-aged women (fig. 2-2). In those with no history of hypertension or diabetes, risk of coronary heart disease was lowest at a BMI under 21. It is important to note that a BMI of 21 is below the current range of desirable weight. At a BMI of 29 or over, risk was more than doubled as compared to a BMI of under 21. At a BMI of 27.3, the criterion for overweight used in the Third National Health and Nutrition Examination Survey (NHANES III), risk was 84% higher than for those with the lowest body weight. Weight gain after age 18 of even 5 to 7.9 kg (11 to 17 pounds) increased risk by 25% as compared to women gaining or losing 4.9 kg or less (10 pounds).

A 27-year follow-up of Harvard alumni[33] who had a mean age of 47 when first examined found no evidence of increased mortality among lean men. In fact, the lowest mortality was observed in the men with a BMI under 22.5, a level about 20% below the average for men of comparable age and height (see fig. 2-2). The alumni with the highest BMI, 26 or greater, had the same mortality risk as the lightest men with a BMI under 22.5 after 12 years of follow-up. However, after 27 years of follow-up, the heaviest men had a mortality risk 32% above the lightest men. Men at the heaviest weight were most at risk for death attributed to cardiovascular disease and for death before age 50.

The effect of obesity in adolescence on morbidity and mortality in middle and old age emphasizes the importance of both prevention and intervention in young people. A follow-up study of overweight adolescents[44] after 55 years, when they had reached 73 years of age, reported that men who were obese as adolescents had a risk of death from coronary heart disease that was 2 times higher, a risk of death from colon cancer that was 9 times higher, and a risk of cerebrovascular disease that was 13 times higher than their normal weight peers. In contrast, women who were overweight as adolescents had no increase in mortality risk; however, many had arthritis and they were eight times more likely to have difficulty with Activities of Daily Living.

The influence of race on the relationship between BMI and mortality was evaluated in a 15-year study of more than 5,000 African Americans between the ages of 30 and 70.[71] Because these people were members of a prepaid health maintenance organization (HMO), information about possible underlying disease was available for review. After controlling for smoking and the early years of follow-up, no relationship between BMI and mortality was evident in women across the entire range of severe underweight to severe overweight. In men relative risk increased significantly with overt obesity. Thinness, when unrelated to cigarette smoking, did not increase risk.

The relationship between obesity as defined by BMI and the incidence of coronary heart disease and total mortality in African American women requires further evaluation. A 25-year follow-up of women in the Charleston Heart

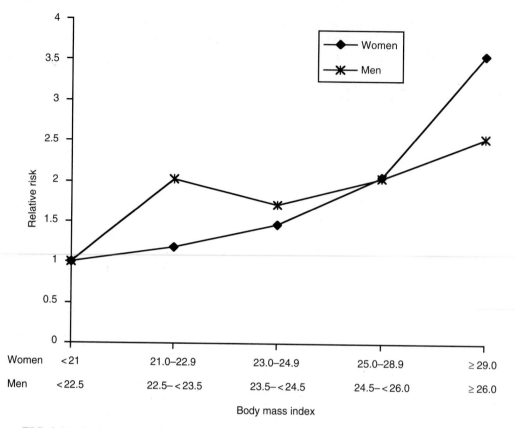

FIG. 2-2   Body Mass Index and Cardiovascular Risk in Men and Women. A below-average body mass index (BMI) is most favorable for long-term cardiovascular health; a BMI even within the average range increases risk.

Data from Willett, W.C., and others: Weight, weight change, and coronary heart disease in women. Risk within the 'normal' weight range, J.A.M.A. 273:461, 1995, and Lee, I.M., and others: Body weight and mortality. A 27-year follow-up of middle-aged men, J.A.M.A. 270:2823, 1993.

Study[62] found that BMI was a predictor of coronary disease in white women but not African American women.

The **waist-to-hip ratio,** or proportion of abdominal to gluteal fat, is associated with the risk of cardiovascular disease in all age groups. Individuals with more abdominal or upper body fat (which produces a larger waist-hip ratio) are more likely to develop hypertension or diabetes and have a greater risk of stroke, regardless of their total body fat. In a five-year follow-up study[15] of nearly 42,000 Iowa women, ages 55 to 69, a 0.15 unit increase in the waist-to-hip ratio (an example would be a 15 cm or 6-inch increase in waist measurement in a woman with a 100 cm or 40-inch hip measurement) was associated with a 60% greater risk of death. Folsom and coworkers[15] consider the waist-to-hip ratio a better measure of risk than BMI and recommend its use in routine health monitoring.

Cardiovascular Disease in Women

Each year 2.5 million women in the United States are hospitalized for cardiovascular illness and 500,000 die from coronary heart disease.[70] Because men are younger when coronary heart disease becomes evident, this disease has traditionally been viewed as a man's disease, and consequently clinical trials have focused on risk reduction in men but not women. Although women develop risk for heart disease about ten years later than men, the average 55-year-old woman can have the same risk of heart attack as the average 55-year-old man.

Prior to menopause estrogen imparts some protection against cardiovascular disease through its effect on serum lipoprotein levels.[3] In the presence of estrogen HDL cholesterol is increased and LDL cholesterol remains in the desirable range. Following menopause HDL cholesterol drops somewhat and LDL cholesterol begins to rise. In postmenopausal women receiving estrogen or hormone replacement therapy, LDL cholesterol remains at former levels although plasma triglycerides increase significantly. Estrogen also appears to increase blood flow in the carotid arteries, which benefits women with clinical atherosclerosis. Although few clinical trials have been conducted, available evidence from a prospective study of 48,470 nurses over a 10-year period indicated that estrogen-treated women had only half the risk of coronary heart disease of untreated women.[3] Another important finding was that women at low risk benefited as much from estrogen therapy as women at high risk. In a study of older women[3] whose average age was 73, estrogen offered the greatest protection against fatal or nonfatal heart disease or stroke in the oldest women; risk in the estrogen users was about half that of the nonusers. This was true regardless of existing risk factors including known heart disease, hypertension, overweight, or cigarette smoking.

Barrett-Connor and Miller[3] emphasized the need for clinical trials that evaluate strategies for the prevention of heart disease in women. They pointed out that no other prescription regimen has been given on such a large scale without demonstrated proof of efficacy through clinical trials as has estrogen replacement therapy. Issues related to estrogen use include increased risk of breast or endometrial cancer and increased serum triglycerides.

Cardiovascular Disease in Ethnic Groups

African Americans, Hispanic Americans, and Native Americans are at particular risk for conditions contributing to the development of coronary heart disease.[31,36] Hypertension and subsequent renal failure or stroke are more prevalent among African Americans than among white Americans.[31] The causes of increased hypertension among African Americans are likely to be both genetic and environmental. Hypertension is prevalent among black populations in Africa, suggesting a genetic link. Dietary factors and poor medical management may also be involved. African American women are more likely to be obese than white women and have a higher risk of hypertension.

Native Americans and Mexican Americans have the same degree of obesity as black Americans but are not as likely to develop hypertension.[36] In spite of their obesity, their blood pressure and serum cholesterol remain low. However, obese Native Americans and Mexican Americans have a higher incidence of diabetes. Blood pressures are lower in Asian Americans and Pacific Islanders compared to white Americans. Hypertension is prevalent in Cuban and Puerto Rican men and women, although data are limited. Minority group approaches to intervention need to be evaluated in clinical trials.

Prevention of Cardiovascular Disease

Large-scale clinical trials have tested dietary and drug interventions on reducing the number of deaths from coronary heart disease. Several primary prevention trials using drug therapy reported that deaths from coronary heart disease were lower among men receiving aggressive intervention to lower their serum cholesterol, but in some cases total mortality was the same or even higher in those who received therapy as compared to those who did not.[66] The Multiple Risk Factor Intervention Trial[43] emphasized dietary treatment and followed 7,000 men for 10.5 years. In that study mortality rates for coronary heart disease among those receiving dietary treatment were 11% lower, and mortality rates for all causes were 8% lower compared to those not receiving dietary treatment. This effect was observed four years after the treatment program was completed. It appears that the benefits of intervention are ongoing and may not become evident until years later. In fact, the full benefit of treatment may not be apparent for 10 to 20 years.

Continuing research is being directed toward dietary and lifestyle patterns that prevent the formation of atherosclerotic plaques or lead to the regression of existing plaques. A comprehensive regimen consisting of a low-fat vegetarian diet, stress management techniques, prescribed exercise, and regular group sessions to provide social support proved to be successful in reducing the size of existing atherosclerotic lesions in middle-aged men and women.[51] Daily use of one aspirin tablet may lower risk of myocardial infarction based on aspirin's ability to prevent the formation of blood clots that can block the passage of blood through a coronary artery.

Occurrence of Cancer

Cancer is the second leading cause of death among people over age 65 and by the year 2000 is expected to replace heart disease as the leading cause of death in the United States.[46] The anticipated emergence of cancer over heart disease as the leading cause of death is based on the consistent decline in deaths from heart disease over the past 40 years. This decline was brought about in part by public education and lifestyle modification designed to reduce the prevalence of risk factors that lead to coronary heart disease. Unfortunately, the lifestyle factors associated with cancer (except for cigarette smoking) are just beginning to receive attention. As Nissinen and Stanley[46] have pointed out, cancer research is now at the stage where cardiovascular research was 30 years ago. Epidemiologic studies have revealed some associations between diet and cancer, but the evidence is often conflicting. This has led to considerable debate over whether there is sufficient evidence to make specific dietary recommendations.

Breast cancer has increased in incidence over the past 15 years, and its association with dietary fat remains an issue.[72] The decline in reported cases of stomach cancer has been attributed to the increased use of refrigeration in food storage and lower consumption of salted and pickled foods.[72] The incidence of colon cancer has remained relatively unchanged despite public education about eating foods high in fiber. Dietary components being evaluated in relation to cancer risk include total kilocalories, fat, fiber, iron, selenium, calcium, ascorbic acid, beta carotene, and vitamins E and A.

Dietary Factors and Cancer Risk

Development. The sequence of events that transform a normal cell into cancerous tissue include three steps: initiation, promotion, and progression.[69] Dietary influences may interact in any of these steps. The **initiation** step in carcinogenesis is an irreversible genetic alteration that gives a normal cell the potential for uncontrolled growth. This genetic damage may result from an environmental toxin, a free radical molecule, or unknown causes. In the **promotion** step the abnormal cell is stimulated to grow and produce a cancer. Nutrients that act as antioxidants and can prevent cellular damage by free radical molecules may offer some protection against cancer initiation or promotion. The last and most serious step in cancer development is the **progression** step in which the tumor cells metastasize and colonize new cancer sites in the body.

Genetic and environmental factors, including diet, appear to be involved in the development of cancer. In animal models high-fat diets promote tumor growth; however, both the total energy intake and the type of fat influence this response. In certain animals diets high in energy that lead to rapid growth and enhanced cell proliferation increase tumor development, whereas in other animals with similar energy intakes, no tumors develop. This evidence supports the concept of a genetic influence on cancer development.[69]

Dietary fat. Ongoing human epidemiologic studies evaluating dietary fat intake and cancer incidence have produced inconclusive results. Many factors contribute to the differences in findings among studies.[11] The food records obtained may not be valid representations of actual food intake or the particular type of fat consumed. Food patterns may have changed between the time of the initial survey and the intervening years of follow-up. A further complicating factor is that high-fat diets are likely to be high in energy as well. Little work has been done on dietary intake at older ages and cancer incidence.

Dietary fat has been most closely associated with cancers of the breast and the colon. A study of over 89,000 nurses, age 34 to 59,[24] revealed no significant association between total dietary fat or type of fat and breast cancer after 11 years of follow-up. Similarly, the risk of breast cancer was not related to the intake of meat, eggs, cheese, and milk among more than 27,500 Seventh-Day Adventist women in California studied between 1960 and 1980.[59] Although Seventh-Day Adventists are less likely to eat meat (on the average, 55% had meat less than once a week), most of the women ate cheese and eggs at least one to three times a week and drank one to two glasses of milk a day. Mean fat intake was 38% of total energy; saturated and polyunsaturated fats contributed 11% and 18%, respectively, of total kilocalories.

Hunter and coworkers[24] pooled information from seven prospective studies in the United States, Sweden, Canada, and the Netherlands that included 337,819 women ages 28 to 76. They identified 4,980 cases of breast cancer. Among these women fat intake ranged from less than 20% of total energy to more than 45% of total energy. When the women in the highest quintile of total fat intake were compared with the women in the lowest quintile, their risk of breast cancer was increased by 5%. Relative risk was similar when evaluated on the basis of saturated, monounsaturated, or polyunsaturated fat intake. Women consuming a diet containing less than 20% fat had no reduction in risk. Those workers concluded that lowering fat intake in middle age is unlikely to influence risk of breast cancer.

Colon and rectal cancer have been associated with high intakes of dietary fat, particularly animal fat.[11] In the group of nurses described above, intake of animal fat was significantly related to incidence of colon cancer.[74] Women who ate beef, pork, or lamb five to six times a week had a risk nearly twice that of women who ate chicken with the skin removed or fish. A low intake of fiber from fruit appeared to contribute to risk, but this association was not statistically significant. Among Seventh-Day Adventist men and women,[59] consumption of animal foods, including dairy products and eggs, was unrelated to colon cancer; however, the use of low-fat dairy products may have contributed to this finding. Colon cancer appears to be more strongly linked to intake of red meat than intake of fat. Men with prostate cancer were found to be consuming higher levels of linolenic acid primarily obtained from red meat.[72]

Dietary fiber. Dietary fiber has been promoted as a means of reducing the risk of colorectal cancer.[11] Possible mechanisms by which dietary fiber may exert a protective effect include 1) reducing exposure to carcinogens by acting as a diluent and increasing fecal bulk, 2) reducing exposure to carcinogens by decreasing transit time, or 3) increasing the excretion of fecal bile acids that enhance the risk of cancer. Certain fiber components such as pectin decrease intestinal cell proliferation and may thereby reduce risk. Fiber-rich foods, rather than fiber per se, provide a more consistent protective effect against colorectal cancer, suggesting that other factors (e.g., carotenoids or ascorbic acid) may be involved.[11] Fiber intake was not associated with incidence of colon cancer in nearly 48,000 health professionals followed for six years.[16]

Dietary minerals. Epidemiologic studies have reviewed dietary intakes of calcium, iron, and selenium in relation to cancer risk.[11] A high intake of calcium lowers the secretion of bile acids thought to promote colon cancer; however, further work is needed to determine the physiologic importance of this observation. A recent committee concluded that insufficient evidence was available to justify a recommendation to increase calcium intake for colon cancer prevention.[11]

Iron catalyzes the production of high energy oxygen molecules considered to be potential carcinogens; consequently, iron status has been evaluated in respect to cancer risk. Individuals with extremely high iron stores may be at greater risk, but there is no association between dietary iron and the development of cancer.[4]

Dietary vitamins. Increasing evidence suggests that ascorbic acid, vitamin E, and the carotenoids decrease the risk of cancer. These substances function as antioxidants and protect tissues against oxidative damage from highly reactive free radicals. Ascorbic acid is the primary antioxidant in blood plasma; it protects vitamin E in cell membranes and complements the action of the carotenoids. Apart from its role as a precursor of vitamin A, beta carotene can interfere with carcinogenesis at both the initiation and promotion steps.[11]

Low intake of vegetables and fruits and low plasma levels of beta carotene have been associated with the subsequent development of lung cancer. A study of 872 men ages 40 to 59 who were followed for 25 years[7] revealed an inverse relationship between intake of ascorbic acid and the incidence of lung cancer. Ascorbic acid in amounts of 70 mg or more a day appeared to offer some protection against cancer, even among smokers.

Prospective studies evaluating intake of antioxidant vitamins and incidence of breast or colon cancer have produced mixed results. In the Nurses Study[23] large intakes of vitamin C and vitamin E from food and supplements did not offer protection against breast cancer over an eight-year follow-up. At the same time intake of total vitamin A or preformed vitamin A at the RDA level or higher reduced risk by 10% to 20%. Surprisingly, vitamin A supplements were of no benefit to those women with low vitamin A intake from food. Carotenoids with vitamin A activity contributed to the reduction in risk. In 751 men with a mean age of 61, supplements of vitamin C, vitamin E, beta carotene, or all three, had no effect on the incidence of colorectal cancer after four years.[19]

Available evidence does not support the use of concentrated vitamin supplements as a preventive measure against cancer. Conversely, the liberal use of carotenoid-containing fruits and vegetables appears to have a positive role in cancer prevention. Following the Five A Day rule for fruits and vegetables seems to be a practical way to lower cancer risk.

NUTRIENT INTAKE AND LIFE SPAN

Limited research now exists to provide a basis for general dietary recommendations that will extend life and years of physical well-being.

Available studies as described earlier have focused on particular nutrients and specific diseases or causes of death. Longitudinal studies evaluating the overall dietary pattern of individuals or their health and lifestyle practices and their subsequent morbidity and mortality have been few.

Longitudinal Studies of Diet and Health

The Michigan study. A longitudinal study of 103 older Michigan women evaluated over a 24-year period[54] suggested that the nutrient quality of the diet influenced both physical well-being and length of life. After seven years mortality was higher in those women consuming diets containing less than 40% of the RDA for one or more nutrients. The nutrients most frequently deficient were calcium, vitamin A, and ascorbic acid.

A follow-up after 24 years revealed that the survivors who ranged in age from 64 to 90 years had reduced the quantity and improved the quality of the food they ate.[28] Energy intake decreased from 1,683 kcal to 1,297 kcal and fat from 74 g to 51 g. Protein intake did not change. Foods such as sweet, baked items that are high in simple carbohydrate and fat but low in other nutrients were eaten less often. Fruits, vegetables, breads and cereals, and low-fat rather than high-fat dairy foods were emphasized. Fat as a percentage of total kilocalories decreased from 40% to 35%. Reducing dietary fat to 30% of total energy and increasing complex carbohydrates to 55% to 60% of total energy can model successful aging.

The Alameda health study. A longitudinal study begun in 1965[9] is examining behavioral and demographic influences on the incidence of disease and overall mortality in nearly 7,000 residents of Alameda County, California. In both men and women, seven health-related practices decreased risk of death in middle and advanced age:

- not smoking
- drinking no alcohol or only moderate amounts
- regular physical activity
- seven to eight hours of sleep a night

- appropriate relative weight (not more than 10% under or 30% over average weight for height)
- not eating between meals
- regularly eating breakfast

These patterns were particularly consistent among individuals age 70 or older.

As people live longer, they also become increasingly concerned about their ability to remain independent. Not only did the seven health practices described above increase the length of life, they also reduced physical disability in the survivors.[9] Those people who were following six or seven of the health practices when first interviewed were only half as likely to be disabled as those following three or less health practices. The people who followed four or five health practices had about two-thirds the risk of disability as those following three or less.

The Alameda Health Study[9] suggests that patterns of mortality and morbidity, even among the elderly, are not merely a random process. Lifestyle choices over which the individual has some control play a role in exacerbating or reducing risk. Behavior in later life is at least partly responsible for an individual's health status regardless of genetic influences. In pairs of male identical twins, an increase in systolic and diastolic blood pressure and a 50 mg/dl increase in serum triglycerides occurred only in the twin who had a significant weight gain between young adulthood and middle age.[45] These findings emphasize the need for and the potential benefits of intervention strategies directed toward individuals at both younger and older ages. Improving health practices can have a positive effect among those in poor health by preventing further decline. Nutrition education should be an integral part of such an intervention.

What Can We Learn from Centenarians?

Georgia centenarian study. The Georgia Centenarian Study[25] collected nutrition and diet information from 22 centenarians who were living in the community and were mentally able to participate in data collection. Most reported eating breakfast every day, and most had by their recall a reasonably stable body weight over their adult life with less than a 50-pound difference between their minimum and maximum weight. Their mean energy intake was 1,581 kcal with 37% as fat and 13% as saturated fat. On the average the centenarians met the current public health initiative of Five A Day with two servings of fruit and three servings of vegetables a day, with one vegetable a dark green or deep yellow vegetable. These elderly people had a low intake of alcohol, reporting only one alcoholic beverage a week. It is interesting to see that these exceptionally elderly people remained in reasonable health despite a diet relatively high in fat. They avoided excessive weight gain, whether by an active lifestyle or genetic background. Johnson and coworkers[25] suggested that a stable body weight may have decreased their risk of chronic disease or, alternatively, helped them to avoid illnesses associated with weight loss.

What Can We Learn from Other Cultures?

Traditional and evolving food patterns in different geographic regions around the world provide opportunities to study the influence of nutrient intake and lifestyle on the development of chronic disease. As new technology allows rapid communication among all parts of the world, people in rural and urban centers are adopting new food patterns from other cultures and in some cases moving from more active to more sedentary lifestyles. Individuals remaining in locations where traditional patterns are continued can be compared with populations who have adopted new food patterns and enable us to evaluate the effects of such changes on health and well-being. We will examine some examples of changes in nutrient intake, both positive and less appropriate, and health outcomes.

Food patterns in Japan. Life expectancy in Japan has risen dramatically in this century and changes in food intake have been associated with this increase. In Japan in 1960 life expectancy at age 45 was 27 years for men and 32 years for women, similar to the United States. In 1990 Japan had the highest life expectancy at age 45 of any nation in the world, about 33 years for men and 34 years for women.[32]

In 1958 Japan had the highest death rate from cerebrovascular disease in the world, and cerebrovascular disease and stomach cancer were the leading causes of death.[18] The traditional diet in Japan consisted of large amounts of salted rice, along with soybean soup and pickled vegetables, which also added to sodium intake. Red meat and eggs were seldom eaten although fish was included in the diet regularly. Intakes of both fat and saturated fat were low, making up only 11% and 3% of total energy, respectively.[18] Willett[72] suggested that the high salt intake and the low intake of fresh fruits contributed to the high rates of stomach cancer. Very low serum cholesterol, characteristic of the Japanese, and a high sodium intake have been associated with cerebrovascular disease and stroke.

Since that time the Japanese have added meat to their diet, although not to the extent that Americans have, and reduced their intake of salt. The death rate from cerebrovascular disease, accomplished by lowering sodium intake, has dropped by more than half since 1960. A comparison of food intake in men and women age 60 and over in the Japanese village with the shortest life expectancy and the Japanese village with the highest life expectancy revealed that those living longer consumed 1) three times more meat; 2) one and one half times more vegetable protein (primarily soy protein); 3) three times more green vegetables; and 4) one half the amount of salt. Meat intake among the long-lived was still less than 50 g a day (less than a 2-ounce serving), and intake of milk and dairy products was about 150 g a day (about a 5-ounce serving).[18]

Recent evidence suggests that the traditional Japanese diet based on rice and fish is no longer typical among young people. Although Japan continues to enjoy the highest life expectancy in the world, a dramatic decline in the use of fish and reduced intake of eicosapentaenoic acid may be contributing to the fourfold increase in the death rate from ischemic heart disease. Since 1960 fat intake in Japan has continued to rise above the former level of 11%. A recent dietary study of 11-year-olds found their fat intake to equal 34% of total energy.[18] Higher intakes of dietary fat have been accompanied by an increase in serum cholesterol levels. Between 1960 and 1980 mean serum cholesterol rose by 15 mg/dl, and in the last ten years it has continued to increase at a rate of 1 mg/dl a year.[18] This increase in dietary fat can be expected to lead to a growing incidence of atherosclerotic lesions in Japanese children and young adults.

China study. China is one of the few places in the world where it is possible to find a group of individuals who are genetically homogeneous and who have lived in the same place and eaten the same foods throughout their lives. This has provided an opportunity to compare the effect of different eating patterns and nutrient intakes on the development of degenerative diseases and intervention strategies. The Linxian region of China has one of the highest rates of esophageal and stomach cancer in the world.[8,64] People living in this region have low intakes of meat, fruits, most vegetables, and many vitamins and minerals. Staple food items making up the diet are corn, millet, sweet potatoes, and wheat. A study begun in 1985 is examining the effects of specific vitamin and mineral supplements within the range of one to two times the Recommended Dietary Allowance (RDA) on reduction of these cancers.[8,64] The vitamins and minerals being given in different combinations are vitamins A, C, and E, riboflavin, niacin, beta carotene (a precursor of vitamin A), zinc, selenium, and molybdenum. About 29,600 adults are participating in the study. After five years total mortality decreased by nearly 10% in those people given the beta carotene, vitamin E, and selenium, and esophageal cancer incidence dropped by 42%.[64] The incidence of gastric cancer fell by 62% among the people taking vitamin A and zinc.[8] These findings suggest that improved intakes of vitamins and minerals within the range associated with normal food intake contribute to overall health and cancer prevention. It would be interesting to examine specific vitamin and mineral intakes associated with the traditional Japanese diet in light of the high incidence of stomach cancer in that population.

Mediterranean countries. In the geographical regions of Crete, Greece, and southern Italy, the rates of heart disease and stroke traditionally have been among the lowest in the world. In the 1960s mortality rates from coronary heart

TABLE 2-3   *Comparison of Dietary Patterns in the 1960s*

Characteristic	United States	Mediterranean Region (Greece)
Fat (% of total energy)	39	37
Saturated fat (% of total energy)	18	8
Vegetables (g/day)	171	191
Fruits (g/day)	233	463
Legumes (g/day)	1	30
Breads and cereals (g/day)	123	453
Potatoes (g/day)	124	170
Meat (g/day)	273	35
Fish (g/day)	3	39
Eggs (g/day)	40	15

Adapted from Kushi, L.H., Lenart, E.B., and Willett, W.C.: Health implications of Mediterranean diets in light of contemporary knowledge. 2. Meat, wine, fats, and oils, Am. J. Clin. Nutr. 61(suppl):1416S, 1995.

❖

PLANT FOODS IN THE MEDITERRANEAN DIET

vegetables
olives
potatoes
beans, chickpeas, other legumes
nuts, seeds
fruit
Grain products
couscous
bulgur
pasta
polenta
rice

disease were six times higher in the United States than in Greece. Food intake also differed greatly between Americans and Greeks and played a major role in defining disease patterns (see table 2-3).[32] Examination of the food habits in the Mediterranean region led to the characterization of the Mediterranean diet that when accompanied by a high level of physical activity prevented the development of obesity and promoted a high life expectancy.[73] The traditional Mediterranean diet contained a variable amount of fat ranging from less than 25% to more than 35% of total kilocalories, depending on the specific region. The major source of fat was olive oil, high in monounsaturated fatty acids; saturated fat made up less than 7% to 8% of total fat. The major source of energy was complex carbohydrates coming from plant foods (see box). Fresh fruit was the typical dessert and sweet items, usually made with honey, were eaten only a few times a week. Cheese and yogurt were the usual dairy foods as refrigeration was generally unavailable, and these were used in low to moderate amounts. No more than four eggs

were eaten in a week, and red meat was used sparingly. Bread was eaten at all meals with no butter or margarine. Wine was included in the diet in low to moderate amounts and usually consumed with meals.[73]

Since 1960 the use of red meat and the intake of animal fat has increased markedly in Greece and other Mediterranean countries.[65] In a middle class population in Athens, use of pork increased eightfold and use of beef and veal increased nearly sixfold between 1969 and 1989. Conversely, use of beans fell by 80% and use of chickpeas by 60%. Changes in the dietary pattern over time appear to have influenced the development of coronary heart disease and other chronic disease in this region. In a small cohort of 182 older people from rural villages in Greece,[65] researchers found that 149 were following the traditional diet which included 1) a high ratio of monounsaturated to saturated fat, 2) a high intake of legumes, cereal foods, fruits, and vegetables, and 3) a low intake of meat and dairy products. Over a five-year follow-up, the death rate was 26% in the group that continued to follow the traditional pattern, but rose to 45% in the group who had increased their intake of total fat and saturated fat and reduced their use of plant foods.

Many lessons can be learned by evaluating the food patterns of various cultures and their impact on life expectancy and the prevalence of chronic disease. Evidence from the Mediterranean region and Japan suggests that plant foods and grains provide the foundation of a health-promoting diet. Generous intakes of fruits and vegetables decrease risk of both coronary heart disease and cancer. Use of red meat in moderate amounts will provide animal protein and important vitamins and minerals while limiting intake of fat and saturated fat. Occasional use of fish will contribute n-3 fatty acids that may play a role in reducing cardiovascular risk. Use of olive oil, high in monounsaturated fatty acids, rather than saturated fats is a prudent choice. Selection of low-fat dairy foods rather than those high in fat promote bone health without adding excessive amounts of fat. Avoiding foods and condiments high in sodium and limiting foods that are concentrated sources of fat and simple sugars will support lifelong health. The Dietary Guidelines for Americans suggest appropriate food patterns.

Need for Continued Research

Although an optimum nutrient intake, regular physical activity, and an appropriate body weight extend physical well-being and delay the aging process, the mechanisms by which this is accomplished are not understood. Furthermore, the literature on which these conclusions are based is fragmentary, usually involving only small numbers of people observed over short periods of time. Most existing studies have involved primarily white people and future studies should include African American, Hispanic, and other race and ethic groups.

In their comprehensive review of nutrition and aging published nearly 30 years ago, Howell and Loeb[21] called for studies that evaluate the lifelong food intake of individuals in relation to their physical health and chronic disease in advancing years. Such a study should begin in childhood, as food habits early in life influence biochemical processes and the development of chronic disease. Intervention strategies for women and ethnic minorities who have different patterns of disease risk must be defined based on outcomes of clinical trials. Only by such strategies will we learn what dietary and lifestyle patterns are necessary to ensure optimal health throughout life.

Summary

Both the quantitative and qualitative aspects of our diet influence physical well-being, incidence of chronic disease, and length of life. Aging is a multifactorial process involving the interaction of genetic control and environmental insults which eventually overwhelm the organism. A nutritionally adequate diet, restricted only in energy, increases the life span and delays the onset of age-related physiologic

---

❖ ❖ ❖

CASE STUDY

A woman age 59 has been referred to you for counseling because her family has a history of both cardiovascular disease and cancer. She believes that a person's risk of disease is "all in their genes" and doesn't think that what she does will make much difference. She is 5 feet, 5 inches tall and weighs 150 pounds. She is in generally good health although her blood pressure is 150/85. Her total serum cholesterol is 215 mg per dl.

1. What components of her diet would you assess that might increase or decrease her risk of these diseases?

2. What recommendations would you make about her dietary intake?

3. What information would you need about her lifestyle? What might be some helpful suggestions to offer about healthy lifestyle practices for disease prevention?

4. What information or evidence could you provide to convince her of the possible benefits of following a healthy eating and living pattern?

and biochemical changes in experimental animals. Undernutrition during fetal development and in the first year of life appears to lead to pathologic changes which decrease the human life span because of diseases such as coronary heart disease, hypertension, and non-insulin-dependent diabetes mellitus. Research on humans such as epidemiological studies, cohort studies, cross-sectional studies, and clinical trials, are being used to learn how nutrient intake and health practices affect the aging process.

The public health emphasis on reducing total dietary fat has been instrumental in the declining incidence of cardiovascular disease that has occurred since 1960. Elevated blood pressure, inappropriate blood lipoprotein patterns, obesity, smoking, low physical activity, and glucose intolerance continue to be strong predictors of coronary risk in both middle-age and elderly adults. Diets that emphasize fish, antioxidants such as vitamins C and E plus copper, sufficient carotenoids and folate, complex carbohydrates from grain foods, or moderate alcohol use have been associated with a reduced risk of coronary heart disease. Continuing to be physically active and avoiding excessive body fat is strongly correlated with a decreased level of coronary heart disease and stroke in the aging population. The most promising intervention for cardiovascular disease is dietary treatment rather than drugs to lower serum cholesterol, but a healthy lifestyle throughout the life cycle is the best prevention.

Epidemiological studies have revealed some associations between diet and cancer, but the evidence is often conflicting. Limiting dietary fat and increasing consumption of fruits and vegetables rich in carotenoids and ascorbic acid appear to offer some protection against the development of cancer, although other factors present in these foods also may play a role. The Mediterranean diet that emphasizes fruits, vegetables, breads, and cereals has been associated with longevity and good health. Lifestyle practices that appear to support physical well-being into old age are not smoking, little alcohol, regular exercise and sleep habits, appropriate body weight, and regular meals.

REVIEW QUESTIONS

1. Describe the five current theories of aging. What are the characteristics of the genetic theories as compared to the environmental theories? How does the process of aging occur at the organism level, the organ level, and cellular and molecular levels?

2. How does energy restriction influence a) the length of life, b) the incidence of degenerative disease, and c) the occurrence of age-related biochemical changes in animal models? Discuss possible hormonal mechanisms that may bring about these changes.

3. What are the major risk factors for cardiovascular disease in people age 65 or older? Do risk factors differ for older people compared to middle-aged people? Do risk factors differ for older women compared to older men? How might these risk factors be reduced or modified?

4. What evidence exists to suggest that body weight influences human life span? How does obesity contribute to mortality risk in older people? What are possible biases in research studies that may obscure the risk associated with obesity?

5. What are the three steps in the development of cancer? What nutrients are associated with increased and decreased risk of certain cancers? How do they relate to cancer development?

6. List several health practices that appear to increase the length of life and decrease the development of physical disability in older people. How might these practices retard the development of degenerative disease?

SUGGESTED LEARNING ACTIVITIES

1. Review the health practices associated with an increased life span in the Alameda Health Study. Visit a congregate meal site or senior citizens center and interview 10 older people about their general health habits. Compare their health habits to those of the Alameda population.

2. Plan an activity program for an older person that will allow him or her to expend 200 kcal to 250 kcal a day in physical activity.

3. Develop a handout on cardiovascular health issues and positive dietary and health practices for older women. Be sure to use a print size that is easy to read, terms that are easy to understand, and pictures that include all race and ethnic groups.

4. Visit the web site of the Food and Nutrition Information Center of the U.S. Department of

Agriculture at http://www.nal.usda.gov/fnic and look for nutrition education materials that emphasize foods associated with reduction of cancer risk. Make a list of materials that would be helpful to older people living alone who want to reduce their risk of cancer.

REFERENCES

1. Ascherio, A., and others: Dietary intake of marine n-3 fatty acids, fish intake, and the risk of coronary disease among men, New Engl. J. Med. 332:977, 1995.
2. Barker, D.J.P.: The fetal origins of adult disease, Nutr. Today 31(3):108, 1996.
3. Barrett-Connor, E., and Miller, V.: Estrogens, lipids, and heart disease, Clin. Geriatr. Med. 9(1):57, 1993.
4. Beard, J.L.: Are we at risk for heart disease because of normal iron status? Nutr. Rev. 51(4):112, 1993.
5. Beeuwkes, A.M.: Early speculations on diet and longevity. 1., J. Am. Diet. Assoc. 28:628, 1952.
6. Beeuwkes, A.M.: Early speculations on diet and longevity. 2., J. Am. Diet. Assoc. 28:707, 1952.
7. Bloch, G.: Epidemiologic evidence regarding vitamin C and cancer, Am. J. Clin. Nutr. 54:1310S, 1991.
8. Blot, W.J., and others: Nutrition intervention trials in Linxian, China: supplementation with specific vitamin/mineral combinations, cancer incidence, and disease-specific mortality in the general population, J. Natl. Cancer. Inst. 85:1483, 1993.
9. Breslow, L., and Breslow, N.: Health practices and disability: some evidence from Alameda county, Prevent. Med. 22:86, 1993.
10. Byers, T., and Bowman, B.: Brief critical reviews: vitamin E supplements and coronary heart disease, Nutr. Rev. 51(11):333, 1993.
11. Committee on Diet and Health. Food and Nutrition Board: Diet and health. Implications for reducing chronic disease risk, Washington, DC, 1989, National Academy Press.
12. Corti, M.C., and others: HDL cholesterol predicts coronary heart disease mortality in older persons, J.A.M.A. 274:539, 1995.
13. Darby, W.J.: Early concepts on the role of nutrition, diet and longevity. In Prinsley, D.M., and Sandstead, H.H., editors: Nutrition and aging, New York, 1990, Alan R. Liss.
14. Davidson, M., Bulkow, L.R., and Gellin, B.G.: Cardiac mortality in Alaska's indigenous and non-native residents, Intl. J. Epidemiol. 22(1):62, 1993.
15. Folsom, A.R., and others: Body fat distribution and 5-year risk of death in older women, J.A.M.A. 269:483, 1993.
16. Giovannucci, E., and others: Intake of fat, meat, and fiber in relation to risk of colon cancer in men, Cancer Res. 54:2390, 1994.
17. Goldberg, G.R., and Prentice, A.M.: Maternal and fetal determinants of adult diseases, Nutr. Rev. 52(6):191, 1994.
18. Goto, Y.: Changing trends in dietary habits and cardiovascular disease in Japan: an overview, Nutr. Rev. 50(12):398, 1992.
19. Greenberg, E.R., and others: A clinical trial of antioxidant vitamins to prevent colorectal adenoma, New Engl. J. Med. 331:141, 1994.
20. Harris, T., and others: The low cholesterol-mortality association in a national cohort, J. Clin. Epidemiol. 45(6):595, 1992.
21. Howell, S.C., and Loeb, M.B.: Nutrition and aging: A monograph for practitioners, Gerontologist 9(suppl.):1, 1969.
22. Hulley, S.B., and Newman, T.B.: Cholesterol in the elderly. Is it important? J.A.M.A. 272(17):1372, 1994.
23. Hunter, D.J., and others: A prospective study of the intake of vitamins C, E, and A and the risk of breast cancer, New Engl. J. Med. 329:234, 1993.
24. Hunter, D.J., and others: Cohort studies of fat intake and the risk of breast cancer—a pooled analysis, New Engl. J. Med. 334:356, 1996.
25. Johnson, M.A., and others: Nutritional patterns of centenarians, Intl. J. Aging and Human Development 34(1):57, 1992.
26. Kannel, W.B.: Nutrition and the occurrence and prevention of cardiovascular disease in the elderly, Nutr. Rev. 46(2):68, 1988.
27. Kannel, W.B.: Justification for management of blood lipids in the elderly. In Rosenberg, I.H., editor: Nutrition assessment of elderly populations. Measure and function, New York, 1995, Raven Press.
28. Kelley, L., Ohlson, M.A., and Harper, L.J.: Food selection and well-being of aging women, J. Am. Diet. Assoc. 33:466, 1957.
29. Klag, M.J., and others: Serum cholesterol in young men and subsequent cardiovascular disease, New Engl. J. Med. 328:313, 1993.
30. Krumholz, H.M., and others: Lack of association between cholesterol and coronary heart disease mortality and morbidity and all-cause mortality in persons older than 70 years, J.A.M.A. 272:1335, 1994.
31. Kuller, L.H.: Overview. Cardiovascular diseases and stroke in African-Americans and other racial

minorities in the United States, Circulation 83:1463, 1991.

32. Kushi, L.H., Lenart, E.B., and Willett, W.C.: Health implications of Mediterranean diets in light of contemporary knowledge. 2. Meat, wine, fats, and oils, Am. J. Clin. Nutr. 61(suppl):1416S, 1995.

33. Lee, I.M., and others: Body weight and mortality. A 27-year follow-up of middle-aged men, J.A.M.A. 270:2823, 1993.

34. Lumey, L.H., Stein, A.D., and Ravelli, A.C.J.: Timing of prenatal starvation in women and birth weight in their first and second born offspring: the Dutch famine birth cohort study, Euro. J. Obstet. Gynec. Reprod. Biol. 61:23, 1995.

35. Manson, J.E., and others: Body weight and longevity, J.A.M.A. 257:353, 1987.

36. Martinez-Maldonado, M.: Hypertension in Hispanics, Asians, Pacific-Islanders, and native Americans, Circulation 83:1467, 1991.

37. Masoro, E.J.: Dietary restriction and aging, J. Amer. Geriatr. Soc. 41:994, 1993.

38. Masoro, E.J., Shimokawa, I., and Yu, B.P.: Retardation of the aging processes in rats by food restriction, Ann. N.Y. Acad. Sci. 621:337, 1991.

39. McCay, C.M., and others: Retarded growth, life span, ultimate body size and age changes in the albino rat after feeding diets restricted in calories, J. Nutr. 18:1, 1939.

40. Monsen, E.R., editor: Research: successful approaches, Chicago, 1992, The American Dietetic Association.

41. Moordian, A.D.: Theories of aging. In Morley, J.B., Glick, Z., and Rubenstein, L.Z., editors: Geriatric nutrition. A comprehensive review, ed. 2, New York, 1995, Raven Press.

42. Morris, D.L., Kritchevsky, S.B., and Davis, C.E.: Serum carotenoids and coronary heart disease: the lipid research clinics coronary primary prevention trial and follow-up study, J.A.M.A. 272:1439, 1994.

43. Multiple Risk Factor Intervention Trial Research Group: Mortality rates after 10.5 years for participants in the multiple risk factor intervention trial, J.A.M.A. 263(13):1795, 1990.

44. Must, A., and others: Long-term morbidity and mortality of overweight adolescents, New Engl. J. Med. 327:1350, 1992.

45. Newman, B., and others: Nongenetic influences of obesity on other cardiovascular disease risk factors: an analysis of identical twins, Am. J. Public Health 80:675, 1990.

46. Nissinen, A., and Stanley, K.: Unbalanced diets as a cause of chronic diseases, Am. J. Clin. Nutr. 49:993, 1989.

47. Paffenbarger, R. S., and others: Changes in physical activity and other lifeway patterns influencing longevity, Med. Sci. Sports Exerc. 26(7):857, 1994.

48. Paffenbarger, R.S., and others: The association of changes in physical-activity level and other lifestyle characteristics with mortality among men, New Engl. J. Med. 328:538, 1993.

49. Posner, B.M., and others: Healthy People 2000: The rationale and potential efficacy of preventive nutrition in heart disease: the Framingham Offspring-Spouse Study, Arch. Intern. Med. 153(13):1549, 1993.

50. Psaty, B.M., and others: Risk ratios and risk differences in estimating the effect of risk factors for cardiovascular disease in the elderly, J. Clin. Epidemiol. 43(9):961, 1990.

51. Reversing heart disease through diet, exercise, and stress management: an interview with Dean Ornish, J. Am. Diet. Assoc. 91:162, 1991.

52. Ridker, P.M., and others: Association of moderate alcohol consumption and plasma concentration of endogenous tissue-type plasminogen activator, J.A.M.A. 272:929, 1994.

53. Rowe, J.W.: Aging processes. In Abrams, W.B., Beers, M.H., and Berkow, R., editors: Merck manual of geriatrics, ed. 2, Whitehouse Station, NJ, 1995, Merck Research Laboratories.

54. Schlenker, E.D.: Nutritional status of older women, Ph.D. dissertation, Michigan State University, East Lansing, 1976.

55. Serdula, M.K., and others: Alcohol intake and subsequent mortality: findings from the NHANES I follow-up study, J. Stud. Alcohol 56:223, 1995.

56. Sherman, S.E., and others: Does exercise reduce mortality rates in the elderly? Experience from the Framingham Heart Study, Am. Heart J. 128:965, 1994.

57. Sherman, S.E., and others: Physical activity and mortality in women in the Framingham Heart Study, Am. Heart J. 128:879, 1994.

58. Slattery, M.L., and Randall, D.E.: Trends in coronary heart disease mortality and food consumption in the United States between 1909 and 1980, Am. J. Clin. Nutr. 47:1060, 1988.

59. Snowdon, D.A.: Animal product consumption and mortality because of all causes combined, coronary heart disease, stroke, diabetes, and cancer in Seventh-Day Adventists, Am. J. Clin. Nutr. 48:739, 1988.

60. Srinath, V., and others: Diet in the prevention and treatment of atherosclerosis: A perspective for the elderly, Clin. Geriatr. Med. 11(4):591, 1995.

61. Stampfer, M.J., and others: A prospective study of plasma homocyst(e)ine and risk of myocardial infarction in US physicians, J.A.M.A. 268:877, 1992.

62. Stevens, J., and others: Body mass index and body girths as predictors of mortality in black and white women, Arch. Intern. Med. 152:1257, 1992.

63. Sytkowski, P.A., Kannel, W.B., and D'Agostino, R.B.: Changes in risk factors and the decline in mortality from cardiovascular disease. The Framingham Heart Study, New Engl. J. Med. 322:1635, 1990.

64. Taylor, P.R., and others: Prevention of esophageal cancer: the nutrition intervention trials in Linxian, China, Cancer Res. 54(Suppl.):2029s, 1994.

65. Trichopoulou, A., and others: Diet and survival of elderly Greeks: a link to the past, Am. J. Clin. Nutr. 61:1346S, 1995.

66. U.S. Department of Health and Human Services: Second report of the expert panel on detection, evaluation, and treatment of high blood cholesterol in adults, NIH Publication No. 93-3095, Washington, DC, September, 1993, U.S. Government Printing Office.

67. Van Itallie, T.B., and Lew, E.A.: Health implications of overweight in the elderly. In Prinsley, D.M., and Sandstead, H.H., eds.: Nutrition and aging, New York, 1990, Alan R. Liss.

68. Vijg, J., and Wei, J.Y.: Understanding the biology of aging: the key to prevention and therapy, J. Am. Geriatr. Soc. 43:426, 1995.

69. Visek, W.J.: Diet and cancer. In Prinsley, D.M., and Sandstead, H.H., eds.: Nutrition and aging, New York, 1990, Alan R. Liss.

70. Wenger, N.K., Speroff, L., and Packard, B.: Cardiovascular health and disease in women, New Engl. J. Med. 329(4):247, 1993.

71. Wienpahl, J., Ragland, D.R., and Sidney, S.: Body mass index and 15-year mortality in a cohort of black men and women, J. Clin. Epidemiol. 43(9):949, 1990.

72. Willett, W.C.: Diet and health: what should we eat? Science 264:532, 1994.

73. Willett, W.C., and others: Mediterranean diet pyramid: a cultural model for healthy eating, Am. J. Clin. Nutr. 61(suppl):1402S, 1995.

74. Willett, W.C., and others: Relation of meat, fat, and liver intake to the risk of colon cancer in a prospective study among women, New Engl. J. Med. 323(24):1664, 1990.

75. Willett, W.C., and others: Weight, weight change, and coronary heart disease in women, J.A.M.A. 273:461, 1995.

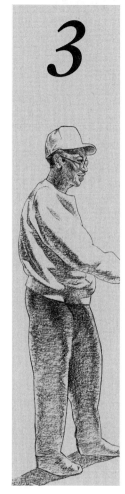

3

Nutrient Requirements and Metabolism

✦✦✦

Objectives

After studying the chapter, the student should be able to:

✔ *Understand how the recommended dietary allowances (RDAs) for older adults were established and why the recommendations may be unrealistic*

✔ *Recognize the need for an adequate energy intake in older people and understand how energy intake influences protein status*

✔ *Identify appropriate food sources of carbohydrate, protein, and fat for the older person*

✔ *List the methods of evaluation useful in determining the protein requirements or status of older adults*

✔ *Understand how age-related changes in protein metabolism affect the protein requirement*

INTRODUCTION

The **Recommended Dietary Allowances** (RDAs), as applied to older adults, continue to be controversial. In past years research defining the specific requirements of older people was lacking, and current recommendations for older adults have been extrapolated from those developed for younger adults. Moreover, the influence of the aging process on the physiologic roles and metabolism of the macronutrients is not well understood. We do know that inappropriate intakes of fat and saturated fat accelerate degenerative changes associated with aging and the development of chronic disease. At the same time research suggests that omega-3 fatty acids play a positive role in promoting good health. New methods for evaluating protein synthesis and loss in various body compartments have added to the present understanding of protein needs and the role of exercise in the preservation of lean body mass. Foods high in complex carbohydrates usually are good sources of important vitamins, minerals, and fiber and should represent a major portion of the energy intake. In this chapter we will discuss the roles of carbohydrate, fat, and protein and the metabolic basis for dietary recommendations for older adults.

RECOMMENDED DIETARY ALLOWANCES

Recommendations for Older Adults

The RDAs were developed to be an estimate of the nutrient needs of all healthy people.[13] For younger age groups research studies are available to serve as a basis for these recommendations. Because research studies with older adults have been limited, the RDAs for people over age 50 have been extrapolated from those developed for adults ages 25 to 50. For many nutrients, including protein and most vitamins and minerals, the recommended intakes are the same for younger adults ages 25 to 50 and older adults ages 51 and over (see appendix A). Exceptions include the iron allowance for women and the thiamin, riboflavin, and niacin allowances for men and women. The RDA for iron drops from 15 mg to 10 mg for women after age 50 because menstruation and the associated iron loss has ceased. The requirements for thiamin, riboflavin, and niacin are lower in response to the lower energy intake expected in people over age 50. Before 1989 the Food and Nutrition Board suggested a further adjustment in energy intake for those age 76 and older, based on the reduced physical activity expected of people in this age group. However, a low level of physical activity should not be encouraged or considered normal for older adults, and downward adjustments in energy intake should be handled on an individual basis.

Limitations of the Recommended Dietary Allowances

The RDAs have many limitations when applied to older people. Factors that contribute to these problems include 1) the heterogeneity among aging people, 2) the physiologic changes associated with the aging process, 3) individual health status and presence of chronic disease, and 4) the heavy use of prescription and over-the-counter drugs by this age group.[43] People continue to change in body composition, physiologic function, and metabolic adaptation as they age. Epidemiologists and government census specialists have recognized the significant differences that continue to develop as people age and for this reason no longer use the broad category of 65 years and over.[3] Aging changes are complicated further by chronic disease and treatment with multiple medications. Blumberg[3] considers it unrealistic to assume that all individuals beyond age 50 have similar nutrient requirements. The nutrient needs of a healthy person in his 70s who swims regularly and takes no medications differ markedly from those of a frail 90-year-old who is homebound with serious cardiac and renal disease.

Physiologic changes such as altered digestion or absorption, brought about by the decreased secretion of hydrochloric acid or intrinsic factor, increase the need for particular nutrients. Estrogen withdrawal after menopause alters calcium absorption and metabolism and thereby raises the calcium requirement. Reduced kidney function in some older adults indicates that excessive amounts of protein should be avoided.

Another concern about the RDAs for older adults is the interrelation between particular nutrients and degenerative diseases. Chronic disease influences nutrient requirements, both as a result of the disease process itself and in relation to the therapeutic drugs prescribed to manage the condition. Older renal patients on hemodialysis can have elevated requirements for the water soluble vitamins.[11] Diuretics prescribed in the management of hypertension can deplete body stores of potassium, magnesium, zinc, pyridoxine, or folic acid, depending on the particular drug (see chapter 10). For the older individual in poor health, the RDAs may not provide a realistic estimate of nutrient needs.

Approaches to Dietary Recommendations

Opinions differ widely about the criteria for specific RDAs for older age groups. For example, should nutrient requirements be based on

TABLE 3-1   *Status of Current RDAs and ESADDIs for Older Adults**

Current Recommendation	Nutrient
Level too high	Magnesium, chromium, vitamin A
Level too low	Protein, calcium, vitamin D, riboflavin, vitamin B-6, vitamin B-12
Insufficient information for change	Phosphorus, iodine, manganese, fluoride, molybdenum, vitamin K, niacin, pantothenic acid, biotin

*RDA = Recommended Dietary Allowance
ESADDI = Estimated Safe and Adequate Daily Dietary Intake
Data from Wood, R.J., Suter, P.M., and Russell, R.M.: Mineral requirements of elderly people, Am. J. Clin. Nutr. 62:493, 1995; and Russell, R.M., and Suter, P.M.: Vitamin requirements of elderly people: an update, Am. J. Clin. Nutr. 58:4, 1993.

existing age-associated changes in body composition and physiologic and metabolic function, or should optimal body composition and function be defined for particular age groups and nutrient intakes designed to maintain them?[3] A second issue is related to disease risk. Should nutrient recommendations be at levels known to prevent deficiency or address optimal levels associated with maximal reduction of chronic disease risk?[21] Current research suggests that supplementation with vitamin B-6 and vitamin E can reverse the age-associated decline in immune response although long-term evaluations are required for confirmation. Similarly, older people who consume generous amounts of vitamin C and beta carotene have a reduced incidence of cataracts. Future RDAs may present a range of intake for a particular group that will allow individualization of a recommendation according to age, sex, health status, or level of physical activity. Blumberg[3] has pointed out that we already use this approach in dietary recommendations for individuals with particular risk for cardiovascular disease.

Researchers at the Human Nutrition Research Center on Aging in Boston propose that nutritional information developed over the past decade justifies the development of an RDA category for people age 70 and over.[39,56] They also cite evidence to support the idea that current RDAs for older adults may not be appropriate (table 3-1). While the RDAs for protein and several vitamins and minerals seem to be too low, the recommended levels of other nutrients would seem to be too high. Issues surrounding the requirements for these nutrients will be discussed in this and later chapters.

In contrast to these proposals others view the available research information as too limited to allow specific recommendations for the elderly and see no reason to suggest that healthy older people should consume a diet different from that recommended for younger people.[16] Also, the extreme individual differences that exist among physically impaired older people would imply that one set of standards would not be applicable to all in an older age group. Hegsted[16] points to the need to develop standards that will help individuals with diet planning. In his opinion the RDAs tend to encourage the use of supplements, since individuals are unprepared to select diets that will provide the levels of nutrients assumed to be required.

A reasonable approach is the evaluation of older people as individuals, considering their general health, level of physical activity, and degree of chronic disease. It is important that we prevent nutrient depletion but also avoid providing excessive levels of nutrients that may result in adverse or toxic effects.[14] Detailed study of the nutrient requirements of older people is a continuing need. A special area for emphasis might be nutrient requirements after age 75, when physiologic limitations increase and nutrient needs are most influenced by long-term drug use. An important group for study is the healthy elderly, from whom we might learn what levels of nutrient intake promote successful aging.

DIETARY CARBOHYDRATE AND FIBER

Carbohydrate Intake

Foods high in complex carbohydrates include fruits, vegetables, legumes, and breads and cereals. These foods contribute energy, fiber, iron and other trace minerals, and important vitamins and vitamin precursors to the diet. Whole-grain breads and cereals are a better choice than more refined products as they contain higher amounts of fiber, vitamins, and minerals. High-sucrose carbohydrate foods are poor sources of fiber and micronutrients.

Data from the Third National Health and Nutrition Examination Survey (NHANES III)[51] indicate that carbohydrate contributes substantially to the energy intake of people age 60 and over. Median carbohydrate intake varied from 237 g to 209 g in the men ages 60 to 69 and 80 and over, respectively. Comparable values for women were 185 g and 173 g. It is interesting to note that the amount of carbohydrate in the diet did not decrease proportionately with the decrease in total energy intake. Median energy intakes decreased by 234 kcal in the men and 208 kcal in the women over this age range, whereas kilocalories from carbohydrate decreased by 104 kcal and 48 kcal in the men and women, respectively. Carbohydrate intake is lower in older women than in older men and lower in African American and Mexican American elderly than in white elderly. For the most part these differences in carbohydrate intake reflect differences in energy intake.

Current guidelines of the U.S. Department of Agriculture and U.S. Department of Health and Human Services recommend that 55% or more of total kilocalories be supplied by carbohydrate.[47] Generous intakes of complex carbohydrate foods increase dietary levels of important vitamins, minerals, and fiber and decrease dietary levels of fat. In the NHANES III study[51] older women were more likely to approach this goal than older men. Percent of energy from carbohydrate ranged from 47 to 52 among the men. African American men between the ages of 60 and 69 had the lowest proportion of kilocalories from carbohydrate, and Mexican American men

ages 70 to 79 had the highest. In women energy intake from carbohydrate ranged from 51% to 57% with white and African American women ages 80 and over and Mexican American women ages 70 to 79, meeting the standard of 55% or more. In the Boston Nutritional Status Survey[41] of economically advantaged elderly, carbohydrate supplied only 48% to 49% of total energy.

It appears that living situation does not necessarily influence the proportion of kilocalories consumed as carbohydrate. In a study of Dutch women[24] residing in nursing homes, assisted-living residences, or in their own homes, percent of energy as carbohydrate was 45 to 46.5. Age and sex may influence the type of carbohydrate consumed. In the Boston study[41] the oldest volunteers (ages 80 and older) consumed proportionately more kilocalories from cookies and sugars (includes candy and syrups), and the women consumed relatively more of these items than the men. Individuals eating more high sucrose items were also more likely to attain their recommended RDA for energy. For the Dutch women described above, living situation did not influence intakes of sugar, but did influence intakes of complex carbohydrates. Women living independently ate more complex carbohydrates than those who were institutionalized. The institutionalized women were older and chewing problems or chronic disease may have influenced food choices.

The Body's Need for Carbohydrate

Glucose is a major energy source for many body tissues, including the brain and nervous system. Because other dietary components can be converted to glucose, there is no absolute dietary requirement for carbohydrate under most circumstances.[13] However, when dietary carbohydrate is very limited, stored triglycerides are broken down at a rapid rate, the oxidation of fatty acids is enhanced, and ketone bodies begin to accumulate. **Very-low-carbohydrate diets** advocated for weight loss that substitute protein for carbohydrate are inappropriate and dangerous for older individuals. An excessive intake of protein, with subsequent increases in nitrogenous waste, puts additional stress on the renal system. Fluid and electrolyte balance, already precarious in older people with advanced cardiac or renal disease, can be further distorted by very-low-carbohydrate diets. Older people trying to lose weight should be advised to avoid such regimens. Diets in which 60% to 70% of total kilocalories come from carbohydrate and monounsaturated fat have been found to support improved glycemic control in certain non-insulin-dependent diabetics.[29]

Dietary Fiber

Individuals of all ages are being encouraged to eat generous amounts of plant foods high in fiber. Foods high in **dietary fiber** are associated with appropriate serum lipoprotein patterns and decreased incidence of cardiovascular disease, diabetes, and colon cancer. The Food and Nutrition Board's Committee on Diet and Health[47] suggests that people eat five or more servings of a combination of fruits and vegetables and six or more servings of a combination of legumes and breads and cereals every day. The National Cancer Institute[49] recommends that people eat 20 g to 30 g of dietary fiber each day. Unfortunately, median intakes of the older adults interviewed in the NHANES III study[49] were generally below this goal. Older white men had about 15 g of dietary fiber a day and older white and Mexican American women about 13 g. Older African American men and women had even lower intakes, ranging from 10 g to 12 g, with the exception of men ages 80 and over whose intake fell to 7 g. Mexican American men ages 60 to 79 came the closest to the recommended level of intake with 17 g to 18 g of dietary fiber. The centenarians who participated in the Georgia study[20] consumed only 11 g of dietary fiber a day. Although the centenarians averaged 16 servings of fruit and 23 servings of vegetables each week (about 5.5 servings a day), they had less than one serving a day of a whole-grain bread or cereal.

Health status may influence the amount of fiber eaten. The institutionalized women in the Dutch study[24] had only 14 g of dietary fiber a day; the women in the assisted-living residence had 20 g, and the women living independently had 27 g. The women living independently who were younger and in better health had

three times the amount of fresh fruit, two times the amount of vegetables, and more bread than the institutionalized women. Breads and cereals are popular foods with older people although whole-grain items are less commonly used and should be encouraged. A recent evaluation of older people in Oklahoma[17] found that individuals consuming 20 g or more of dietary fiber each day had higher intakes of copper, magnesium, selenium, potassium, and iron. Appropriate intakes of dietary fiber, obtained from foods, help to maintain normal bowel function. Fiber supplements should be used with caution; in excessive amounts they contribute to bowel dysfunction.

LIPID INTAKE AND METABOLISM
Fat Intake

Recent national surveys indicate that older people are consuming levels of total fat and saturated fat above those recommended for adults of all ages. But the proportion of fat in the diets of older adults did decrease markedly between the NHANES II study[52] and the NHANES III study[51] (table 3-2). A point of concern to nutrition educators, however, should be the fact that absolute intakes of total fat and saturated fat decreased by only 2 g in men and actually increased in women over this period. This indicates that total kilocalories from fat have not decreased to any extent; in fact total energy intake increased with added amounts of carbohydrate and protein in the diet. In the NHANES III study the proportion of kilocalories supplied by fat did not change with age among people ages 60 and over. Women consumed less total fat than men.

The Georgia centenarians[20] living in the community continued to consume high levels of fat into advanced age. It would be interesting to study the serum lipoprotein profiles of the centenarians who appear to have aged successfully despite their fat intakes above recommended levels. Cholesterol intakes fell within suggested amounts for both the general population of older people and the Georgia centenarians.

TABLE 3-2 Differences in Fat Intakes of Older Population Groups

Age (years)	NHANES II (1976–1980)		NHANES III (1988–1991)		Georgia Centenarians
	Men 60–69	Women 60–69	Men 60–69	Women 60–69	100+
Total fat (g)	82	53	80	59	71
Fat (% of kcal)[1]	38	36	33	33	42
Saturated fat (g)	29	18	27	20	25
Saturated fat (% of kcal)[1]	13	13	11	11	15
Cholesterol (mg)[1]	415	262	312	210	290

[1]Recommended Levels:
  No more than 30% of total kcal from fat
  Less than 10% of total kcal from saturated fat
  No more than 300 mg of cholesterol

Data from U.S. Department of Health and Human Services: Energy and macronutrient intakes of persons ages 2 months and over in the United States: Third national health and nutrition examination survey, Phase I, 1988–91, Advance Data from Vital and Health Statistics, Number 255, Oct. 24, 1994, Hyattsville, MD, National Center for Health Statistics; U.S. Department of Health and Human Services, U.S. Department of Agriculture: Nutrition monitoring in the United States: an update report on nutrition monitoring, DHHS Pub. No. (PHS) 89-1255, Washington, DC, 1989, U.S. Government Printing Office; and Johnson, M.A., and others: Nutritional patterns of centenarians, Intl. J. Aging Hum. Develop. 34(1):57, 1992.

Intakes of polyunsaturated fatty acids were about 7% of total kilocalories in all older age and gender groups evaluated in the NHANES III study.

Essential Fatty Acids

Essential fatty acid requirements. Dietary fat is a source of both energy and the essential fatty acids necessary to maintain health. The two classes of dietary essential polyunsaturated fatty acids are represented by **linoleic acid,** an n-6 polyunsaturated fatty acid, and **alpha-linolenic acid,** an n-3 polyunsaturated fatty acid.[44] These fatty acids and their metabolites play an important role in the structure and function of every cell in the body and in recent years have been proposed as factors in reducing risk of chronic disease. Linoleic acid itself carries out few of the functions of an essential fatty acid, but it is metabolized to other substances including arachidonic acid which bring about the effects associated with the omega-6 essential fatty acids.[18] The first step in the conversion of linoleic acid to its important derivatives requires the enzyme delta-6-desaturase. This enzyme is present in lower amounts in older people[28] and in patients with diabetes mellitus. Reduced levels of this enzyme have been associated with the development of diabetic complications, including diabetic neuropathy.[18] Alpha-linolenic acid, an omega-3 fatty acid, has been identified recently to be an essential fatty acid. It also requires the delta-6-desaturase enzyme for the first step in the conversion to eicosapentaenoic acid and docosahexaenoic acid. The conversion of alpha-linolenic acid to eicosapentaenoic acid and docosahexaenoic acid occurs at a very slow rate, and elderly people in particular have a limited capacity to complete these metabolic steps.[44] Both eicosapentaenoic acid and docosahexaenoic acid are found in fatty fish and dietary intake of these acids from fish is important in meeting body needs. These fatty acids, whether synthesized by the body from available alpha-linolenic acid or supplied in the diet, may play a role in reducing the risk of cardiovascular disease, although further work is needed to clarify this effect.[18]

Overt essential fatty acid deficiency is seldom identified in adults, although it has been described in patients maintained on parenteral feedings that did not contain fat, and in individuals with serious fat malabsorption problems.[44] At present there are no RDAs assigned to either linoleic acid or alpha-linolenic acid. According to the Food and Nutrition Board,[13] a linoleic acid intake equal to 1% to 2% of total energy intake will prevent clinical or biochemical signs of deficiency. Several countries in Europe have recommended that at least 0.5% of total energy be supplied as omega-3 fatty acids, and a recent panel of experts has proposed a level of 1% of energy from omega-3 fatty acids in nutrition formulas.[2] Further work should address the need for a specific RDA for eicosapentaenoic acid and docosahexaenoic acids within the omega-3 group and possibly for arachidonic acid within the omega-6 group.

Intakes of essential fatty acids. Information regarding the usual intakes of particular classes of essential fatty acids by older people is sparse. Most dietary surveys report intakes of polyunsaturated fatty acids in total. As noted earlier, polyunsaturated fatty acids supplied 7% of the total energy for the older participants in the NHANES III study.[51] Intakes of polyunsaturated fatty acids were in the range of 3.6% to 4.6% of total energy in the Boston Nutritional Status Survey of healthy older people.[22] Witte-Foster and colleagues[55] did evaluate linoleic acid intake in a survey of older women in Iowa. The young-old women with a mean age of 72 ate 8 g of linoleic acid daily which supplied 5% of their total kilocalories, whereas the old-old women with a mean age of 88 ate only 7 g which still supplied 5% of their total energy intake.

Institutionalized older people can have a very low intake of linoleic acid despite a high intake of fat. In a French nursing home,[1] linoleic acid intake was only 4 g a day, although fat provided more than 40% of total energy. Younger people living in that region who ate similar types of food got 12 g of linoleic acid a day on a similar intake of fat. The older institutionalized subjects had lower concentrations of both linoleic acid and arachidonic acid in their serum lipids, compared to the young subjects. According to

Asciutti-Moura and coworkers,[1] the decreased levels of arachidonic acid in the serum lipids of the older adults could relate to a decreased ability to metabolize linoleic acid to arachidonic acid. An enzyme needed for this conversion requires vitamin B-6 as a cofactor, and this enzyme activity level is reduced if vitamin B-6 status is poor. Vitamin B-6 status was not evaluated in these older people.

A comparison of the fatty acid composition of serum lipoproteins in younger women ages 24 to 35 and older women ages 79 to 90 found the proportion of linoleic acid in cholesterol esters and phospholipids to be lower in the older women.[23] Although the linoleic acid intake of the older women was somewhat lower than that of the younger women (2% versus 3% of total energy), these values were not significantly different, and the intake of the older women fell within the range of intake believed to be sufficient to prevent essential fatty acid deficiency. Lecerf and coworkers believed that this change in lipid composition was not related to diet. The changes in fatty acid composition observed in the older women were similar to age-related degenerative changes described in animal studies. The fall in plasma content of linoleic acid among the elderly women, however, was not accompanied by the appearance of other metabolites that serve as biological markers of essential fatty acid deficiency. Phospholipid concentrations of linoleic acid and docosahexaenoic acid did not differ between older people with eye disorders and their matched controls, as compared to people of middle age.[42]

In healthy elderly men in Denmark,[33] higher plasma levels of total polyunsaturated fatty acids and linoleic acid were associated with a lowered immune response. Those workers[33] concluded that a low fat diet (less than 30% of total kilocalories as fat) that is also low in linoleic acid and the n-6 polyunsaturated fatty acids may be prudent for elderly people and optimal immune function.

It appears that further work is needed to establish optimum recommended dietary levels of essential fatty acids for older adults. Future nutrition surveys should define intakes of the two classes of essential fatty acids in healthy older people. As all population groups continue to lower their fat intake in response to public health initiatives, it will become increasingly important that dietary advice focus on foods that will ensure appropriate intakes of essential fatty acids.

PROTEIN REQUIREMENTS IN THE OLDER ADULT
Uncertainties in Protein Requirements

Evaluating protein requirements is an intensive process requiring substantial resources on the part of the researchers and a high degree of commitment on the part of the individuals being studied. Consequently, relatively few studies have evaluated the protein requirements of older people. Because protein requirements are related to protein synthesis and breakdown in skeletal muscle and body organs, changes in body composition can influence protein needs. Emotional stress, infection, and chronic diseases, which increase protein requirements, are common in older people. Also, a low-calorie diet influences the utilization of dietary protein. These factors can compromise protein status and make the older individual vulnerable to protein loss.

The Body's Need for Protein

Protein needs of adults. Protein metabolism continues as a dynamic process throughout adult life. Although physical growth has ceased, sufficient protein must be consumed to replace body nitrogen losses, which include (1) desquamated cells from the gastrointestinal tract and skin, (2) body secretions, including perspiration or digestive enzymes lost through the gastrointestinal tract, and (3) nitrogenous end products of body metabolism excreted in the urine. Proteins oversee the maintenance of cell and organ function in their roles as enzymes, hormones, and mediators of immune responses.[45] Thus age-related changes in protein availability and synthesis could have far-reaching consequences for physical well-being.

In the older individual, positive nitrogen balance can occur as part of the repletion of body protein stores after an illness, period of malnutrition, or stress. Strength training that increases muscle mass is associated with nitrogen retention and a positive nitrogen balance. When nitrogen excretion exceeds nitrogen intake, as occurs in infection, after surgery, in debilitating illness, or with glucocorticoid therapy, protein depletion ensues.[60] Nitrogen balance measurements reflect the sum total of nitrogen gain or loss; however, they do not provide answers as to the relative gain or loss of individual tissues. An adult is seldom in nitrogen equilibrium which indicates a net gain or loss of zero, but rather has fluctuating periods of nitrogen accretion and loss that on the average produce a net balance.

Loss of body protein. Even well-nourished adults appear to lose body protein as a function of age. Both longitudinal and cross-sectional studies have demonstrated a progressive decline in body potassium over the course of adult life. Potassium is more highly concentrated in the muscle than in the nonmuscle portion of the fat-free body. This led Cohn and coworkers[10] to the conclusion that the nonmuscle protein mass (made up of the brain, lungs, and organs in the abdominal cavity) generally is less affected by age-related protein losses. In contrast, skeletal muscle decreased by 46% in their subjects between the ages of 20 and 80. This estimate of the age-related decline in skeletal muscle agrees with other workers who reported that skeletal muscle made up 25% of body weight at birth, increased to 45% of body weight in the young adult, and declined to 27% of body weight beyond age 70.[58] This loss in muscle tissue is believed to contribute to the decrease in maximum oxygen consumption observed in older as compared to younger men.

The loss in body muscle and protein content has led to different interpretations of the protein requirement of older people.[26] First, this decrease in active metabolic tissue could reduce the need for protein and amino acids. An opposing point of view is that an inadequate intake of protein and amino acids contributes to protein loss, and increased amounts of protein are required to maintain appropriate body function and reestablish protein reserves. As we will see in later sections, protein intake, hormonal changes, and physical activity all play a role in the maintenance or loss of muscle protein in older adults.

Age-related changes in protein metabolism. Body proteins are in a constant state of synthesis and breakdown, referred to as **protein turnover.** Using labeled amino acids such as glycine or leucine, it is possible to estimate whole body protein turnover as influenced by age, sex, body composition, or diet. Comparisons between younger and older men and women[54] indicate that younger people have higher rates of whole-body protein turnover, and men have higher rates than women; however, when protein turnover is calculated on the basis of lean body mass, the differences between older and younger people and men and women are minimal.

Protein intake also influences whole-body protein turnover in older individuals. When protein provided 21% of total kilocalories, protein synthesis and breakdown, measured in g of protein per day, were significantly higher than when protein provided only 12% of total kilocalories.[30] Reducing the level of protein turnover is a means by which the body can conserve protein and adapt to a lower protein intake.[9] Pannemans and coworkers[30] also observed lower protein turnover among older women as compared to older men in their research, and this difference remained after adjustments for total fat free mass and protein intake per unit of fat-free mass. Both estrogen and testosterone stimulate protein synthesis, but women experience a significant loss of estrogen at menopause whereas, in men, testosterone concentrations decrease gradually with advancing age.

Strength or resistance training influences protein synthesis and breakdown in people of all ages.[57] Two weeks of resistance training brought about an increase in muscle protein synthesis that was equal in younger and older participants. An equally important observation was that muscle protein breakdown did not increase along with muscle protein synthesis, resulting in a net gain in muscle protein. This observation prompted those workers[57] to suggest that a resistance training program in older people may elevate their protein requirement. Fiatarone and

coworkers[12] observed no effect on outcome of a 15 g protein supplement given to elderly participants in a resistance training program; however, those individuals were receiving appropriate levels of protein prior to and during the exercise program. Resistance training has been shown to restore muscle tissue and function in older individuals (see chapter 5).

The loss of muscle mass that occurs with normal aging results in a greater contribution of the visceral organs, including the liver, kidney, and heart to whole-body protein metabolism. Young and coworkers[58] propose that muscle protein turnover accounts for only 20% of whole body protein turnover in older men as compared to 30% in younger men. The visceral organs have a higher rate of protein metabolism than skeletal muscle. This higher rate of metabolism must be considered when evaluating the nutritional needs of a debilitated older person with low muscle mass and body weight, because in this individual the visceral organs will contribute in a major way to energy and protein needs.

The nutritional significance of the age-related reduction in muscle mass and its relative contribution to total body protein metabolism is unclear. It is known that skeletal muscle serves as a protein reserve and plays an important role in metabolic adaptation in periods of stress such as illness, infection, surgery, or reduced food intake.[60] A reduced muscle mass increases the vulnerability of the older person to unfavorable nutritional consequences when protein requirements are elevated and food intake interrupted.

PROTEIN REQUIREMENTS IN OLDER PEOPLE
Methods for Evaluating Protein Requirements

Protein requirements can be evaluated using two different approaches. The **factorial method** evaluates all possible routes of nitrogen loss and establishes a level of protein intake that is expected to replace those losses. Body nitrogen is lost through the skin, urine, and feces in the form of desquamated cells, secretions, and metabolic waste products, even when no protein is provided in the diet. These losses, referred to as obligatory nitrogen losses, represent the minimum amount of nitrogen that must be replaced each day.

The second approach for determining protein requirements is the **balance method.** In a balance study, individuals are fed graded amounts of protein to determine the minimum level of protein that will maintain the individual in nitrogen equilibrium or zero nitrogen balance. Neither method is ideal when applied to older people. Although it appears that healthy elderly people can adapt to lower levels of dietary protein, obligatory nitrogen losses may still be higher than those of younger people. Also, protein requirements will still be higher in older people with nitrogen losses similar to younger people, if the older people use dietary proteins less efficiently.[26]

Nitrogen balance studies, although the method of choice, have limitations. Observations can be influenced by the prior intake of the older subject. An individual who has been on a low protein diet and has poor protein reserves is more likely to retain protein and reach equilibrium on a lower protein intake than an individual whose protein status has been optimum. Balance studies also are likely to use test diets that can differ markedly from the usual food pattern. Because of the cost and intense commitment required of participants, the time period allowed for adjustment may be relatively short. Whether older persons require a longer period of time to adapt to a new dietary pattern or level of nutrient intake is unclear.

Nitrogen Balance Studies

The protein requirements of older people have been evaluated using various levels and types of protein. Overall, these studies suggest that the current RDA for protein, 0.8 g/kg body weight, is not adequate to maintain nitrogen balance in healthy older people or in those who, although fit for their age, have chronic diseases and are taking prescription drugs (fig. 3-1).[6,15]

In a recent double blind evaluation of protein requirements conducted at the Human Nutrition Research Center on Aging in Boston,[6] 12 healthy men and women ranging in age from 56

to 80 years were studied. Each was assigned a diet that provided either the recommended level of protein (0.8 g/kg body weight) or twice the recommended level (1.6 g/kg body weight). Over 77% of the protein provided came from milk and eggs. Individuals remained on the diet for 11 days. All volunteers lived in a metabolic ward for the duration of the study and were provided with a sufficient level of kilocalories to meet calculated energy needs. On the lower level of intake (0.8 g/kg body weight), three of the six subjects were in negative nitrogen balance, and lost 6 mg to 14 mg of nitrogen per kg of body weight per day. All subjects receiving the higher protein intake were in positive nitrogen balance. Prediction equations based on these subjects indicated that the mean protein intake required to achieve nitrogen balance was 1 g/kg of body weight per day.

An earlier study evaluated the adequacy of the current RDA for protein (0.8 g/kg body weight) over a 30-day period in a somewhat older group.[15] The men had a mean age of 75 years and the women a mean age of 78. Although free of diabetes or other endocrine disorders, these older people had heart disease, hypertension, and gastrointestinal problems, including peptic ulcer and diverticulosis, and were typical of the older population with chronic diseases. After 30 days, four of the eight women and three of the seven men were still in negative nitrogen balance. In the women hemoglobin levels dropped from 13.7 to 13 g/dl over the study period. Older women appear to be more vulnerable to protein loss as suggested by this decrease in hemoglobin. This probably results from their reduced muscle mass and their diminished reserve of protein and amino acids.

Campbell and coworkers,[6] after comprehensive review of all available data, concluded that the mean protein requirement of older adults is 0.91 g/kg body weight compared to the value of 0.6 g/kg body weight set by the 1985 Joint FAO/WHO/UNU Expert Committee (fig. 3-1). The Food and Nutrition Board[13] in establishing a safe protein intake for all older people increased the value of 0.6 g/kg by 25% to set an RDA of 0.8 g/kg. Based on a protein requirement of 0.91 g/kg, Campbell and coworkers[6]

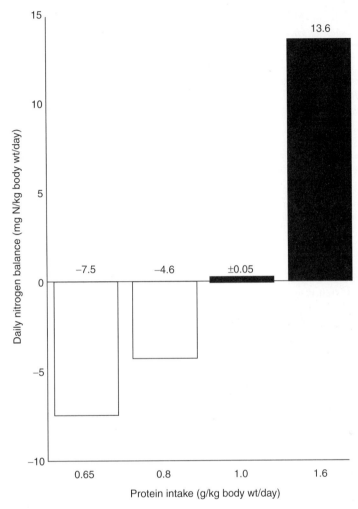

FIG. 3-1   Retention and Loss of Nitrogen in Healthy Older People Given Increasing Amounts of High Quality (Egg and Milk) Protein. The level of protein required for nitrogen balance in older people has been calculated to be at least 1 g per kg of body weight.

Data from Campbell, W.W., and others: Increased protein requirements in elderly people: new data and retrospective reassessments, Am. J. Clin. Nutr. 60:501, 1994, and Uauy, R., Scrimshaw, N.S., and Young, V.R.: Human protein requirements: nitrogen balance response to graded levels of egg protein in elderly men and women, Am. J. Clin. Nutr. 31:779, 1978.

suggest that the safe protein intake for elderly adults is 1.0 to 1.25 g/kg body weight. These levels are 25% to 56% above the current RDA.

Adaptation to changes in protein intake. Protein intake is marginal in many older people. In a study of 1,156 New England elderly people above 70 years of age,[31] about one-fifth had protein intakes that did not meet 75% of the RDA. Major considerations when setting recommended intakes for older people are their reduced protein reserves and decreased ability to adapt to changes in protein availability.

TABLE 3-3   *Influence of Protein Intake on Body Composition and Functional Responses in Older Women*

	Low Protein Diet (0.45 g/kg body wt)	Adequate Protein Diet (0.9 g/kg body wt)
Lean body mass	↓	No change
Cellular immune response	↓	No change
Muscle strength	↓	↑
Muscle power	↓	↑
Serum albumin	No change	↑
Serum total protein	No change	↑

Data from Castaneda, C., and others: Elderly women accommodate to a low-protein diet with losses of body mass, muscle function, and immune response, Am. J. Clin. Nutr. 62:30, 1995.

Adaptation is the process by which an individual reaches a new steady state in response to a change in food or nutrient intake.[8] This implies that body functions are maintained at former levels in the new steady state. A term that more likely describes this process in older people is **accommodation,** in which losses occur in important functions as a result of an inadequate protein intake.[8]

Changes in function that occur as a result of accommodation became apparent in 12 healthy elderly women given a low protein diet (0.45 g/kg body weight) or an adequate protein diet (0.92 g/kg body weight) for nine weeks.[8] The women eating the low protein diet experienced losses in lean tissue, immune response, and muscle function (table 3-3). These losses became apparent after only three weeks on the low protein diet and continued to increase in severity as the diet continued. Loss of lean body mass measured by whole body dual energy x-ray absorptiometry reached almost 2 kg over the nine-week period, and calculated losses of body potassium indicated that much of the tissue lost was muscle tissue. Antigen responses to hypersensitivity skin tests decreased by 50% in the low protein group, paralleling changes associated with **protein energy malnutrition** (PEM). Muscle function, strength, and power were measured in the dominant hand, by the chest press, and in leg extensor muscles. Losses in muscle function in the dominant hand and in immune response became apparent before the loss of lean body mass and may serve as early indicators of marginal protein status. Serum albumin levels were unchanged in the low protein group, suggesting the limited value of this measurement in assessing marginal protein deficiency. An unexpected finding was the observed increase in serum immunoglobulins, albumin, muscle strength, and power in the women on the higher protein intake. These findings suggest that the protein status of these women may have been less than optimal prior to the beginning of the study.

This report has significant implications for clinicians and public health nutritionists. Many older people in the United States and throughout the world are existing on marginal protein intakes. It does appear that over time older people can adjust to a lower protein intake and reduce their nitrogen loss. Castaneda and coworkers[8] reported that nitrogen losses in elderly women eating the low protein diet fell from 1 g of nitrogen per day at the end of three weeks to 0.35 g per day at the end of nine weeks. However, as described above, this was accompanied by a loss of muscle mass and functional capacity. These results urge renewed study of the relation of protein intake to the loss of lean body mass now attributed to normal aging.

Health status and protein intakes. An evaluation of nitrogen balance in elderly British men and women living in their own homes[4] and eating self-selected diets indicated that both protein intake and health status influence long-term protein status. Chronically ill older people may never adapt to a diet marginally deficient in protein. The healthy elderly people in this study maintained nitrogen equilibrium on intakes of about 1 g of protein per kg of body weight. At the same time the housebound elderly who had various chronic diseases including lung disease, heart disease, and osteoarthritis were eating only about 0.65 g to 0.69 g of protein per kg of body weight and were losing 1 g to 1.7 g of nitrogen per day. These losses were occurring on intakes of about 80% of the RDA. Even those housebound elderly consuming 0.8 g of protein per kg of body weight (100% of the RDA) were losing those amounts of nitrogen. The long-term consequences of nitrogen loss on health status are indicated by the fact that when approached about a year later regarding another study, the health of the housebound subjects had deteriorated to the point that they were unable to participate. It is pertinent that the housebound elderly were not all receiving daily meal delivery. Bunker and coworkers[4] questioned whether their deterioration in health status might have been prevented or slowed with more food.

Factors Influencing Protein Requirements and Utilization

Energy intake and nitrogen balance. The classic studies in protein metabolism described the protein-sparing action of carbohydrate and emphasized the need for sufficient kilocalories to promote the appropriate utilization of dietary protein and amino acids. An older study by Zanni and coworkers[61] indicated that nitrogen balance in older men fed marginal levels of protein (0.59 g/kg of body weight) could be improved by increasing energy intake. Those men were consuming 45 kcal/kg of body weight as compared to the energy intake of 30 kcal/kg currently recommended by the Food and Nutrition Board.[13] Alternatively, energy intake did not influence nitrogen balance in the elderly British healthy and housebound subjects described above.[4] It is of interest that the healthy women studied by Castaneda and coworkers[8] required additional kilocalories to maintain their body weight when consuming the diet marginal in protein (0.45 g/kg of body weight). Their daily energy intake increased from 1,862 kcal to 2,139 kcal, an increase from 27 kcal/kg to about 31 kcal/kg of initial body weight. In spite of this increase in energy intake, changes in body composition and function occurred; however, added kilocalories may play a role in the accommodation process.[9] Unfortunately, it is likely that many older people with marginal protein intake also have inadequate energy intake.

Prior protein intake. The metabolic response to a particular type or level of protein is influenced by the protein intake of the previous months as well as the current intake. As long as three months may be required to adapt to a low protein intake when previous intake was liberal. An individual with marginal protein status and limited protein reserves will respond with a strongly positive nitrogen balance when placed on a high protein diet, as protein stores are being replenished.[15] Conversely, a well-nourished individual may not demonstrate protein retention regardless of the level and quality of protein fed. These responses are evident in the well-nourished elderly placed on the low and high protein diets described in figure 3-1.

Individual variability. Protein requirements vary among individuals of a particular age and sex as well as within the same individual from one time to another. Physiologic stress, such as inflammation and infection, increases protein requirements and can result in substantial nitrogen losses, mediated in part by the stress response of the glucocorticoid hormones.[36] Emotional stress can be detrimental to nitrogen balance, and even liberal protein intakes may not prevent nitrogen loss when emotional upset is severe. Swanson[46] described an older woman living alone who went from negative to positive nitrogen balance on an equivalent amount of protein when a grandson came to live with her and her psychologic outlook improved. Many older people endure constant emotional stress from declining health and fear of losing independence, financial problems, or loneliness after the death of a spouse. The long-term impact of such psychologic distress on nitrogen balance has not been evaluated.

Amino Acid Requirements

The protein requirement includes the need for the nine essential amino acids that cannot be synthesized by the body. Information about the amino acid requirements of older people is sparse, although some evidence suggests that the need for several of the essential amino acids may change with age. The requirement for tryptophan appears to be somewhat lower and the threonine requirement somewhat higher per unit of lean body mass. In general, the requirements for certain essential amino acids actually may be somewhat higher if calculated on the basis of active metabolic tissue.[58] In light of the fact that animal protein makes up about 65% of the total protein in the average American diet, all essential amino acids are likely to be available in adequate amounts when protein intake is adequate.[13]

Plasma Amino Acid Levels

The fasting plasma amino acid profile can provide useful information about an individual's nutritional status.[38] A dietary intake deficient in protein or any single essential amino acid is reflected in changes in plasma amino acid levels. PEM results in a lower ratio of essential amino acids to nonessential amino acids in the plasma. Studies of healthy older people[5,34] consuming adequate amounts of protein suggest that plasma amino acid levels are not influenced by age. Plasma levels of essential amino acids were similar in healthy younger men and healthy older men[5] with protein intakes of more than 1 g per kg of body weight. Alternatively, another group of apparently healthy older men living in the community[38] had lower plasma levels of methionine, threonine, phenylalanine, and the branched-chain essential amino acids (leucine, isoleucine, and valine). Although none of the older men with lower plasma essential amino acid levels had a serum albumin level below 3.5 g/dl, protein nutrition may still have been marginal, based on their lower ratio of essential to nonessential amino acids. Lower than normal

levels of the branched-chain amino acids could influence the variability in patients' responses to levodopa, a drug used to treat Parkinson's disease. Levodopa competes with the branched-chain amino acids for transport across the blood-brain barrier. Low levels of the branched-chain amino acids will indirectly promote increased uptake of levodopa by the brain.[38]

Hormonal Control of Protein Metabolism

Protein metabolism and lean body mass are influenced by several of the endocrine hormones. Growth hormone, testosterone, insulin, the glucocorticoids, and thyroid hormone all play a role.[36] Cytokines, produced by the immune system, bring about changes in protein synthesis and, indirectly, changes in muscle mass. Growth hormone, insulin, and testosterone are anabolic hormones and promote protein synthesis. On the other side, the glucocorticoids and cytokines promote protein catabolism and are responsible for the body's initial response to inflammation, infection, or trauma.[19] Thyroid hormone increases both protein synthesis and degradation but also is required for the synthesis of growth hormone in the pituitary gland. Under most circumstances these hormones are in balance and support protein synthesis, appropriate growth, and preservation of lean body mass. In aging or disease, this balance can be disrupted, resulting in changes in protein metabolism and total muscle mass. The influence of these hormones on age-related changes in body composition will be discussed in chapter 5. At this time we will focus on the actions of particular hormones and the cytokines on protein synthesis and catabolism.

Insulin and protein metabolism. The major hormone controlling the utilization and retention of amino acids is insulin. The rise in plasma levels of both glucose and amino acids after a meal containing carbohydrate and protein stimulates the secretion of insulin from the beta cells of the pancreas. Insulin promotes the movement of plasma amino acids into the skeletal muscle for protein synthesis and inhibits the breakdown of existing muscle proteins and subsequent flow of amino acids into the peripheral circulation. Insulin plays an important part in promoting the movement of the branched-chain amino acids from the plasma into the skeletal muscle. The **branched-chain amino acids** have a particular role in the control of protein metabolism.[59] The branched-chain amino acids carry amino groups into the skeletal muscle and regulate protein synthesis and breakdown. When the branched-chain amino acids are in short supply, the breakdown of protein is curtailed in an effort to conserve body protein. When the amino acid pool increases, protein synthesis is stimulated.

Normal aging is associated with reduced sensitivity of skeletal muscle and adipose cells to the action of insulin and transport of glucose. This resistance of peripheral tissues to the action of insulin contributes to the deterioration in glucose tolerance observed in many older people. Recent work has looked at whether the influence of insulin on amino acid metabolism is similarly changed in later years. In contrast to the age-related decline in the effect of insulin on glucose metabolism, plasma amino acid levels and protein metabolism appear to continue to remain sensitive to insulin action into advanced age.[25]

Growth hormone. Growth hormone is an important anabolic hormone that influences protein metabolism throughout life. It promotes the movement of amino acids into the cell and stimulates protein synthesis and cell growth. Growth hormone also increases the use of fatty acids for energy rather than the use of carbohydrate or amino acids. Growth hormone improves nitrogen balance, and the age-related decline in circulating levels of this hormone may play a part in the reduced ability of older people to maintain nitrogen equilibrium.

Glucocorticoids. The **glucocorticoids** (cortisol and cortisone) are secreted by the adrenal cortex in response to stress that occurs after trauma, infection, surgery, or in almost any debilitating disease. The glucocorticoids cause a breakdown of cellular proteins and the movement of those amino acids out of the cell and into the plasma. Amino acids are deaminized and the carbon skeletons used for glyconeogenesis, and urinary nitrogen increases. Although there is disagreement as to the occurrence of age-related changes in glucocorticoid concentrations under basal conditions, many physiological circumstances commonly existing in older people stimulate glucocorticoid secretion.

Cytokinins. Interleukin 1-β is a **cytokinin** that induces the early reactions to infection often referred to as the acute phase response.[36] Clinical components of the acute phase response include the mobilization of amino acids from muscle protein, resulting in weight loss and negative nitrogen balance. Secretion of both the glucocorticoids and growth hormone is enhanced. Roubenoff and Rall[36] pointed out that this mobilization of amino acids may serve a useful purpose because the proliferation of important proteins and cells of the immune system and the repair of damaged tissue require an ample supply of amino acids. Thus, interleukin 1-β promotes disease resistance while at the same time bringing about significant losses of muscle protein. At present there is no evidence to suggest that elderly people have higher levels of interleukin 1-β under normal conditions; however, long-term illness and continued secretion of cytokinins could lead to serious depletion of protein reserves.

PROTEIN INTAKE AND PROTEIN STATUS
Factors Influencing Protein Intake

The protein intake of many older people is adequate based on the current RDA, although gender, age, and ethnic group influence the amount of protein eaten. In the NHANES III study,[51] men had higher protein intakes than women and were more likely to meet their RDA. Men ages 60 to 69 had a median protein intake of 78 g of 124% of their RDA, but intake dropped to 64 g or about 100% of the RDA by the age of 80. Among the women ages 60 to 69, median intake was 60 g or 120% of the recommended level, but by age 80 and over intake fell below the RDA (the oldest women consumed 49 g or 99% of their RDA). Intakes were lower in older African Americans and Mexican Americans than in older white people and were lowest among African American and Mexican American elderly ages 80 and over. Among the oldest

African Americans, median intake was about 90% of the RDA, and in the oldest Mexican American group it was 82% to 95% of the RDA.

Earlier in this chapter we discussed research evidence that supports raising the RDA for older people from 0.8 g per kg body weight to at least 1 g per kg body weight. This represents an increase of 20% in the amount of protein to be consumed. Using 120% of the current RDA as a standard, about half of the men and women ages 60 to 69 examined in the NHANES III study are consuming an optimal level of protein. In the older age groups, less than half of those examined are meeting even the current RDA. Ryan and coworkers,[40] who collected food intake records from 474 older people in different geographical regions of the United States, reported that 10% of the women ages 65 to 74 and nearly 20% of the women above age 74 consumed less than two-thirds of the current RDA for protein. Among the men of similar ages, 17% and 6% respectively ate foods providing less than two-thirds of the RDA. The authors did not comment on the fact that protein intake increased with age in the men (a lower percentage of those ages 75 and over consumed less than two-thirds of the RDA), whereas it decreased with age in the women.

Comparing protein intakes in the older people interviewed by Ryan and coworkers[40] with the subjects who participated in the Boston Nutritional Status Survey[41] points to income level as a significant factor in dietary protein status. Significant numbers of the older people representing all income levels studied by Ryan and coworkers were consuming less than two-thirds of the RDA for protein. In contrast, only 3% of the middle to upper income men and 2% of the women in the Boston study ate foods providing less than two-thirds of the RDA. In the NHANES II study,[50] 10% of all older men and women ages 65 to 74 had less than two-thirds of the RDA for protein, but 18% of low income older adults had less than this amount. In the Boston institutionalized population who had their food provided, less than 2% of the 266 individuals studied had protein intakes below two-thirds of the RDA.[41]

Living situation and food availability could influence protein intake. In a Dutch study[24] protein intake ranged from 55 g in institutionalized older women to 67 g in women residing in assisted-living facilities to 77 g in women living independently. For the Dutch women total energy intake appeared to influence the absolute amount of protein consumed. All of the women consumed about 16% of their total kilocalories as protein; however, the women living independently consumed more food overall than the others. Energy intake ranged from 1,410 kcal in the institutionalized women to 1,697 kcal in those residing in assisted-living to 1,888 kcal in the women living in their own homes. The women living independently consumed a slightly greater proportion of their protein from animal sources (29%) as compared to the institutionalized women (25%) and those in assisted living (27%).

In the United States meat is a major contributor to dietary protein, making up about 20% of total intake, and beef contributes about 13% of total intake. Milk and milk products make up about 18%.[48] In the Boston study[48] protein sources other than meat or dairy products influenced the overall level of intake. Older people whose protein intake fell below 0.8 g/kg of body weight had lower intakes of poultry and fish than those with protein intakes of 1.6 g/kg. The people with lower intakes of protein ate more grains and breads, vegetables, and mixed dishes than those with higher intakes. Older individuals with limited incomes might be encouraged to include in their diet more milk and milk products and legumes, which are less expensive sources of high-quality protein than meat, fish, or poultry. The older Dutch women living independently who had higher intakes of protein than their institutionalized counterparts consumed 1.5 times more milk and milk products.

Energy Intake and Protein Status

The greatest deterrent to optimum protein status in older people may be their relatively low energy intake. As described in table 3-4, the median energy intakes of both men and women ages 60 and older are only 68% to 84% of the recommended level.[51] Nevertheless, protein continued to provide about the same proportion of total kilocalories despite decreasing food intake. When energy intake is limiting, dietary essential

TABLE 3-4   *Median Intake of Energy and Protein Compared to the RDA*

	Protein (% RDA)	Protein (% of kcal)	Energy (% RDA)
Men			
50–59 yr	140	16	96
60–69 yr	124	16	84
70–79 yr	111	16	78
80 and over	102	16	74
Women			
50–59 yr	118	16	81
60–69 yr	120	17	78
70–79 yr	111	17	73
80 and over	98	16	68

Data from U.S. Department of Health and Human Services: Energy and macronutrient intakes of persons ages 2 months and over in the United States: Third national health and nutrition examination survey, Phase I, 1988–91, Advance Data from Vital and Health Statistics, Number 255, Oct. 24, 1994, Hyattsville, MD, National Center for Health Statistics.

and nonessential amino acids may be used to meet energy needs which, if continued, will contribute to a deteriorating protein status.

Even apparently well-nourished older people with no clinical or biochemical evidence of poor protein status may have energy intakes that fall below 30 kcal/kg body weight, the level recommended for men and women ages 51 and over.[13] In an older Boston population with mean protein intakes of 1 g/kg of body weight,[27] energy intake was only 25 kcal/kg among the men and 24 kcal/kg among the women. In the housebound elderly British women[4] who were losing large amounts of body nitrogen, energy intake fell to 19 kcal/kg. The impact of low energy intake on the increased need for dietary protein observed in even healthy older people is an important area for study.

Serum Albumin Levels in Older People

Serum albumin levels and age. Albumin is the primary protein synthesized in the liver, and it has two major functions. First, albumin transports many substances, including hormones, long-chain fatty acids, metal cations such as

calcium, and drugs. Second, it maintains osmotic pressure and appropriate fluid distribution in body compartments.[32] Although serum albumin at times has been considered to be a marker of protein status, albumin synthesis and degradation are also influenced by disease. No doubt both issues contribute to our lack of understanding of the influence of age on serum albumin levels. Although decreases in serum albumin have been reported in older people, these evaluations generally did not control for protein status or health conditions that influence serum albumin levels.[32]

Healthy older people with adequate intakes of protein and energy appear to maintain normal serum albumin into advanced age.[7,35,53] An ongoing longitudinal study of about 1,100 men between the ages of 39 and 90[7] reported only a slight decrease in serum albumin over this age range (fig. 3-2). Only one man in the study had a serum albumin below 3.5 g/dl. (Serum albumin levels below 3.5 g/dl indicate declining protein status.) Multiple regression analysis indicated that less than 5% of the variation in serum albumin among these men could be explained on the basis of age. The rate of decline in serum albumin in these men was 0.05 g/dl per decade. Romero and coworkers[35] monitored serum albumin levels in 139 healthy elderly men and women from New Mexico over a 13-year period and found the rate of change to be –0.002 g/dl per year in the men and +0.0001 g/dl in the women. In the SENECA study[53] of over 900 older people in 11 countries in Europe, less than 2% had serum albumin below 3.5 g/dl. Protein intake was statistically correlated with serum albumin; however, in the opinion of those authors it was not biologically relevant. Other researchers[37] have reported a statistical relationship between total energy intake and serum albumin levels in older women.

Overall, serum albumin does not appear to be an appropriate marker to evaluate visceral protein status. Serum albumin does decrease in long-term PEM. Albumin synthesis is reduced in liver disease, and albumin losses are accelerated in renal disease and gastrointestinal disease. Serum albumin levels fall in conditions accompanied by an expanded fluid volume, which occurs in congestive heart failure and renal disease. Rall

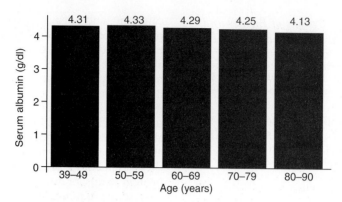

FIG. 3-2 Mean Serum Albumin Levels According to Age. Serum albumin levels did not change with age in healthy men.

Data from Campion, E.W., deLabry, L.O., and Glynn, R.J.: The effect of age on serum albumin in healthy males: report from the normative aging study, J. Gerontol. 43:M18, 1988.

and coworkers[32] pointed out that the acute phase response to infection and inflammation that involves an increase in liver synthesis of proteins for body defense mechanisms results in a decrease in albumin synthesis. Albumin is perceived to be a less essential protein when body homeostasis is threatened. Assessment of protein status and management of older people with PEM will be discussed in chapters 11 and 12, respectively.

Summary

Because little is known about the nutrient requirements of older people, the RDAs for those over age 50 have been extrapolated from those developed for younger people. Energy requirements decrease with advancing age, and iron requirements are lower in women after menopause. Since factors such as changing physiology or medications affect an older person, nutrient recommendations could be made on the basis of age, sex, health status, and level of physical activity. Although there is no established recommendation for carbohydrate, older people are encouraged to get 55% of their kilocalories from carbohydrate foods, with emphasis on complex carbohydrates rich in fiber. The essential fatty acids are vital to cell structure and function and may reduce the risk of chronic disease. Although there is no RDA, it is recommended that 1% to 2% of energy be supplied by linoleic acid and 0.5 to 1% of energy be supplied by omega-3 fatty acids; some researchers suggest that this recommendation is too low.

Throughout life, protein is needed for synthesis of enzymes and hormones and for maintenance of cell and organ structure and function. Factors such as emotional stress, infection, chronic diseases, and changes in body composition affect protein needs, with the result that the elderly are particularly vulnerable to protein loss. The loss of body protein with age is reflected in the decrease of skeletal muscle from 45% of body weight in a young adult to 27% in a 70-year-old. Protein metabolism tends to shift to the visceral organs and the ability of skeletal muscle to serve as a protein reservoir is weakened.

Although nitrogen balance studies require an adaptation period and complete diet control, this method is the best for determining protein requirements in the elderly. Recent research suggests that the current RDA for protein, 0.8 g per kg body weight, is not adequate to maintain nitrogen balance in healthy older people. After a comprehensive review of all data, the recommendation is that the safe protein intake for elderly adults is 1.0 g to 1.25 g per kg body weight. The marginal protein intake seen in

✣ ✣ ✣
CASE STUDY

A man in his early 60s who recently has begun a resistance weight training program to improve his fitness goes to see his doctor and complains of fatigue and low energy. Based on a dietary assessment, his protein intake is 0.8 g per kg body weight and his energy intake is 70% of the RDA. His current body weight is 75 kg.

1. Based on current research, is this an adequate protein intake?
2. What consequences can a low-protein, low-calorie diet have on nutritional status in an older person?

3. What would you recommend to be an appropriate protein intake? What is an appropriate energy intake for this man? Outline a three-day menu listing the appropriate servings of protein and energy foods, keeping fat at a level of 30% or less of total kilocalories. Calculate the total protein and energy intake.
4. What exercise recommendations would you make to help him accomplish his fitness goals without experiencing negative side effects?

many older people results in accommodation, with losses in immune function and muscle function. Another common problem in the elderly is an insufficient energy intake, so that protein and amino acids are not used appropriately. Healthy older people with adequate protein and energy intakes maintain normal levels of serum albumin although albumin levels decrease in long-term PEM and in certain diseases.

When 1 g of protein per kg body weight is used as the standard, less than half of those over age 60 are consuming an optimal level of protein. A low income level, living in an institution, and a high level of chronic disease may be significant factors for low dietary protein.

REVIEW QUESTIONS

1. How were the recommended dietary allowances (RDAs) for older adults established? What are the limitations of the current RDAs? What is the feasibility of specific RDAs for older people?
2. How much carbohydrate should older adults consume? What specific health benefits are associated with foods high in complex carbohydrates? Are diets that are very low in carbohydrates recommended for older adults?
3. How is the metabolism of essential fatty acids altered in the elderly? What changes in serum lipoprotein composition may be related to dietary polyunsaturated fat, and what are the implications for health?
4. What methods are used to measure protein status and requirements in older adults? How does

aging affect protein status? What level of dietary protein is recommended for older persons? What evidence is there that the RDA for protein is inadequate?
5. What are some hormonal changes typically associated with aging, and how might these changes affect protein status?

SUGGESTED LEARNING ACTIVITIES

1. Compare and contrast the RDAs for protein of a 21-year-old college student with a 70-year-old retired college professor. Plan a three-day diet, using a computer nutrient analysis program, to meet the RDAs of each. Each diet should contain 55% carbohydrate, 15% protein, and 30% fat.
2. Illustrate the steps in the conversion of linoleic and alpha-linolenic acid to their metabolic end products. Note steps in which an enzyme or a metabolite may be altered with aging or disease.
3. Prepare answers to the following questions which were asked by older adults attending a lecture on weight loss at a senior center.
   (a) Is there any reason to include fat in my diet?
   (b) How can I decrease caloric intake from fat and not be deficient in protein?
   (c) Why shouldn't I cut calories by avoiding foods high in carbohydrate?
4. Contact the director of a local senior center and ask if you can conduct a taste test on 10 different liquid nutritional supplements. Develop an instrument for rating each supplement by taste, smell, texture, and overall desirability.
5. Plan a three-day diet for a 90-year-old woman who is housebound and edentulous and has protein-energy malnutrition.

REFERENCES

1. Asciutti-Moura, L.S., and others: Fatty acid composition of serum lipids and its relation to diet in an elderly institutionalized population, Am. J. Clin. Nutr. 48:980, 1988.
2. Bjerve, K.S.: Requirements of adults and elderly, World Rev. Nutr. Diet. 66:26, 1991.
3. Blumberg, J.: Nutrient requirements of the healthy elderly—should there be specific RDAs? Nutr. Rev. 52(8):S15, 1994.
4. Bunker, V.W., and others: Nitrogen balance studies in apparently healthy elderly people and those who are housebound, Br. J. Nutr. 57:211, 1987.
5. Caballero, B., Gleason, R.E., and Wurtman, R.J.: Plasma amino acid concentrations in healthy elderly men and women, Am. J. Clin. Nutr. 53:1249, 1991.
6. Campbell, W.W., and others: Increased protein requirements in elderly people: new data and retrospective reassessments, Am. J. Clin. Nutr. 60:501, 1994.
7. Campion, E.W., deLabry, L.O., and Glynn, R.J.: The effect of age on serum albumin in healthy males: report from the normative aging study, J. Gerontol. 43:M18, 1988.
8. Castaneda, C., and others: Elderly women accommodate to a low-protein diet with losses of body mass, muscle function, and immune response, Am. J. Clin. Nutr. 62:30, 1995.
9. Castaneda, C., and others: Protein turnover and energy metabolism of elderly women fed a low-protein diet, Am. J. Clin. Nutr. 62:40, 1995.
10. Cohn, S.H., and others: Improved models for determination of body fat by in vivo neutron activation, Am. J. Clin. Nutr. 40:255, 1984.
11. Descombes, E., Hanck, A.B., and Fellay, G.: Water soluble vitamins in chronic hemodialysis patients and need for supplementation, Kidney Int. 43:1319, 1993.
12. Fiatarone, M.A., and others: Exercise training and nutritional supplementation for physical frailty in very elderly people, New Eng. J. Med. 330(25):1769, 1994.
13. Food and Nutrition Board: Recommended dietary allowances, ed. 10, Washington, DC, 1989, National Academy of Sciences.
14. Freeland-Graves, J.H., and Bales, C.W.: Dietary recommendations of minerals for the elderly. In Bales, C.W., editor: Mineral homeostasis in the elderly, New York, 1989, Alan R. Liss.
15. Gersovitz, M., and others: Human protein requirements: assessment of the adequacy of the current Recommended Dietary Allowance for dietary protein in elderly men and women, Am. J. Clin. Nutr. 35:6, 1982.
16. Hegsted, D.M.: Recommended dietary intakes of elderly subjects, Am. J. Clin. Nutr. 50:1190, 1989.
17. Hermann, J.R., Hanson, C.F., and Kopel, B.H.: Fiber intake of older adults: relationship to mineral intakes, J. Nutr. Elderly 11(4):21, 1992.
18. Horrobin, D.F.: Fatty acid metabolism in health and disease: the role of Δ-6-desaturase, Am. J. Clin. Nutr. 57(suppl.):732S, 1993.
19. Jeevanandam, M., Petersen, S.R., and Shamos, R.F.: Protein and glucose fuel kinetics and hormonal changes in elderly trauma patients, Metabolism 42(10):1255, 1993.
20. Johnson, M.A., and others: Nutritional patterns of centenarians, Intl. J. Aging Hum. Develop. 34(1):57, 1992.
21. Lachance, P., and Langseth, L.: The RDA concept: time for a change? Nutr Rev. 52(8):266, 1994.
22. Lamon-Fava, S., and others: Effects of dietary intakes on plasma lipids, lipoproteins, and apolipoproteins in free-living elderly men and women, Am. J. Clin. Nutr. 59:32, 1994.
23. Lecerf, J., and others: Variations in the fatty acid composition of lipid classes from lipoproteins in elderly women, Atherosclerosis 98:241, 1993.
24. Löwik, M.R.H., and others: Institutionalized elderly women have lower food intake than do those living more independently (Dutch Nutrition Surveillance Survey), J. Am. Coll. Nutr. 11(4):432, 1992.
25. Marchesini, G., and others: Insulin resistance in aged men: relationship between impaired glucose tolerance and decreased insulin activity on branched-chain amino acids, Metabolism 36:1096, 1987.
26. Munro, H.N.: Protein nutriture and requirements of the elderly. In Munro, H.N., and Danford, D.E., editors: Nutrition, aging, and the elderly, New York, 1989, Plenum Press.
27. Munro, H.N., and others: Protein nutriture of a group of free-living elderly, Am. J. Clin. Nutr. 46:586, 1987.
28. Nestel, P. J.: Dietary fat for the elderly: what are the issues? In: Munro, H., and Schlierf, G., editors: Nutrition of the elderly, New York, 1992, Raven Press.
29. New recommendations and principles for diabetes management, Nutr. Rev. 52(7):238, 1994.
30. Pannemans, D.L.E., Halliday, D., and Westerterp, K.R.: Whole-body turnover in elderly men

and women: responses to two protein intakes, Am. J. Clin. Nutr. 61:33, 1995.

31. Posner, B.M., and others: Nutritional risk in New England elders, J. Gerontol. 49(3):M123, 1994.

32. Rall, L.C., Roubenoff, R., and Harris, T.B.: Albumin as a marker of nutritional and health status. In Rosenberg, I.H., editor: Nutritional assessment of elderly populations, measure and function, New York, 1994, Raven Press.

33. Rasmussen, L.B., and others: Effect of diet and plasma fatty acid composition on immune status in elderly men, Am. J. Clin. Nutr. 59(3):572, 1994.

34. Research Group on Aging (GERBAP): Extensive laboratory assessment of nutritional status in fit, health-conscious, elderly people living in the Paris area, J. Am. Coll. Nutr. 11(4):432, 1992.

35. Romero, L.J., Hunt, W.C., and Garry, P.J.: Serum albumin results from a longitudinal study of community-dwelling healthy elderly in the New Mexico aging process study. In Rosenberg, I.H., editor: Nutritional assessment of elderly populations, measure and function, New York, 1994, Raven Press.

36. Roubenoff, R., and Rall, L.C.: Humoral mediation of changing body composition during aging and chronic inflammation, Nutr. Rev. 51(1):1, 1993.

37. Roubenoff, R., Grimm, L.W., and Roubenoff, R.A.: Albumin, body composition, and dietary intake in chronic inflammation. In Rosenberg, I.H., editor: Nutritional assessment of elderly populations, measure and function, New York, 1994, Raven Press.

38. Rudman, D., and others: Fasting plasma amino acids in elderly men, Am. J. Clin. Nutr. 49:559, 1989.

39. Russell, R.M., and Suter, P.M.: Vitamin requirements of elderly people: an update, Am. J. Clin. Nutr. 58:4, 1993.

40. Ryan, A.S., Craig, L.D., and Finn, S.C.: Nutrient intakes and dietary patterns of older Americans: a national study, J. Gerontol. 47(5):M145, 1992.

41. Sahyoun, N.: Nutrient intake by the NSS elderly population. In Hartz, S.C., Russell, R.M., and Rosenberg, L.H., editors: Nutrition in the elderly. The Boston nutritional status survey, London, 1992, Smith-Gordon and Company.

42. Sanders, T.A.B., and others: Essential fatty acids, plasma cholesterol, and fat-soluble vitamins in subjects with age-related maculopathy and matched control subjects, Am. J. Clin. Nutr. 57:428, 1993.

43. Schneider, E.L., and others: Recommended dietary allowances and the health of the elderly, New Engl. J. Med. 314:157, 1986.

44. Simopoulos, A.P.: Omega-3 fatty acids in health and disease. In Prinsley, D.M., and Sandstead, H.H., editors: Nutrition and aging, New York, 1990, Alan R. Liss.

45. Stadtman, E.R.: Protein modification in aging, J. Gerontol. 43:B112, 1988.

46. Swanson, P.: Adequacy in old age. Part 1. Role of nutrition, J. Home Econ. 56:651, 1964.

47. Thomas, P.R.: Improving America's diet and health: from recommendation to action, Washington, DC, 1991, National Academy Press.

48. Tucker, K., and Rush, D.: Food choices of the elderly. In Hartz, S.C., Russell, R.M., and Rosenberg, L.H., editors: Nutrition in the elderly. The Boston nutritional status survey, London, 1992, Smith-Gordon and Company.

49. U.S. Department of Health and Human Services: Dietary intake of vitamins, minerals, and fiber of persons ages 2 months and over in the United States: Third national health and nutrition examination survey, Phase I, 1988–91, Advance Data from Vital and Health Statistics, Number 258, Nov. 14, 1994, Hyattsville, MD, National Center for Health Statistics.

50. U.S. Department of Health and Human Services: Dietary intake source data: United States, 1976–80, DHHS Publication No. (PHS) 83-1681, Washington, DC, 1983, U.S. Government Printing Office.

51. U.S. Department of Health and Human Services: Energy and macronutrient intakes of persons ages 2 months and over in the United States: Third national health and nutrition examination survey, Phase I, 1988–91, Advance Data from Vital and Health Statistics, Number 255, Oct. 24, 1994, Hyattsville, MD, National Center for Health Statistics.

52. U.S. Department of Health and Human Services, U.S. Department of Agriculture: Nutrition monitoring in the United States: an update report on nutrition monitoring, DHHS Pub. No. (PHS) 89-1255, Washington, DC, 1989, U.S. Government Printing Office.

53. Van Staveren, W.A., and others: Serum albumin and dietary protein in the Euronut SENECA project. In Rosenberg, I.H., editor: Nutritional assessment of elderly populations, measure and function, New York, 1994, Raven Press.

54. Welle, S., and others: Utility of creatinine excretion in body-composition studies of healthy men

and women older than 60 y, Am. J. Clin. Nutr. 63(2):151, 1996.

55. Witte-Foster, S.R., Garcia, P.A., and Dove, C.R.: Lipid profiles, serum immunoglobins, dietary intake, and drug use of older rural Iowa women, J. Am. Diet. Assoc. 91:679, 1991.

56. Wood, R.J., Suter, P.M., and Russell, R.M.: Mineral requirements of elderly people, Am. J. Clin. Nutr. 62:493, 1995.

57. Yarasheski, K.E., Zachwieja, J.J., and Bier, D.M.: Acute effects of resistance exercise on muscle protein synthesis rate in young and elderly men and women, Am. J. Physiol. 265(Endocrinol. Metab. 28):E210, 1993.

58. Young, V.R.: Protein and amino acid metabolism with reference to aging and the elderly. In Prinsley, D.M., and Sandstead, H.H., editors: Nutrition and aging, New York, 1990, Alan R. Liss.

59. Young, V.R., and Bier, D.M.: Amino acid requirements in the adult human: how well do we know them? J. Nutr. 117:1484, 1987.

60. Young, V.R., Munro, H.N., and Fukagawa, N.: Protein and functional consequences of deficiency. In Horwitz, A., and others, editors: Nutrition in the elderly, New York, 1989, Oxford University Press.

61. Zanni, E., Callaway, D.H., and Zezulka, A.Y.: Protein requirements of elderly men, J. Nutr. 109:513, 1979.

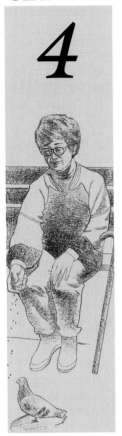

4

Nutrient Digestion and Absorption

✦✦

Objectives

After studying the chapter, the student should be able to:

✔ *Recognize the significance and prevalence of gastrointestinal discomfort in older people*

✔ *Understand the difficulties in defining changes that occur in the aging gastrointestinal tract*

✔ *Distinguish between age-related physiological changes in the gastrointestinal tract and those caused by disease or lifestyle effects*

✔ *Identify factors that contribute to malabsorption of macronutrients in older people*

Aging changes in the gastrointestinal tract could have important implications for the nutritional status of older adults, although many healthy older adults experience no change in gastrointestinal function even beyond age 80. However, incomplete digestion and the resulting impaired absorption of nutrients will lead to nutrient deficiencies, regardless of the adequacy of intake. If changes in the functional capacity of the gastrointestinal tract cause physical discomfort, the older person may eat less, also increasing the possibility of nutrient deficiency. For these reasons gastrointestinal symptoms reported by older individuals should not be ignored.

AGING AND GASTROINTESTINAL FUNCTION
Level of Function

Function in the gastrointestinal tract is generally well preserved into advanced age. Many older studies describing changes in the gastrointestinal tract were performed on hospitalized patients or on individuals in long-term care facilities.[56] The extensive reserve capacity of the organs that make up the gastrointestinal system is primarily responsible for the preservation of generally adequate function in healthy older people. No change in the dietary requirement of any particular nutrient is justified based on available evidence regarding age-related changes in the gastrointestinal tract. Yet, altered taste, hypochlorhydria, and decreased blood flow to the liver are changes of clinical importance.[59]

Of all organ systems the gastrointestinal tract is the most common source of chronic discomfort in older people, and some gastrointestinal disorders, including diverticulosis and atrophic gastritis, are more common among older than younger adults. Holt[27] pointed out that gastrointestinal disease can be more difficult to diagnose in older patients with several concomitant disorders that can distort the usual features of the primary disease. Clinical signs may be atypical because of age-related differences in gastrointestinal motility or the localized perception of pain induced by medications or changes in the central nervous system.

Gastrointestinal distress does not necessarily indicate malabsorption; individuals with no symptoms may absorb nutrients poorly, whereas others with constant gastrointestinal discomfort may absorb nutrients normally. Because of the potential impact of gastrointestinal disorders on nutritional status and the fact that gastrointestinal symptoms often signal organic disease, all complaints need to be investigated carefully.

Prevalence of Problems

As with many chronic conditions, chronic digestive disorders increase with age. Among the people participating in the National Health Interview Surveys from 1990 to 1992, the age gradient was especially steep for gastric ulcers, presence of diverticula in the intestine, and gallbladder stones.[74] While only 5 per 1,000 men and 11 per 1,000 women in the general population reported having diverticulosis, this increased to 28 per 1,000 men and 49 per 1,000 women age 65 and older. Gallbladder stones were a problem for 11 of every 1,000 older people as compared to 4 of every 1,000 people in the general population.[74]

Older women are more likely to have gallbladder disease, but older men are more likely to have ulcers. More than twice as many older men than younger men have gastric ulcers, and older black people are more likely to have gastric ulcers than older white people. In contrast, gallbladder stones and diverticulosis are reported by fewer black elderly than white elderly. It is important to recognize, however, that these reports are based on general interviews and did not include physical examinations. The lower reporting of some chronic digestive conditions by black elderly may relate to fewer physician visits for the diagnosis of these problems rather than reduced incidence.[74]

In a random sample of Minnesota elderly,[71] 328 responded to a mail questionnaire about gastrointestinal symptoms. Twenty-four percent reported chronic constipation associated with abdominal pain, and 13% experienced frequent diarrhea. Heartburn was a common problem, occurring at least once a week among 22% of the respondents, and frequent abdominal distension was reported by 20%. Talley and coworkers[71] commented that only 23% of those with chronic problems had sought medical advice. The relative importance of digestive disorders to the health care system is apparent in the fact that gastrointestinal biopsies and cholecystectomies are among the five most common inpatient surgical procedures performed on elderly women. A comprehensive assessment of community-living elderly[40] revealed that 24% had undiagnosed gastrointestinal disease, 31% had undiagnosed cardiovascular disease, and 21% had undiagnosed hypertension.

Eating problems and symptoms of digestive distress do increase with age in older adults. Nevertheless, data collected in the Georgia Centenarian Study[7,31] suggest that most older people living in the community have adequate gastrointestinal function (table 4-1). Although chewing, biting, and bowel problems (constipation or diarrhea) were most frequent in the centenarians, food intolerance was more frequent in those ages 60 to 89 (48% versus 5%). This suggests that gastrointestinal dysfunction is more closely related to chronic diseases than to aging, although both factors probably are involved.

Basis of Problems

Unfortunately, digestive symptoms are often nonspecific, and it is not always possible to determine a specific organic cause or disease. A wide variety of commonly used prescription and over-the-counter drugs, including digitalis,

TABLE 4-1 Percentage of Older People Reporting Problems of the Gastrointestinal Tract*

	Ages 60–69 (n = 46)	Ages 80–89 (n = 44)	Ages 100+ (n = 19)
Any illness that interferes with eating?	13	14	26
Any trouble biting or chewing certain foods?	17	16	37
Any foods not eaten because they disagree with you?	48	48	5
Any abdominal pain or discomfort in the last month?	4	9	5
Any trouble swallowing in the last month?	2	2	5
Any vomiting in the last month?	2	5	0
Any problems with your bowels (diarrhea or constipation)?	17	25	37
On a special diet?	9	16	16

*People answering yes to each question; preliminary data from the Georgia Centenarian Study.
Modified from Bowman, B.A., Rosenberg, I.H., and Johnson, M.A.: Gastrointestinal function in the elderly. In: Munro, H., and Schlierf, G., editors: Nutrition of the elderly, Nestle Nutrition Workshop Series, Vol. 29, New York, 1992, Raven Press.

anticonvulsants, diuretics, and aspirin, can cause gastrointestinal distress. McRae[40] emphasized that digestive complaints may be indicative of another underlying problem. He related an incident involving a 76-year-old woman who complained of abdominal pain after eating and had a recent history of weight loss. Failing eyesight had forced her to discontinue her many community activities, and depression, anorexia, and abdominal discomfort followed. General stress is often revealed in the form of digestive disturbance in people of all ages. Mental and emotional stress can lead to gastric upset or a change in bowel habits. The interaction of age-related changes in the structure, motility, and secretion of the gastrointestinal tract, influenced by psychologic or physical stress, can initiate digestive disorders or exacerbate existing organic disease.

The Oral Cavity

A healthy **oral cavity** is disease free and comfortable and functions adequately for eating.[39] Unique structures in the oral cavity assist in the complex process of eating, which involves moistening, masticating, tasting, and swallowing food.
  Moistening the food. Mucins, lubricating substances in the saliva, soften the food so it can be more easily chewed and bind the food particles together in a bolus to be swallowed.

  Masticating the food. Chewing crushes the food and prepares it for swallowing. Chewing efficiency depends on the number of teeth and their condition and the length of time that the food is chewed. Optimum chewing efficiency allows an older person to select a wider variety of food. The movement of food within the mouth also stimulates the taste buds and releases odors that stimulate the olfactory receptors.
  Tasting the food. Sensory receptors that produce taste are found on the tongue and roof of the mouth. Tasting requires saliva to dissolve the substances in food that produce taste and bring them in contact with the taste buds.
  Swallowing the food. Swallowing is a complicated process by which food is moved from the oral cavity into the esophagus and down to the stomach. For swallowing to occur normally, food must be moistened and formed into a bolus.

Oral Health Problems

Tooth loss, gum diseases, or reduced flow of saliva are some of the oral health problems that influence food choices and may adversely affect nutrient intake.

Dental Problems

Healthy gums, teeth, and supporting structures make an important contribution to an individual's quality of life. The ability to chew and enjoy favorite foods adds much to the older person's pleasure in eating and desire to eat. In past years the loss of all teeth (becoming **edentulous**) was viewed as a normal consequence of aging. Limited knowledge of the cause or treatment of gum disorders and lack of technical expertise in repair of dental cavities resulted in the loss of teeth even before middle age. A survey of 1,156 New Englanders age 70 and over[46] revealed that 38% were edentulous. A comparison of the current dental status of people age 75 and over with available statistics for that age cohort when they were middle aged indicates that they actually lost their teeth 30 years ago.[9] The relative proportion of edentulous older people will continue to decline as younger age groups benefit from prevention strategies for dental disease and tooth loss. Being edentulous at older ages is associated with early tooth loss. People who begin to lose teeth early in life are more likely to lose all of their teeth later. Socioeconomic status is also related to being edentulous in older age. Among those with fewer than eight years of school, 51% were edentulous as compared to only 29% of those with 12 or more years of school.[9]

Dental caries were considered at one time to be a childhood disease because most tooth surfaces became decayed early in life and teeth were subsequently lost.[9] Improved dental hygiene has decreased the incidence of caries overall; however, with more older people retaining their teeth, caries have become a lifelong problem. In the study of the New England elderly,[16] 28% of the women and 34% of the men had untreated dental caries. Decay on the crown of the tooth was more frequent than decay below the gum line (root decay). Root decay occurs in older people with gum problems that expose the root surface to plaque.

Periodontal disease, responsible for 30% of tooth loss in elderly people, is both treatable and preventable.[17] **Periodontal disease** refers to inflammation of the gums, bone, and ligaments surrounding and supporting the teeth. Periodontal disease is caused by infection and, left untreated, can threaten the overall health status of debilitated elderly people.[6,17] As is true for dental caries, periodontal disease results from the accumulation of plaque on the surface of the

tooth, which attracts particles of food and bacteria that produce a low-grade infection in the adjacent gums (gingiva). This condition is called gingivitis and causes tenderness and bleeding. If it is allowed to continue, pus forms, with swelling of the gums and pain. When the inflammation spreads to the ligaments and bone, teeth loosen and are lost.

In both the upper (**maxilla**) and lower (**mandible**) jaws, bone is eroded throughout maturity. As is true for bone elsewhere in the skeleton, bone resorption and deposition are highly synchronized during periods of growth and development and change in rates after maturity, with resorption exceeding deposition. In fact the jaw (**alveolar**) bone is one of the first bones in the body to begin to lose bone mineral and matrix.[39] The rate of loss is four times more rapid in the mandible than the maxilla. This loss of bone contributes to the development of periodontal disease and loss of teeth, but at the same time periodontal disease accelerates loss of alveolar bone. When alveolar bone resorption is excessive, the bone ridge may not accommodate the use of a denture without pain in the nerve tissues beneath the bone.

A major problem associated with the need for treatment of dental caries or periodontal disease or the purchase of dentures is meeting out-of-pocket costs.[17] Medicare does not cover dental expenses, and most dental insurance plans available from employers do not continue past retirement.

Changes in Taste and Smell

The senses of both taste and smell respond to chemical stimuli and cooperate closely to produce the sensory perception of food.[43,78] Complaints of loss in taste or disordered taste often involve changes in both these senses. The sense of smell (**olfaction**) contributes to the flavor of foods and beverages. The response that we call **taste** is actually the result of three different sensations: taste, smell, and mouth feel. Receptors on the tongue and oral cavity produce the sensations of salty, sweet, sour, or bitter. Other receptors in the mouth produce sensations of texture or temperature. Volatile elements from the food move from the back of the mouth up into the nasal cavity where they act on the olfactory receptors. In aging, sensory losses can involve taste, smell, or sensitivity to touch within the mouth.

Olfactory or taste sensations can be lost in several ways.[78] Head trauma from falls causes olfactory loss, and in older people losses related to head trauma are often permanent. Chronic or repeated respiratory infections can result in cumulative losses in smell. The nerves that control taste pass through the inner ear; thus ear infections as well as respiratory infections can lead to temporary or permanent changes in taste. In Bell's palsy (a loss in function of the facial nerve occurring in the elderly) taste can be affected. Medications and systemic metabolic abnormalities can affect taste. Interestingly, all receptors within a taste bud are in direct contact with microvilli. Taste substances in the blood can diffuse through the capillary wall and stimulate the taste receptor.[78] Individuals treated with radiation for cancer of the head or neck usually experience some degree of sensory loss. Patients with Parkinson's disease or senile dementia of the Alzheimer type (SDAT) have olfactory loss.[43]

Little is known about the life history of sensory function within individuals. Data now available were obtained from cross-sectional studies and indicate that olfactory losses are more substantial than losses in taste.[78] The ability to recognize odors declines dramatically, although taste remains robust in many older people. The effects of long-term infections, decayed teeth and periodontal disease, or heavy use of prescription drugs may play a greater role than aging itself in the deterioration of sensory perception.

Xerostomia

Xerostomia, or dry mouth, is a common problem among older people. One study estimated that 16% to 28% of older people in the community have dry mouth.[4] Xerostomia can arise from several causes. A decrease in the secretion of saliva may be related to changes in sensory receptors that stimulate saliva flow or to changes in the central nervous system. Prescription drugs, including antidepressants, antihypertensive agents, and bronchodilators, decrease salivary secretion. In a group of institutionalized elderly people, 60% of the women reported dryness of the mouth and on the average they took five medications a day.[4] Radiation and chemotherapy treatment for head and neck cancers result in xerostomia. Problems with lubricating, masticating, tasting, and swallowing food are critical effects of this condition. Saliva also plays an important role in lubricating and maintaining the teeth and oral mucosa, destroying harmful microorganisms and neutralizing potentially toxic substances taken into the mouth. Infections, ulcers in the oral cavity, and rampant tooth decay are consequences of dry mouth.[39]

Xerostomia is an important risk factor for inadequate nutrient intake. Using artificial salivas or hard, sugarless candy may help to relieve discomfort. When possible, therapeutic drugs that do not affect salivary gland function might be substituted for those that induce or exacerbate xerostomia.[39] (Dietary intervention to assist the individual with oral or gastrointestinal problems will be discussed in chapter 12.)

Dysphagia

Dysphagia is derived from the Greek words *dys* meaning disordered and *phagia* meaning to eat. It is characterized by difficulty in swallowing and passing food from the oral cavity to the stomach. Dysphagia in older people is caused by changes in the central nervous system and a breakdown in neuromuscular control. Recent medical evidence suggests that dysphagia is the result of pathologic processes, not aging.[68] The severity of dysphagia will vary with the severity of the disease. Medical conditions, such as a stroke, Parkinson's disease, or organic brain syndrome, damage the nerves that control the muscles involved in swallowing and tongue movement.[18] Diabetic neuropathy can lead to swallowing disorders. Reduced salivary secretion contributes to dysphagia when food has not been moistened sufficiently to form a bolus, and discrete food particles must pass from the throat into the esophagus. The incidence of dysphagia increases with age. It is estimated that 30% to 50% of institutionalized older people have swallowing disorders.[68]

Dysphagia has serious implications for both nutritional and physical health. This condition limits the type and quantity of food and liquids consumed, contributing to malnutrition or dehydration. The most immediate danger is choking with aspiration of food into the lung and development of pneumonia. Thus, care in feeding and the selection of appropriately prepared foods are paramount.

Gastrointestinal Problems

Adverse food reactions. An **adverse food reaction** is any unfavorable reaction after food has been eaten. Two types of adverse food reactions, food allergy reactions and food intolerance reactions, have different causes. Food allergy reactions (sometimes referred to as food sensitivity) involve an abnormal immune response; food intolerance reactions are related to other factors. Food intolerance reactions are more common and can be caused by toxins in the food (such as salmonella), a pharmacologic substance in the food (such as caffeine in coffee), physiologic abnormalities like a lactase deficiency, or particular circumstances in an individual.[60]

Food sensitivity reactions. A variety of mechanisms in the gastrointestinal tract prevent foreign proteins from entering the body.[60] Gastric acid and protein-digesting enzymes act to break down foreign proteins, and antibodies secreted by the immune system enter the intestine and bind with foreign proteins and prevent their absorption. Food sensitivity is an abnormal reaction between specific glycoproteins in foods and the immune system, resulting in the secretion of food-specific antigens and T cells. Only a few foods, including shellfish, peanuts, and wheat, account for the majority of food sensitivity reactions.

Gluten-sensitivity enteropathy. Gluten-sensitivity enteropathy, formerly referred to as celiac disease, is caused by gliadin, a protein substance found in gluten.[14] Gliadin is a component of wheat, oats, rye, and barley. Although this disorder is more common in young adults, increasing numbers of cases are being diagnosed in people age 70 and over.[34] Injury to the mucosa of the small intestine caused by gliadin (gluten) sensitivity results in profound malabsorption of fat, protein, vitamins, and minerals. Diarrhea, with steatorrhea and weight loss, are the classic symptoms and are sometimes accompanied by severe anemia and osteomalacia. However, many older patients have more subtle symptoms, such as general gastrointestinal complaints, mild anemia, or low serum folate levels.[12] Malaise or loss of general well-being is present in 80% of patients with gluten-sensitivity enteropathy, although this is often so insidious in onset that in the elderly it is overlooked or assumed to be related to aging. Loss of appetite, fatigue, and anemia in older people are more likely to lead to tests for cancer than for gastrointestinal disease.[14] Gluten-sensitivity enteropathy has been associated with increased risk of cancer and other diseases related to the immune system, including diabetes and thyroid disease.

Gluten-sensitivity enteropathy is treated with dietary management which involves removing all gluten-containing products from the diet; oral supplements of vitamins and minerals may be required.

Food intolerance. Perceived discomfort in the gastrointestinal tract after eating a particular food influences whether a person will eat that food again or eat foods considered to be similar. Older adults report a higher frequency of food intolerance than younger adults, although severe symptoms of intolerance, including nausea, vomiting, or diarrhea, are relatively infrequent.[71]

Vegetables are sometimes singled out as foods causing gastrointestinal distress because they contain fiber or undigestible carbohydrates, such as raffinose, that lead to gas production. Zimmerman and Krondl[80] studied food intolerance in older people receiving home-delivered meals in Toronto. Forty percent of the recipients had one or more perceived food intolerances. Vegetables were the most frequently cited foods causing symptoms. The vegetables most poorly tolerated included cauliflower, cabbage, brussels sprouts, onions, and corn. Carrots, peas, and broccoli, although poorly tolerated when raw, were well tolerated cooked. Celery and lettuce were the only raw vegetables well tolerated by those with food intolerance. Burping was the most common symptom reported, followed by flatulence, heartburn, and abdominal pain. Zimmerman and Krondl[80] emphasized that many well-tolerated vegetables, including raw vegetables, were not being included in home-delivered meals because planners believed them to cause discomfort. It is important to note that broccoli, spinach, carrots, and yams—all good sources of folic acid or the carotenoids—were well tolerated when cooked.

Lactose intolerance arising from the lack of the enzyme lactase, which is required to break down lactose, is more common in African American elderly than white elderly. Bloating, distension, and diarrhea are the most common adverse effects that occur after eating foods with lactose. That reaction can lead to an avoidance of dairy foods, resulting in low calcium intake. (Lactose intolerance will be discussed in detail later in this chapter.)

Perceptions of food intolerance could be influenced by factors unrelated to the food item. Many prescription and over-the-counter medications have unfavorable side effects, including nausea, vomiting, and constipation. Procainamide, used to treat cardiac arrhythmias, sometimes causes nausea and vomiting; methotrexate used in cancer treatment often causes diarrhea; and haloperidol, an antipsychotic drug, can lead to constipation. Many drugs are taken with meals; thus, it is difficult to discern the true cause of subsequent distress. Also, poor dental status and poor mastication of food could slow the normal digestive process.

Dyspepsia. Dyspepsia is characterized by a nonspecific set of symptoms that may include abdominal pain, bloating, fullness, sensations of gas, or heartburn.[53] Abdominal discomfort after eating can have many causes. Drugs, including nonsteroidal anti-inflammatory drugs, digitalis, levodopa, or aspirin, can irritate the gastric mucosa. Overconsumption of food or alcohol may be at fault. Alterations in gastric motility can contribute to dyspepsia and reflux of gastric contents into the esophagus. Discomfort from burning sensations or from distension often leads to constant swallowing to relieve the distress. However, swallowing air often increases the discomfort. Psychologic and emotional stress and anxiety cause gastric distress. Report-

ing of frequent indigestion increases with age. In a national survey[74] the frequency of this problem was double in people over age 64 as compared to the general population. Fewer African Americans report frequent indigestion, irrespective of age.

Although chronic dyspepsia can signal the presence of ulcers or other serious organic disorder, many individuals have chronic dyspepsia with no identifiable cause. Those with nonulcer dyspepsia have a similar rate of gastric emptying, and their levels of gastric acid and intestinal gas are no higher than those without symptoms. Efforts to identify particular personality types that are more likely to have nonulcer dyspepsia have been unsuccessful.[53]

Symptoms can be reduced by avoiding caffeine-containing foods, alcohol, aspirin, and other known stomach irritants. Severe gastric distress is treated with H_2-blockers, drugs that reduce the secretion of gastric acid.[44] Indigestion is not a normal consequence of advancing age. Chronic dyspepsia in an older person must be evaluated carefully for possible organic disease.

Diverticular disease. Diverticular disease occurs almost exclusively in people over age 40 and increases in both incidence and severity with age. Incidence is estimated to be as high as 30% by age 50, and by age 70 over half of the population has diverticular disease.[15] **Diverticulosis** is identified by the pouchlike projections that appear along the inner wall of the colon, particularly where the colon joins the rectum. **Diverticulitis** is a complication of diverticulosis. Diverticulitis, inflammation of the diverticula, results from the perforation of the wall of the diverticula. Bleeding may occur and in the worst case, abscesses may form if fecal material passes into the peritoneal cavity. For about 85% of patients, diverticulosis is asymptomatic; symptoms from uncomplicated diverticulosis include diarrhea or constipation, flatulence, and heartburn.

It has been theorized that diverticula are caused by increases in intraluminal pressure that result when diets are low in fiber and bulk, and the intestinal wall becomes less elastic. Although this idea is popular, intraluminal studies have not demonstrated increased luminal pressure in older people with or without diverticula in their colon.[15] Bran and other bulk-forming agents have been used successfully to treat elderly people with radiologically confirmed diverticular disease when sufficient fluid is provided. Diverticular disease is associated with varicose veins and ischemic heart disease in older people.

Problems in Bowel Function

Prevalence of constipation. Constipation is one of the most common gastrointestinal problems in the United States and accounts for more than 2.5 million physician visits a year.[41] Evaluation is difficult because we lack a standard definition for this condition. **Constipation** is a chronic problem involving decreased frequency of bowel movements, difficult passage of stools, passage of hard stools, or a sensation of incomplete emptying of the bowel. Normal bowel habits range from three bowel movements a week to two bowel movements a day. A common definition of constipation is less than three bowel movements a week.[13,61]

Unfortunately, many individuals who have normal bowel function consider themselves to be constipated. Among the 15,000 individuals between the ages of 12 and 74 who were evaluated in the first National Health and Nutrition Examination Survey (NHANES I),[61] 31% of those with four to six bowel movements a week reported constipation. Both age and race influence constipation (fig. 4-1).[74] Individuals age 65 and over appear to be the most affected by this condition as prevalence rates were about 50% higher than for those below age 65. Black elderly are more likely to report this condition than white elderly. In a random sample of 209 older Baltimore adults ranging in age from 65 to 93,[79] 30% reported being constipated at least once a month. At the same time only 3% reported a stool frequency of fewer than three per week. Among these older people, having to strain to pass stools was regarded as a primary symptom of constipation.

Causes of constipation. Constipation can have many causes. Normal bowel habits may be interrupted by a change in the diet or activity level or after a bout with diarrhea resulting from a viral infection or food poisoning. Irritable bowel syndrome or spastic colon, often

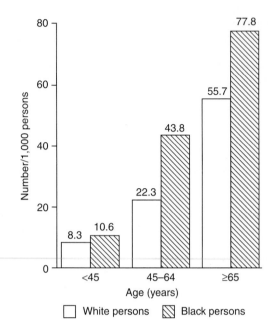

FIG. 4-1   Prevalence of Constipation According to Age and Ethnic Group. Black adults and older people ages 65 and over are the most likely to report frequent constipation.

Data from U.S. Department of Health and Human Services: Current estimates from the National Health Interview Survey, 1993, Vital and Health Statistics, Series 10, No. 190, DHHS Pub. No. (PHS) 95-1518, Hyattsville, MD, 1994, U.S. Government Printing Office.

associated with stress, can result in alternating patterns of diarrhea and constipation. Certain metabolic conditions lead to constipation. Hypothyroidism or hyperthyroidism, abnormal serum calcium or potassium levels, reduced or excessive secretion of the adrenocorticoid hormones, or dehydration can cause constipation. Degenerative neurologic disorders, including Parkinson's disease or neural damage resulting from a stroke, contribute to constipation. Sluggish bowel movements can be a sign of depression in both younger and older adults. Many medications are potential causes of constipation. Various drugs used to treat hypertension, depression, and Parkinson's disease and narcotics used to control pain can alter bowel habits. Calcium and iron supplements and antacids containing aluminum add to the problem. Low dietary fiber and fluid intakes may contribute to constipation but are also common among older people with normal bowel function.[13,72]

Individuals who have used laxatives for a long period and become dependent on these drugs may not be able to establish normal bowel function. A less common but serious cause of constipation is obstruction of the lower bowel as a complication of cancer.[44] Constipation accompanied by blood in the stool, severe cramps, a tender distended abdomen, or markedly narrow stools requires immediate medical evaluation.

AGING AND PHYSIOLOGIC CHANGES IN THE GASTROINTESTINAL TRACT

Our understanding of the normal physiology of the gastrointestinal tract is limited for both younger and older adults.[62] Functional and noninvasive tests to define normal activity and changes occurring in healthy older adults are generally lacking. Nevertheless, it is likely that changes associated with the aging process influence gastrointestinal function in some people. Disorders in gastrointestinal function could arise from changes in muscle fibers, muscle innervation, or brain and hormonal control.[54,59] Although gastrointestinal function may be normal under usual conditions, older people are less able to compensate for changes in the type or amount of food eaten, or for the effects of pathogens or chronic disease. Saltzman and Russell[59] emphasize the importance of separating age-related changes in the gastrointestinal tract from those due to chronic disease.

Physiologic Changes in the Esophagus

The **esophagus** transports food from the mouth to the stomach. The upper esophageal sphincter allows the passage of food from the throat (pharynx) into the esophagus. The lower esophageal sphincter controls the movement of food into the stomach. Normal motor activity in the esophagus consists of orderly peristaltic waves that move from the upper esophageal sphincter through the smooth muscle in the esophageal wall to the lower esophageal sphincter. The peristaltic wave terminates with the closing of the lower sphincter, preventing backflow from the stomach into the esophagus.[63]

In some older individuals, normal peristaltic waves do not occur or their amplitude is decreased, resulting in delayed esophageal emptying.[42] Consequently, the esophagus becomes dilated as food accumulates and continuing muscle contractions are both painful and ineffective in propelling the food bolus forward. Studies of healthy older men and younger men indicate that esophageal function is not impaired in healthy aging people.[1,50,51] The amplitude and duration of the peristaltic waves moving food through the upper esophageal sphincter were similar in both groups, and one report suggested that the amplitude and duration of the peristaltic waves were actually greater in the older as compared to the younger men.[51,64] Shaker and Lang[63] considered this increase to be a positive response to the reduced size of the upper esophageal sphincter opening in older people. Older men also responded with peristaltic waves of greater force to a swallow of mashed potatoes as compared to water.[65] It did appear, however, that receptors in the esophagus of the older men were less sensitive to the presence of food and required greater stimulation to produce waves of typical amplitude and duration. This change in sensitivity may contribute to the disordered esophageal motility observed in some elderly.

Another problem can be gastroesophageal reflux or the backflow of stomach contents into the esophagus. This happens when the lower esophageal sphincter is weakened. Irradiation therapy for head or neck cancer often causes weakening of this sphincter. Because the gastric contents are very acidic, they damage the mucosal lining of the esophagus, produce heartburn, and have been associated with precancerous lesions.[44,47] **Gastric reflux** is a more serious problem for older people because the esophagus is less sensitive to refluxed food or liquid. In younger people the reflux of gastric contents is more likely to stimulate swallowing and peristaltic waves that return these contents to the stomach.[64]

Physiologic Changes in the Stomach

Bowman and coworkers[7] suggest that the most striking effect of aging on gastrointestinal function occurs in the stomach. Changes in the gastric mucosa affect the secretion of hydrochloric acid, which is important for the absorption of various nutrients such as calcium and iron and the control of bacterial microflora. The gastric mucosa also secretes intrinsic factor, necessary for the absorption of vitamin B-12.

Changes in the gastric mucosa. The populations of cells that make up the gastric mucosa renew at varying rates. In young adults the daily loss of cells from the mucosal surface is balanced by the proliferation of new cells. Decreased rates of cell division, changes in cell maturation or differentiation, or increased rates of cell loss alter the integrity of the gastric mucosa, resulting in atrophy or ulceration and diminished functional capacity.[3]

Atrophic gastritis is a chronic inflammation of the stomach accompanied by deterioration of the mucosal lining. Among 359 older people in Boston (257 lived in the community and 102 were institutionalized), the prevalence of atrophic gastritis increased with age.[35] Twenty-four percent of those ages 60 to 69 and 37% of those ages 80 to 99 had this condition. A consequence of atrophic gastritis is decreased or no secretion of hydrochloric acid (hypochlorhydria or achlorhydria).

Various explanations, including alterations in cell division, autoimmune responses, and actions of particular drugs, have been offered for the age-related increase in atrophic gastritis.[3,59] One logical consideration is a possible decrease in cell proliferation.[3] It has been reported that the blood supply to the gastric mucosa is diminished in older age, and energy metabolism and the production of high-energy intermediates is slowed in human mucosal cells. These changes in delivery to and use of nutrients by the mucosa could influence the rate of cell proliferation. However, a recent study suggested that the number of parietal cells actually

increased with age in normal older people; thus, it would appear that cell numbers are not the only factor involved.[19]

One type of atrophic gastritis that occurs in older people is related to **altered immune response.** This involves a decrease in the immunoglobulins known to protect the mucosal surface and an increase in the autoimmune factors that damage mucosal tissues.[3] *Helicobacter pylori,* a microorganism associated with both gastritis and peptic ulcers, is being studied as a possible cause of atrophic gastritis in older people. The basis for the increased presence of this bacteria in the stomach of elderly people is not clear; however, it is not the result of a decrease in gastric acid.[3]

Nonsteroidal anti-inflammatory drugs (NSAIDs) such as ibuprofen or indomethacin, used to treat arthritis and chronic pain, are a possible cause of gastritis, blood loss from the gastrointestinal tract, and peptic ulcers in older people. Increased use of NSAIDs is related to the increased incidence of peptic ulcer in people over age 60.[22] Studies with animals suggest that in older age the gastric mucosa is less able to repair an injury resulting from particular drugs or bacteria.[3]

Changes in gastric motility. Gastric motility changes little with age in healthy people. The sequential contractions, responsible for moving the gastrointestinal contents along the tract, are controlled partly by the inherent innervation of the smooth muscle and partly by the autonomic nervous system. The gastrointestinal hormones secretin and cholecystokinin also help to regulate gastrointestinal motility.[25]

Gastric motility is evaluated on the basis of gastric emptying time in individuals fed a test meal. When older people with no gastrointestinal disease were fed a high-carbohydrate test meal, gastric emptying time was somewhat slowed (136 minutes as compared to 81 minutes in younger people).[59] Gastric motility is slowed in elderly people with neuropathy of the autonomic nervous system, which occurs in diabetes, Parkinson's disease, or chronic alcoholism. Radiation therapy in cancer treatment causes a decline in gastric motility.[48] Older individuals empty liquids from the stomach less rapidly than younger individuals, whereas the emptying of solid foods seems to occur at the same rate in all adults.[58] Delayed gastric emptying influences the absorption of drugs with delayed onset of pharmacologic action.[48]

Physiologic Changes in the Small Intestine

Intestinal mucosa. Relatively little information is available describing age-related changes in the intestinal mucosa of humans. General health and nutritional status appear to be more important than age in determining cell morphology and function in the small intestine.[3] Little difference in cell structure or in the number of villi per unit area appears to exist between older well-nourished adults and young controls. Animal studies indicate that mucosal cells take longer to mature, which may suggest differences in the level of enzyme activity in those cells; however, this has not been confirmed in humans.[3] Animal work also indicates that the proliferation of cells in the crypt of the villi actually increases in older age, although these cells never differentiate into specialized cells. Increased proliferation of cells in the crypt has been related to increased cancer risk.[3]

A significant change that occurs in the small intestine of older individuals with atrophic gastritis is the colonization of bacteria, primarily lactobacilli and streptococci.[29] When normal levels of hydrochloric acid are secreted by the gastric mucosa, only limited numbers of bacteria are found in the proximal small intestine. When secretion of hydrochloric acid is absent or extremely limited, **bacterial overgrowth** of the small bowel may ensue.

Bacterial overgrowth has important implications for nutritional status. Bacteria compete for the available B vitamins and may induce vitamin deficiencies. Certain bacteria interfere with the absorption of fat and other macronutrients. The impact that uncontrolled bacterial overgrowth can have on nutritional status was evaluated in a study of institutionalized and underweight older people whose diets were monitored.[26] After treatment with antibiotics, 13 of the 16 began to gain weight on intakes equal in kilocalories to those consumed previously. Only 2 of the 16

had been consuming less than 1,600 kcal per day. Since there was no control group in this study, improvement may have been related to cures of general low grade infections that also prevented weight gain. Recent studies[57] with both healthy elderly and older people admitted to an acute care hospital indicate that bacterial overgrowth related to hypochlorhydria alone does not result in clinical malabsorption. Healthy elderly absorbed fat and carbohydrate normally, although Saltzman and coworkers[57] reported that two subjects had low serum vitamin B-12 levels and might have been vitamin B-12 deficient. In the hospital patients, hemoglobin and serum folate, vitamin B-12, and albumin levels were similar in those with bacterial overgrowth or normal levels of intestinal bacteria.

Intestinal motility. There appears to be no change of clinical importance in the motility of the upper bowel in healthy older people. When older individuals who were free of gastrointestinal disease were given a test meal consisting of whole-wheat bread, scrambled eggs, and orange juice, transit time from the mouth to the entrance to the colon did not differ from young controls.[77] Slower transit through the small intestine may be beneficial, for if digested food passes too rapidly, important nutrients may not be absorbed.

Physiologic Changes in the Colon

The functions of the colon are to complete the absorption of water, electrolytes, and bile acids and to act as a reservoir for fecal matter until it is excreted. Morphologic changes in the colon include some degree of mucosal atrophy and change in the mucus-secreting cells.[12,66] The inner smooth muscle layer of the colon wall weakens as collagen fibers are lost and replaced with connective tissue. The major structural change in the aging colon is diverticulosis; the major functional change is constipation. A recent study[37] provided interesting evidence to suggest that lifestyle, rather than aging, contributes to functional changes in the colon. Nine active elderly men who were accustomed to exercising for two hours a day, three days per week, were asked to discontinue this activity for two weeks. Gastrointestinal transit time was measured before and after the rest period. Mean colon transit time increased from 11 hours to 20 hours during the period of physical inactivity. Exercise may be an important therapeutic measure for maintaining intestinal motility in older people.

Physiologic Changes in the Pancreas

It is likely that advancing age leads to some degree of morphological and functional change in the pancreas. The pancreas is smaller and weighs less in people over age 70; however, this may relate to the smaller body size of older people. In any case the functional reserve of this organ is so great that 90% of its secretory capacity can be lost before clinical consequences become apparent.[12] Pancreatic disease or chronic pancreatitis usually causes the organ's failure to support normal digestion and absorption. Chronic pancreatitis is a frequent complication of long-term alcohol abuse. Pancreatic insufficiency results in steatorrhea, diabetes, and weight loss.

Physiologic Changes in the Liver and Gallbladder

Liver function. The liver is one of the largest organs in the body, and blood flow to the liver represents almost one-third of the resting cardiac output.[25] Liver size decreases with age, and this change in liver weight reflects the loss of parenchymal cells that carry on general liver function.[11] This age effect on liver function is extremely important because older people take more drugs than any other segment of our society and most drugs are metabolized and excreted by the liver.[59] **Cytochrome 450 enzymes** that metabolize drugs appear to have decreased activity in aging adults, although some studies have reported no change in enzyme levels. The fact that 20% of older people experience at least one adverse drug reaction in their lifetime points to the importance of the liver in drug metabolism. Albumin synthesis declines slightly and is unrelated to protein malnutrition.[11]

The influence of chronic diseases on liver function has received little attention. Chronic alcohol use, protein energy malnutrition, obesity, diabetes mellitus, and hypothyroidism can alter the flux of fatty acids delivered to the liver and the balance in fatty-acid oxidation, storage, and excretion in liver cells.[11] In general, fat accumulation in the liver produces only an enlargement of this organ and not a change in function.

Gallbladder function. Diseases of the gallbladder and bile ducts account for about one-third of the abdominal surgeries performed in people over age 70.[36] The development of gallstones or calculi in the gallbladder is extremely common in older people. The prevalence of gallstone disease is higher in women than in men, and in white people than in African Americans. Prevalence rates in white women increase from 15% among those ages 40 to 49 to 30% among those ages 60 to 69.[36] Most of the time gallstone disease is asymptomatic and unrecognized. Biliary colic or intense, unexpected pain lasting one or several hours is the only symptom of uncomplicated gallstones. Biliary complications such as obstruction of the bile duct are rather infrequent. Treatments that dissolve gallstones now offer alternatives to surgery for the older individual with a recurring or acute problem.

Gallstones consist of condensed cholesterol, bile pigments, and calcium salts. Several factors contribute to the rise in occurrence of gallstones in later life.[11] First, increased secretion of cholesterol and decreased secretion of bile acids by the liver increase the cholesterol saturation of bile and the likelihood of precipitation of a gallstone. Also, the gallbladder contracts less efficiently, resulting in an increased amount of bile remaining in the gallbladder. Finally, longstanding obesity or long-term use of clofibrate or estrogen increase risk of gallstones. The effect of estrogen likely contributes to the increased incidence of gallbladder problems in women.

AGING AND DIGESTIVE SECRETIONS
Problems in Evaluation

Studies evaluating digestive secretion in older people have been few and the results inconsistent. In some cases findings were probably influenced by the selection of institutionalized or hospitalized older people as subjects. Previous diet influences the levels of digestive enzymes. The effect of age may differ if the level of secretion is measured under basal rather than stimulated conditions.

Although the volume of several digestive secretions appears to decrease in older adults (table 4-2), the functional significance of these changes is not understood. Digestive secretions normally are produced in amounts substantially above what is required, allowing a margin of safety. Any degree of malabsorption caused by changes in digestive secretions is also influenced by individual dietary habits. Eating one or two very large meals rather than several smaller meals is more likely to result in some degree of malabsorption if enzyme levels are significantly reduced. The form in which a nutrient is consumed (e.g., heme versus inorganic iron) influences the digestive secretions required. Chronic use of antacids may raise the pH in the stomach and alter digestive function. Thus, older people must be evaluated individually if malabsorption is suspected.

Digestive Secretions in the Oral Cavity

Generally salivary gland function is well preserved into advanced age in healthy adults. Parotid salivary flow, under both basal and stimulated conditions, was similar in young (age 39 or younger), middle-aged (age 40 to 59), and older (age 60 or older) men in the Baltimore Longitudinal Study of Aging.[5] Salivary flow does not necessarily decrease despite the fact that the salivary glands in older people have about one-third fewer fluid-secreting cells. According to Baum,[5] either the remaining fluid-secreting cells become more efficient and increase their output, or the salivary glands have a significant reserve capacity that is used in later life.

A recent study[76] evaluated the amylase concentration in the saliva of older adults living in a retirement community. The enzyme concentration was actually higher in the older adults than in the younger controls. It may be that the proportion of water in the salivary fluid is reduced in older age, thereby increasing the concentration of enzyme. Chronic disease or particular medications rather than aging may be responsible for the decreased salivary secretion in some older adults.[4] Diabetes with associated neuropathy has been evaluated as a possible influence on salivary secretion. However, older diabetics in good glucose control and nondiabetics of similar age had no differences in parotid or submandibular secretion under basal or stimulated conditions. It appears that dry mouth in even well controlled diabetics is caused by osmoregulation in compensation of increased urine flow.[4] There has been no research describing the effects of salivary amylase and lingual lipase on the digestion of dietary fat and carbohydrate in older people.

Digestive Secretions in the Stomach

Hydrochloric acid. The major components of gastric juice are hydrochloric acid, pepsinogen, intrinsic factor, and mucus. The reduction in acid secretion in older people parallels the decrease in the number of parietal cells in the gastric mucosa. **Hypochlorhydria,** caused by the loss of a variable number of cells, can range from mild to severe.[29] If all parietal cells are lost, no hydrochloric acid is secreted, even with chemical stimulation. Although the prevalence of atrophic gastritis with reduced acid secretion increases with age, many healthy older people have gastric acid levels similar to younger people, and in some older people, acid secretion is actually higher. Among 41 healthy men ranging in age from 44 to 71 years,[23] acid secretion under basal, meal-stimulated, and gastrin-stimulated conditions was significantly higher than in younger men ages 23 to 42 years. It should be noted, however, that the mean age of the older men was 57 years, suggesting that a reasonable number were of middle age. Serum gastrin levels tended to be higher in healthy octogenarians with hypochlorhydria than in those with normal acid secretion.[30] **Gastrin** is the gastric hormone that stimulates secretion of gastric juice. This finding indicates that low acid secretion is the result of changes in the gastric mucosa and parietal cells, and not a breakdown in hormonal control. Animal studies have demonstrated an

TABLE 4-2 *Age-Related Changes in Digestive Hormone and Secretion Levels*

	Digestive Function	Level of Secretion
Hormones		
Gastrin	Stimulates flow of gastric enzymes and hydrochloric acid	No change; may increase in some individuals
Secretin	Stimulates secretion of pancreatic juice rich in bicarbonate and promotes production of bile by the liver	No change observed
Cholecystokinin (CCK)	Stimulates secretion of pancreatic juice rich in enzymes and bicarbonate and causes ejection of bile from the gallbladder to the duodenum	Increased
Secretions		
Saliva	Moistens food and aids in mastication and swallowing	Generally no change; decreased in some individuals
Salivary amylase	Breaks down starch to dextrins and some maltose	No change; may increase in some individuals
Hydrochloric acid	Activates pepsinogen to pepsin for protein digestion; causes some breakdown of sucrose to glucose and fructose; brings about release of vitamin B-12 from proteins	Decreased to some extent in many individuals; may be increased in others
Pepsin	Breaks down complete proteins to peptides and peptones	May decrease in volume
Pancreatic juice	Contains pancreatic amylase, pancreatic lipase and trypsin for digestion of carbohydrates, lipids, and proteins, respectively; contains bicarbonate which neutralizes the acidity of chyme	May decrease in volume
Pancreatic amylase	Breaks down starch and glycogen to maltose	May decrease in volume
Trypsin	Splits peptide bonds to form small polypeptides and amino acids	No change observed
Pancreatic lipase	Hydrolyzes triglycerides to monoglycerides, fatty acids, and glycerol	May decrease in volume
Bile	Emulsifies lipids to smaller fat particles for digestion; combines with lipids and fatty acids to form micelles	No change
Disaccharidases	Breaks down disaccharides to monosaccharides	Lactase—decreased Maltase—unchanged Sucrose—unchanged

age-related decrease in acid secretion in response to a fixed amount of gastrin.[3]

When evaluating the sources of hydrogen ions in the gastrointestinal tract, it is important to remember that eating acid foods will provide hydrogen ions.[29] Also, complete digestion of 30 g of triglycerides will produce 100 mEq of fatty acids. Decreases in gastric acid secretion do not appear to influence gastric motility although the possibility of a relationship remains controversial. A significant rise in pH decreases the absorption of folic acid and adversely affects the absorption of iron and calcium.

The secretion of increased levels of gastric acid by some elderly people has been evaluated in relation to the increased incidence of peptic ulcers in this age group. Evaluation of basal and maximal levels of gastric acid secretion in 427 peptic ulcer patients between 12 and 73 years revealed no differences based on age.[45] The evaluation considered the high acid secretion observed across all ages to play a role in the development of ulcers in these patients. Others believe that a reduction in the mucus-secreting cells in older people offers less protection against mucosal damage.[3] An age-related defect in the secretion of somatostatin may play a role. **Somatostatin,** a hormone secreted by the stomach, acts in opposition to gastrin by suppressing acid release by the parietal cells and restraining the secretion of gastrin. Animal studies[33] suggest that while gastrin secretion is well preserved into advanced age, somatostatin secretion is diminished. In addition, *Helicobacter pylori,* previously thought to be benign, has been found to penetrate the protective layer of mucus and inflict damage on the mucosa. Another area of current research is the clinical significance of the age-related decrease in prostaglandins, which protect the gastric and duodenal mucosa.[3]

Pepsinogen. There has been no recent work evaluating pepsinogen secretion and activation in elderly people. In an older study the pepsin activity in the gastric juice was reported to be 25% lower in people over age 60.[55] This reduced activity could relate to reduced synthesis of the pepsinogen enzyme precursor by the chief cells of the gastric mucosa, or reduced conversion of pepsinogen to pepsin. The conversion to pepsin requires hydrogen ions which are reduced in number in older people with atrophic gastritis. Pepsin levels were not related to age in a group of patients with peptic ulcers.[45] The effect of decreased pepsin activity on protein digestion is unknown.

Intrinsic factor. Reduced secretion of intrinsic factor can limit absorption of vitamin B-12. According to Russell,[56] however, a more important limitation on vitamin B-12 absorption is the loss of gastric acid, which reduces the bioavailability of this vitamin. Also, some evidence suggests that the proliferating bacteria can bind the vitamin released from food. (The absorption of vitamin B-12 will be discussed further in chapter 6.)

Digestive Secretions in the Small Intestine

Digestive secretions that act on food in the small intestine include disaccharidases synthesized in the brush border of the mucosa, amylase, lipase, proteases, and bicarbonate secreted by the pancreas, and bile secreted by the liver and stored and released by the gallbladder. A well-recognized change in disaccharidase secretion is the decrease in the enzyme lactase in older adults. This results in a decreased tolerance for milk and other dairy products high in lactose. At the same time it appears that brush border concentrations of sucrase and maltase are unchanged.

Pancreatic secretions remain the same under basal conditions or when first stimulated with secretin or cholecystokinin; however, with continued stimulation, pancreatic secretion is lower in older people.[59] Duodenal contents obtained by aspiration from older adults indicated lower levels of bicarbonate, lipase, amylase, and chymotrypsin.[59] Nevertheless, the majority of older adults do not report any abdominal discomfort after meals or show signs of fat malabsorption. Gullo and coworkers[24] evaluated pancreatic function using a water-soluble ester that is hydrolyzed by pancreatic enzymes. When compared on the basis of age, pancreatic function did not differ between those ages 66 to 79 and those ages 80 to 88.

Bile salts seem to be secreted in normal amounts in healthy older people. The response time and rate of emptying of the gallbladder after a meal containing fat are similar in young and elderly adults (60 to 82 years).[32] The aging gallbladder does become less sensitive to cholecystokinin so that increased levels are required to bring about contraction. In response to this situation, the duodenal mucosa appears to secrete greater amounts of cholecystokinin; consequently, the actual sequence of gallbladder emptying is similar in adults of all ages.[56]

The ability of the gastrointestinal mucosa to adapt to certain nutrition conditions such as an abrupt change in nutrient intake is being evaluated using animal models.[3, 20] This has important implications for older individuals who have an acute illness or undergo surgery. The disaccharidases found in the brush border of the small intestine decrease at similar rates in both young and old animals when food is withheld. Upon refeeding, however, older animals demonstrated an exaggerated response with a strong proliferation of cells representing uncontrolled growth. This observation requires further study in terms of its relevance to aging humans and potential cancer risk.

AGING AND NUTRIENT ABSORPTION

Factors Influencing Nutrient Absorption

Nutrient absorption depends on many factors, including the completeness of digestion, integrity of the intestinal mucosa, presence of competing or inhibiting substances, and blood supply to the absorptive surface. In healthy older people digestion is reasonably complete, and nutrients are presented in the molecular or ionic form necessary for absorption. Structural changes in the cell membrane cause a decline in the transport capacity of aging cells in other organs, and this effect may occur in intestinal mucosal cells as well.[12]

Decreased blood perfusion to the small intestine will influence the rate or degree of nutrient absorption. Reduced blood flow lowers the concentration gradient between the mucosal cell and the portal vein, slowing absorption. Evidence for this concept comes from work evaluating drug absorption.[52] The compounds affected most by the level of blood flow were those with the highest absorption rates. When uptake occurred by passive diffusion, the degree of absorption did not change when blood flow fell to 10% of normal. The rate of uptake of lipid soluble compounds decreased by half when blood flow fell by 35%. In light of the fact that splanchnic blood perfusion to the intestinal region drops by almost 50% in older age groups, the influence of blood flow rate on the absorption of specific nutrients should be examined. Current evidence suggests that the absorption of carbohydrate, fat, and protein generally is unaffected in healthy older people at normal levels of intake.[55,56,59]

Absorption of Carbohydrate

Glucose absorption. Carbohydrate absorption in older people has been studied using **D-xylose** excretion levels in the urine and hydrogen levels in expired air after a high carbohydrate meal. D-xylose is absorbed by an active transport mechanism similar to the one for glucose and galactose. Since D-xylose is not metabolized, the rate and completeness of absorption of a test dose can be measured by serum levels and renal excretion.[2] Serum levels of D-xylose at either one or two hours after ingestion of the test dose did not differ in older adults ages 56 to 86 compared to young controls.[2] Urinary excretion of D-xylose was slowed in direct proportion to increasing age. It has since been determined, however, that the decline in D-xylose excretion is caused by changes in renal function common in older people, not by changes in carbohydrate absorption.

Carbohydrate absorption has been studied in older people with bacterial overgrowth resulting from atrophic gastritis or treatment with a gastrointestinal drug (omeprazole) that inhibits gastric acid secretion.[57] D-xylose serum levels following a dose of 25 g of D-xylose were well within the normal range, indicating that the capacity for carbohydrate absorption is unchanged in these patients. In contrast, glucose transport in duodenal tissue obtained from biopsies was about one-third lower in older people with confirmed bacterial overgrowth as compared to normal elderly people.[75] Examination of the mucosal tissue revealed no histological changes or changes in enzyme levels that would explain the reduced transport. The subjects in this study were referred for biopsy on the basis of gastrointestinal symptoms; therefore, other disorders could have influenced this finding. All had normal anthropometric measurements and no overt signs of malnutrition.

A confounding factor in studies evaluating the effect of bacterial overgrowth on carbohydrate digestion and absorption has been the use of hydrogen breath tests to establish the presence of bacterial overgrowth. Although these noninvasive tests have been reported to have a specificity and sensitivity as high as 90%, hydrogen breath tests identified only 6% of older people with bacterial overgrowth that was confirmed by aspiration of intestinal contents.[57] All of these elderly subjects were hypochlorhydric as a result of atrophic gastritis or omeprazole treatment. The bacterial overgrowth caused by reduced gastric acid may differ in number and types of organisms and in clinical significance from bacterial overgrowth caused by decreased intestinal motility or blind loop syndrome.[38,63] Also, any detrimental effects of bacterial overgrowth have less impact on the nutritional status of healthy elderly as compared to those with complicating medical conditions.

Changes in the permeability of the intestinal mucosa, whether caused by disease or injury, influence the absorption of both small and large molecules. Conditions such as gluten-sensitive enteropathy result in such changes. When this occurs, the passive absorption of large molecules increases, whereas the absorption of small molecules decreases. Mannitol and lactulose, poorly metabolized sugars, differ in their molecular size and routes of absorption. Mannitol, a large molecule, is absorbed through pores in the membrane, and lactulose, a small molecule, is absorbed at the tips of the villi. The ratio of urinary excretion of lactulose to mannitol after ingestion of a test dose is a confirmed measure of intestinal mucosal integrity.[58]

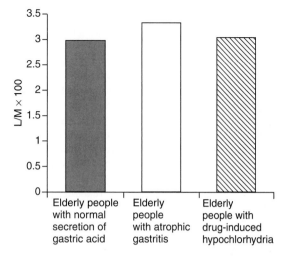

FIG. 4-2　Intestinal Permeability in Older People with Reduced Gastric Acid Secretion. The urinary excretion of a test dose of lactulose and mannitol is a measure of intestinal permeability. The lactulose to mannitol ratio was the same in elderly people with atrophic gastritis, those with drug-induced hypochlorhydria, and elderly control subjects.

Saltzman, J.R., and others: Bacterial overgrowth without clinical malabsorption in elderly hypochlorhydric subjects, Gastroenterology 106:615, 1994. © American Gastroenterological Association. (Used with permission.)

A comparison of subjects ages 20 to 39 years, 40 to 59 years, and 60 years and over at the Human Nutrition Research Center on Aging in Boston[58] indicated no change in the urinary lactulose to mannitol ratio (L/M) with age. Older people excreted a smaller proportion of both molecules based on changes in renal function. It is interesting to note that bacterial overgrowth resulting from reduced gastric acid does not adversely affect intestinal permeability (fig. 4-2). Although the ratio was a bit higher in the older subjects with atrophic gastritis, this difference was not significant. Saltzman and coworkers[58] concluded that bacterial overgrowth resulting from reduced gastric acid is reasonably benign as compared to bacterial overgrowth related to other medical problems.

Lactose absorption. Reduced levels of lactase in the small intestine and gastrointestinal distress after drinking milk have been implicated in the relatively low consumption of milk and other dairy products by many older people. The lactase activity of some people in adulthood is very similar to that in infancy and childhood, whereas in others it drops to low levels. Lactose maldigestion is more prevalent among African American than among white adults.[49]

The inability to digest lactose relates to both ethnic background and age. When given 1½ cups of milk (16.5 g lactose), adults age 50 and over had a higher incidence of maldigestion (46%) than adults below age 50 (26%).[49] Maldigestion was based on breath hydrogen analysis over a five-hour period after drinking the milk. Half of the African Americans maldigested lactose but only 17% of the whites. In the African Americans the problem increased with age. Below age 50, lactose maldigestion was 2.5 times more prevalent among African Americans as compared to whites; at age 50 and over, it was 3.5 times more prevalent among African Americans. Sixty-three percent of those with lactose maldigestion reported some symptoms after drinking milk but only 3% complained of severe symptoms. In that study all subjects were served a breakfast consisting of eggs, toast, fresh fruit, juice, and coffee, supplying about 128 g of carbohydrate, one hour following consumption of the milk. The additional food could have exacerbated symptoms in the lactose maldigesters. Asians also have a high prevalence of lactose maldigestion. In a comparison of young and elderly Asian American maldigesters,[69] the most reported symptom was flatulence, with few reporting abdominal cramps or diarrhea.

An evaluation of 21 healthy adults[70] suggested that factors other than physiologic responses to lactose may be important to the appearance of symptoms after drinking a glass of milk. These subjects who all reported severe lactose maldigestion were tested in a double-blind trial over two weeks. Every morning they drank one cup of lactose-hydrolyzed milk or one cup of milk that was sweetened with aspartame to simulate the taste of the lactose-hydrolyzed milk. There was no significant difference in the severity of symptoms of bloating, abdominal pain, diarrhea, or flatulence after either beverage; in

fact, relatively few symptoms were reported. Those authors concluded that some people mistakenly attribute distress following a meal to milk or dairy products when other foods may be the actual cause.

Milk is a significant source of calcium in older adults, even to age 100 and over. Analysis of food frequency records obtained from 241 participants in the Georgia Centenarian Study[21] indicated that milk provides about half of the servings from the dairy group (table 4-3). It is interesting that servings of milk did not differ by age or ethnic group. African American elderly had about five servings (five cups) of milk a week as did white elderly. Ice cream and cheese, other than cottage cheese, were the next most popular dairy foods. Yogurt was used rather sparingly by this group. It appears that many older whites and African Americans can comfortably consume small amounts of milk at one time, and use of milk and other dairy products should be encouraged. Milk is a good choice because it is fortified with vitamin D which is necessary for calcium absorption.

Expectation of discomfort, regardless of the cause, could be an important consideration in the consumption of dairy products by older adults. Enzyme preparations that can be added to milk products to break down the lactose are commercially available.

Absorption of Fat

Currently there is no evidence to suggest that fat digestion or absorption is altered in healthy older people.[28] When fat absorption is impaired in older adults, two different factors may be involved. First, the older individual could have decreased secretion of pancreatic lipase or bile salts because of altered pancreatic, hepatic, or gallbladder function. Second, bacterial overgrowth in the small intestine, including bacteria with the ability to split bile salts, effectively reduces the bile salts available to form the micelles necessary for fat absorption. Among 114 adults ranging in age from 19 to 91 who were given 100 g of fat a day, fat malabsorption was not evident.[2] In those ages 20 to 60, fecal fat was 3.3 g per day; in those ages 60 to 70 it was 2.5 g; and in the oldest group, ages 70 to

TABLE 4-3   *Consumption of Dairy Foods by Older People (number of servings per week)*

	All Cheeses	Ice Cream	Total Milk	Total Dairy Foods
People ages 60–69	2.6	1.3	5.1	9.6
People ages 100 and over	2.1	2.0	6.0	10.3
White elderly	2.5	1.6	5.4	10.0
African American elderly	2.4	1.9	5.2	9.6

Data from the Georgia Centenarian Study.
Serving sizes: milk, 8 oz. glass; cheese, 2 oz.; cottage cheese, ½ cup; ice cream, one scoop; yogurt, 1 cup.
Modified from Fischer, J.G., and others: Dairy product intake of the oldest-old, J. Am. Diet. Assoc. 95:918, 1995.

91, it was 2.9 g. Fat absorption in all age groups was above the normal value of 95%. These subjects also were given a labeled dose of bile salts, and over a six-hour-period, their expiration of labeled carbon dioxide was monitored to test for the action of intestinal bacteria on bile salts. There was no evidence of an age-associated increase in the splitting of bile salts by intestinal microorganisms. This was true as well for older people with atrophic gastritis or drug-induced hypochlorhydria and confirmed bacterial overgrowth.

Even debilitated older people absorb a high percentage of their dietary fat, and high-fat formulas can be effective in supplying kilocalories to severely undernourished patients. Older individuals with a mean age of 64 who were fed 350 g of fat a day by nasogastric tube absorbed 93% of the fat delivered.[67] Although fecal fat reached a level of 23 g a day, fat excretion still represented less than 10% of the fat received. Over the 22-day test period these patients gained an average of 5 kg, and nitrogen retention reached 4.9 g per day. Simko and Michael[67] concluded that a high absorptive reserve is maintained into old age, even with complicating disease. Although the amount of fat fed to these patients would not be appropriate over an extended period, it provided an available and usable source of energy for short-term rehabilitation. The ability of malnourished elderly to absorb a high percentage of the fat delivered to the gastrointestinal tract may be enhanced if the fat is given in small amounts over a 24-hour period.

In general older people can tolerate and digest normal amounts of dietary fat and even high levels when it is distributed over several meals. When fat does appear in the stool, it usually is in the form of neutral fat or triglyceride, indicating that the amount of pancreatic lipase needed to digest the fat is the limiting factor. Normally, neutral fat constitutes only a minor portion of fecal fat, with fatty acids the predominant form.

Absorption of Protein

Despite the importance of protein to health, evaluation of the effectiveness of protein digestion and absorption in older people has been limited, although there is no evidence to indicate that these processes are impaired. Healthy older men and women with a mean age of 77 who were consuming self-selected diets[8] supplying 0.97 g of protein per kilogram of body weight absorbed 85% of their protein intake. Absorption fell to 81% in housebound older adults of similar age with a high level of chronic disease. Recent nitrogen balance studies[10] reported an apparent digestibility of 85% to 91% in older Boston people consuming diets containing 0.8 to 1.6 g of protein per kilogram of body weight. In older debilitated patients receiving a liquid diet containing protein derived from casein and soybeans,[67] 88% of the protein was absorbed. This group received 81 g of protein a day delivered by nasogastric tube over a 24-hour period, thus presenting the gastrointestinal tract with small amounts of protein at a time.

❖ ❖ ❖
CASE STUDY

An 82-year-old woman, recently widowed, visited her local free health care clinic complaining of chronic stomach pain and recent weight loss. Following a diagnostic examination which consisted of physical and biochemical assessment, no organic cause of her symptoms was identified.

1. Based on the above information, what are possible causes of her symptoms?
2. What additional information about her socioeconomic or living situation would aid in determining the causes of her symptoms?

3. What do you need to know about her recent food pattern?
4. Develop a plan for counseling this client including your approach and general recommendations.
5. What health professionals might you consult with or use as possible referrals in this situation?

The amount of protein consumed may influence overall digestion and absorption in older people. At protein levels exceeding 1.5 g of protein per kilogram of body weight, the amount of nitrogen in the feces of older subjects exceeded that in younger subjects.[55,59] Rosenberg and coworkers[55] concluded that older adults may tolerate high protein diets less well than younger adults, but they noted that very few individuals have been studied. There is no evidence to suggest that healthy elderly people or elderly people with superimposed chronic disease cannot effectively digest and absorb available protein and amino acids.

Absorption of Vitamins and Minerals

Age-related changes in the absorption of vitamins and minerals are receiving increased attention. For the most part these nutrients are being studied in a clinical context considering changes in metabolism, relationships in prevention of chronic disease, and prevalence of deficiency. For this reason the absorption of specific vitamins and minerals is discussed in chapters 6 and 7.

Issues in Malabsorption

When malabsorption of the macronutrients occurs in older people, several factors usually are involved. Pancreatic insufficiency, gluten-sensitive enteropathy, bacterial overgrowth associated with a blind loop in the intestine,

complications of surgery, high use of medications, or chronic disease can contribute to impaired digestion and absorption.

General malabsorption in older people is often associated with structural or functional changes in the gastrointestinal tract. Chewing problems limit food mastication and reduce the surface area exposed to the action of digestive secretions. Laxatives that produce inappropriately rapid transit of the food bolus through the gastrointestinal tract reduce the relative amount of nutrients absorbed. The presentation of smaller amounts of food and nutrients at one time may maximize function. Spreading food intake over three meals may be advantageous, rather than eating one or two large meals. These considerations should be shared with older people in nutrition counseling.

Summary

Functional disturbances of the gastrointestinal tract increase with age. Factors such as dental problems, taste perception changes, xerostomia, and dysphagia may all result in food avoidance and, thus, diminished nutrient intake. Digestive symptoms reported by older people are often nonspecific and may be due to food sensitivity reactions, food intolerance, gluten-sensitive enteropathy, or constipation. Although many physiological changes in the gastrointestinal tract occur in older people, it is important to separate age-related changes from those resulting from chronic disease or medication and lifestyle effects.

It is believed that digestion can proceed normally despite a significant reduction in digestive enzymes because of the vast reserve capacity of the pancreas and other secretory organs. The most common age-related change in digestive secretions occurs in the stomach as a result of atrophic gastritis, with loss of parietal cells and a decline in the secretion of hydrochloric acid. The subsequent rise in pH has implications for the absorption of various nutrients, including vitamin B-12, and bacterial overgrowth. Current evidence suggests that the absorption of carbohydrates, fat, and protein is not affected by age.

REVIEW QUESTIONS

1. Why is it a common belief that gastrointestinal function drastically declines with advancing age? What functional changes occur in the gastrointestinal tract with aging? Are there any gender differences in these changes?
2. Define *xerostomia* and *dysphagia*. How common are these two problems in older people? What dietary alterations might be necessary when they occur?
3. What are some of the most common causes of dyspepsia in the older person? What is the difference between chronic indigestion and nonulcer dyspepsia?
4. How common are complaints of constipation in the older population? How is constipation defined, and what dietary measures are recommended to alleviate the problem?
5. What are the major changes in function and digestive secretions in the mouth, esophagus, stomach, intestinal tract, pancreas, liver, and gallbladder in older people? How do these changes affect the digestion and absorption of carbohydrate, protein, fat, vitamins, and minerals?
6. What factors should be considered before applying the results of a study designed to examine gastrointestinal function in a population of older hospitalized patients to a healthy, free living population of older people?

SUGGESTED LEARNING ACTIVITIES

1. Select one of the following medications and present a 15-minute oral drug report, emphasizing the nutrient/drug interactions, effects on the gastrointestinal tract, and possible associated gastrointestinal symptoms:
   - procainamide
   - ibuprofen
   - methotrexate
   - haloperidol
2. Plan a two-day menu for a 77-year-old man who is experiencing dysphagia following a stroke.
3. Interview five clients receiving home-delivered meals in a program nearby and prepare a list of foods which are avoided by these clients. Write a report including why each food is avoided, which major nutrients these foods contain, and whether or not these nutrients are provided in adequate amounts by other food selections.
4. Prepare a one-page educational tool on the benefits of stress reduction and exercise on the gastrointestinal health of older people. Include examples of an appropriate exercise regimen and stress reduction techniques.

REFERENCES

1. Adamek, R.J., and others: Long-term esophageal manometry in healthy subjects. Evaluation of normal values and influence of age, Dig. Dis. Sci. 39:2069, 1994.
2. Arora, S., and others: Effect of age on tests of intestinal and hepatic function in healthy humans, Gastroenterology 96:1560, 1989.
3. Atillasoy, E., and Holt, P.R.: Gastrointestinal proliferation and aging, J. Gerontol. 48(2):B43, 1993.
4. Atkinson, J.C., and Fox, P.C.: Salivary gland dysfunction, Clin. Geriatr. Med. 8(3):494, 1992.
5. Baum, B.J.: Salivary gland fluid secretion during aging, J. Am. Geriatr. Soc. 37:453, 1989.
6. Berkey, D.B., and Shay, K.: General dental care for the elderly, Clin. Geriatr. Med. 8(3):579, 1992.
7. Bowman, B.A., Rosenberg, I.H., and Johnson, M.A.: Gastrointestinal function in the elderly. In: Munro, H., and Schlierf, G., editors: Nutrition of the elderly, Nestle Nutrition Workshop Series Vol. 29, New York, 1992, Raven Press.
8. Bunker, V.W., and others: Nitrogen balance studies in apparently healthy elderly people and those who are housebound, Br. J. Nutr. 57:211, 1987.
9. Burt, B.A.: Epidemiology of dental diseases in the elderly, Clin. Geriatr. Med. 8(3):447, 1992.
10. Campbell, W.W., and others: Increased protein requirements in elderly people: new data and retrospective reassessments, Am. J. Clin. Nutr. 60:501, 1994.

11. Caraceni, P., and Van Thiel, D.H.: The effect of age on the liver. In: Morley, J.E., Glick, Z., and Rubenstein, L.A., editors: Geriatric nutrition. A comprehensive review, ed. 2, New York, 1995, Raven Press.

12. Cashman, M.D.: The aging gut. In: Chernoff, R., editor: Geriatric nutrition. The health professional's handbook, Gaithersburg, MD, 1991, Aspen Publications.

13. Castle, S.C.: Constipation: endemic in the elderly, Med. Clin. N. Am. 73:1497, 1989.

14. Connon, J.J.: Celiac disease. In: Shils, M.E., Olson, J.A., and Shike, M., editors: Modern nutrition in health and disease, ed. 8, Philadelphia, 1994, Lea and Febiger.

15. Deckmann, R.C., and Cheskin, L.J.: Diverticular disease in the elderly, J. Am. Geriatr. Soc. 40:986, 1993.

16. Douglass, C.W., and others: Oral health status of the elderly in New England, J. Gerontol. 48:M39, 1993.

17. Ellen, R.P.: Considerations for physicians caring for older adults with periodontal disease, Clin. Geriatr. Med. 8(3):599, 1992.

18. Ergun, G.A., and Miskovitz, P.F.: Aging and the esophagus: common pathologic conditions and their effect upon swallowing in the geriatric population, Dysphagia 7:58, 1992.

19. Farinati, F., and others: Changes in parietal and mucous cell mass in the gastric mucosa of normal subjects with age: a morphometric study, Gerontology 39:146, 1993.

20. Ferraris, R.P., and Vinnakota, R.R.: Regulation of intestinal nutrient transport is impaired in aged mice, J. Nutr. 123:502, 1993.

21. Fischer, J.G., and others: Dairy product intake of the oldest-old, J. Am. Diet. Assoc. 95:918, 1995.

22. Fries, J.F., and others: Toward an epidemiology of gastropathy associated with nonsteroidal anti-inflammatory drug use, Gastroenterology 96:647, 1989.

23. Goldschmiedt, M., and others: Effect of age on gastric acid secretion and serum gastrin concentrations in healthy men and women, Gastroenterology 101:977, 1991.

24. Gullo, L., and others: Aging and exocrine pancreatic function, J. Am. Geriatr. Soc. 34:790, 1986.

25. Guyton, A.C., and Hall, J.E.: Textbook of medical physiology, ed. 9, Philadelphia, 1996, W.B. Saunders.

26. Haboubi, N.Y., Cowley, P.A., and Lee, G.S.: Small bowel bacterial overgrowth: a cause of malnutrition in the elderly, Eur. J. Clin. Nutr. 42:999, 1988.

27. Holt, P.R.: General perspectives on the aged gut, Clin. Geriatr. Med. 7:185, 1991.

28. Holt, P.R., and Balint, J.A.: Effects of aging on intestinal lipid absorption, Am. J. Physiol. 264(Gastrointest. Liver Physiol. 27):G1, 1993.

29. Holt, P.R., Rosenberg, I.H., and Russell, R.M.: Causes and consequences of hypochlorhydria in the elderly, Dig. Dis. Sci. 34:933, 1989.

30. Husebye, E., and others: Fasting hypochlorhydria with gram positive gastric flora is highly prevalent in healthy old people, Gut 33:1331, 1992.

31. Johnson, M.A., and others: Nutritional patterns of centenarians, Inter. J. Aging Human Develop. 34(1):57, 1992.

32. Khalil, T., Poston, G.J., and Thompson, J.C.: Effects of aging on gastrointestinal hormones. In: Prinsley, D.M., and Sandstead, H.H. editors: Nutrition and aging, New York, 1990, Alan R. Liss.

33. Kogire, M., and others: Effects of aging on gastrin and somatostatin secretion from isolated perfused rat stomach, Dig. Dis. Sci. 38:303, 1993.

34. Kowlessar, O.D.: Malabsorption syndromes. In: Abrams, W.B., and Berkow, R., editors: Merck manual of geriatrics, Rahway, NJ, 1990, Merck Sharp and Dohme Research Laboratories.

35. Krasinski, S.D., and others: Fundic atrophic gastritis in an elderly population, effect on hemoglobin and several serum nutritional indicators, J. Am. Geriatr. Soc. 34:800, 1986.

36. Krasman, M.L., Gracie, W.A., and Strasius, S.R.: Biliary tract disease in the aged, Clin. Geriatr. Med. 7:347, 1991.

37. Liu, F., Kondo, T., and Toda, Y. Brief physical inactivity prolongs colonic transit time in elderly active men, Int. J. Sports Med. 14:465, 1993.

38. MacMahon, M., and others: Small intestinal bacterial overgrowth—an incidental finding, J. Am. Geriatr. Soc. 42:146, 1994.

39. Martin, W.E.: The oral cavity and nutrition. In: Morley, J.E., Glick, Z., and Rubenstein, L.Z., editors: Geriatric nutrition. A comprehensive review, ed. 2, New York, 1995, Raven Press.

40. McRae, T.D.: Common complaints of the elderly. In: Reichel, W., editor: Care of the elderly. Clinical aspects of aging, ed. 4, Baltimore, 1995, Williams and Wilkins.

41. Merkel, I.S., and others: Physiologic and psychologic characteristics of an elderly population with chronic constipation, Am. J. Gastroenterol. 88:1854, 1993.

42. Meshkinpour, H., Haghighat, P., and Dutton, C.: Clinical spectrum of esophageal aperistalsis in the elderly, Am. J. Gastroenterol. 89:1480, 1994.

43. Murphy, C.: Nutrition and chemosensory perception in the elderly, Clin. Rev. Food Sci. Nutr. 33(1):3, 1993.

44. Norton, R.A.: Gastrointestinal disease in the aged. In: Reichel, W., editor: Care of the elderly. Clinical aspects of aging, ed. 4, Baltimore, 1995, Williams and Wilkins.

45. Pilotto, A., and others: Effect of age on gastric acid, pepsin, pepsinogen group A, and gastrin secretion in peptic ulcer patients, Gerontology 40:253, 1994.

46. Posner, B.M., and others: Nutritional risk in New England elders, J. Gerontol. 49(3):M123, 1994.

47. Räihä, I., and others: Prevalence and characteristics of symptomatic gastroesophageal reflux disease in the elderly, J. Am. Geriatr. Soc. 40:1209, 1992.

48. Räihä, I., and Sourander, L.: GI motility disorders: diagnostic workup and use of prokinetic therapy, Geriatrics 48(11):57, 1993.

49. Rao, D.R., and others: Prevalence of lactose maldigestion. Influence and interaction of age, race, and sex, Dig. Dis. Sci. 39(7):1519, 1994.

50. Ren, J., and others: Effect of age and bolus variables on the coordination of the glottis and upper esophageal sphincter during swallowing, Am. J. Gastroenterol. 88:665, 1993.

51. Ren, J., and others: Effect of aging on the secondary esophageal peristalsis: presbyesophagus revisited, Am. J. Physiol. 268:G772, 1995.

52. Richey, D.P.: Effects of human aging on drug absorption and metabolism. In: Goldman, R., and Rockstein, M., editors: Physiology and pathology of human aging, New York, 1975, Academic Press.

53. Richter, J.E.: Functional disorders of the gastrointestinal tract. In: Abrams, W.B., and Berkow, R., editors: Merck manual of geriatrics, Rahway, NJ, 1990, Merck Sharp and Dohme Research Laboratories.

54. Roberts, D., Gelperin, D., and Wiley, J.W.: Evidence for age-associated reduction in acetylcholine release and smooth muscle response in the rat colon, Am. J. Physiol. 267(Gastrointest. Liver Physiol. 30):G515, 1994.

55. Rosenberg, I.H., Russell, R.M., and Bowman, B.B.: Aging and the digestive system. In: Munro, H.N., and Danford, D.E., editors: Nutrition, aging, and the elderly, New York, 1989, Plenum Press.

56. Russell, R.M.: Changes in gastrointestinal function attributed to aging, Am. J. Clin. Nutr. 55:1203S, 1992.

57. Saltzman, J.R., and others: Bacterial overgrowth without clinical malabsorption in elderly hypochlorhydric subjects, Gastroenterology 106:615, 1994.

58. Saltzman, J.R., and others: Changes in small-intestine permeability with aging, J. Am. Geriatr. Soc. 43:160, 1995.

59. Saltzman, J.R., and Russell, R.M.: Gastrointestinal function and aging. In: Morley, J.E., Glick, Z., and Rubenstein, L.Z., editors: Geriatric nutrition. A comprehensive review, ed. 2, New York, 1995, Raven Press.

60. Sampson, H.A.: Food allergy. In: Shils, M.E., Olson, J.A., and Shike, M., editors, Modern nutrition in health and disease, ed. 8, Philadelphia, 1994, Lea and Febiger.

61. Sandler, R.S., and others: Demographic and dietary determinants of constipation in the U.S. population, Am. J. Public Health 80:185, 1990.

62. Schuster, M.M.: Influence of aging on gastrointestinal disorders. In: Abrams, W.B., and Berkow, R., editors: Merck manual of geriatrics, Rahway, NJ, 1990, Merck Sharp and Dohme Research Laboratories.

63. Shaker, R., and Lang, I.M.: Effect of aging on the deglutitive oral, pharyngeal, and esophageal motor function, Dysphagia 9:221, 1994.

64. Shaker, R., and others: Effect on aging, position, and temperature on the threshold volume triggering pharyngeal swallows, Gastroenterology 107:396, 1994.

65. Shaker, R., and others: Effect on aging and bolus variables on pharyngeal and upper esophageal sphincter motor function, Am. J. Physiol. 264:G427, 1993.

66. Shamburek, R.D., and Farrar, J.T.: Disorders of the digestive system in the elderly, New Engl. J. Med. 322:438, 1990.

67. Simko, V., and Michael, S.: Absorptive capacity for dietary fat in elderly patients with debilitating disorders, Arch. Intern. Med. 149:557, 1989.

68. Sonies, B.C.: Oropharyngeal dysphagia in the elderly, Clin. Geriatr. Med. 8(3):569, 1992.

69. Suarez, F.L., and Savaiano, D.A.: Lactose digestion and tolerance in adult and elderly Asian-Americans, Am. J. Clin. Nutr. 59:1021, 1994.

70. Suarez, F.L., Savaiano, D.A., and Levitt, M.D.: A comparison of symptoms after the consumption of milk or lactose-hydrolyzed milk by people with self-reported severe lactose intolerance, New Engl. J. Med. 333:1, 1995.

71. Talley, N.J., and others: Prevalence of gastrointestinal symptoms in the elderly: a population-based study, Gastroenterology 102:895, 1992.

72. Towers, A.L., and others: Constipation in the elderly: influence of dietary, psychological, and physiological factors, J. Am. Geriatr. Soc. 42:701, 1994.

73. U.S. Department of Health and Human Services: Normal human aging: the Baltimore longitudinal study of aging, NIH Publication No. 84-2450, Washington, DC, 1984, U.S. Government Printing Office.

74. U.S. Department of Health and Human Services: Trends in the health of older Americans: United States, 1994, DHHS Publication No. (PHS) 95-1414, Hyattsville, MD, 1995, U.S. Government Printing Office.

75. Wallis, J.L., and others: Duodenal brush-border mucosal glucose transport and enzyme activities in aging man and effect of bacterial contamination of the small intestine, Dig. Dis. Sci. 38:403, 1993.

76. Wand, C.H., and Woolfold, C.A.: Salivary amylase activity of the aged, Gerontology 36:193, 1990.

77. Wegener, M., and others: Effect of aging on the gastrointestinal transit of a lactulose-supplemented mixed solid-liquid meal in humans, Digestion 39:40, 1985.

78. Weiffenbach, J.M., and Bartoshuk, L.M.: Taste and smell, Clin. Geriatr. Med. 8(3):543, 1992.

79. Whitehead, W.E., and others: Constipation in the elderly living at home, J. Am. Geriatr. Soc. 37:423, 1989.

80. Zimmerman, S.A., and Krondl, M.M.: Perceived intolerance of vegetables among the elderly, J. Am. Diet. Assoc. 86:1047, 1986.

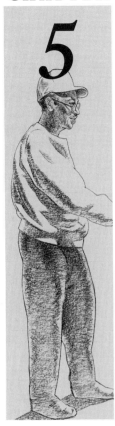

CHAPTER

5

Body Composition, Energy, and Physical Activity

✦✦

Objectives

After studying the chapter, the student should be able to:

✔ *List existing methods of measuring body composition and understand their limitations when applied to older people*

✔ *Recognize the influence of aging on body composition*

✔ *Identify the factors affecting body composition in older people*

✔ *Understand the effect of physical activity on body composition in older people*

✔ *Calculate the energy requirement in older people*

Both health professionals and the general public are concerned with the amounts of fat and muscle in our bodies. Early researchers recognized a relationship between body constituents and health and disease and examined cadavers to determine the size and content of various body compartments. In the nineteenth century, as the chemical elements were being identified, many were found in body tissues and fluids. The discovery of naturally occurring isotopes and the recent development of bioelectrical conductivity measurements have made it possible to evaluate body compartments in living people. Body composition can provide an indication of nutritional status and level of physical fitness and point to changes that reflect disease processes, not normal aging. Assessment of changes in body composition can help to quantify the effects of a nutrition intervention or exercise program. Decreases in body muscle contribute to the decrease in energy requirements observed in older people. Energy balance in older age groups is complicated further by the age-related decline in physical activity. These relationships are important clinically when assisting an older individual with weight management.

BODY COMPARTMENTS
Definitions

To evaluate body composition, we must divide the body into compartments according to chemical, anatomic, or fluid characteristics. The **chemical model** organizes the body into four compartments according to their water, mineral, protein, and fat content. The **tissue model** includes five compartments: skeletal muscle, adipose tissue, bone, blood, and other (which includes organs and lymph).[33]

Both direct and indirect methods are used to measure body compartments. Direct measurements can be used to quantify particular compartments; for example, dilution methods provide a measure of total body water, and sophisticated instruments can evaluate body calcium, located primarily in the bone. However, no practical methods are available to directly measure the size of some body compartments. Instead, we must rely on indirect methods of calculation based on direct measurements and established biological relationships between body compartments.[34]

Body protein cannot be measured directly, but total body nitrogen can be measured; body protein is estimated by multiplying the value for body nitrogen by 6.25. This calculation is based on the fact that proteins are on the average 16% nitrogen.[23] It is important to remember that some proteins are higher in nitrogen and some proteins are lower. Direct measurements are always preferred because formulas established for and based on healthy young adults are less appropriate for healthy or malnourished older adults. Both the absolute and relative sizes of the body compartments are influenced by the aging process and by disease. It is imperative that we learn how aging influences the biological relationships between body compartments and formulas used for indirect measurement of body composition. Several body compartments that are important to our study of aging adults are discussed below.

Fat-Free Mass

The **fat-free mass (FFM)** is equal to total body weight minus weight of body fat. Body components included in the FFM are water, protein, and minerals. The intracellular and extracellular fluids, muscle, vital organs, protein components of adipose cells, and the skeleton are included in the FFM. A term used less often is lean body mass (LBM). LBM designates the compartment remaining when the ether-extractable fat from the adipose tissue is subtracted from total body weight. LBM does include the structural lipids in cell membranes and nerves, although this lipid is rather small in amount compared to the amount of triglyceride stored in adipose tissue.[29] FFM is a rather heterogeneous tissue and is determined by both direct and indirect measurements. Total body water, total body potassium, and total body calcium can be measured directly.[14] These values can be used to calculate muscle mass and bone mineral.

Body Cell Mass

Body cell mass (BCM) is the term used to describe the body compartment that includes the active energy-using cells of the body.[29] BCM includes the cells in muscle, vital organs, blood, and brain. Cells in bone and connective tissues, which have slow turnover rates, are excluded. BCM is calculated on the basis of total body potassium and includes the tissues that account for most of the body's oxygen consumption. BCM is a useful concept because it includes tissues that are directly influenced and altered by nutrient intake and physical activity over days or weeks.

Total Body Water

On a weight basis, water is the most abundant constituent in the body, making up about 60% of body weight in young adult men and 50% in young adult women.[29] About 55% of **total body water (TBW)** is intracellular, and about 45% is extracellular. Extracellular water consists of plasma, lymph, and the interstitial fluid bathing the cells. Sodium is the primary electrolyte in the extracellular fluid, and potassium is the primary electrolyte in the intracellular fluid. Eighty-five percent of the sodium in the body is found in the extracellular compartment; 98% of the potassium in the body is found in the cells.

TBW is relatively easy to measure, since an isotope-labeled tracer dose of water will reach equilibrium with both intracellular and extracellular water in several hours. TBW can be calculated according to the volume of labeled water given and the final equilibrium concentration. Specific isotopes or dyes can be used to estimate total extracellular fluid volume, allowing intracellular fluid volume to be calculated by difference.

Body Fat

Fat is stored in the adipose tissue in the form of triglycerides (neutral fat) and can account for as much as one half of total body weight. Adipose tissue consists of about 83% triglyceride, 2% protein, and 15% water. Total body fat can be estimated using anthropometric measurements, computed tomography (CT), and neutron activation systems. Total body fat also can be calculated using equations derived from the measurements of FFM and BCM.

Influences on Body Compartments

Body compartments are constantly subject to changes in volume resulting from external or internal influences. External influences, such as increases or decreases in energy intake or strength training, lead to changes in FFM and body fat. Internal influences include the aging process or pathologic changes related to disease.

A shift in the size of one compartment effects a change in the size of others. TBW will be altered if FFM decreases or increases. Since adipose tissue contains less water than does FFM, an increase in fat at the expense of muscle decreases total body water. A loss of bone mineral as a consequence of aging decreases the size of the FFM but not of the BCM, which is made up of highly metabolically active cells. Our next step is to review current methods for evaluating body composition and consider the appropriateness of each with the older adult.

METHODS FOR EVALUATING BODY COMPOSITION
Limitations of Existing Methods

Early researchers studied body composition by chemically analyzing human cadavers for water, fat, nitrogen, and specific minerals. Highly specialized methods have since been developed to evaluate body composition as a function of age, sex, level of nutrition, or state of health. Because many of these methods are based on relationships between body water and body electrolyte content in young adults, they may not hold true in older adults. Methods based on physical measurements do not take into account the possible movement of body fat from one location to another, nor do external dimensions always reflect accurately internal changes in tissue composition caused by normal aging or chronic disease. Research methods that assess the size and composition of body compartments need to be validated in healthy older adults. Methods to assess body composition that are reasonably accurate, inexpensive, and noninvasive are urgently needed for clinical evaluation of older people in community and health care settings.

Current methods used to evaluate body composition and their limitations when applied to older people are described in table 5-1. Except for anthropometric and body density measurements, these methods have been used with relatively few older people, and reference standards for older age groups are just being developed. Many of these methods are invasive to the individual and require medical supervision or depend on highly specialized, expensive equipment available in few locations. Because of the effort and travel required of the individuals who have participated in these studies, only fairly healthy older people have been examined, and there is little information about those over age 85.[12] For frail elderly people, methods that involve intense cooperation from the participant (e.g., determination of body density by underwater weighing) are both stressful and difficult.

In general, the methods that provide direct measurement of a body compartment or constituent are more likely to yield appropriate estimates in older people. Direct methods include dilution measurements, whole body counting, computed tomography, dual-energy x-ray absorptiometry (DEXA), and neutron activation analysis. Body water, minerals, and nitrogen can be directly measured using one or a combination of these methods, which allow estimation of compartment size with very little use of

TABLE 5-1 *Methods for Evaluating Body Composition in Older People*

Method	Basis of Measurement	Usefulness with Older People
Dilution methods	Estimates body fluid volumes using stable isotope tracers such as O^{18} or B^{82} or Evans blue dye; calculation based on assumption that FFM is 73% water	Fat-free tissue will vary in water content in fatter individuals, and fat will be underestimated; method is inappropriate for older people who are dehydrated or edematous
K^{40} counting	Uses whole body scintillation counter to measure the naturally occurring radioactive isotope K^{40}; lean tissue is believed to have a relatively constant potassium concentration	Potassium concentration is higher in muscle than in connective tissue; older people have less muscle mass and more connective tissue; whole body potassium concentration often is lower in older people, presenting problems with interpretation
Excretion of muscle metabolites (creatinine)	Urinary creatinine derived from creatine phosphate is a valid index of lean body mass using height as a standard for body size	Age-related changes in height and kidney function influence creatinine-height index; requires 24-hour urine collection
Neutron activation	Individual is exposed to a carefully controlled flow of neutron irradiation raising the activity level of nitrogen, calcium, sodium, potassium, and chloride which can then be quantified in a whole body scintillation counter	Only minimal assumptions are required (protein = nitrogen value × 6.25); not influenced by edema or reduced bone calcium; requires expensive and highly sophisticated equipment
Dual-energy x-ray absorptiometry	Beams of x-ray directed into the body pass through different tissues at different levels of intensity and reductions in intensity are recorded by the system's detectors; will differentiate bone, fat, and fat-free, mineral-free tissue	Low level of radiation allows repeated measurements; provides correct analysis for people with differing bone densities and muscle mass; may underestimate fat in body trunk; requires expensive equipment

Technique	Description	Comments
Imaging techniques (computed tomography, magnetic resonance imaging)	A technique that uses x-ray or radio waves to produce an image and quantify total volumes of muscle, fat, and specific organs	Requires fair amount of radiation; not adversely affected by level of hydration, mineral density, or muscle wasting in older people
Density measurement	Body density is determined by weighing an individual first in air and then completely submerged in water to obtain an estimate of water displacement; equations are based on standard densities (fat = 0.9 g/cc; FFM = 1.1 gm/cc)	Can be unsuitable for frail older people; older people may be dehydrated or edematous, leading to inappropriate calculations; standard value used for proportion of bone mineral is inaccurate for older women with bone loss
Whole body electrical conductivity (TOBEC)	Lean tissues with a high water content conduct electricity better than fat tissue; measures the change in electrical conductivity pattern when a person is placed in a chamber with oscillating electromagnetic waves	Can overestimate LBM in a person with considerable body fat; estimate is improved by including an accurate height measurement in calculations; no radiation exposure; expensive apparatus required
Bioelectrical impedance	A weak electrical current is passed through the body (between right hand and right foot); the resistance to the current flow is proportional to total body water and lean body mass	Problems similar to those noted with TOBEC; no radiation exposure; fairly inexpensive apparatus; offers promise for routine use if specific equations can be developed for use with older people
Anthropometric measurements	Direct measurement of body height, weight, skinfold thicknesses, and circumferences allow calculation of body fat using available formulas	Does not provide valid estimate of internal fat; assumptions and equations may not hold true for older person in whom the regional fat pattern is individualized; equipment is inexpensive and portable

established formulas that may introduce error when used with older people.[33]

Overestimation and Underestimation of Body Compartments

Body density methods. Body composition methods that rely on standard formulas describing the hydration of body tissues appear to underestimate FFM and overestimate body fat in older people.[3,33] Measuring body density by underwater weighing provides estimates on only two body compartments, body fat and FFM, and neither compartment is measured directly. Standard prediction equations are required to calculate the volume of both FFM and fat.

Early work with cadavers and animals determined that FFM is about 73% water.[3] Neutron activation studies at Brookhaven National Laboratory with healthy men and women between the ages of 26 and 93 indicated an age-related trend in the water content of FFM.[33] For 20-year-olds the FFM was about 72% water, whereas for 80-year-olds the FFM was about 74% water. The standard value used in prediction equations to represent the density of the FFM has been 1.1 g per cubic cm. In that study the true value for younger people was 1.101 g per cubic cm and for older people, 1.098 g per cubic cm.

Several factors could contribute to this decrease in density of the FFM in older people.[3] An increase in body water, which has a density of 1 g per cubic cm, would lower the overall density of the FFM. An increase in adipose tissue, which occurs with aging, effectively increases the relative water content of the FFM because adipose cells, when their fat has been removed, have a water content of 98%; the only other constituent remaining in the cell is a small amount of protein (2%). Other cells that make up the fat-free tissue are about 73% water, because their protein content is higher. The density of the FFM also will decrease if bone mineral is lost. When the body density relationships were developed, the FFM was believed to be 6% to 7% bone mineral.[43] Intensive studies of older and younger adults using DEXA indicate that the relative contribution of bone mineral to the FFM can be quite variable (4% to 8%), depending on age, sex, or ethnic group.[43] Younger women have more bone than older women, and African Americans have more bone than white people. The density of the FFM in African American adults of all ages is higher than that of white adults based on their greater amounts of bone mineral. It is likely that all of these factors contribute to the decrease in the density of the FFM in older people.

Even a small error in the density of the FFM will lead to a significant error when calculating the volume of body fat. Ninety-eight older people had their body composition evaluated using body density methods or DEXA. The percentage of body fat in both the men and women was 2% higher when calculated by body density measurement equations.[3] Differences within individuals were even more striking. In three women the level of body fat calculated from the density measurement was 6% higher than by DEXA; for several men it was 8% higher. Conversely, the FFM was higher by one kg in both sexes when measured by DEXA than when calculated from body density measurements.

Dual-energy X-ray absorptiometry (DEXA) methods. The x-ray methods initially developed in the 1980s have been modified to become **dual-energy x-ray absorptiometry** with a greater precision and accuracy for evaluating bone mineral density and fat or lean soft tissue. Nevertheless, this method is not yet poised to become the gold standard for determining body composition.[60] Studies with neonatal animals who have a higher level of hydration in their lean tissue than adults (this is also true in human infants) revealed significant errors; lean tissue was slightly underestimated whereas fat tissue was overestimated. Thus, it appears that DEXA is not appropriate for older patients with congestive heart failure or kidney or liver disease who retain higher than normal levels of fluid. The positioning of fat on the body also contributes to error with this method. Body fat located on the trunk region is underestimated because the bony ribs and spine interfere with the x-ray beam penetrating soft tissues. Snead and coworkers[67] documented the underestimation of upper body fat by measuring the body composition of younger people before and after placing 2 kg packets of lard on the chest or the legs. When placed on the legs, 96% of the added fat was identified as fat; total body fat was measured to be 10.8 kg before and 12.8 kg after the fat was placed. In contrast only 55% of the added fat was identified as fat when it was placed on the chest; body fat was measured to be 10.8 kg before and 11.9 kg after. Because fat accumulated in aging tends to be added on the trunk rather than the extremities, data obtained by DEXA may not present a true estimation of body fat.

Clinical significance. Gains or losses of body water, potassium, and protein in particular body compartments become especially important when estimating body composition in individuals with metabolic disorders. In patients with electrolyte disturbances, severe renal disease, or cancer, body water can shift to other compartments, and body potassium may be lost.[66] Thus, estimates based on these constituents have a high degree of error. In these individuals, body nitrogen and calcium are better measures of body compartments than body potassium or total body water.[14]

Body Composition Methods for Nutrition Screening

Rapid, inexpensive body composition methods are needed for use in nutrition screening and clinical intervention. To this end efforts are under way to improve the estimates of body compartments obtained by bioelectrical impedance and anthropometric measurements. Several studies[3,16] have compared results obtained by DEXA, body water dilution techniques, and density measurements with these less expensive methods. Estimates of body fat determined by bioelectrical impedance in people above age 60 were highly correlated with values obtained by the more expensive methods; however, the prediction equations developed with younger populations overestimated the FFM by about 6 kg in older adults.[16] Despite these problems, bioelectrical impedance measurements, which require only a few minutes with no discomfort to the client, hold promise for use in clinical settings.

A current area of research with bioelectrical impedance is the comparison of body trunk measurements and arm or leg measurements. In young people the arm and leg account for 85% of total body impedance although they account for only 35% of total body volume.[11] This suggests that the trunk contributes very little to the total body resistance. Substantial changes in body composition in aging occur in the trunk and little is known about the possible influence of such fat deposition on the flow of current.[11]

The influence of chronic diseases on impedance methods must also be considered. Impedance measurements obtained on the arm or leg may be adversely affected by edema or fluid accumulation resulting from heart or renal disease or untreated hypertension. Standard equations developed for use with impedance equipment may not apply when the amounts of muscle and fat are decreased relative to the amount of bone, which occurs in protein-energy malnutrition, cancer cachexia, or other wasting syndromes. The combined use of bioelectrical impedance and anthropometric measurements improved the estimates of body compartments in cancer patients evaluated in a hospital setting.[26] Conversely, extreme obesity with large fat deposits on the upper arm may alter impedance measures and their interpretation.[11] Skin texture, which changes with age, has been mentioned as a factor in bioelectrical impedance measurements. Bioelectrical impedance methods have special potential for the assessment of older people who are paraplegic or confined to bed or chair.[11] Measurement of a body segment such as an arm or leg could provide an estimate of hydration, body water distribution, or fatness. For this to be possible, standards must be developed consistent with age-related changes in body compartments in both health and disease conditions.

Anthropometric measurements also offer promise as a low-cost, practical method for evaluating changes in body size or body composition in the elderly. Body measurements usually are included in physical examinations and nutrition assessments; body weight, height, circumferences, and skinfold thicknesses are most commonly used. But the collection of anthropometric measurements in older people presents special problems.[11] Most measurements are taken in a standing position, and many elderly people are unable to stand, or stand erect, for an extended period of time. An elderly patient may be chair-bound or bedridden because of a hip or other fracture. Frail or seriously ill individuals are often too weak to stand. Recumbent knee height can be used to estimate stature in older people who are not ambulatory. Expensive equipment such as a bed or wheelchair scale would have to be available to weigh these individuals. Skinfold and circumference measurements along with knee height can be used to estimate body weight.

When body weight measurements are available, they can be influenced by abnormal levels of fluid, muscle, or fat. Fluctuations in body water because of fluid retention or dehydration will significantly alter body weight (remember, two cups of water weigh one pound). Congestive heart failure or kidney disease with increased extracellular or intracellular fluid will mask a weight loss caused by protein-energy malnutrition, cardiac cachexia, or undiagnosed cancer. An older person of normal body weight may have a critically low muscle mass but high body fat.

Skinfold thicknesses have been used as indicators of body fatness. The use of skinfold thicknesses evolved from the physiologic finding that in young adults about half of all body fat is subcutaneous (found directly under the skin). Prediction equations for total body fat based on four skinfold thicknesses—triceps, biceps, suprailiac, and subscapular—in 237 elderly people (60 to 87 years of age) provided estimates of body fat that differed from density measurements.[56] In women the prediction equations were more likely to underestimate body fat, and the error increased with increasing body fat. For men, the opposite was true; body fat was overestimated.

Age-related changes in total body fatness and increased deposition of internal fat rather than subcutaneous fat present problems with the interpretation of fatness estimates based on skinfold thicknesses. Minten and coworkers,[45] following evaluation of anthropometric measurements

obtained from 515 Dutch elderly, concluded that body weight and skinfold thicknesses did not provide consistent measures of fatness in the men over age 75 and in the women over age 70. Those workers[45] suggested that circumference measurements of the waist or hip might provide a more appropriate estimate of total body fat. Data from 424 independent-living elderly people in Texas[40] indicate that arm and waist circumferences have promise as predictors of chronic disease risk. Waist measurements may be of particular value based on the known association of abdominal obesity and chronic disease.

Standards of Evaluation

Evaluation and interpretation of anthropometric measurements require a set of reference values against which to compare individual values. Measurements obtained from older people need to be compared with reference values developed from people of similar age and ethnic group as both the level and distribution of fat and muscle will differ. A major limitation of anthropometric methods is the small amount of available reference data for people above age 80 and for older members of African American, Asian, and Hispanic groups.[11] Consequently, reference standards for an older population usually are the average values obtained from that age group and may not represent the ideal. However, the mere survival of these individuals suggests that even average values present a reasonable basis for comparison. (Discussion of specific anthropometric measurements and their use in nutritional assessment can be found in chapter 11.)

FACTORS AFFECTING BODY COMPOSITION
Genetic Influence

One's proportion of body fat is controlled to some extent by genetic factors. Bouchard and coworkers[6] suggested that distribution of body fat is influenced more by genetic factors than is total body fat. Females at all ages have a higher percentage of body fat than males and a smaller proportion of FFM. Among 700 healthy men and women ages 23 to 30, body fat based on body density measurements was 17% in men and 29% in women.[2] Body fat continues to increase with age in both sexes. Women have more body fat regardless of their level of physical activity, although women characterized as physically fit have less fat. Increases in body fat from youth to middle age were reported in women even before the advent of laborsaving devices, when housekeeping and farm chores required heavy physical labor. In a study conducted with rural women nearly 30 years ago,[48] body fat evaluated by density and anthropometric techniques rose from 26% to 39% between the ages of 18 and 67 years. Interestingly, the percentages of body fat in the young women measured 30 years ago are very similar to the young women described above. Ethnic origin influences body composition. Asians[76] and African Americans[54] have higher proportions of body fat than white adults of similar body weight and different patterns of fat distribution.

Physical Activity

Physical exercise influences the accumulation of body fat in individuals of all ages. Physically active older men had less body fat (24% versus 27%) and more lean body mass (62 kg versus 57 kg) than inactive men of similar age and body weight.[24] In fact, the physically active older men, some of whom were long-distance runners, had a lower percentage of body fat than inactive younger men. Older women enrolled in a 26-week walking program[4] decreased their skinfold thicknesses 6% to 8%. Physical activity also brings about positive changes in fat pattern. In an older adult physical fitness program, participants showed a decrease in abdominal fat and waist-to-hip ratio, even though their total body fat was unchanged.[65]

Nutrient Intake

Prevailing wisdom once held that a gain in body weight or body fat represented a simple excess of energy intake over energy expenditure. We have come to realize that many factors relating to the type of food consumed and the individual's physiologic status influence the gain or loss of body fat. Consumption of kilocalories in the form of fat rather than carbohydrate may

accelerate the accretion of body fat. The conversion of dietary carbohydrate to storage fat through the synthesis of fatty acids requires 23 of every 100 kcal consumed; in contrast, dietary fatty acids can be converted to triglycerides and deposited directly in adipose tissue at a cost of only 3 kcal per 100 kcal consumed.[7] Current work also suggests that individuals may differ in their sensitivity to the satiety-producing effect of fat.[59]

AGE-RELATED CHANGES IN BODY COMPOSITION
Longitudinal Versus Cross-Sectional Studies

Advances in methodology allow us to evaluate more precisely the size and composition of body compartments and the changes in these compartments that occur throughout adulthood. There is general agreement that body compartments change as a function of age, although the degree of change among individuals varies considerably. Unfortunately, we lack longitudinal evaluations that would tell us exactly when and at what rate these changes occur. We are also lacking long-term research studies that relate changes in body composition to lifelong diet, exercise, or lifestyle patterns.

Most available data on body composition come from cross-sectional studies. Cross-sectional comparisons of body compartments in individuals of different ages are complicated by secular and age-related changes. Each succeeding generation is taller and heavier; thus, older people tend to be shorter and may weigh less than younger people, regardless of age-related changes. Ideally, the effect of the aging process on body composition should be evaluated on the basis of longitudinal changes observed in the same individual. These data are being recorded in the Baltimore Longitudinal Study of Aging (BLSA) for future evaluation.[71]

Changes in Body Compartments

A general characteristic of age-related changes in most individuals is a loss of FFM and a gain in fat.[22] Bartlett and coworkers[2] evaluated

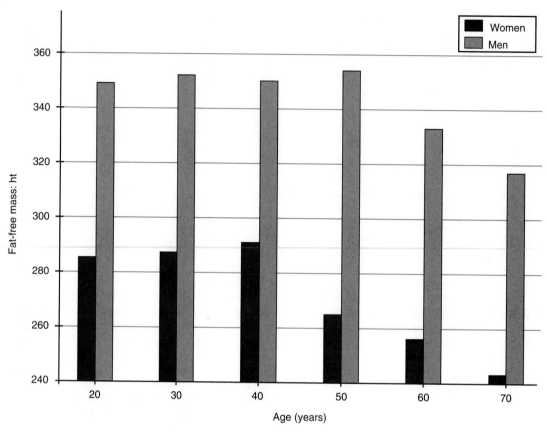

FIG. 5-1 Ratio of Fat-Free Mass to Height According to Age. In men the ratio of fat-free mass to height declines after age 50; in women it declines from about age 40. The decrease in the ratio of fat-free mass to height indicates a loss of fat-free tissues.

Data from Barlett, H.L., and others: Fat-free mass in relation to stature: ratios of fat-free mass to height in children, adults, and elderly subjects, Am. J. Clin. Nutr. 53:1112, 1991.

813 adults by density methods and found different trends for changes in FFM and body fat over adulthood. Although body fat increased consistently from age 25 to age 65 and over (from 17% to 29% in men and from 29% to 38% in women), FFM did not change appreciably until middle age. After age 45 FFM fell from 62 kg to 55 kg in the men and from 48 kg to 39 kg in the women. Because older people tend to be shorter in stature than younger people, the decrease in FFM might have related to the size of the older subjects and not represent an actual loss in FFM at older ages. To investigate this

possibility Bartlett and colleagues[2] calculated a ratio of FFM to height (g per cm) to correct for differences in body size (fig. 5-1). Overall loss in FFM is higher in women, as the FFM-to-height ratio declined by 15% in women and only 9% in men. Both bone mineral and muscle undergo accelerated loss following menopause in women. The influence of both aging and hormone levels on these changes will be discussed in following sections.

A study from Italy[49] has provided insight regarding continuing changes in body composition to age 100 and beyond. Paolisso and coworkers[49]

TABLE 5-2   *Body Composition in Adults, Older Adults, and Centenarians*

	Below Age 50		Age 75 and Over		Age 100 and Over	
	Men	Women	Men	Women	Men	Women
Body height (cm)	178	175	177	173	162	159
Body weight (kg)	71.4	67.1	70.1	64.5	61.4	55.5
Body mass index	22.5	21.9	22.4	21.6	23.4	22.0
Fat-free mass (kg)	56	51	48	40	41	37.8
Body fat (%)	25	30	30	35	33	37
Waist-hip ratio	0.83	0.80	0.85	0.83	0.82	0.78

Modified from Paolisso, G., and others: Body composition, body fat distribution, and resting metabolic rate in healthy centenarians, Am. J. Clin. Nutr. 62:746, 1995.

compared body composition and fat distribution in younger adults (below age 50), older adults (75 to 99 years of age), and centenarians (100 years of age and over). All were in good health, had no signs of edema or dehydration, and were not using drugs that could affect fluid or electrolyte balance. As described in table 5-2, body height, body weight, and fat-free mass continued to decline with age in both men and women. At the same time percentage of body fat increased. FFM and body weight were significantly lower in the centenarians as compared with both the adults below age 50 and those ages 75 to 99. It is interesting to note that the centenarians of both sexes had a lower (more favorable) waist-to-hip ratio than their counterparts in either age group. It appears that the waist-to-hip ratio increases as age and body mass index (BMI) increase. This trend was reversed in the centenarians, perhaps by lifestyle factors, hormone patterns, or genetic influences. Because these data represent a cross-sectional evaluation, it is not known if the centenarians enjoyed lower waist-to-hip ratios throughout their adult life and so avoided the increased mortality risk associated with higher ratios or if they lost abdominal fat as they continued to age.

Although total body fat increased throughout the life span, even in the centenarians, subcutaneous fat measured on the upper arm (triceps) and the trunk (chest) decreased. This would suggest a greater deposition of internal fat, which is not obvious using skinfold measurements. Body compartments in the centenarians as measured by bioelectrical impedance and anthropometric methods were strongly correlated. However, bioelectrical impedance has been shown to underestimate body fat located on the upper body; hence, their percentage of body fat may be higher than reported. Longitudinal studies of elderly groups, including centenarians, will allow further evaluation of changes in body compartments in extreme old age and potential benefits of intervention.

Hormone Secretion and Changes in Body Compartments

Hormonal changes and changes in lifestyle have been implicated in the age-related loss of muscle and bone mineral and the gain in body fat.[15,62] Secretion patterns of the sex steroid hormones, estrogen and testosterone, and growth hormone are altered at older ages. These hormones are known to strongly influence protein metabolism, fat deposition, and bone mass in both men and women. Age-related reductions in the secretion of growth hormone and the sex steroid hormones are believed to contribute to the less favorable alterations in body composition that occur at older ages. An active area of research is the use of hormone replacement to reverse the degenerative changes of aging.

Estrogen replacement therapy has been studied to the greatest extent in relation to the prevention of bone loss and possibly cardiovascular disease in women. Clinical trials of growth hormone replacement have as a goal increasing lean body mass and decreasing total body fat in older men and women. (The use of estrogen replacement therapy in prevention of cardiovascular disease and bone loss is discussed in chapters 2 and 12.)

Male Sex Steroid Hormones

Men, as compared to women, experience a more gradual decline in production of their gonadal hormones. Nevertheless, by age 50, over half have testosterone levels below those seen in young men.[46] This decline in testosterone levels has been associated with the decreased ability of older men to maintain positive nitrogen balance. Also, elderly men with very low testosterone levels are more at risk for hip fracture. Short-term testosterone therapy improves muscle mass and muscle strength in older men and, surprisingly, decreases serum LDL-cholesterol levels. Unfortunately, testosterone replacement therapy has undesirable side effects, including gynecomastia (breast enlargement) and accelerated enlargement of the prostate gland.[46]

Female Sex Steroid Hormones

Women experience a dramatic change in the secretion of estrogen with the onset of menopause and cessation of ovarian function. The loss of estrogen at menopause contributes to alterations in calcium absorption and bone metabolism and may play a role in the accelerated loss of skeletal muscle observed in postmenopausal women.[1] Body potassium is used as an indicator of total muscle mass because it is the major cation within the cell and is active in muscle contraction. In women the rate of loss of body potassium is greatest during the first three years after menopause, just as the accelerated loss of bone mineral occurs immediately after estrogen withdrawal.[1] Beyond that time potassium and calcium losses continue, although at a slower rate. Aloia and coworkers[1] suggested that muscle mass may be lost first and contribute to the loss of bone mineral through reduced mechanical stress on the skeleton. Although menopause and the change in hormonal secretion could bring about these changes in body composition, it is possible that increasing age also has an influence.

Based on a study of 373 early postmenopausal women in Denmark,[77] it appears that menopause and aging exert separate effects on specific body compartments. The women ranged in age from 50 to 60 years and were measured using DEXA. Body fat, lean tissue mass (fat-free, mineral-free soft tissues), and bone mineral were evaluated according to years since menopause and total age. As described in figure 5-2, age rather than menopause influenced body fat mass. The relationship between age and increased abdominal fat remained significant even after the obese subjects were removed from the calculation. In contrast, years since menopause was a significant predictor of total lean tissue in these women. Reduced energy expenditure and inappropriate energy intake could contribute to the increase in body fat. Estrogen deficiency would appear to be a major factor in the loss of lean body mass. Estrogen replacement therapy may have value for preserving muscle mass and preventing the increase in abdominal fat that contributes to health risk.

Growth Hormone

Growth hormone is secreted by the anterior lobe of the pituitary gland in response to growth hormone-releasing factor produced in the hypothalamus. Growth hormone controls the production and release by the liver and other tissues of insulin-like growth factor (formerly referred to as somatomedin C). Insulin-like growth factor (IGF) is responsible for the effects of growth hormone in target tissues.[15] Plasma levels of growth hormone and IGF decline with age even in healthy older adults. Growth hormone levels declined 14% per decade in healthy, nonobese men between the ages of 21 and 71.[15] IGF plasma levels fall 30% to 40% over adulthood. Low growth hormone and IGF levels in younger persons result in atrophy of the lean body mass and an increase in body fat, including abdominal fat. Thus, it has been suggested that the characteristic and unfavorable changes in body

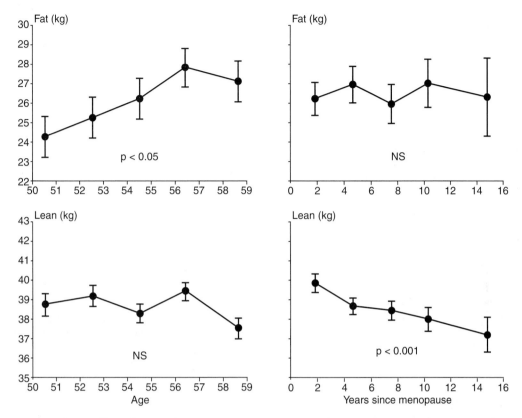

FIG. 5-2   Effect of Age and Years Since Menopause on Body Fat and Lean Tissue Mass. Total body fat increases significantly with age but is not influenced by years since menopause; in contrast, lean tissue decreases significantly following menopause but is not influenced by age.

Wang, Q., and others: Total and regional body-composition changes in early postmenopausal women: age-related or menopause-related?, Am. J. Clin. Nutr. 60:843, 1994. © American Society for Clinical Nutrition. (Reprinted with permission.)

composition associated with aging may relate to the diminished secretion of these hormones.

The administration of growth hormone to older men not only increased their plasma growth hormone and IGF levels but also brought about changes in their body composition.[62] After six months of hormone replacement, lean body mass had increased by 9% and adipose tissue had decreased by 15%. Mean body weight increased by only 1 kg over this period, whereas lean body mass increased by almost 5 kg and body fat decreased by about 3.5 kg. Body composition was unchanged in

control subjects of similar age who did not receive the hormone therapy. Those researchers noted that six months of growth hormone administration reversed the changes that occur over 10 to 20 years of aging.

Continued research has not supported the expectations raised by early studies. Controlled clinical trials with both men and women have produced conflicting results and raise serious questions regarding the efficacy of growth hormone as a means of reversing or preventing the changes of normal aging. A six-month trial conducted with 27 healthy elderly women (mean age of 67)[35] resulted in no increase in lean body mass or decrease in body fat based on density measurements; however, a 9% decline in total body fat (2.7 kg) was calculated on the basis of skinfold thickness measurements. Those researchers[35] pointed out that sodium retention and edema occur with high dosages of growth hormone. Even at lower dosages, subtle changes in fluid shifts between the intracellular and extracellular compartments could confound body composition measurements. In comparison, a short-term study (four weeks) with women who were somewhat older (mean age of 72 years)[69] did report significant increases in lean body mass from 1.2 kg to 3.3 kg as measured by DEXA. Several of the women in this study were also receiving estrogen replacement therapy which may have contributed to the anabolic effects observed.

The effect of growth hormone on lean body mass is pertinent because loss of muscle mass and muscle strength have been implicated in the prevalence of falls and ensuing disability among elderly people. In younger people exercise is a physiologic stimulus for the release of growth hormone; likewise, it has been suggested that decreased activity in advancing age may contribute to both the reduced secretion of growth hormone and loss of muscle. Available data[61] indicate that physical exercise does not influence growth hormone levels in the elderly. In fact, a comparison of sedentary and physically fit older men indicated the opposite: plasma levels of IGF were inversely related to kilocalories per kg of physical exercise per week.[61] Another area of interest has been the potential use of growth hormone replacement to augment the muscle response to strength training in older people. Unfortunately, increases in muscle strength with resistance exercise tended to plateau after about 12 weeks; further gains over the next 10 weeks were similar in growth hormone-treated and control older men.[68]

Growth hormone also has a role in control of bone remodeling. Growth hormone activates osteoblasts, the cells which produce bone matrix and sequester bone mineral. In older women receiving growth hormone replacement therapy, bone mass was preserved.[35]

Growth hormone replacement therapy has a high prevalence of side effects, including edema, joint pain and swelling, and carpal tunnel syndrome. Available studies have reported unequivocal results likely related to small sample sizes and differences in levels and time period of hormone replacement. The clinical usefulness of growth hormone replacement on a long-term basis remains to be defined. On a short-term basis, growth hormone may prove beneficial in promoting nitrogen retention in older individuals with catabolic illnesses, shortening the duration of protein loss and supporting recovery.

Physical Activity and Changes in Body Compartments

For most people physical activity is a personal choice and offers an opportunity for the prevention of age-related changes in body compartments. Older people who remain physically active can, at least to some extent, prevent the accumulation of excessive body fat while maintaining more appropriate levels of fat free mass. This was demonstrated by Kohrt and coworkers,[39] who evaluated healthy sedentary and healthy fit younger and older people. The older male athletes averaged about six hours of exercise training a week, and the older female athletes about five hours. All had been training regularly for at least 10 years. Although running was the primary activity in both age groups, many of the older athletes engaged in cycling, swimming, weight-lifting, and walking. Body composition was determined by density and skinfold thickness measurements.

As described in table 5-3, the older sedentary men and women had an average of 10.1 kg and 12.2 kg more fat than their young counterparts.[39] In contrast, the older trained men and women differed in fat mass by less than half as much (4.3 kg for the men and 5.5 kg for the women) from the younger trained men and women. It is interesting to note that the older trained women whose BMI was about the same as the sedentary young women (21.5 versus 21.4) still had a higher percentage of body fat (25.3% versus 24%). FFM was lower in the older groups, regardless of training. Although training did not eliminate the age-related

TABLE 5-3   *Effect of Exercise on Body Composition in Older and Younger Adults*

	Sedentary		Trained	
	Young	**Old**	**Young**	**Old**
Men				
Age (yrs)	26	64	26	62
Body weight (kg)	76.5	81.9	69.6	65.9
Body mass index	24.0	26.4	21.7	22.1
Body fat (kg)	13.7	23.8	7.1	11.4
Fat-free mass (kg)	62.8	58.0	62.5	54.6
Women				
Age (yrs)	25	64	27	57
Body weight (kg)	59.3	68.8	56.8	58.5
Body mass index	21.4	25.5	20.3	21.5
Body fat (kg)	14.6	26.8	9.5	15.0
Fat-free mass (kg)	44.7	42.0	47.3	43.6

Modified from Kohrt, W.M., and others: Body composition of healthy sedentary and trained, young and older men and women, Med. Sci. Sports Exerc. 24:832, 1992.

increase in body fat (estimated to occur at a rate of about 2% per decade), it did prevent undesirable fat accumulation in the upper trunk and abdominal region. Despite increases in total body fat, abdominal skinfold measurements for the older trained men and women were less than or equal to those of their young, sedentary counterparts. The older trained individuals in this study had a minimum of 2.5 hours of training per week. This is the equivalent of 30 minutes a day, five days a week, an exercise level that should be possible for the majority of healthy older people.

Physical Activity and Muscle Mass

The principal component affected by the age-related decrease in FFM is skeletal muscle. Some authors refer to the age-related loss in skeletal muscle as **sarcopenia** (*sarco* is a Greek derivative meaning "related to the flesh").[18] The age-related loss in muscle strength is the result of this loss in muscle mass and not a loss in the functional ability of remaining muscle cells.

Physical inactivity and loss of muscle fibers. The 50% decrease in muscle mass occurring over adulthood has been documented by computed tomography and by counting individual muscle fibers in a muscle biopsy. Computed tomography revealed a reduced cross section of muscle area as well as a decrease in the density of muscle fibers and an increase in intramuscular fat.[18] One factor contributing to the decrease in muscle mass is a sedentary lifestyle with muscle atrophy related to a lack of use. Similar changes—atrophy of the skeletal muscle and loss of muscle strength—occur in young people when muscle activity is significantly reduced by bed rest or immobilization. Evans and Campbell[18] considered decreased amounts of physical activity to be the major contributor, and age to be of secondary importance, to the changes in physical capacity that begin to take place in middle age.

Skeletal muscle is made up of two types of fibers. Those muscles that maintain posture contain primarily type I fibers. Most other muscles contain both type I and type II fibers. The muscle fiber type that is used depends on the level of muscle force required. For slow, low-intensity exercise, typical of most day-to-day activities, such as shopping, meal preparation, or personal care, most of the muscle force needed comes from type I fibers. For higher-intensity exercise—running, cycling, pushing against a resistance force—both type I and type II fibers participate. Type II fibers are lost to a greater extent than type I fibers, and this loss is significantly related to loss in muscle strength.[17]

Endurance training and muscle fibers. Endurance training involves prolonged, rhythmic exercise such as walking or cycling; strength training involves generating force against a resistance, as in lifting or lowering heavy weights. These two types of training have very different effects on body composition in older people. Endurance training lowers body fat but does not significantly increase muscle mass.[17] Older endurance-trained athletes have a lower proportion of body fat than sedentary individuals of similar age but not an increased muscle mass.

Strength training and muscle fibers. Strength training leads to hypertrophy of both type I and type II muscle fibers and an increase in muscle mass. This occurs in both younger and older adults who begin a strength training regimen. A 10-week program of weight training enhanced both muscle size and muscle strength in 100 frail nursing home residents with an average age of 87.[19] Eighty-three participants had been unable to walk without the use of a cane, walker, or wheelchair, and 66 had at least one fall in the previous year. Muscle strength in the knee and hip was directly related to total body potassium (a measure of cell mass including muscle mass). Muscle strength more than doubled in those enrolled in the exercise program, and the cross-sectional area of the midthigh muscle increased. Of practical importance was the substantial improvement in walking speed, stair-climbing ability, and overall physical activity. Four participants who had used a walker required only a cane after the resistance training. Increased spontaneous physical activity could reflect a reduced fear of falling after the resistance training or greater ease in moving to an upright position. The muscle strength of older people is strongly dependent on the preservation of muscle mass.

Some reversal of muscle atrophy is possible with regular strength training despite advanced age or poor functional status; however, the training must be continued to maintain any gains in muscle mass achieved. Four weeks after a trained group of older people resumed a sedentary lifestyle, their gains in muscle strength began to deteriorate.[20] The fact that muscle status could be improved in frail elderly people emphasizes the potential for reversing or preventing age-related muscle loss in middle-aged adults or those recently retired.

CURRENT TRENDS IN BODY MEASUREMENTS
Changes in Body Stature

Age and secular influences. Older age groups are shorter in stature than younger age groups as a result of actual losses in height as well as secular influences. **Secular changes** refer to changes occurring over time as each succeeding generation increases in height. The classic work of Trotter and Gleser[70] evaluated the relative influence of age changes versus secular changes on body height by measuring the length of the long bones (the femur and tibia) in 855 cadavers. Bone length does not change as a result of the aging process; therefore, differences in bone length between generations result from secular influences. Age-related losses in height are caused by the vertical shrinking and collapse of the vertebrae in the spinal column and curvature of the spine, as seen in lordosis or kyphosis.

Trotter and Gleser[70] found that both secular and age-related factors contributed to the differences in stature across age cohorts. Age-related changes were most prominent among white women who lost 7.8 cm in height over adulthood. White women are also most at risk for osteoporosis, which contributes to loss in stature. African American women and white and African American men lost 2.6 to 3.5 cm in height. The average rate of loss across all groups was 0.6 cm per decade between ages 20 and 90;

however, losses occurred most rapidly after age 50, with only slight losses occurring before age 40. Within specific age and sex groups, individuals will differ in their loss of height. A 10-year longitudinal study of 11 women between the ages of 48 and 77 revealed no change in height in two of the participants (ages 56 and 77) and losses of 0.5 to 2.0 cm in the other nine.

An ongoing longitudinal study of 220 older people over age 65[13] has suggested that actual losses in height may be greater than previously reported. Based on six years of observation, the rate of decline in this population is about 0.5 cm per year and is constant in all age and sex groups. If continued, these losses will translate to 4 to 5 cm per decade. A continual loss in stature has serious implications for the selection of an appropriate body weight standard for an older individual.

Stature of adults in the United States. According to measurements obtained in the NHANES II study,[41] both sex and age influence standing height. Men are taller than women of the corresponding age. Standing height decreased by 2.2 inches between the ages of 18 and 74 in both African American men and white men. In white women standing height decreased by 2.1 inches and in African American women by 1.8 inches over this age range. The ethnic group to which an individual belonged appeared to have little influence on standing height at any age. African American women have a greater bone mineral mass than white women at all ages, and they have less risk of osteoporosis and damage to the vertebrae. Loss of bone in the vertebrae contributes in a major way to the loss in height in older men and women.

Changes in Body Mass Index (BMI)

All adult age groups in the United States are becoming both larger and heavier. In men and women mean BMI increases until age 59 and then declines.[41] Of particular concern is the continuing escalation in the proportion of adults who are overweight. A comparison of data from the NHANES I, II, and III studies points to the increasing numbers of middle-aged and older adults who have a higher than desirable amount

of body fat (fig. 5-3).[41] Between the NHANES II and NHANES III studies, the mean body weight of adults ages 20 through 74 increased by about 3.6 kg (nearly 8 lb). Over this time period mean height increased by less than 1 cm (less than a half inch). Overweight in the NHANES studies is defined as a BMI greater than or equal to 27.8 for men and 27.3 for women. By this definition 41% of those ages 60 to 74 are overweight. Over half of all women ages 50 to 59 are overweight. This is of particular concern in view of the finding that a BMI above 27 in middle age carries a twofold risk of mobility limitations in later years.[42] (Prevalence of overweight in white, African American, and Hispanic elderly examined in NHANES III will be discussed in chapter 9.)

ENERGY REQUIREMENTS AND EXPENDITURE
Defining the Energy Requirement

Defining the energy requirement of an older individual is complicated at best. Loss of muscle mass and a decrease in physical activity lower the energy requirement, and energy intake may have to be reduced to prevent unwanted weight gain. At the same time protein, vitamin, and mineral needs remain the same or may even increase. For example, it appears that the requirement for vitamin B-6 is higher in elderly people than previously thought, and increased intakes of calcium may retard bone loss in older men and women. The continuing need for important micronutrients coupled with the declining need for energy emphasizes the importance of nutrient density in food selection for older adults.

One approach used to define the energy needs of older adults has been to survey apparently healthy older people and determine their intakes of kilocalories.[36] This approach assumes that the intakes of the individuals surveyed are appropriate for maintaining health and well-being, and recommendations are developed based on those intakes. James and coworkers[36] suggested a proactive approach to the development of energy requirements for older adults. This entails defining what the energy expenditure of a

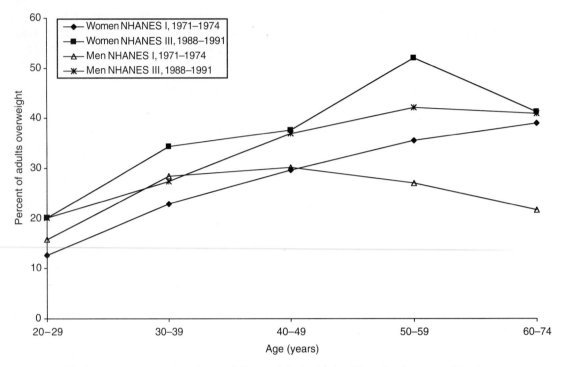

FIG. 5-3   Increase in Prevalence of Overweight in Adults. There has been a striking increase in the percentage of overweight adults between the NHANES I study (1971–1974) and the NHANES III study (1988–1991).

Data from Kuczmarski, R.J., and others: Increasing prevalence of overweight among U.S. adults. The National Heath and Nutrition Examination Surveys, 1960 to 1991, J.A.M.A. 272(3):205, 1994.

healthy, active older person of appropriate size and body composition *should be*. The appropriate energy expenditure of that individual or population then becomes the recommended level of kilocalories to be consumed.

Components of the Energy Requirement

The components of the energy requirement of adults can be classified as those that are biologic, those related to the social aspects of physical activity, and those that are medically desirable (see box).[36] The biologic components of energy expenditure include the support of normal body functions, the maintenance of tissues, and the energy cost associated with digesting and metabolizing food and nutrients. The energy required for digestion and metabolism usually is defined as the **thermic effect of food (TEF).**

Another major component of energy expenditure is physical activity, and this component, in contrast to the energy expended for biologic functions, is under voluntary control. Thus, an individual may increase physical activity as a means of achieving energy balance. The energy expended in physical activity can involve gainful employment, food preparation, household chores, or personal care. Energy expenditure is sometimes associated with social activities or recreation that enhances a person's sense of well-being. The third component of the energy requirement is health-related and refers to the prescriptive, high-intensity exercise and conditioning required for cardiovascular fitness and maintenance of muscle mass.

New research methods allowing the direct assessment of total energy expenditure have spurred new interest in the evaluation of energy

❖

COMPONENTS OF ENERGY EXPENDITURE

- **Biologic**
  Basal requirements
  Thermic effect of food
- **Physical activity**
  Occupational (economic)
  Socially desirable activities
     Household and meal chores
     Personal chores
     Recreational activities
- **Medically desirable**
  High-intensity exercise for cardiovascular fitness

Adapted from James, W.P.T., Ralph, A., and Ferro-Luzzi, A.: Energy needs of the elderly, a new approach. In Munro, H.N., and Danford, D.E., editors.: Nutrition, aging, and the elderly, New York, 1989, Plenum Press.

needs in all age groups, including the elderly. In most people, energy balance is regulated by remarkably sensitive mechanisms. For an individual with an energy requirement of 2,000 kcal, a discrepancy of only 2% between energy intake and expenditure would result in a positive or negative energy balance of 40 kcal a day (equal to three saltine crackers) or a weight change of about 40 lb. over a 10-year period.[64] Saltzman and Roberts[64] pointed out that relatively few people experience this magnitude of weight change, which implies that energy regulation is even more sensitive than 2%. At present we know little about the influence of the aging process on energy regulation.

Resting Energy Expenditure (REE)

Resting energy expenditure and basal metabolism. In most older individuals the **resting energy expenditure (REE)** makes up the largest share of the **total energy expenditure (TEE)**. In the older sedentary adult, the REE usually represents 60% to 75% of the TEE.[58] The REE is measured on an individual who is at rest and under conditions of **thermal neutrality,** which means the person is neither perspiring nor shivering.[23] The REE is the energy required to:

1. Carry on the vital processes of the body, including renal, cardiovascular, pulmonary, and neural function,
2. Maintain electrolyte gradients and body temperature, and
3. Support necessary chemical reactions in the body under resting conditions.

The REE is more commonly used as an estimate of the involuntary energy expenditure than is basal metabolism, although the two are closely related. An individual's basal metabolism is measured immediately upon waking in the morning and 12 hours after the last meal. Thus, basal metabolism is measured after digestion and absorption have been completed, and does not include the energy expenditure associated with the TEF. The REE, although measured with the individual at rest, may include energy expenditure from the TEF from the last meal. In most cases the basal metabolism and the REE of an adult differ by less than 10%.[23]

Factors influencing resting energy expenditure. The REE is influenced by age, sex, body size, body composition, thyroid status, and prior exercise. Thyroid hormones to a great extent regulate REE. Both age and sex differences in REE relate to body composition and amount of FFM. Women have lower resting energy needs per unit of height and weight than men of similar age because women have a higher proportion of body fat and a lower proportion of FFM than men.[36] Individuals with a larger body size and a greater surface area for heat loss have a higher REE. Studies with twins[5] suggest that genetic influences account for 40% to 50% of the individual variability in REE and may contribute to the tendency to develop obesity that exists within families. Among Pima Indian families[5] in Arizona, the resting energy metabolism varied by about 500 kcal per day in individuals from different families who were similar in age, sex, and build but varied by only 60 kcal in similar individuals from the same families.

Age and resting energy expenditure. It has long been recognized that REE declines with age. Records from the BLSA[71] suggest that basal metabolic needs decline by 3% to 4% per decade after age 40. James and coworkers[36] concluded that basal needs expressed on the basis of body weight decline by 24% in men and 15% in women between the ages of 20 and 60 years. These age-related decreases in resting energy requirements are believed to result from the loss of muscle mass and the increase in body fat that occur over adulthood. REE, when calculated on the basis of FFM, total body water, or total body potassium, is remarkably similar in younger and older individuals. Among healthy, physically active older men,[9] basal energy needs were 13% lower than in younger men when calculated on the basis of body weight. When expressed per unit of body potassium, basal energy needs were similar. In that study the total body potassium was 12% lower in the older compared to the younger men.

Factors other than changes in FFM and body fat also contribute to the lower REE in older people. A comparison of young men (mean age = 23) and older men (mean age = 68) at the Human Nutrition Research Center on Aging in Boston[57] indicated an age effect on REE per unit of FFM (fig. 5-4). This suggests that the aging process alters in some way the metabolic activity of lean tissue contained in the FFM. Differences in FFM between younger and older people cannot fully account for the lower REE in older people. Vaughan and coworkers[72] evaluated both basal metabolic rate and sleeping metabolic rate in healthy young and older men and women. Although sleeping metabolic rate was similar in both age groups when adjusted for sex and FFM, the basal metabolic rate remained lower in the older group. In other words the younger people increased their energy expenditure (by 12%) moving from the sleeping to the basal state (awake but resting), whereas the older individuals did not.

Researchers have evaluated the involvement of a variety of factors in this decline in REE.[52] Dietary intake or alterations in thyroid hormone levels do not influence this change. Decreases in maximum aerobic capacity (VO_2 max) appear to be related to the lowered REE in older men but the mechanism is unknown. Poehlman and coworkers[52] suggested that VO_2 max may be a biological marker for an energy-consuming reaction within the cell that is altered as physical activity declines. Specific biochemical pathways

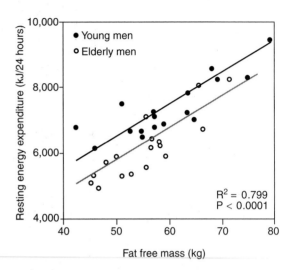

FIG. 5-4 Resting Energy Expenditure and Fat-Free Mass in Younger and Older Men. Elderly men have a lower resting energy expenditure per kg of fat-free mass as compared to younger men.

Roberts, S.B., and others: Influence of age on energy requirements, Am. J. Clin. Nutr. 62(suppl.):1053S, 1995. © American Society for Clinical Nutrition. (Reprinted with permission.)

within the cell could be involved; decreased activity levels of Na-K transport enzymes are believed to make a small contribution to the age-related decline in REE.

It is noteworthy that the decline in REE becomes apparent at different ages in men and women and is associated in women with menopause.[52] In men the reduction in REE begins at age 40; in women the significant decline begins after age 50. The REE also falls at a faster rate in men as compared to women (11 kcal a day each year versus 5.5 kcal a day each year). Menopause and subsequent estrogen deficiency are significant and independent factors contributing to the decline in REE in women.

Sympathetic nervous system and resting energy expenditure. Plasma norepinephrine concentrations are elevated in older people as a result of the enhanced secretion of norepinephrine by the neural tissues. This enhanced secretion may be caused by the increase in abdominal and visceral fat in older people; percentage of body fat is a predictor of plasma norepinephrine levels regardless of age. Sympathetic nervous system hormones do play a role in lipolysis and increased oxidation of fat. Poehlman and colleagues[52] observed high levels of plasma norepinephrine in physically active older men participating in an eight-week exercise (cycling) program. REE increased by 10%, and the increased REE was associated with the enhanced secretion of norepinephrine. The role of these hormones in energy metabolism in aging requires further study.

Thyroid hormone and resting energy expenditure. Thyroid hormone controls the rate of energy metabolism in the cell; however, age-related decreases in REE do not reflect a thyroid hormone deficiency. In general, levels of thyroxine (T_4) remain unchanged in older people although levels of triiodothyronine (T_3) may be somewhat lower.[27] Less T_4 is secreted by the aging thyroid gland, but it is believed that this is a homeostatic response to the loss of metabolically active muscle tissue. Serum levels of thyroid stimulating hormone (TSH), secreted by the anterior lobe of the pituitary gland, are not influenced by age; elevated serum TSH levels are indicative of thyroid failure and hypothyroidism.[27]

Hypothyroidism and hyperthyroidism are serious conditions in older people. Both are more commonly found in women and institutionalized elderly people. The incidence of hypothyroidism increases with age. Hypothyroidism is found in 4% to 7% of older people compared to 1% of younger people.[46] Healthy elderly people over the age of 60 sometimes have elevated serum TSH levels despite normal serum T_4 levels. Low T_3 levels are associated with declining health status or low energy intake.[28] Unfortunately, mild hypothyroidism is not always recognized in older people because many of the characteristic symptoms—lethargy, constipation, or limited tolerance to cold—often are assumed to be typical of older people.

Hyperthyroidism is an equally serious condition in the aged, since excessive thyroid hormone increases the work of the heart, causing tachycardia and arrhythmias. Weight loss, tremors, and muscle weakness, first noticed when climbing stairs, occur frequently. In contrast to younger hyperthyroid patients, older people with hyperthyroidism do not always have increased appetites, and they may be apathetic or withdrawn. Because the signs and symptoms of thyroid disorders may be overlooked in clinical evaluations, older individuals should undergo periodic screening of blood thyroxine levels.[27]

Predicting Resting Energy Expenditure

Simple prediction equations use body height, weight, age, and sex to estimate REE. Such equations can overestimate or underestimate REE in older people, depending on the particular group. Among 40 healthy older people between the ages of 51 and 82,[25] actual REE was significantly different from predicted REE (1,512 kcal versus 1,420 kcal). Although the mean REE was underestimated by only about 6%, the REE of particular individuals was overestimated or underestimated by 10% to 20%. The researchers were impressed with the stability of the REE in their older subjects. Individual measurements taken six months apart differed by less than 20 kcal.

A primary concern is the reliability of prediction equations in malnourished elderly people. The major difficulty in using prediction equations with a poorly nourished cancer patient or elderly individual with cardiac cachexia lies in the estimate of the lean tissue mass. In the normal individual the lean tissue mass is directly proportional to body size. In a malnourished individual both body fat and lean tissue are lost; however, the muscle component of the lean body tissue is preferentially lost, whereas visceral organs remain relatively intact. Because the visceral component of the lean body tissue is responsible for 60% to 70% of the REE, prediction equations based on body weight can underestimate the REE of a malnourished patient by as much as 18%.[26]

Compiled data from several sources suggest that older men and women have a basal energy need of about 20 kcal per kilogram of body weight per day.[36] The basal energy requirement of an individual who is lighter in weight could be somewhat higher when calculated per kilogram of body weight, since visceral tissues with a higher level of metabolic activity will constitute a greater proportion of the lean body tissue.

The prediction equations used by the Food and Nutrition Board[23] for the calculation of REE and the Recommended Dietary Allowances (RDA) were developed by an Expert Committee of the World Health Organization. These prediction equations include body weight, height, and age and are specific for men and women.

Men over age 60   REE (kcal/day) = (13.5 × body wt in kg) + 487

Women over age 60   REE (kcal/day) = (10.5 × body wt in kg) + 596

Poehlman and coworkers[52] studying older healthy men and women developed and field-tested age- and gender-specific equations for the prediction of REE using different sets of variables. In men body weight, leisure time activity, age, and chest skinfold predicted REE with an error of estimate of ±42 kcal a day. For women body weight, height, and menopausal status could predict REE with an error of estimate of ±66 kcal a day. Further work is required to validate these equations with large population groups; however, this is an attempt to apply more specific measures of body fat and physiologic status to calculation of REE.

Thermic Effect of Food (TEF)

The TEF is the increase in energy expenditure above the REE that occurs for several hours after a meal is eaten. The TEF represents the energy expended in digesting, transporting, metabolizing, and storing food and nutrients. Although it accounts for only about 10% of the total daily energy expenditure, this can vary according to the energy source in the meal and its metabolic fate. Protein brings about the highest TEF, carbohydrate has a moderate effect, and fat has little or no measurable thermic effect.

The influence of age on the TEF is not understood. Test meals have led to similar increases in energy expenditure in younger and older adults when adjusted for differences in body composition.[73] The relationship between physical activity and TEF remains undefined, with one report[52]

suggesting that younger and older men with high fitness levels have a higher TEF following a test meal. No differences were observed in a comparison of younger and older men and women in whom physical activity levels were determined by questionnaire.[73] This suggests that any existing differences relate to body composition rather than physical activity.

Physical Activity and Energy Expenditure

In developing the energy requirement of an older adult, two major benefits result from including appropriate amounts of physical activity. First, the increased energy expenditure associated with the exercise contributes to overall nutritional status by allowing the intake of additional food supplying important protein, vitamins, and minerals. Second, physical training contributes to cardiovascular fitness, the maintenance of muscle mass and muscle strength, and improved functional ability to continue housekeeping tasks and personal care.

Nutritional Benefits of Physical Activity

Regular exercise patterns have been associated with improved dietary intake although findings differ among groups. Nutrient intake was evaluated in a physically fit group of elderly women who exercised about 1.5 hours a day and in a sedentary group, all with a mean age of 73.[8] Energy intake was significantly higher in those who exercised regularly whether calculated per day (2,062 kcal versus 1,631 kcal) or per kilogram of body weight (37 kcal per kg of body weight versus 24 kcal per kg). The women with the higher energy intake also had higher intakes of protein, fiber, zinc, magnesium, iron, calcium, folic acid, and all of the B complex vitamins with the exception of vitamin B-12. It is also likely that women with a strong orientation toward health and fitness will choose their foods more carefully than other women of similar age.

In contrast, no significant differences in energy and nutrient intake existed between physically active and sedentary older Dutch women,[74] although the active women did tend to make more appropriate food choices. They ate more vegetables, fruits, legumes, and nonalcoholic drinks than the sedentary women. The sedentary women had a significantly higher BMI (29.1) as compared to the active women (who had a BMI of 24.7) and a higher percent of body fat based on skinfold thicknesses and bioelectrical impedance measurements. Those authors pointed out that an age-related decrease in physical activity coupled with an energy surplus might have contributed to this obesity.

Endurance training and resistance training have been shown to increase energy intake and expenditure in older people. In older men and women completing an eight-week endurance training[50] program, mean energy intake increased from 1,878 kcal to 2,212 kcal a day, and analysis of energy substrates indicated that oxidation of fat increased by 22%. Body weight, body fat, and FFM did not change with training. Energy requirements increased by 15% in elderly people[10] completing 12 weeks of resistance training. Those participants lost about 2 kg of body fat with a commensurate increase in body water. Others have observed no increase in energy expenditure with a supervised endurance training program meeting several times each week. In that case participants had reduced activity on the days that they did not attend the program.[30] Older people who increase their energy needs by increasing their physical activity should be encouraged to choose additional servings of fruits, legumes, whole-grain breads and cereals, and low-fat dairy products, all high in important vitamins and minerals.

Physiologic and Health Benefits of Physical Activity

Physical exercise improves the response and recovery of the cardiovascular and respiratory systems, increases muscle strength, and can positively alter body composition and serum lipoprotein levels in older people. Exercise programs consisting of three to four sessions of 30 to 60 minutes each week that include walking, calisthenics, cycling, or jogging improve aerobic capacity and physical strength.[21] Water exercises are appropriate for older people with osteoarthritis or recovering from joint or muscle injuries, as the buoyancy of the water reduces the stress on the knee and hip joints.[63] The American Heart Association Committee on Exercise and Cardiac Rehabilitation[21] supports the idea that even low-intensity activities such as walking, golf, badminton, dancing, or housework, if performed daily, can have long-term health benefits and lower the risk of cardiovascular disease.

Schwartz and coworkers[65] evaluated improvements in aerobic capacity and body composition in older men ages 60 to 82 and younger men ages 24 to 31 enrolled in a six-month endurance training program. The older men began their program exercising at only 50% to 60% of their maximal heart rate, but after four months all were able to exercise for 45 minutes at 85% of their maximal heart rate. The older men also began with a lower aerobic capacity but achieved a 20% increase in their maximal aerobic capacity for about the same degree of improvement as the younger men. In contrast, only the older men demonstrated changes in body composition with a 2.5 kg loss in body weight, a 2.4 kg loss in body fat, and a 2.3% loss in total body fat. These changes in body fat content become physiologically significant when evaluated according to body fat distribution. It was evident by computed tomography that fat was preferentially lost from abdominal and chest fat deposits; thus, a rather small loss in body weight and body fat contributed to a reduction in cardiovascular risk. Although FFM did not change in the older men, thigh muscle mass increased significantly. The length of an exercise program is an important consideration, since changes in body composition were not observed after three months of training but became evident by the end of six months.

Endurance training also leads to metabolic changes in skeletal muscle that diminish the risk of chronic disease.[44] After 12 weeks of walking, jogging, and calisthenics, older men had higher levels of muscle glycogen, with an increased sensitivity of tissues to insulin and a greater ability to metabolize glucose.

The increased functional capacity and muscle strength resulting from endurance and resistance exercise can contribute immeasurably to the older adult's ability to remain independent. Increased muscle strength decreases the risk of falls and decreases the risk of bone fracture if falls do occur. Regular physical activity helps to maintain alertness and effectiveness and increases bone strength (see chapter 12). Even moderate exercise, if consistent, can lead to improved cardiorespiratory fitness with decreased fatigue in the older person. Through continued physical activity, a 70-year-old person can achieve an aerobic capacity equal to that of a sedentary 30-year-old.[32] However, no strenuous exercise regimen should be undertaken without a medical evaluation beforehand and professional supervision.

Developing an exercise program. The older person must enjoy the exercise planned and feel reasonably safe from injury or the exercise program is likely to be abandoned. For those with muscular or skeletal problems, walking at a comfortable pace with a cane or walker, if needed, is appropriate exercise. In elderly people walking is less likely than jogging to result in injuries to the hip, leg, or foot.[53] Women appear to be more susceptible to injuries while jogging than men. Decreased bone mass in women may contribute to their reduced ability to adapt to high-impact exercise such as jogging. Abrupt, overly strenuous activity for those who have been sedentary is dangerous for both the heart and the large muscles.

Allowing for individual differences and gradually increasing activity when conducting a group exercise program increases the probability of success. Although some older people enjoy doing exercises or walking and jogging in a group, others prefer to exercise by themselves. The sedentary older individual with stiff joints and awkward movements might find group activities embarrassing but may attend sessions to hear about exercises that could be done at home. The cost of equipment must be considered when planning exercise activities. A stationary bicycle or other exercising equipment offers the advantage of exercising indoors and allows the individual to stop and rest when necessary, but such a purchase may be prohibitive.

Activities requiring no financial expenditure are more likely to be adopted by older clients.

Arm and hand exercises are possible for people who can no longer walk. Flexing the arm and finger muscles can reduce stiffness and promote self-feeding or recreational pursuits such as arts or crafts or playing a musical instrument. Improving arm muscle strength may allow the older person to use a bar to pull up to a sitting position. These activities can be presented in the context of nutrition education or as a group social activity.

Physical activity counseling. Healthy older people are more likely to begin and continue regular exercise than less healthy people of similar age. With this in mind, Harris and coworkers[32] recommend physical activity counseling with older adults. The obvious health benefits of even a moderate level of physical activity should be presented to an older person. Benefits result from an increased energy expenditure of even 500 kcal per week. A gradual increase in activity is important when working with someone who is beginning an exercise program. Most injuries among those exercising for health reasons are caused by excessive activity after a long period of muscle disuse. Such risk is minimized by seeking the advice of an exercise science professional in selecting an appropriate activity and gradually increasing the intensity and duration.

Physical activities are more likely to be continued if they are easy to perform and convenient and provide social support. Walking programs fulfill all of these requirements and, as a low-impact activity, are a safe way to begin exercise if an individual has been sedentary. Walking can be done alone or with a senior citizens group or indoor mall walking club and demands no particular time schedule. It does not cause excessive discomfort and when begun on a gradual basis carries little risk. Exercise programs have shown mixed results; some report measurable increases in lean body mass and bone mineral, improvement in lipoprotein patterns, or decreases in body fat[4] whereas others have not.[31,47] However, regular walking habits will increase energy expenditure. Physical activity counseling should be incorporated into nutrition counseling and health promotion programs for older adults.

TABLE 5-4 Recommended Energy Intake for Adults Over Age 50

	Men	Women
Body weight (kg)	77	65
REE (kcal/day)	1,530	1,280
Total energy allowance (kcal/day)	2,300	1,900
Range to allow for individual differences (± 20%)	1,840–2,760	1,520–2,280

Adapted from Food and Nutrition Board: Recommended dietary allowances, ed. 10, Washington, DC, 1989, National Academy Press.

Recommended Dietary Allowance for Energy

At one time the RDAs for energy divided the population above age 50 into two categories; those ages 51 to 75, and those ages 76 and over.[23] The recommended intake of kilocalories for the latter group was adjusted downward to accommodate the anticipated decrease in physical activity in the oldest age group. The 1989 RDA grouped all individuals over the age of 50, promoting the concept that a further decrease in energy expenditure is neither inevitable nor desirable (table 5-4).

The recommended energy allowances[23] are based on the median height and weight for each age and sex group as reported in the NHANES II study. Thus, the body weights used in these calculations are actual body weights and are higher than desirable weights. The REE was calculated using the prediction equations of the World Health Organization presented on page 112. The TEF was considered to represent only about 5% to 10% of the energy value of the food eaten and to contribute little to the overall energy requirement.

The recommended energy intakes for those over age 50 are based on light to moderate activity levels and represent 1.5 times the basal requirement. Such an activity level might include eight hours of rest, 13 hours of very light physical activity (activities involving sitting or standing), and three hours of light activity (activities involving walking on a level surface at 3 mph).

Underestimation of Total Energy Expenditure (TEE)

Recent studies[37,57] evaluating TEE in healthy older people have provided strong evidence that current recommendations significantly underestimate the energy needs of elderly people. These studies were made possible by the development of a new method, the doubly labeled water method, which allows the direct measurement of total energy expenditure in free-living individuals.[57] As noted earlier, estimates of energy needs in older adults traditionally relied on the reported energy intakes from food records of healthy older people in the community. Studies comparing energy expenditure based on food intake records with actual energy expenditure using the doubly labeled water method indicate that food intake records seriously underestimate energy intake and, subsequently, energy requirements. Self-reported food intake based on three-day diet records obtained from 137 older men and women[37] demonstrated that women underestimate their energy intake to an even greater degree than older men. On average the men underreported their intake by 12% (311 kcal) and the women by 24% (527 kcal). Although mean BMI was 24.3 in the older women, within the range for normal weight, those with a higher proportion of body fat underestimated their energy intake by the greatest amount. Those researchers pointed out that women experience a high level of social pressure to remain slim and consume less food and may be more likely to underestimate their food intake. Degree of adiposity was not related to underreporting of energy intake in the men.

Several studies[57,58] have been conducted at the Human Nutrition Research Center on Aging in Boston using the doubly labeled water method. This method involves the use of naturally occurring, stable isotopes of oxygen and hydrogen. The elimination rates of these isotopes is related to the production of carbon dioxide, which is a measure of energy expenditure. Using this method it is possible to calculate TEE over a period of several weeks. Eighteen healthy men with a mean age of 68, a body weight of 79 kg, and a BMI of 25.2 were evaluated over a ten-day metabolic period and one month following, using the doubly labeled water technique.[57] All food was provided but the subjects maintained their normal lifestyle and activities. Table 5-4 shows that the mean body weight of these men was close to the median body weight used to calculate the RDA, yet the TEE of the Boston men was 2,690 kcal, or 390 kcal higher than the recommended intake of 2,300 kcal for their age and sex.

It also appears that older people overestimate the degree of exertion associated with various physical activities.[57] These elderly men reported an average of about a half hour of strenuous activity a day which approximates the amount of strenuous activity provided for in the current RDA, but nonstrenuous activities such as walking were reported as strenuous activities in their activity records. The men reported only four minutes a day of truly strenuous activity (activities with an energy expenditure of greater than five times the REE). Actual REE in these men was 1,481 kcal as compared with the estimated value of 1,530 kcal used for the RDA calculation. Those workers[57] suggest that the RDA underestimates the energy cost of physical activity and in particular, nonstrenuous physical activity. When comparing younger and older men, nonstrenuous physical activity is responsible for 38% of the age-related decline in TEE and strenuous physical activity for only 16%.

Evaluation of energy balance in 11 healthy, elderly English women (mean age was 73)[55] yielded similar findings regarding the energy requirement. Both the TEE and level of physical activity of those women exceeded the standards used in Great Britain to estimate the energy requirement. Mean body weight equaled 60 kg and TEE 2,201 kcal, characteristics similar to many younger women in Great Britain and the United States. Actual basal metabolic rate was 1,221 kcal as compared to the predicted value of 1,235 kcal. Evaluation of energy intake and expenditure suggested that

an activity factor of 1.8 was appropriate for estimating the TEE in these women (1.5 is the activity factor used for calculating the TEE according to the RDA). There is evidence that the energy cost of standard activities is higher in older than younger people.[75] Middle-aged women (mean age was 42) and older women (mean age 72) had similar energy expenditures when sitting quietly without any movement; however, the additional energy expenditure when walking was about a third higher in the older group (4 kcal per minute versus 3 kcal per minute).[75] It is noteworthy that the TEE in the older English women described earlier[55] whose body weight was 60 kg was 2,201 kcal, whereas the RDA for older women whose body weight is 65 kg is 1,900 kcal (table 5-4); however, the English women walked on average about 10.5 hours a week.

Older women, even those above age 80, have more hours of light activity involving walking than do older men (table 5-5).[36] Older women may continue their usual routine of household tasks, or this increased activity may reflect a better health status among older women who may be caring for spouses in poorer health. Physical activity does drop in both sexes beyond age 80. Nevertheless, the current RDAs for energy need to be evaluated in light of new findings.

Particular segments of the elderly population whose energy requirements need further attention are those with chronic or acute illness. In a study of elderly patients admitted to the hospital[38] with cardiovascular disease, bone disease, respiratory disease, or disorders of the central nervous system, actual TEE exceeded predicted energy expenditure and energy intake in 15 of the 19 patients evaluated. The mean energy deficit was 310 kcal but rose as high as 812 kcal in men. For seven patients (three women and four men), the actual REE exceeded the predicted level. Elderly patients with a malignancy, congestive heart failure, and chronic obstructive lung disease can have an elevated REE.[51] These issues need to be considered when developing an energy recommendation for an older person in the hospital or at home.

TABLE 5-5   *Daily Activity (in Hours) of Older Men and Women**

Age (years)	Men		Women	
	60–69	80+	60–69	80+
Sleeping/resting	9.4	11.3	9.4	11.4
Sitting	7.7	8.4	7.2	8.4
Standing	3.6	2.0	2.0	1.0
Walking/moving about	3.2	2.4	5.3	3.1

*Due to rounding, totals may not equal 24 hours.
Adapted from James, W.P.T., Ralph, A., and Ferro-Luzzi, A.: Energy needs of the elderly: a new approach. In Munro, H.N., and Danford, D.E., editors: Nutrition, aging, and the elderly, New York, 1989, Plenum Press.

Issues in Defining the Energy Requirement

Critical issues relating to the energy requirement of older people are (1) the energy intake required for optimum rather than maintenance levels and (2) the regulation of energy balance. Less than optimal energy intakes decrease utilization of protein, result in decreased REE and sense of well-being and over time can result in weight loss. Conversely, an energy surplus or reduced sensitivity of the mechanisms that allow the body to adapt to fluctuations in energy intake contribute to the age-related increase in body fat. Roberts and coworkers[58] evaluated adaptive responses to overfeeding and underfeeding in young and elderly subjects. TEE, REE, and body composition were evaluated following an increase of 1,000 kcal a day or decrease of 788 kcal below the energy intake required for weight maintenance. There appeared to be no spontaneous increase in physical activity or thermogenesis (an energy wasting mechanism) in either age group in response to overfeeding. On the average, 85% to 90% of the excess energy was added to the body mass and the remaining kcal could be accounted for in the energy costs of depositing protein and fat. Younger and older men also demonstrated similar responses to underfeeding, with weight loss accounting for 64% of the energy deficit and decreases in REE and TEE accounting for the remainder. These studies[58] were conducted in normal weight older men with a BMI of 24.3; findings could differ in obese older men or lean or obese older women. Those researchers concluded that energy balance on a day-to-day basis may be maintained through control of nutrient intake rather than adaptations in energy expenditure, but voluntary physical exercise also plays an important role in long-term energy balance.

Older overweight individuals should be encouraged to (1) avoid items high in fat or sugar and low in nutrient density, (2) limit the number of servings of nutrient-dense foods that are high in kilocalories and fat, and (3) increase physical activity to increase energy expenditure. Any attempt to prevent unwanted weight gain or accomplish weight loss that does not include an exercise component will probably have very limited success. Exercise using 150 to 200 kcal per day will help in weight control. Physical activity to stimulate appetite and improve well-being is also appropriate for the underweight older adult. For this individual a diet moderate in fat (35% of total kilocalories) will allow more servings of nutrient-dense items higher in fat. Intervention strategies for both overweight and underweight elderly people are described in chapter 12.

Summary

Estimates of body composition can be used to indicate nutritional status, physical fitness, and the possibility of disease. Evaluation of body

❖ ❖ ❖

CASE STUDY

A recently retired 66-year-old woman, in good health and with no physical limitations, has gained 10 pounds in the last year and wishes to change this trend. Body fat analysis using bio-electrical impedance revealed a 32% body fat composition.

1. How would you determine the site of her body fat stores?

2. How might the site of her body fat stores influence her overall health status?
3. What factors would you explore that may be related to her weight gain?
4. What specific suggestions would you give her to decrease body fat and increase muscle mass?

composition in older people is difficult because standards and methods developed for younger adults are not always appropriate for older adults. Whole body counting, body density measurements, and neutron activation and dilution techniques provide reasonable estimates of body fat and lean tissue but require expensive equipment, highly trained personnel, and in some cases extensive cooperation on the part of the client. Anthropometric measurements, although practical and safe, may be unreliable due to changes in skinfold compressibility and the age-related movement of body fat from the extremities to the trunk. Bioelectrical impedance appears to be a promising clinical tool to estimate body fat when used with standards appropriate to the elderly.

Advancing age is accompanied by an increase in body fat and a loss of lean body mass, particularly muscle mass. Since this pattern is less evident among aging individuals with moderate caloric intakes and continuing physical exercise, lifestyle and overconsumption of kilocalories are contributing causes. Although body composition changes are related to hormone levels and genetic factors, an appropriate exercise program can reduce body fat and increase muscle mass in the elderly. Loss of lean body mass with a consequent drop in resting energy metabolism and decreasing physical activity lead to a decline in the total energy expenditure of the older individual. At the same time protein, vitamin, and mineral requirements remain unchanged or may increase. Nutrition counseling should stress the selection of nutrient-dense foods and development of a physical activity program.

REVIEW QUESTIONS

1. What are the problems associated with methods most often used to estimate body composition in the elderly?
2. How does aging influence body composition, specifically fat-free mass, total body water, body fat, and body weight?
3. What are the beneficial effects of physical exercise on body composition in aging adults? What types of exercise are best suited to older people? What factors influence adherence to an exercise plan?
4. What factors contribute to the resting energy expenditure (REE) in older people? What is the best method for determining REE in older people? What method is the most practical to the clinician working with older adults?
5. What are the implications for meal planning for older adults, based on the fact that total energy expenditure changes as people age?
6. What nutritional suggestions can be made to the older person who is overweight? Will exercise help weight reduction in the older person? If so, how much and what type of exercise is recommended?

SUGGESTED LEARNING ACTIVITIES

1. Visit a nutrition assessment laboratory, and view a demonstration of body composition analyses. Research the pros and cons of estimating body fat by use of skinfold calipers, bioelectrical impedance, dual-energy x-ray absorptiometry, and density measurements.
2. Talk with physical training specialists employed by different physical fitness centers or health clubs about resistance training programs they would recommend for men and women over 60 years of age.

3. Write a lesson plan for a 20-minute class to be presented at a senior citizens center on the advantages of strength training for older adults.
4. Visit a facilitated living center for senior citizens. Tour the recreational facilities, and estimate residents' kilocalories expended for a reasonable time of participation in each activity. Does the center offer a variety of activities suitable for different levels of physical fitness and various physical limitations?

REFERENCES

1. Aloia, J.F., and others: Relationship of menopause to skeletal and muscle mass, Am. J. Clin. Nutr. 53:1378, 1991.
2. Bartlett, H.L., and others: Fat-free mass in relation to stature: ratios of fat-free mass to height in children, adults, and elderly subjects, Am. J. Clin. Nutr. 53:1112, 1991.
3. Baumgartner, R.N., and others: Body composition in elderly people: effect of criterion estimates on predictive equations, Am. J. Clin. Nutr. 53:1345, 1991.
4. Bergman, E.A., and Boyungs, J.C.: Indoor walking program increases lean body composition in older women, J. Am. Diet. Assoc. 91:1433, 1991.
5. Bogardus, C., and others: Familial dependence of the resting metabolic rate, New Engl. J. Med. 314:96, 1986.
6. Bouchard, C., and others: Genetic effect in resting and exercise metabolic rates, Metabolism 38:364, 1989.
7. Bray, G.A.: Obesity. In Brown, M.L., editor: Present knowledge in nutrition, ed. 6, Washington, DC, 1990, International Life Sciences Institute, Nutrition Foundation.
8. Butterworth, D.E., and others: Exercise training and nutrient intake in elderly women, J. Am. Diet. Assoc. 93:653, 1993.
9. Calloway, D.H., and Zanni, E.: Energy requirements and energy expenditure of elderly men, Am. J. Clin. Nutr. 33:2088, 1980.
10. Campbell, W.W., and others: Increased energy requirements and changes in body composition with resistance training in older adults, Am. J. Clin. Nutr. 60:167, 1994.
11. Chumlea, W.C., and others: Bioelectric and anthropometric assessments and reference data in the elderly, J. Nutr. 123(2II):449, 1993.
12. Chumlea, W.C., and Baumgartner, R.N.: Status of anthropometry and body composition data in elderly subjects, Am. J. Clin. Nutr. 50:1158, 1989.
13. Chumlea, W.C., and others: Distributions of serial changes in stature and weight in a healthy elderly population, Human Biol. 60:917, 1988.
14. Cohn, S.H., and others: Improved models for determination of body fat by in vivo neutron activation, Am. J. Clin. Nutr. 40:255, 1984.
15. Corpas, E., Harman, S.M., and Blackman, M.R.: Human growth hormone and human aging, Endocr. Rev. 14(1):20, 1993.
16. Deurenberg, P., and others: Assessment of body composition by bioelectrical impedance in a population ages > 60 y, Am. J. Clin. Nutr. 51:3, 1990.
17. Evans, W.J.: Exercise, nutrition, and aging, Clin. Geriatr. Med. 11:725, 1995.
18. Evans, W.J., and Campbell, W.W.: Sarcopenia and age-related changes in body composition and functional capacity, J. Nutr. 123(2II):465, 1993.
19. Fiatarone, M.A., and others: Exercise training and nutritional supplementation for physical frailty in very elderly people, New Engl. J. Med. 330:1769, 1994.
20. Fiatarone, M.A., and others: High-intensity strength training in nonagenarians: effects on skeletal muscle, J.A.M.A. 263:3029, 1990.
21. Fletcher, G.F., and others: Statement on exercise benefits and recommendations for physical activity programs for all Americans, Circulation 86(1):340, 1992.
22. Flynn, M.A., and others: Total body potassium in aging humans: a longitudinal study, Am. J. Clin. Nutr. 50:713, 1989.
23. Food and Nutrition Board: Recommended dietary allowances, ed. 10, Washington, DC, 1989, National Academy Press.
24. Forbes, G.B.: Human body composition: growth, aging, nutrition, and activity, New York, 1987, Springer-Verlag.
25. Fredrix, E.W.H.M., and others: Resting and sleeping energy expenditure in the elderly, Eur. J. Clin. Nutr. 44:741, 1990.
26. Fredrix, E.W.H.M., and others: Estimation of body composition by bioelectrical impedance in cancer patients, Eur. J. Clin. Nutr. 44:749, 1990.
27. Gambert, S.R.: Endocrinology and aging. In: Reichel, W., editor: Care of the elderly. Clinical aspects of aging, ed. 4, Baltimore, 1995, Williams and Wilkins.
28. Goichot, B., and others: Thyroid hormone status and nutrient intake in the free-living elderly. Interest of reverse triiodothyronine assessment, Eur. J. Endocrinol. 130:244, 1994.
29. Going, S.B., and Lohman, T.G.: Aging and body composition. In: Watson, R.R., editor: Handbook

of nutrition in the aged, ed. 2, Boca Raton, FL, 1994, CRC Press.

30. Goran, M.I., and Poehlman, E.T.: Endurance training does not enhance total energy expenditure in healthy elderly persons, Am. J. Physiol. 263(Endocrinol. Metab. 26):E950, 1992.

31. Grediagin, M.A., and others: Exercise intensity does not affect body composition change in untrained, moderately overfat women, J. Am. Diet. Assoc. 95:661, 1995.

32. Harris, S.S., and others: Physical activity counseling for healthy adults as a primary preventive intervention in the clinical setting, J.A.M.A. 261:3590, 1989.

33. Heymsfield, S.B., and others: Body composition and aging: a study by in vivo neutron activation analysis, J. Nutr. 123(2II):432, 1993.

34. Heymsfield, S.B., and Waki, M.: Body composition in humans: advances in the development of multicompartment chemical models, Nutr. Rev. 49(4):97, 1991.

35. Holloway, L., and others: Effects of recombinant human growth hormone on metabolic indices, body composition, and bone turnover in healthy elderly women, J. Clin. Endocrinol. Metab. 79:470, 1994.

36. James, W.P.T., Ralph, A., and Ferro-Luzzi, A.: Energy needs of the elderly, a new approach. In Munro, H.N., and Danford, D.E., editors: Nutrition, aging, and the elderly, New York, 1989, Plenum Press.

37. Johnson, R.K., Goran, M.I., and Poehlman, E.T.: Correlates of over- and underreporting of energy intake in healthy older men and women, Am. J. Clin. Nutr. 59:1286, 1994.

38. Klipstein-Grobusch, K., and others: Energy intake and expenditure in elderly patients admitted to hospital with acute illness, Brit. J. Nutr. 73:323, 1995.

39. Kohrt, W.M., and others: Body composition of healthy sedentary and trained, young and older men and women, Med. Sci. Sports Exerc. 24(7):832, 1992.

40. Kubena, K.S., and others: Anthropometry and health in the elderly, J. Am. Diet. Assoc. 91:1402, 1991.

41. Kuczmarski, R.J., and others: Increasing prevalence of overweight among U.S. adults. The national health and nutrition examination surveys, 1960 to 1991, J.A.M.A. 272(3):205, 1994.

42. Launer, L.J., and others: Body mass index, weight change, and risk of mobility disability in middle-aged and older women. The epidemiologic follow-up study of NHANES I, J.A.M.A. 27(14):1093, 1994.

43. Lukaski, H.C.: Soft tissue composition and bone mineral status: evaluation by dual-energy x-ray absorptiometry, J. Nutr. 123(2II):438, 1993.

44. Meredith, C.N., and others: Peripheral effects of endurance training in young and old subjects, J. Appl. Physiol. 66:2844, 1989.

45. Minten, V.K.A.M., and others: Inconsistent associations among anthropometric measurements in elderly Dutch men and women, J. Am. Diet. Assoc. 91:1408, 1991.

46. Morley, J.E.: Nutrition and the endocrine system. In: Morley, J.E., Glick, Z., and Rubenstein, L.Z., editors: Geriatric nutrition: a comprehensive review, New York, 1995, Raven Press.

47. Nieman, D.C., and others: Physical activity and serum lipids and lipoproteins in elderly women, J. Am. Geriatr. Soc. 41:1339, 1993.

48. Ohlson, M.A., and others: Anthropometry and nutritional status of adult women, Hum. Biol. 28:189, 1956.

49. Paolisso, G., and others: Body composition, body fat distribution, and resting metabolic rate in healthy centenarians, Am. J. Clin. Nutr. 62:746, 1995.

50. Poehlman, E.T., and others: Effects of endurance training on total fat oxidation in elderly persons, J. Appl. Physiol. 76(6):2281, 1994.

51. Poehlman, E.T., and others: Increased resting metabolic rate in patients with congestive heart failure, Ann. Intern. Med. 121:860, 1994.

52. Poehlman, E.T., Arciero, P.J., and Goran, M.I.: Endurance exercise in aging humans: effects of energy metabolism, Exerc. Sport Sci. Rev. 22:251, 1994.

53. Pollock, M.L., and others: Injuries and adherence to walk/jog and resistance training programs in the elderly, Med. Sci. Sports Exerc. 23(10):1194, 1991.

54. Prothro, J., and Rosenbloom, C.A.: Body measurements of black and white elderly persons with emphasis on body composition, Gerontology 41:22, 1995.

55. Reilly, J.J., and others: Energy balance in healthy elderly women, Brit. J. Nutr. 69:21, 1993.

56. Reilly, J.J., and others: Prediction of body density from skinfold thickness in elderly subjects: are the existing equations valid?, Ann. Hum. Biol. 21(6):613, 1994.

57. Roberts, S.B., and others: Influence of age on energy requirements, Am. J. Clin. Nutr. 62(suppl.):1053S, 1995.

58. Roberts, S.B., and others: Energy expenditure, aging, and body composition, J. Nutr. 123:474, 1993.

59. Rolls, B.J., and Hammer, V.A.: Fat, carbohydrate, and the regulation of energy intake, Am. J. Clin. Nutr. 62(suppl.):1086S, 1995.

60. Roubenoff, R., and others: Use of dual-energy x-ray absorptiometry in body-composition studies: not yet a "gold standard," Am. J. Clin. Nutr. 58:589, 1993.

61. Rudman, D., and Mattson, D.E.: Serum insulin-like growth factor I in healthy older men in relation to physical activity, J. Am. Geriatr. Soc. 42:71, 1994.

62. Rudman, D., and others: Effects of human growth hormone in men over 60 years old, New Engl. J. Med. 323:1, 1990.

63. Ruoti, R.G., Troup, J.T., and Berger, R.A.: The effects of nonswimming water exercises on older adults, J. Orth. Sports Phys. Ther. 19(3):140, 1994.

64. Saltzman, E., and Roberts, S.B.: The role of energy expenditure in energy regulation: findings from a decade of research, Nutr. Rev. 53(8):209, 1995.

65. Schwartz, R.S., and others: The effect of intensive endurance exercise training on body fat distribution in young and older men, Metabolism 40:545, 1991.

66. Simons, J.P.F.H.A., and others: The use of bioelectrical impedance analysis to predict total body water in patients with cancer cachexia, Am. J. Clin. Nutr. 61:741, 1995.

67. Snead, D.B., Birge, S.J., and Kohrt, W.M.: Age-related differences in body composition by hydrodensitometry and dual-energy x-ray absorptiometry, J. Appl. Physiol. 74(2):770, 1993.

68. Taaffe, D.R., and others: Effect of recombinant human growth hormone on the muscle strength response to resistance exercise in elderly men, J. Clin. Endocrinol. Metab. 79:1361, 1994.

69. Thompson, J.L., and others: The effects of recombinant human insulin-like growth factor-I and growth hormone on body composition in elderly women, J. Clin. Endocrinol. Metab. 80:1845, 1995.

70. Trotter, M., and Gleser, G.: The effect of aging on stature, Am. J. Phys. Anthropol. 9:311, 1951.

71. U.S. Department of Health and Human Services: Normal human aging: the Baltimore Longitudinal Study of Aging, NIH Publication No. 84-2450, Washington, DC, 1984, U.S. Government Printing Office.

72. Vaughan, L., Zurlo, F., and Ravussin, E.: Aging and energy expenditure, Am. J. Clin. Nutr. 53:821, 1991.

73. Visser, M., and others: Resting metabolic rate and diet-induced thermogenesis in young and elderly subjects: relationship with body composition, fat distribution, and physical activity level, Am. J. Clin. Nutr. 61:772, 1995.

74. Voorrips, L.E., van Staveren, W.A., and Hautvast, J.G.A.J.: Are physically active elderly women in a better nutritional condition than their sedentary peers?, Eur. J. Clin. Nutr. 45:545, 1991.

75. Voorrips, L.E., and others: Energy expenditure at rest and during standardized activities: a comparison between elderly and middle-aged women, Am. J. Clin. Nutr. 58:15, 1993.

76. Wang, J., and others: Asians have lower body mass index (BMI) but higher percent body fat than do whites: comparisons of anthropometric measurements, Am. J. Clin. Nutr. 60:23, 1994.

77. Wang, Q., and others: Total and regional body-composition changes in early postmenopausal women: age-related or menopause-related?, Am. J. Clin. Nutr. 60:843, 1994.

CHAPTER

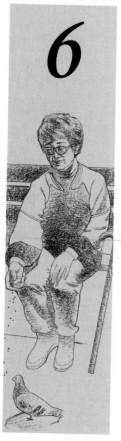

6

Vitamins in Aging

❖❖

Objectives

After studying the chapter, the student should be able to:

✔ *Identify gastrointestinal and associated physiologic alterations which influence the absorption of vitamins in the older person*

✔ *Outline the requirements of fat-soluble and water-soluble vitamins in the elderly*

✔ *Understand the role of vitamins in health promotion and prevention of chronic disease*

✔ *Recognize chronic disease conditions common in the elderly and their effect on vitamin needs and status*

✔ *Understand the importance of functional biochemical indices to evaluate vitamin status in the elderly*

Vitamin requirements and metabolism are receiving increasing attention as epidemiologic findings suggest that intakes of particular vitamins reduce the risk of certain degenerative diseases. Vitamins that act as antioxidants appear to have a role in preventing coronary artery disease and cancer. Current work is exploring the actions of particular vitamins in relation to immune function, the formation of cataracts, and the development of osteoporosis, all problems associated with aging. Physiologic processes, including neural function, formation of red blood cells, and tissue repair, require specific vitamins. At the same time vitamin requirements may increase in advancing age as a conse-

quence of less efficient absorption or utilization or enhanced excretion. The potential for vitamin toxicity may increase in older people with compromised kidney function who ingest inappropriate types or amounts of vitamin supplements. Research exploring these relationships is continuing, although much remains to be learned. The current recommended intakes of vitamins can be found in appendix A.

FAT-SOLUBLE VITAMINS
Factors Influencing Absorption

Digestive secretions. Dietary fat, essential for the absorption of the fat-soluble vitamins, usually is consumed in the form of triglycerides which must be broken down into monoglycerides or free fatty acids for absorption to take place. The **fat-soluble vitamins** (A, D, E, and K) become associated with lipid globules in the stomach and then join with bile salts in the intestinal lumen to form **micelles.** The micelles carry both fatty acids and the fat-soluble vitamins to the mucosal surface, where absorption occurs. Pancreatic lipase, required for the digestion of dietary fat, is usually present in sufficient amounts in older adults to allow this process to proceed normally. Bile salts secreted by the liver and stored in the gallbladder are necessary for the formation of micelles. Older people with pancreatic or liver disease can have problems absorbing both fat and the fat-soluble vitamins. For those unable to absorb sufficient lipid, fat-soluble vitamins can be administered in water miscible emulsions either orally or intramuscularly.

Dietary constituents. Dietary fat has two important functions in the absorption of fat-soluble vitamins. First, lipids transport the vitamins from the stomach into the small intestine; second, lipids delay gastric emptying and ensure the delivery of only small amounts of fat at a time, thereby promoting formation of micelles. At least 5 g of dietary fat a day are required to support absorption of the fat-soluble vitamins.[17] Polyunsaturated fatty acids, compared to saturated fatty acids, lower absorption of the fat-soluble vitamins. It also appears that the absorption of vitamin A is depressed by the presence of peroxidized fat.[17] Peroxidized fat arising from the oxidation of polyunsaturated fatty acids may be detrimental to vitamins D, E, and K as well. Highly concentrated supplements of fat-soluble vitamins have potential for creating nutrient imbalances as well as toxicity.

Vitamin A and Carotenoids

Vitamin A is supplied to the body as preformed vitamin A found only in animal foods and as vitamin A precursor carotenoids found in vegetables and fruits. Vitamin A is important for visual function, the maintenance of epithelial tissues, and resistance to infection.

Absorption of vitamin A. Preformed vitamin A is present in animal foods and vitamin

supplements in the form of retinyl esters. Retinyl esters are hydrolyzed through digestion to yield retinol, the form of vitamin A that enters the mucosal cell.[17] In the mucosal cells of the small intestine, retinol is reesterified into retinyl esters and incorporated into the triglyceride-rich chylomicrons, which enter the lymph and then the general circulation.

The removal of vitamin A esters from the plasma after absorption is slowed in older adults. Krasinski and coworkers[32] administered 3,000 retinol equivalents (RE) in the form of retinyl esters to healthy older adults (mean age = 65) and younger adults (mean age = 32) in Boston. Plasma retinyl esters were measured in both groups for eight hours. The increase in plasma retinyl esters above fasting levels was similar in both groups for the first four hours after ingestion of the vitamin A, but the older group had significantly higher levels for hours five through eight (fig. 6-1). When the vitamin A was consumed along with a high fat meal it became apparent that the postprandial rise in plasma retinyl esters occurred in parallel to the rise in the plasma chylomicrons. The slowed removal of retinyl esters from the plasma in older adults is related to the delayed removal of this lipid fraction. The slowed removal of chylomicrons may be caused by decreased levels of lipoprotein lipase enzyme. This enzyme, located on the endothelial surface of the capillary, hydrolyzes the triglyceride in the chylomicron and allows the fatty acids to move into the cell. When the triglyceride has been removed, the chylomicron remnant containing the retinyl esters is taken from the plasma by the liver. Plasma retinyl esters are the major postprandial metabolites of vitamin A.

Older people also can effectively utilize vitamin A precursors as a source of vitamin A. Older subjects given a test dose of beta carotene had an increase in plasma retinyl esters.[38] This indicated that beta carotene was not only absorbed, but also converted to retinol in the intestinal mucosa and esterified for assimilation in the chylomicrons.

Metabolism of vitamin A. An evaluation of vitamin A status in 562 healthy Boston adults between 60 and 98 years of age confirmed the

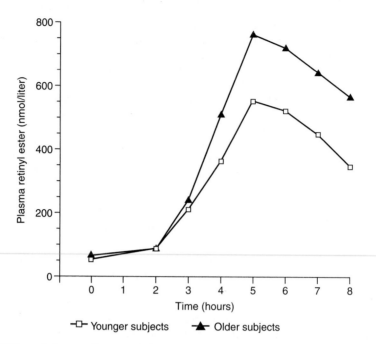

FIG. 6-1   Effect of Age on Postprandial Plasma Retinyl Ester (Vitamin A) Levels. Mean plasma retinyl ester levels in older people, age 50 and over (▲), and younger people, under age 50 (□), given 3,000 retinol equivalents of vitamin A. Mean levels at five hours and beyond are significantly higher in the older group.

Reproduced from Krasinski, S.D., and others: Postprandial plasma retinyl ester response is greater in older subjects compared with younger subjects, J. Clin. Invest. 85:883, 1990, by copyright permission of The American Society for Clinical Investigation.

high bioavailability of retinyl esters, the form of vitamin A contained in vitamin supplements.[33] Plasma retinol levels were similar in those who took vitamin A supplements and those who did not, but plasma retinyl ester levels were more than doubled in those taking daily supplements containing 5,000 to 10,000 IU; levels nearly tripled in those taking daily supplements containing more than 10,000 IU. In those older people taking more than 10,000 IU a day, the fraction of total plasma vitamin A (retinol plus retinyl esters) circulating as retinyl esters was 13%. It is generally accepted that a retinyl ester fraction greater than 10% indicates chronic vitamin A toxicity.

Several researchers[33,73] have evaluated serum aspartate aminotransferase enzyme levels in elderly people consuming concentrated vitamin A supplements over a period of years. An elevated serum aspartate aminotransferase level is a clinical indicator of liver damage and might be expected in hypervitaminosis A. Although serum enzyme levels appeared to increase in proportion to the concentration of vitamin A supplements consumed, elderly people taking vitamin A supplements over a period of years do not always have elevated levels.[73] Other conditions associated with an aging population, including heart disease or liver problems caused by alcohol abuse, also lead to abnormally high serum aspartate aminotransferase levels. When inappropriate enzyme levels are observed in liver function tests, vitamin A supplement use should be considered as a possible cause.

Many older people consume concentrated supplements of both vitamin A and vitamin E. It has been shown in animals that vitamin E decreases the activity of hepatic retinyl ester hydrolase, the enzyme required to mobilize retinyl esters stored in the liver.[33] This relationship has not been demonstrated in older human subjects; nevertheless, it suggests that concentrated vitamin E supplements could exacerbate the risk associated with prolonged use of vitamin A supplements in excess of the recommended dietary allowance (RDA).

Vitamin A requirements. Total vitamin A intake includes both preformed vitamin A found in animal products and the vitamin A precursor carotenoids found in fruits and vegetables. Unfortunately, analytical methods that can ascertain the specific carotenoids present in a particular food item have only recently been perfected. Consequently, food composition tables based on International Units (IU) still include carotenoids since found to have little or no vitamin A activity. Beta carotene is the carotenoid with the highest vitamin A activity, and it is used as a standard. The Food and Nutrition Board[17] recommends the use of retinol equivalents (RE) based on established conversion factors for expressing vitamin A activity. The 1989 RDAs expressed in retinol equivalents are 1,000 RE for men and 800 RE for women over age 50.

Vitamin A intake and biochemical status. Mean intake of vitamin A in older men and women tends to exceed the RDA. In the Third National Health and Nutrition Examination Survey (NHANES III)[78] mean intakes equaled 1,306 RE in men ages 60 to 69, 1,322 RE in those ages 70 to 79, and 1,207 RE in those ages 80 and over. Mean intakes were a bit lower among the women, 1,097 RE in the 60- to 69-year-old group, 1,155 RE in the 70- to 79-year-old group, and 1,083 RE in the oldest group. Mean intakes of vitamin A tend to skew to the right as a result of the exceedingly high intakes among those consuming foods exceptionally rich in vitamin A (liver) or carotenoids (e.g., carrots, broccoli) or vitamin supplements.

Despite the fact that mean vitamin A intake equals or exceeds the RDA in most older populations, many elderly individuals have poor intakes. In healthy participants in the Boston Nutritional Status Survey, 14% to 32% consumed less than two-thirds of the RDA for vitamin A based on food intake.[76] Those consuming diets

high in milk, cereal, and fruit servings were more likely to have adequate intakes of vitamin A; those whose diets were based on bread and poultry were more likely to be deficient. Frail older people, those with physical problems, or those with mouth problems such as xerostomia are more likely to have low intakes. Ethnic background influences vitamin A intake. More than half of the older African Americans and Mexican Americans surveyed in the NHANES III consumed less than 67% of the RDA.[78]

Plasma vitamin A levels tend to increase until about age 40 in men and age 60 in women and then plateau. In the Baltimore Longitudinal Study of Aging (BLSA)[21] only 1 of 285 older adults had a plasma level indicative of deficiency. Older men had higher plasma retinol levels than older women but plasma levels did not correlate with total vitamin A or retinol intakes in either sex. A four-year study of 200 healthy white elderly people in New Mexico[19] reported no changes over that period; mean plasma retinol levels were 57 µg/dl in the men and 59 µg/dl in the women. Only two individuals, one man and one woman, consumed less than half of the RDA for vitamin A; almost half consumed 2,000 RE of vitamin A a day (two to two and a half times the RDA). The older men taking a supplement had significantly higher plasma retinol levels than those who were not.

Although fairly simple to determine, plasma vitamin A levels do not always identify older individuals at risk of deficiency. Among 30 institutionalized older people over age 80,[10] dietary intakes met or exceeded recommended levels for all but four subjects, and plasma retinol levels were above 30 µg/dl for all but two subjects. Nevertheless, response to a test dose of 450 RE of vitamin A indicated that 7 of the 30 had depleted liver stores. Some workers suggest, however, that such tests should be replicated several times to obtain a true indication of vitamin A stores in elderly people.

Chronic disease, infection, and weight loss are associated with depletion of liver vitamin A stores. Liver content of retinyl esters measured at autopsy was higher in older people who died suddenly of a heart attack or stroke compared to those of similar age who had long-term illnesses or wasting diseases.[62] Vitamin A requirements are substantially increased during serious infection because of urinary losses of retinol and retinol-binding protein. Patients with pneumonia or sepsis may lose the equivalent of 50% of the RDA a day.[74]

There is a need for functional tests that will detect declining vitamin A status before deficiency becomes overt. Visual abnormalities can be detected when serum levels range from 20 to 40 µg/dl. It is important to use fasting blood samples when evaluating vitamin A status in light of the elevated postprandial rise in plasma vitamin A levels in elderly groups.

Roles of the carotenoids. At one time the major function of the carotenoids was thought to be as precursor of vitamin A. It has since been recognized that carotenoids have a unique role as antioxidants, independent of their vitamin A activity. Recent attention has been directed to the relationship between carotenoid intake and incidence of cardiovascular disease, cancer, and degenerative changes in the eye. Unfortunately, randomized trials have produced mixed results. A Finnish trial, performed with heavy smokers, failed to demonstrate a protective effect of beta carotene in the prevention of cardiovascular disease or lung cancer; in fact, lung cancer incidence was actually higher in the beta carotene supplement users.[51] In contrast Morris and coworkers[45] found that men with the highest plasma carotenoid levels had a cardiovascular risk only 65% that of men with the lowest plasma carotenoid levels. Factors that contribute to different findings among studies are the source and type of carotenoids consumed. Several trials have fed beta carotene supplements whereas others have estimated carotenoid intakes based on the use of fruits and vegetables that contain many specific carotenoids, not only beta carotene. The Eye Disease Case Control Study found that reduced risk of macular degeneration was related to use of spinach and collard greens which are high in lutein and zeaxanthin.[66] Other unknown components in fruits and vegetables may also contribute to the observed health benefits of these foods.

Beta carotene is considered safe at intakes ranging from 15 to 50 mg per day.[2] It does appear, however, that older people both absorb beta carotene and convert a portion of the amount absorbed to retinol. In light of the elevated levels of serum aspartate aminotransferase enzyme in some elderly people who ingest concentrated vitamin A supplements over a period of years, this age group may have increased susceptibility to vitamin A overload. Older people might be better advised to consume generous amounts of food sources rich in vitamin A and carotenoids instead of supplements.

Vitamin E

Vitamin E functions as an important antioxidant in trapping free radicals and preventing related tissue damage. Vitamin E has long received attention as a possible elixir for delaying the onset and severity of age-related physical changes or chronic disease. Only recently has research been initiated to provide experimental evidence to support or dispel these claims.

Absorption of vitamin E. Currently there is no evidence to suggest that the absorption of vitamin E (alpha-tocopherol) is influenced by age. Vitamin E deficiency, when it is identified, is often associated with serious fat malabsorption. Alpha-tocopherol is absorbed and utilized more efficiently than gamma- or beta-tocopherol by both younger and older people.[17]

Vitamin E requirements. The vitamin E requirement in tocopherol equivalents (TE) is influenced by the level of intake of polyunsaturated fatty acids (PUFA). The RDA is designed to maintain the suggested ratio of 0.4 mg TE per gm of PUFA.[17] In general, foods high in PUFA, such as vegetable oils, are also high in vitamin E; thus, as intakes of PUFA rise, so should intakes of vitamin E. However, this is not always the case. Chicken, a food recommended as a substitute for protein foods high in saturated fat, has a relatively high content of PUFAs but a low content of vitamin E and a ratio of only 0.2 mg TE per gm PUFA. Fats and oils are the major contributors of vitamin E in the older adult's diet (31%) followed by breads, cereals, and bakery products (28%), vegetables (7%), and eggs (4%).[46]

For individuals using fish oil supplements, the relationship between vitamin E and PUFA intakes becomes important. In older women given 2 g of fish oil high in omega-3 fatty acids daily, the reduction in plasma triglyceride levels and improvement in the ratio of polyunsaturated to saturated fatty acids were accompanied by a significant increase in the peroxidation of serum lipids.[43] The fish oil capsules consumed contained 3 IU of vitamin E per gm of lipid. Plasma vitamin E levels did not change over the three-month period of supplementation, although the ratio of plasma vitamin E to plasma omega-3 fatty acids declined significantly.

As we continue to stress the need to reduce intakes of items high in saturated fatty acids and suggest substitutions that contain increased amounts of PUFAs or omega-3 fatty acids, it is also important to encourage increased intakes of fruits and vegetables that will add to the total vitamin E intake without adding more fat.

Vitamin E intake and biochemical status. Surveys of community-living and institutionalized older adults have not revealed significant numbers who are deficient in vitamin E; nevertheless, plasma levels do decrease in both men and women beyond age 60. In the Boston study[22] plasma α-tocopherol fell from 32 μmol/L to 21 μmol/L in men and from 32 μmol/L to 26 μmol/L in women between the ages of 60 and 90. Plasma levels were 23% lower in institutionalized elderly men and women who had median plasma levels of 20 μmol/L and 23 μmol/L, respectively. This report suggests that many elderly, particularly institutionalized elderly, may be at risk for vitamin E deficiency (plasma levels between 12 μmol/L and 23 μmol/L place an individual at risk). Evaluation of the dietary, supplemental, and plasma α-tocopherol levels in 131 Kentucky adults[55] over age 65 indicated a strong relationship between total intake and plasma levels. Thirty-five percent of the subjects were taking vitamin E supplements which provided intakes over 10 times higher than the level of vitamin provided in the diet (90.3 mg versus 7.8 mg). Based on dietary intake alone, 37% were consuming less than two-thirds of the RDA for vitamin E; when supplements were included, the number with deficient intakes fell to 25%.

Dietary data from the NHANES III study[78] indicate that vitamin E is a nutrient of concern for the older population. Median intake was 7.49 mg TE for older white men, 5.43 mg TE for older African American men, and 6.60 mg TE for older Mexican American men ages 60 to 69. The equivalent values for white, African American, and Mexican American women were 6.31 mg TE, 4.48 mg TE, and 4.21 mg TE. The recommended intakes are 10 mg TE for men and 8 mg TE for women.[17] This means that more than half of all the older people surveyed had intakes well below the RDA.

Role of vitamin E in disease prevention. Vitamin E as a potent biological antioxidant has been evaluated for its ability to delay chronic disease. The possible relationship of vitamin E with cardiovascular disease in both men[59] and women[72] was the subject of two major reports involving nearly 40,000 men and 87,000 women in the health professions. The men, ages 40 to 75 years,[59] were free of coronary heart disease when the study began. After four years of follow-up it was apparent that the men taking in more than 60 IU of vitamin E a day reduced their risk of developing coronary heart disease by over one-third, as compared to the men taking in less than 7.5 IU of vitamin E. Findings were very similar among the middle-aged and older women who were followed for eight years.[72] Those with the highest vitamin E intakes had about a 40% decrease in risk. In the women's study higher intakes were obtained from supplements, either multivitamin preparations containing about 30 IU of vitamin E or vitamin E tablets containing about 100 IU each. In both men and women supplements had to be used for at least two years to make an impact on coronary risk. Based on the Iowa Women's Health Study[8] of 32,215 women between the ages of 55 and 69, vitamin E may also lower an individual's risk of colon cancer. Total vitamin E intake equaled 36 IU a day for those who developed colon cancer over four years of follow-up; daily intake was 66 IU among those who remained free of colon cancer.

There is no one biological explanation for the protective effect of vitamin E. It is likely that the action of vitamin E in preventing the oxidation of LDL-cholesterol and subsequent vascular damage is a factor in the prevention of coronary disease. At the same time supplementation with 800 mg a day of α-tocopherol improved cell-mediated immune function in healthy older people.[44] A 30-day clinical evaluation of the elderly people consuming the 800 mg supplement revealed no unwanted side effects on hepatic or renal function, hematologic status, or normal serum constituents as a result of the supplementation. Nevertheless, the long-term effects of vitamin E supplements in excess of 80 to 100 times the RDA are unknown. General recommendations for vitamin E supplementation levels must await further study.

Vitamin D

Vitamin D traditionally was considered to be a vitamin; however, it acts as a hormone. A **hormone** is a chemical substance produced in one organ of the body that regulates an activity in another organ of the body. Major functions of vitamin D are the regulation of blood calcium levels, the absorption of calcium in the intestine, and the mobilization of calcium from the bone.

Sources of vitamin D. Vitamin D can be supplied to the body through food or supplements, or it can be synthesized in the skin. Skin synthesis is an important source of vitamin D in people of all ages. The form of vitamin D commonly used in food fortification and also produced in the skin is vitamin D_3, cholecalciferol. Vitamin D_3 is synthesized in the skin by the irradiation of 7-dehydrocholesterol, a sterol naturally found in skin cells. The concentration of 7-dehydrocholesterol and the quantity and quality of ultraviolet radiation are major factors in the control of vitamin D_3 synthesis.

Aging influences vitamin D_3 synthesis in several ways. First, older people have a lower concentration of 7-dehydrocholesterol in their skin compared to younger people. Under similar lighting conditions, individuals age 80 synthesized less than half the amount of vitamin D_3 synthesized by individuals age 20.[24] Second, older people with some degree of physical disability spend most of their time indoors and thus have limited exposure to ultraviolet light. Dietary vitamin D is found in relatively few foods. Milk, fortified to the level of 400 IU per quart, is the most common source. Unfortunately, many older people do not drink milk, and other commonly used dairy products such as yogurt and cheese usually do not contain added vitamin D.

Absorption of vitamin D. The effect of aging on vitamin D absorption is not clear-cut. Experiments with physiologic doses of vitamin D indicate that absorption is less efficient in the elderly; however, experiments using pharmacological doses (50,000 IU) found absorption patterns to be similar in young and healthy older adults.[11] Vitamin D is not well absorbed by those with general malabsorption problems. Absorption of an orally administered dose of vitamin D was less than 4% when the flow of bile into the small intestine was interrupted.[11]

Metabolism of vitamin D. Vitamin D obtained from food, supplements, or endogenous synthesis undergoes two biochemical reactions in the conversion to its biologically active form. In the liver, vitamin D is hydroxylated to 25-hydroxyvitamin D [25(OH)D]. In the kidneys, 25(OH)D is hydroxylated to 1,25-dihydroxyvitamin D [1,25(OH)$_2$D], also referred to as calcitriol. It is 1,25(OH)$_2$D that is responsible for the metabolic actions attributed to vitamin D.[17]

Serum levels of vitamin D metabolites are influenced by age, vitamin D availability, parathyroid hormone (PTH) secretion, and kidney function. In general, serum levels of 25(OH)D are similar in younger and older adults if vitamin D intakes are adequate; they differ among national and cultural groups, influenced by food fortification policies and geographical differences.[41] Studies with healthy older people indicate that serum 25(OH)D levels tend to decrease with advancing age, whereas serum levels of the active metabolite calcitriol tend to increase up to age 65 and then plateau.[13] Eastell and coworkers[13] consider this increased production of calcitriol to be a response to an increased intestinal resistance to the action of vitamin D. When calcium absorption declines because of intestinal resistance, serum calcium levels also decline, triggering the secretion of increased amounts of PTH. PTH attempts to restore serum calcium levels to normal by increasing the production of calcitriol, which should increase calcium absorption.

At times institutionalized or hospitalized older people given supplements of vitamin D respond with increased serum levels of 25(OH)D but no increase in serum levels of calcitriol.[18] This finding has been attributed to a deficiency of 1-α-hydroxylase, the enzyme in the kidney that is necessary for the conversion of 25(OH)D to the active dihydroxy metabolite calcitriol. The activity level of 1-α-hydroxylase decreases with age, and the magnitude of the decrease is proportional to the age-related decrease in renal function (see chapter 13). The glomerular filtration rate at which this enzyme level becomes critical to vitamin D function is 50 ml per min.[18] The glomerular filtration rate reported in healthy older men ages 75 to 84 in the BLSA was 97 ml per min.[79] Thus it would seem that renal function must be greatly impaired before the loss of 1-α–hydroxylase becomes clinically important. Despite this finding, Rudman and colleagues[61] observed that bone fractures in institutionalized elderly men were more frequent among those with low blood levels of calcitriol and high blood urea nitrogen levels. It is likely that changes in renal function and hypovitaminosis D account for the wide variability in serum vitamin D metabolite levels observed in older populations.

Intake, sun exposure, and vitamin D requirements. Dietary intakes of vitamin D seldom equal the RDA of 5 μg (200 IU) in older groups. A recent review[29] described mean intakes of 240 IU among residents in a senior housing project and 301 IU in older Iowa women. Median intakes of vitamin D were 235 IU and 150 IU among healthy elderly men and women, respectively, in New Mexico.[29] Institutionalized elderly in New York had an average intake of 379 IU a day but individual intakes ranged from 55 IU to 1,006 IU.[52] Vitamin D intakes in Asian and European elderly have been reported to be as low as 1 μg (40 IU) a day.[41]

Because sunlight exposure and skin synthesis make an important contribution to vitamin D status, serum concentrations of 25(OH)D vary seasonally in those with some sun exposure. Krall and coworkers[30] evaluated dietary vitamin D,

serum 25(OH)D levels, and PTH concentrations in 333 healthy white postmenopausal women in Boston. Their mean age was 58. These women had low dietary intakes of calcium (408 mg a day) and vitamin D (112 IU a day); each is about 50% of the RDA. Vitamin D intake was higher, 427 IU, in those taking supplements. The inverse relationship between serum PTH and 25(OH)D levels was dependent upon vitamin D intake (see table 6-1). When vitamin D intake was greater than 220 IU per day, serum PTH and 25(OH)D levels did not vary with the season. When intake fell below 220 IU, serum 25(OH)D levels were highest between August and October, when sun exposure could be expected to be relatively high, and lowest between March and May, after the cold winter months. Serum 25(OH)D levels dropped about one-third between the summer and late winter examination periods while serum PTH levels rose over that period.

When vitamin D intake or synthesis is not sufficient to maintain the serum 25(OH)D and calcium absorption levels needed to provide sufficient calcium to maintain normal blood calcium levels, PTH secretion increases, and bone calcium is mobilized to restore blood calcium levels to normal. A major goal for the maintenance of bone health in older women is to prevent a rise in serum PTH levels and the subsequent loss of bone mineral. Krall and others[30] concluded that a daily dietary intake of more than 220 IU of vitamin D a day would prevent a seasonal increase in PTH levels and the potential mobilization of skeletal calcium. In older women age 70 and over[64] with intakes of 343 IU of vitamin D a day (about 175% of the RDA), dietary vitamin D was directly related to serum 25(OH)D levels and inversely related to serum PTH levels, regardless of high or low exposure to sunlight.

Older people with chronic disease appear to require vitamin D intakes of 10 μg (400 IU) to maintain appropriate serum levels of vitamin D metabolites. In a group of 109 nursing home patients,[52] none with vitamin D intakes of 400 IU daily had serum 25(OH)D levels below 15 ng/ml, whereas 46% with intakes between 200 IU and 400 IU a day did fall below this level.

TABLE 6-1   *Seasonal Variations in Serum Parameters in Older Women*
with Low Intakes of Vitamin D

	August–October	November–February	March–May
Age (yrs)	58	59	60
Calcium intake (mg/day)	440	412	381
Serum total calcium (mmol/l)	2.34	2.30	2.29
Serum parathyroid hormone (ng/l)	30*	34	37
Serum 25(OH)D (nmol/l)	93*	75	63

*The August–October levels differ significantly from the March–May levels.
Modified from Krall, E.A., and others: Effect of vitamin D intake on seasonal variations in parathyroid hormone secretion in postmenopausal women, New Engl. J. Med. 321:1777, 1989.

Serum 25(OH)D levels below 15 ng/ml are associated with increased secretion of PTH and subsequent mobilization of bone calcium. Regression analysis indicated a 2.0 ng/ml rise in serum 25(OH)D level for every 100 IU increase in vitamin D intake. Among these older people fluid milk accounted for about half of the dietary vitamin D. Without milk, 72% would have taken in less than 200 IU a day. This dependence on milk as a source of vitamin D needs to be addressed in light of the recent report that many samples of fluid milk contain less than 400 IU per quart.[24] State and local public health units need to monitor this situation.

While it appears that a daily intake of 10 μg (400 IU) is necessary to maintain appropriate vitamin D metabolite levels, it is ill-advised for older individuals to consume more than 10 μg of vitamin D in light of its known toxic effects. It is also important that the Food and Nutrition Board[17] reevaluate the appropriateness of the current RDA for vitamin D (5 μg) for both healthy and physically compromised elderly people.

Vitamin K

Vitamin K has long been recognized as essential for the synthesis of proteins that play an important role in blood clotting. Vitamin K is also required for the carboxylation of osteocalcin, a protein component of the bone matrix. Carboxylation of the osteocalcin must occur for mineral deposition and bone formation to proceed

normally. Increased levels of noncarboxylated osteocalcin have been associated with increased risk of hip fracture in elderly people. A study of 51 women over age 81[23] with hip fractures reported that many had reduced serum levels of vitamin K as compared to control women of similar age; in fact, several of the women with fractures had undetectable levels of serum vitamin K.

Few studies exist that describe the usual dietary intakes and normal blood levels of vitamin K in adults of any age. It has been estimated that current dietary intakes of vitamin K range from 300 to 500 μg per day, levels five to ten times the estimated requirement.[17] Since the major dietary sources of phylloquinone are green vegetables, intakes may be less in older people who eat few vegetables because of cost, chewing problems, or personal preference. Based on the established relationship between vitamin K and bone health, dietary sources of this vitamin should receive increased attention in dietary counseling of elderly clients.

WATER-SOLUBLE VITAMINS
Factors Influencing Absorption

The water-soluble vitamins, in contrast to the fat-soluble vitamins, do not require another major nutrient for their absorption. However, other substances or secretions within the gastrointestinal tract influence the movement of particular vitamins across the mucosal cell and into the blood. For several water-soluble vitamins absorption is enhanced in an acid environment and reduced in older people with achlorhydria. Hydrochloric acid is sometimes necessary for the release of a vitamin from its food component; riboflavin and vitamin B-12 are examples. Thiamin and vitamin B-6 are more stable in an acid environment and can lose activity at a higher pH. The presence of alcohol impedes the uptake of several of the B complex vitamins, including thiamin and folic acid.

Both prescription and over-the-counter drugs can interfere with the absorption of water-soluble vitamins. Several anticonvulsant drugs, phenytoin and phenobarbital, reduce the absorption of folic acid. Aspirin binds with folic acid and also can cause a loss of vitamin C. Health professionals providing nutritional care for older adults need to be aware of the impact of particular drugs on nutrient absorption and provide appropriate nutritional advice (see chapter 10).

Ascorbic Acid

The association of ascorbic acid with antioxidant functions that may help prevent the development of atherosclerotic plaques, cataracts, or cancer has brought attention to this vitamin. Ascorbic acid also participates in other important biochemical reactions, including the formation of collagen, the synthesis of neurotransmitters, wound healing, and immune function.

Absorption of ascorbic acid. In general ascorbic acid is highly absorbed; at levels of intake usually supplied in food (20 to 120 mg per day), absorption is 90% or higher.[17] There is no evidence to suggest that ascorbic acid absorption in healthy older adults differs from that in young adults with similar ascorbic acid status. Low blood levels reported in elderly nursing home residents usually are related to low ascorbic acid intake, not impaired absorption.

Metabolism of ascorbic acid. Controlled studies by Blanchard and coworkers[4,5] evaluating ascorbic acid absorption, tissue uptake, and excretion in young and elderly men and women indicate that ascorbic acid status rather than age influences these processes. All subjects consumed a vitamin C-restricted diet supplying less than 10 mg of ascorbic acid daily for several weeks until plasma ascorbic acid levels fell to 0.4 mg/dl;

then, all were given a 500 mg supplement daily for three weeks. Vitamin C metabolism was evaluated in both the depleted and supplemented stages.

After administration of a 500 mg test dose, depleted subjects, regardless of age, had lower plasma levels of ascorbic acid than supplemented subjects, and they excreted a smaller amount of ascorbic acid in the urine. In depleted subjects 96% of the test dose entered tissue storage sites, compared to about 48% in the supplemented individuals. This was as expected, since absorbed ascorbic acid would be taken up more rapidly by the tissues in depleted individuals. Conversely, supplemented subjects excreted about 40% of the test dose, although excretion was somewhat slowed in the older group. Vitamin C urinary excretion is controlled by glomerular filtration and active reabsorption in the kidney tubule. At plasma concentrations up to 1.4 mg per dl, about 97% of the ascorbic acid in the glomerular filtrate is reabsorbed. Above this threshold ascorbic acid spills over into the urine.

Ascorbic acid requirements. The pharmacokinetics and metabolism of ascorbic acid appear to differ between men and women, regardless of age, as a result of the differences in body composition between the sexes.[3] In nonsmoking older men and women on controlled intakes ranging from 30 to 280 mg a day, plasma ascorbic acid levels were significantly lower in men at all levels of intake (see table 6-2).[80] Women reached a plasma level of about 1 mg per dl on an intake of about 90 mg a day; in contrast, older men required an intake of 150 mg a day. On intakes of 60 mg, the current recommended allowance for both sexes, the older men had marginal plasma ascorbic acid levels of 0.5 mg per dl, suggesting risk of vitamin C deficiency. In men plasma levels remained about 1 mg per dl regardless of increasing intake.

The total body pool of ascorbic acid is believed to reach a maximum at 20 mg per kg body weight with a steady-state plasma level of 1 mg per dl. These standards were developed on young adult men, and no comparable data are available for women or older people of either sex. It does appear that older men require more than two times the current RDA to maintain

TABLE 6-2   *Ascorbic Acid Intake and Resulting Plasma Levels in Older Men and Women*

Total Ascorbic Acid Intake mg/day*	Plasma Ascorbic Acid Level mg/dl	
	Men	Women
45	0.28	0.50
60	0.50	0.90
90	0.79	1.09
150	1.05	1.27
280	1.09	1.43

*RDA = 60 mg

Modified from VanderJagt, D.J., Garry, P.J., and Bhagavan, H.N.: Ascorbic acid intake and plasma levels in healthy elderly people, Am. J. Clin. Nutr. 46:290, 1987.

this steady state. This increased requirement is not the result of hormonal differences or renal handling of the vitamin.[53] The increased need for ascorbic acid in men can be explained, at least in part, by their greater size and higher proportion of fat-free mass and lower proportion of body fat. In the studies described above, the women actually received more vitamin per unit of body weight.[3] Future research should equalize ascorbic acid dosages on the basis of body weight or fat-free mass. In the meantime, older men should consume at least the recommended level on a daily basis.

Ascorbic acid intake and biochemical status. In older people socioeconomic status, living situation, gender, and ascorbic acid status are related. Among older economically advantaged people in Boston,[76] only 5% had ascorbic acid intakes falling below two-thirds of the RDA. Biochemical status was generally adequate; only one person had a plasma level indicative of deficiency (less than 0.2 mg per dl), while 6% of the men and 3% of the women had marginal status (0.2 to 0.4 mg per dl). On the other hand, in a population of New England elderly (n = 1154) above age 70[57] with low incomes and declining health, about one-fifth were consuming less than 75% of the RDA.

Functional disability may be a significant risk factor for vitamin C deficiency. Elderly Dutch women residing in a nursing home[37] had a mean ascorbic acid intake of 54 mg, those in an assisted living situation had 97 mg, and those living independently had 132 mg. Deficient plasma vitamin C levels were identified in 35%, 4%, and 0% of the women in institutionalized care, assisted care, and independent housing, respectively. Elderly men who smoke and have low intakes of vitamin C-rich foods are the most likely group to have marginal biochemical status.

Current research with ascorbic acid. Ascorbic acid, acting as an antioxidant, may play a role in preventing degenerative changes associated with aging. Macular degeneration, a change in the retina of the eye, is the leading cause of blindness among people above age 65.[66] Age-related changes in the retina are caused by chemical changes in the polyunsaturated fatty acid structure that result in aggregate molecules and loss of vision. These chemical changes involve oxidation reactions, and current work is evaluating the relationship between an individual's antioxidant status and the development of these conditions.

Increasing ascorbic acid intake has been related to a reduced incidence of cardiovascular disease and might act by reducing blood pressure levels, reducing total serum cholesterol levels, enhancing HDL-cholesterol levels, or reducing serum lipid peroxidation.[20,26,69] Although additional work is needed, two studies of healthy elderly people have reported significant findings. In the BLSA[20] plasma vitamin C was directly related to plasma HDL-cholesterol levels after adjustment for age, sex, obesity, and smoking. In the Boston study[26] older adults with higher plasma ascorbic acid levels had increased HDL-cholesterol and decreased LDL-cholesterol levels and lower blood pressures. Food sources of vitamin C also contribute fiber, potassium, folic acid, and other important nutritional components that may influence these risk factors.

Total intake of ascorbic acid as well as vitamin C-rich fruits and vegetables has been evaluated in epidemiological studies of cancer risk. A prospective study of 11,580 residents of a retirement community,[68] followed for eight years, did find reduced risk of cancer at all sites in women with higher intakes of dietary vitamin C and fruits and vegetables. Men who took vitamin C supplements reduced their risk of bladder cancer, but fruit and vegetable consumption did not influence cancer risk in men. Increased intakes of fruits and vegetables appear to reduce overall cancer risk; however, it is difficult to separate the influence of particular vitamins or other protective substances found in natural foods.

Thiamin

Thiamin participates as a coenzyme in the metabolism of the macronutrients. This vitamin is most closely associated with the breakdown of carbohydrates to yield energy; consequently, the thiamin requirement is related to total energy intake.

Absorption of thiamin. Thiamin absorption or metabolism is not impaired in older people unless associated with alcohol abuse. At physiologic concentrations thiamin is absorbed by an energy-requiring, carrier-mediated process. Folic acid is required for the synthesis of these carrier proteins and so is considered to be essential for thiamin absorption.[70] Among older women in Ireland,[70] however, thiamin status was not influenced by folic acid status either before or after supplementation with folic acid. Polyphenols found in tea and coffee have been described as having antivitamin activity, including antithiamin activity. Thiamin status in the older Irish women was unrelated to polyphenol intake despite high daily use of tea (1,170 g) and coffee (60 g).

Thiamin requirement. The minimum requirement for thiamin is 0.3 mg per 1,000 kcal, although the recommended level is 0.5 mg per 1,000 kcal.[17] Daily intake should not fall below 1 mg even if total energy intake is less than 2,000 kcal. The 1989 RDA suggests 1.2 mg for men and 1 mg for women above age 50.[17] Thiamin plays an important role in the metabolism of neurotransmitters and the control of nerve transmission and fatty acid metabolism; it is needed regardless of energy intake. Thiamin requirements and utilization in alcoholism are discussed in chapter 10.

Thiamin intake and biochemical status. Thiamin intake decreases with age, although

this more likely results from the observed decrease in energy intake rather than from a change in the type of food consumed. In a comparison of healthy elderly, institutionalized elderly, and healthy young adults,[54] daily thiamin intake was significantly lower in the older groups who consumed 1.09 and 0.73 mg, respectively. The younger adults consumed 1.44 mg a day. Despite these differences in total intake, thiamin intake per 1,000 kcal was the same among all three groups, 0.67 mg to 0.71 mg.

Findings from the NHANES III study[78] indicate that dietary thiamin continues to decline beyond age 60. Among the men daily thiamin intake fell from 1.81 mg at ages 60 to 69 to 1.65 mg at age 80 and over. For women in these age categories, intakes declined from 1.42 mg to 1.30 mg. The African American and Mexican American elderly had lower intakes of thiamin than the white elderly. Among 680 generally healthy, independently living older adults in Boston,[76] adequate intakes of thiamin were associated with diets emphasizing servings from the milk, cereal, and fruit groups.

The most appropriate test for the evaluation of thiamin status is the erythrocyte transketolase assay, which measures enzyme activity before and after the addition of thiamin pyrophosphate. The percentage of increase in enzyme activity after the addition of thiamin pyrophosphate indicates the degree of deficiency. The erythrocyte transketolase test is highly sensitive; enzyme activity remains normal on an intake of 0.5 mg of thiamin daily. Estimates of the prevalence of thiamin deficiency have ranged from 2% to 5% in older people in Boston[62] to 28% in older Canadian adults[48] to 48% in older Irish women.[71] Brady and coworkers[9] assessed thiamin adequacy in 38 cardiac clinic patients with congestive heart failure. Of the eight patients with biochemical evidence of thiamin deficiency, four were consuming at least 67% of the RDA.

In most cases thiamin deficiency can be reversed by increasing thiamin intake. In a double-blind study of older Irish women living in their own homes,[71] erythrocyte transketolase activity was restored to normal in those given 10 mg of thiamin a day, whereas enzyme activity remained low in those given a placebo (table 6-3). Also, symptoms of thiamin deficiency (fatigue and

TABLE 6-3   Influence of Thiamin Supplementation on Energy Intake and Well-Being in Older Irish Women

	Placebo Group (n = 40)		Thiamin-Supplemented Group (n = 40)	
	Before	After	Before	After
Number thiamin deficient	19	18	19	0
Energy intake (kcal)	1648	1662	1679	1970
Appetite score	5.9	6.1	6.0	9.5*
Fatigue score	5.0	4.9	5.4	1.2*
General well-being score	4.8	4.8	5.2	8.8*

*The women rated each physical parameter on a scale from 0 (I never have this condition) to 10 (I have this condition all of the time); a high score is appropriate for appetite and general well-being; a low score is appropriate for fatigue.
Modified from Smidt, L.J., and others: Influence of thiamin supplementation on the health and general well-being of an elderly Irish population with marginal thiamin deficiency, J. Gerontol. 46:M16, 1991.

poor appetite) decreased and energy intake increased in those women given thiamin, but not in those given the placebo. Older people who drink alcoholic beverages regularly will have an increased requirement for thiamin. Good sources of dietary thiamin such as whole-grain or enriched bread and cereals, lean pork, legumes, and nuts should be emphasized to older clients.

Riboflavin

The coenzymes of riboflavin participate in many metabolic reactions occurring within the cell. Riboflavin coenzymes act as donors and receptors of electrons in the breakdown of carbohydrates and fats. Riboflavin requirements appear to increase with heavy exercise in both younger and older adults.

Absorption and metabolism of riboflavin. Metabolic studies suggest that the riboflavin requirement is similar in younger and older adults. Among healthy Guatemalan adults above age 60[7] who were depleted and then repleted with riboflavin, the requirement was found to be 1.1 mg to 1.3 mg a day. Differences between men and women related to differences in energy intake. Riboflavin status was evaluated on the basis of urinary riboflavin

excretion and erythrocyte glutathione reductase enzyme activity (this enzyme requires riboflavin as a cofactor). Young people fed equivalent diets under similar conditions had a riboflavin requirement in the same range. Because riboflavin is necessary for the metabolism of carbohydrate, riboflavin needs were evaluated at two levels of carbohydrate intake: a diet in which 57% of the energy was supplied by carbohydrate and a diet in which 68% of total energy was supplied by carbohydrate. Surprisingly, the requirement for riboflavin was lower when 68% of energy was supplied by carbohydrate as compared to 57%. Boisvert and coworkers[7] proposed that the high carbohydrate diet promoted bacterial synthesis of riboflavin in the intestinal lumen.

The current RDA for riboflavin for persons above age 50 is 1.4 mg for men and 1.2 mg for women.[17] Based on the findings described above that suggest that the true requirement lies between 1.1 mg and 1.3 mg per day, the current RDA offers little or no margin of safety. Russell and Suter[62] recommend that the RDA for older adults be raised to the level now recommended for younger adults (1.7 mg for men and 1.3 mg for women). Older women participating in a 10-week exercise program[81] (25 minutes each day, six days each week) required

0.9 mg of riboflavin per 1,000 kcal to maintain appropriate biochemical status. The RDA is based on a standard of 0.6 mg per 1,000 kcal.[17] This apparent increase in the riboflavin requirement as a result of vigorous exercise needs to be investigated further in view of the increasing numbers of older people joining exercise programs.

Riboflavin intake and biochemical status. Dietary intakes of riboflavin vary widely among older groups and can be influenced by age, sex, energy intake, and use of particular food groups. A population study of 2,152 men and women in Beaver Dam, Wis.,[40] reported that men ages 43 to 64 had higher riboflavin intakes than men ages 65 to 84 (median intakes were 1.9 mg and 1.7 mg, respectively). Median intakes of riboflavin were similar in both age groups of women (1.3 mg). Although older women consume less total riboflavin than older men, their intakes are higher when expressed in terms of energy intake. Older Canadian women ranging in age from 65 to 74[75] consumed 1.07 mg of riboflavin per 1,000 kcal whereas the older men had intakes of 0.86 mg per 1,000 kcal. The Food and Nutrition Board[17] recommends that intakes not fall below 0.6 mg per 1,000 kcal. Although this minimum level was exceeded by both the men and women in the Canadian study,[75] 23% of the men were at risk of riboflavin deficiency based on erythrocyte enzyme activity levels, compared to only 7% of the women. In a study of institutionalized (n = 266) and independently living (n = 686) elderly in Boston,[76] biochemical evidence of riboflavin deficiency was present in about 10%.

Riboflavin intake is influenced by use of dairy products and, to a lesser extent, fortified cereal products. This relationship was particularly strong in the cross-sectional study of elderly representing several countries in Europe (SENECA study).[15] The median daily intake of riboflavin was 2 mg in Denmark, where dairy products are consumed frequently; in contrast, intakes below 1 mg were frequent among older people surveyed in Hungary, Belgium, and Greece. Riboflavin intakes tend to be lower in elderly African Americans and Mexican Americans[78] who have lower preferences for dairy products. On the other hand, older lacto-ovo-vegetarian women were more likely to consume the recommended level of riboflavin than were non-vegetarian women of similar age.[49]

One benefit of obtaining riboflavin from dairy products is the contribution these foods make toward meeting the calcium requirement. When the diets of older Bostonians[76] were evaluated according to food types, those with frequent servings of milk, cereal, and fruit had the highest daily intakes of both riboflavin (1.9 mg) and calcium (856 mg).

Niacin

Niacin is a component of the two enzymes NAD (nicotinamide adenine dinucleotide) and NADP (nicotinamide adenine dinucleotide phosphate) which are essential for many metabolic pathways, including glycolysis, the synthesis and oxidation of fatty acids, and the respiratory chain. Niacin requirements and metabolism in aging people have received little attention.

Adequacy of niacin intake varies across population groups. In a national survey of nearly 500 older people,[63] 13% of the men and 11% of the women between the ages of 65 and 74 were consuming less than two-thirds of the RDA. It is interesting to note that niacin intake improved with age in the men, as only 4% of those above age 74 had low intakes. Conversely, niacin intake decreased in the women above age 74 with 18% having intakes below two-thirds of the recommended level. The Food and Nutrition Board[17] notes that some foods such as milk and eggs that are not high in preformed niacin do contain high levels of tryptophan which can be used to synthesize niacin (60 mg tryptophan = 1 mg niacin). However, vitamin B-6 is a required cofactor for this conversion, and vitamin B-6 status is less than optimal in many elderly people. The relative efficiency of this conversion of tryptophan to niacin in the elderly adult has not been evaluated.

Nicotinic acid in high doses (2 g to 6 g a day) has been shown to effectively reduce serum LDL-cholesterol levels and increase serum HDL-cholesterol levels in particular individuals.[12] At the same time side effects, including gastrointestinal distress, jaundice, and cardiac arrhythmias, have been reported in clinical trials.

Slow release nicotinic acid preparations can result in liver damage. Thus older persons should be discouraged from self-medication. The use of nicotinic acid as a drug will be discussed further in chapter 10.

Vitamin B-6 (Pyridoxine)

Vitamin B-6 is an important coenzyme in the metabolism of protein and amino acids, and the requirement for vitamin B-6 increases as the level of protein increases. Vitamin B-6 has a role in immune function and the synthesis of neurotransmitters, issues of great importance to the health and well-being of aging adults. Because the biochemical parameters used in younger people may not be reliable in older people, a major problem is how to evaluate vitamin B-6 status.

Vitamin B-6 absorption and metabolism. Many researchers have reported that older people have decreased levels of plasma pyridoxal phosphate (PLP); however, decreased vitamin intake or metabolic changes, rather than impaired absorption, seem to be the cause. The absorption and utilization patterns of vitamin B-6 were studied in two groups of healthy men ages 20 to 30 and 60 to 70.[16] Each was given an oral dose of isotopically labeled pyridoxine while maintained on a controlled dietary intake. Plasma levels of PLP were similar in both the younger and older men, as was erythrocyte aspartate aminotransferase enzyme activity (used to evaluate vitamin B-6 status in all age groups). Neither the total amount of labeled pyridoxine excreted in the urine nor the pattern of excretion over the three-day recovery period differed with age. Results from this study indicate that the bioavailability of vitamin B-6 is not altered in healthy elderly. Thus, impaired absorption would not seem to be the cause of the decline in plasma PLP levels in some older people.

Plasma PLP is bound to albumin, which protects it from hydrolysis, so a decrease in circulating albumin might be expected to bring about a decrease in plasma PLP. However, the capacity of albumin to bind PLP is believed to be far in excess of the amount of PLP normally found in the plasma. Since PLP is stored in skeletal muscle, Lee and Leklem[34] suggested that differences in vitamin B-6 metabolism between younger and older adults may relate to decreased muscle mass in older age groups. Plasma PLP could be influenced by whole body protein turnover. In elderly adults on a high protein diet, plasma PLP levels tended to decline as protein breakdown increased.[56] This makes sense in that vitamin B-6 is required for many biochemical reactions occurring in protein metabolism.

Vitamin B-6 requirement. Recent work at the Human Nutrition Research Center on Aging in Boston[58] indicates that the vitamin B-6 requirements of healthy elderly men and women are about 1.96 mg and 1.90 mg per day, respectively. These values are based on the amount of vitamin B-6 required to bring about normal excretion levels of xanthurenic acid after administration of a set amount of tryptophan. Vitamin B-6 is a cofactor for several enzymatic steps in the conversion of tryptophan to niacin. When vitamin B-6 is not available in the required amounts, tryptophan metabolism cannot proceed normally and xanthurenic acid, an intermediary metabolite, begins to accumulate and is excreted in the urine. In the Boston study the older subjects were depleted of vitamin B-6 and then fed gradually increasing amounts of the vitamin at two different levels of dietary protein (0.8 and 1.2 g per kg body weight). In contrast to younger individuals in whom protein intake significantly influences vitamin B-6 requirements, the vitamin B-6 requirement in these older individuals did not vary according to protein intake. Older women developed biochemical signs of vitamin B-6 deficiency faster than older men. This could relate to the smaller skeletal mass and vitamin B-6 stores of older women compared to older men.

This study raised serious questions about the sensitivity of widely used biochemical measures of vitamin B-6 status when applied to older people. The tryptophan load test was the most sensitive to vitamin B-6 status. Increases in urinary xanthurenic acid excretion became evident within five days after the implementation of a vitamin B-6 deficient diet, and excretion returned to baseline levels when vitamin B-6 intake became adequate. In contrast, erythrocyte aspartate aminotransferase enzyme activity did not respond to small increases in vitamin B-6 intake after vitamin depletion. Dutch workers[36] have also expressed concern about the lack of sensitivity of this measurement to marginal vitamin B-6 status. They suggested that lower levels of erythrocyte PLP lead to reduced synthesis of the aspartate aminotransferase apoenzyme, thereby introducing a second variable in addition to availability of the vitamin B-6 coenzyme.

This work also points to a discrepancy between the current RDA for vitamin B-6 for people above age 50 and the apparent requirement; this disparity is especially pertinent to women. The apparent requirement of older men was found to be 1.96 mg[58] whereas the RDA, designed to provide a measure of safety, is 2 mg.[17] In women the apparent requirement of 1.9 mg[58] is above the current RDA of 1.6 mg.[17] Moreover, the form of vitamin B-6 fed in the Boston study is highly bioavailable; the vitamin found in dietary sources may be bound to food components and in part unavailable. Thus, a goal for older people should be daily consumption of at least the current RDA. Further work is needed to confirm this apparent age-related increase in vitamin B-6 requirements.

One important consequence of vitamin B-6 deficiency in older people is impaired cell-mediated immunity.[42] Vitamin B-6 depletion resulted in a decreased number of lymphocytes and depressed mitogenic responses in older men and women. These indices were restored to normal following vitamin repletion. Vitamin B-6 deficiency may in fact contribute to the age-related decline in immune function in some older people.

Vitamin B-6 intake and biochemical status. Age, health, sex, and use of supplements influence vitamin B-6 status. Serum vitamin B-6 levels in German, Belgian, and Dutch young people (mean age = 30), healthy elderly people (mean age = 76), and hospitalized elderly people (mean age = 78) are illustrated in figure 6-2.[27] The lowest serum levels were found in the hospitalized elderly. Over half of the hospitalized group had serum vitamin B-6 levels below the normal range as compared to only 9% of the healthy elderly and 1% of the young control subjects. Vitamin B-6 status is also compromised among elderly people at home who have one or

more health problems and marginal vitamin intakes. Manore and coworkers[39] evaluated the vitamin B-6 status in 198 low-income older people in Arizona using three-day dietary records and plasma PLP levels. Thirty-two percent of this population had plasma levels indicating deficiency, and only 5% of those were using supplements. On the other hand, 95% of those with the highest plasma PLP levels were using supplements. Mean intakes from food were 1.5 mg and 1.8 mg a day, respectively, in the groups with low and high plasma levels. Several individuals with low plasma PLP levels were consuming adequate levels of vitamin B-6 (2.5 mg per day); however, they also reported two or more serious health problems (e.g., heart disease, kidney disorders, diabetes). These medical conditions were less common among those with higher plasma vitamin levels. These reports raise questions about the vitamin B-6 status of elderly people with significant chronic disease in spite of appropriate dietary intakes. Prescription drugs used in treating chronic medical conditions can interfere with the absorption or metabolism of vitamins.

For the general elderly population a regular intake of 3 mg of vitamin B-6 (150% to 200% of the RDA) can maintain appropriate serum levels.[6] Among 56 independently living older people in New Jersey,[6] a daily supplement containing 3 mg of vitamin B-6 maintained adequate serum levels regardless of dietary intake. In that study women were more likely to have intakes from food that fell below the current RDA. In view of reported toxicity symptoms and neural dysfunction in people consuming inappropriately high levels of vitamin B-6, it is prudent to avoid supplements containing more than one to two times the RDA (see chapter 10).

Good dietary sources of vitamin B-6 should be emphasized in diet planning with older people. In the NHANES II study,[28] dietary vitamin B-6 was supplied in about equal amounts by animal and vegetable foods. Meat and milk are good sources and also contain high amounts of protein. Fruits, potatoes, and other vegetables and ready-to-eat cereals add to the vitamin B-6 intake without adding significant amounts of additional protein, thus increasing the ratio of

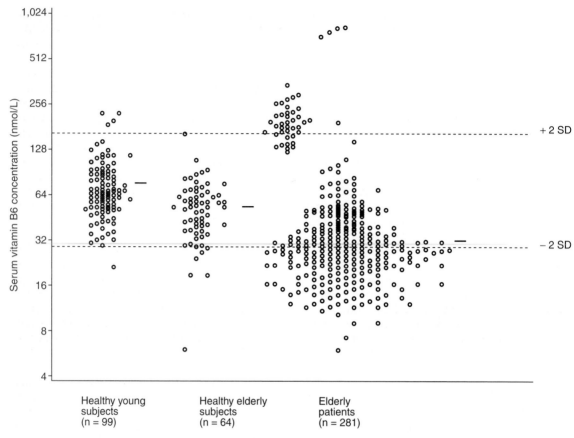

FIG. 6-2 Serum Vitamin B-6 Levels in Healthy Young People, Healthy Elderly People, and Elderly Hospitalized Patients. The dashed horizontal lines represent two standard deviations above and below the mean level of the healthy young people. Hospitalized elderly people are most likely to have low vitamin B-6 levels.

With permission from Joosten, E., and others: Metabolic evidence that deficiencies of vitamin B-12 (cobalamin), folate, and vitamin B-6 occur commonly in elderly people, Am. J. Clin. Nutr. 58:468, 1993. © American Society for Clinical Nutrition.

vitamin B-6 to protein. In the NHANES III study[78] vitamin B-6 intakes were lower in elderly African Americans as compared to elderly white people. Median dietary intakes were 1.83 mg and 1.44 mg in the white men and women ages 60 to 69 and 1.33 mg and 1.16 mg in the African American men and women of similar age. Elderly Mexican American men and women had median intakes of 1.47 mg and 1.13 mg, respectively. The cost of foods high in vitamin B-6 and differences in the use of milk products may contribute to these differences.

Folate

Folate is a general term referring to the family of compounds that have a structure and biologic action similar to folic acid (pteroylglutamic acid). Folate compounds are required coenzymes in the transfer of one carbon fragments from one molecule to another. This reaction is important in the metabolism of nucleic acids, cell division, and protein synthesis.

Absorption of folic acid. About three-fourths of the folates occurring naturally in foods are present as polyglutamates, containing more than one glutamic acid residue per molecule; however, only monoglutamates are absorbed in the small intestine. Pterolypolyglutamate hydrolase enzyme, secreted by the intestinal mucosa, cleaves the polyglutamate molecule to a monoglutamate molecule that is absorbed. Most older people have sufficient hydrolase to release and absorb naturally occurring folates in food. Although age per se does not decrease folic acid absorption, gastrointestinal diseases, such as gluten-sensitive enteropathy, or use of particular drugs, such as phenytoin, can reduce uptake of folic acid.

Poor folic acid status, regardless of cause, can in itself impair folic acid absorption. Folic acid deficiency leads to both structural and functional changes in the upper jejunum, the primary site of folic acid absorption. If mucosal damage is severe, even monoglutamate absorption is depressed. Intestinal changes related to folic acid deficiency are reversed with supplementation.

Folic acid absorption requires an acid environment. Atrophic gastritis (see chapter 4) and the subsequent rise in pH in the proximal small intestine from 6.7 (normal) to 7.1 (atrophic gastritis) impairs folic acid absorption. Absorption of a test dose of folic acid was 51% in healthy elderly people (mean age = 70 years), but only 31% in those with atrophic gastritis (mean age = 72 years).[31] When the folic acid was administered with acid, absorption rose to 54% in those with atrophic gastritis but remained unchanged in those with normal acid secretion. Surprisingly, older people with atrophic gastritis have been found at times to have higher serum levels of folic acid than normal elderly subjects (9.6 ng per ml versus 7.9 ng per ml). It appears that the reduced level of acid in the upper small intestine allows the growth of large numbers of folic acid-synthesizing bacteria, which provide an endogenous source of folic acid.

Liver folic acid content is believed to provide a direct measure of body stores. Liver folic acid stores in 560 liver specimens obtained at autopsy tended to be lower in people who died after age 60.[25] Folic acid levels were also lower in individuals who had long-term illnesses than in those who died accidentally. Only two subjects had liver folic acid levels below 3 ng per g, a level indicating severe deficiency. Although

severe deficiency was not a general problem in that population, older people with long-standing chronic disease would appear to be at greater risk.

Folic acid requirement. The folic acid requirement of older people is receiving increasing attention. Nutrition surveys of adults of various ages conducted prior to 1989 led the Food and Nutrition Board to reduce the recommended intake of folate from 400 µg a day in all adults to 200 µg a day for men and 180 µg a day for women.[17]

Older people have been reported to maintain appropriate biochemical levels on folic acid intakes even lower than the current RDA. Among 270 healthy older adults in New Mexico, about 40% consumed less than 200 µg a day of folic acid; however, only 8% had low serum folic acid levels and only 3% had low red blood cell folic acid levels.[60] In a Boston study of both community-living and institutionalized elderly,[62] less than 3% had plasma folic acid levels below 3 ng per ml, the level associated with deficiency. Of the 2,500 elderly subjects in the SENECA study,[14] none had a plasma folic acid falling below that level. These data suggest that the recommended level of folic acid is sufficient to maintain appropriate storage levels in most healthy people. Folic acid deficiency in chronically ill older people could result from reduced food intake or drugs that interfere with vitamin absorption and metabolism.

Although this evidence provides support for the current RDA, several researchers have observed metabolic changes suggesting folic acid deficiency despite normal plasma levels. Folic acid, along with vitamin B-12, is a required cofactor for the conversion of homocysteine to cysteine. When these cofactors are not present in sufficient amounts, this conversion cannot go forward and homocysteine levels increase markedly. Serum homocysteine levels have been implicated in the accelerated development of vascular disease and increased risk of myocardial infarction. Elderly people with higher intakes and higher plasma levels of folate have lower serum homocysteine concentrations (see fig. 6-3).[67] Among 1,160 adult survivors in the Framingham Heart Study who are now 67 to 96 years, those with daily intakes of about 200 µg of

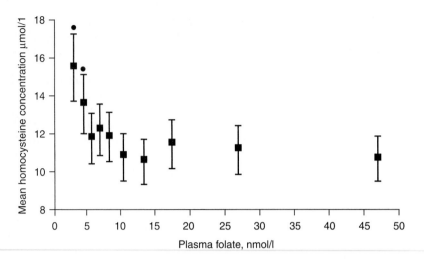

FIG. 6-3   The Relationship Between Plasma Homocysteine Levels and Plasma Folate Levels in Elderly People. Plasma homocysteine levels are significantly higher in those people with plasma folate levels below 5 nmol/l (2.2 ng/ml).

With permission from Selhub, J., and others: Vitamin status and intake as primary determinants of homocysteinemia in an elderly population, J.A.M.A. 270:2693, 1993. © 1993 American Medical Association.

folate (the current RDA for men) had the highest serum homocysteine levels.

Naurath and coworkers[47] in a double blind study evaluated the effect of folic acid, vitamin B-6, and vitamin B-12 supplementation in 180 hospitalized older people with high homocysteine levels. Elevated homocysteine levels returned to normal in 92% of those receiving the vitamins as compared to only 20% of those given the placebo. Many of the subjects who responded to the vitamin supplements had prior serum vitamin levels judged to be adequate by current standards. Folic acid appears to exert the greatest influence on serum homocysteine levels; folic acid supplements reduced plasma homocysteine concentrations by 42%, vitamin B-12 supplements reduced levels by 15%, and vitamin B-6 had no effect.[77] It may be necessary to use serum metabolite levels as well as serum folic acid levels to determine vitamin status and requirements.

Folic acid intake. Income and ethnicity influence folic acid status. In a Florida survey, over one-third of the low income group had folic acid intakes below 100 μg, or 50% of the RDA; this was true for only 3% of the upper income group.[60] Data from the NHANES III study[78] revealed that about half of older African Americans and Mexican Americans have folic acid intakes below the recommended level. In a population of white elderly, about 20% of the men had folic acid intakes below two-thirds of the RDA. Age influences folic acid intake in elderly women as 15% of those ages 65 to 74 had poor intakes as compared to 27% of those age 75 and over.[63] Irregular shopping trips can limit use of citrus fruits and dark green vegetables and lower folic acid intakes. Boiling vegetables for long periods of time can destroy folic acid. Low-cost sources with emphasis on preparation methods that enhance folic acid retention should be stressed in nutrition education programs.

Vitamin B-12

Vitamin B-12 is required for the normal metabolism of neural tissue, and a deficiency results in degenerative changes in the myelin sheath and irreversible neurologic damage. Vitamin B-12 is also required for the replication and metabolism of DNA and the maturation of the red blood cells.

Absorption of vitamin B-12. Intrinsic factor secreted by the chief cells of the gastric mucosa is required for the absorption of vitamin B-12. Lack of intrinsic factor leads to vitamin B-12 deficiency and pernicious anemia (see chapter 12). Vitamin B-12 absorption studies were performed on 76-year-old participants in the Goteborg, Sweden, longitudinal study (n = 38).[50] Among those with normal serum vitamin B-12 levels, urinary excretion of the labeled test dose (representing the vitamin that had been absorbed) ranged from 8.6% to 45.2%. This compared favorably to the reference interval of 10% to 38% absorption established with young people in that laboratory. When the elderly subjects with vitamin B-12 concentrations below normal (below 130 pmol per liter) were tested, only 13 of the 20 had normal absorption.

Russell and Suter[62] suggest that many older people with poor vitamin B-12 absorption have a problem other than lack of intrinsic factor. Atrophy of the gastric mucosa, with decreased production of acid, is a major cause of vitamin B-12 malabsorption. Decreased secretion of hydrochloric acid results in decreased hydrolysis of proteins along with decreased conversion of pepsinogen to pepsin, which also helps break down protein and release protein-bound vitamin B-12. Many older people with apparently normal absorption when tested with free cobalamin (vitamin B-12) are unable to absorb food-bound vitamin B-12.[65] An acid environment also assists in the binding of vitamin B-12 to carrier proteins that facilitate its transfer to intrinsic factor. The absorption of protein-bound vitamin B-12 is increased in achlorhydric patients when 4 oz of cranberry juice is consumed at the same time.[65] A rise in gastric pH also permits bacterial overgrowth that reduces vitamin B-12 availability. Bacteria can bind the vitamin, thereby inhibiting its absorption, or metabolize or alter its structure.

Individuals with atrophy of the gastrointestinal mucosa may require more dietary vitamin B-12 than is currently recommended. When all ability to absorb vitamin B-12 is lost, cobalamin may have to be provided by injection. In light of the potentially devastating effects of vitamin B-12 deficiency on the nervous system and mental function and the high prevalence of atrophic gastritis in the elderly, Russell and Suter[62] consider a dietary intake of 3 µg to be safer for older adults. The current RDA is 2 µg for both men and women.[17]

Vitamin B-12 intake and biochemical status. Information describing dietary intakes of vitamin B-12 in older populations indicates a general level of adequacy, although particular problems may exist. Vitamin B-12 intakes could be limited for low-income or vegetarian older people since it is found only in animal foods which tend to be expensive or consumed in lesser amounts by vegetarians. In a national study representing all income levels,[63] 9% of the men and 20% of the women ages 65 to 74 had vitamin B-12 intakes below two-thirds of the RDA. In that population the incidence of poor intake about doubled to 15% in the men age 75 and over, although the proportion of women with poor intakes was generally the same for all above age 64. Older vegetarian women in California[49] had vitamin B-12 intakes much like nonvegetarian women of similar age. Nevertheless, personal food patterns do influence vitamin B-12 status. In the Boston study,[76] only 3% of the elderly following a milk-cereal-fruit type diet or a meat-potatoes type diet had poor intakes as compared to 11% of those following a bread-poultry type diet.

Serum vitamin B-12 levels decrease with age, even among healthy elderly populations. This was evident in a recent evaluation of elderly members of the Framingham Heart Study (fig. 6-4).[35] Using the generally accepted value of 148 pmol per liter as the lower limit of normal, 5.3% of the elderly subjects but only 1.7% of the young controls had deficient levels. At the same time many of the older subjects had above normal levels of serum methylmalonic acid, a marker of vitamin B-12 deficiency. Methylmalonic acid accumulates when vitamin B-12 is not available to support the biochemical conversion of methylmalonyl coenzyme A to succinyl coenzyme A within the citric acid cycle. Serum methylmalonic acid levels tend to rise above normal when serum vitamin B-12 levels fall

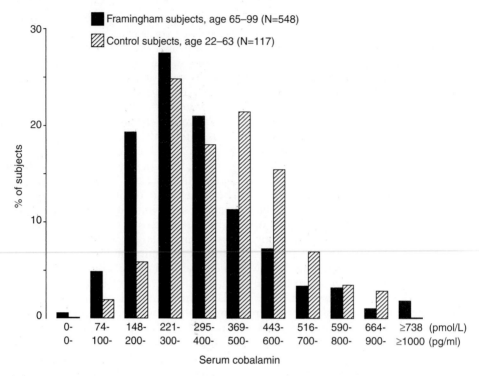

FIG. 6-4 Comparison of Serum Vitamin B-12 (Cobalamin) Levels in Community-Living Elderly People and Younger People. The majority of the elderly people had serum levels at the lower end of the distribution; more of the younger people had serum levels at the middle or the upper end of the distribution.

With permission from Lindenbaum, J., and others: Prevalence of cobalamin deficiency in the Framingham elderly population, Am. J. Clin. Nutr. 60:2, 1994. © American Society for Clinical Nutrition.

below 258 pmol per liter. Because abnormally high serum levels of methylmalonic acid indicate a metabolic deficiency of vitamin B-12, Lindenbaum and coworkers[35] propose that a serum level of 258 pmol per liter, not 148 pmol per liter, be the critical measure of vitamin B-12 adequacy. If this measure was applied to the Framingham elderly, 40.5% would be categorized as deficient, compared to 18% of the young controls. Eleven percent of the elderly subjects had elevated serum methylmalonic acid levels.

In general, reported levels of vitamin B-12 deficiency based on serum vitamin B-12 levels measured in large-scale studies have been 5% or less.[1] Evaluations of small groups of elderly people with a high prevalence of chronic disease have led to estimates of deficiency as high as 29%. Based on the findings of Lindenbaum and coworkers, the true incidence of deficiency may actually be higher. Presently, the analytic procedures for determination of serum methylmalonic acid are both costly and, in many settings, unavailable. It is urgent that clinicians responsible for the care of older adults investigate procedures for the diagnosis of vitamin B-12 deficiency (see also chapter 12).

Summary

Progress continues in assessing the complex issues relating to vitamin needs in aging as we learn more about metabolic status and the physiology of aging. Decreases in gastric secretions, increase in the gastric pH, changes in intestinal

CASE STUDY

The family of an 89-year-old man in good health has noticed changes in his personality and functional ability over the past four months. He can't remember what day it is and has turned from being friendly and gregarious to being sullen and withdrawn. He has complained of burning in his fingers and toes. He likes milk and meat and eats these foods regularly, but seldom eats fruits and vegetables. A recent physical exam and blood test showed no abnormality or evidence of anemia. His family has decided he is becoming senile and may need to enter a nursing home.

1. What might be the basis for this man's change in behavior and cognitive function?

Which nutrients are likely to be low, based on his food preferences?

2. What biochemical assays might you suggest to further examine the cause of his problem?

3. What dietary or physiologic factors might be contributing to this problem? Explain.

4. What treatment strategies, dietary or other, might be appropriate to reverse these changes in function and behavior?

5. Develop a set of dietary recommendations and suggested foods to provide specific nutrients that are likely low in his current diet.

---

epithelium, and decreases in lean body mass and relative energy intakes are compounded by chronic disease factors and use of multiple medications. These changes provide a myriad of variables to delineate in determining vitamin needs.

Reported intakes of vitamin E generally fall short of the RDA, even when including supplement use. A growing body of evidence suggests that the current RDAs for vitamin D, vitamin B-6, vitamin B-12, vitamin C, folate, and riboflavin may not provide a sufficient level for optimum health. Conversely, continued use of vitamin A supplements in excess of the RDA may place older people at risk of vitamin A toxicity. Limited sunlight exposure and low daily intakes coupled with reduced ability to absorb and convert vitamin D to its active form places both sick and healthy elderly at high risk for compromised bone health. Functional tests of enzyme activity or the evaluation of serum metabolite levels are better indicators of vitamin status than serum vitamin levels which may not reflect true vitamin status.

REVIEW QUESTIONS

1. Are the current RDAs for vitamins adequate for most older people? What evidence exists to suggest a decreased or an increased need for some vitamins as we age? Which vitamins are included in this group? Identify circumstances which support

the development and use of age-specific biochemical tests to evaluate vitamin status in the elderly.

2. How do functional changes in the aging gastrointestinal tract influence digestion and the absorption of vitamins? List and determine if fat-soluble or water-soluble vitamins are more affected by gastrointestinal changes in older persons. How can dietary constituents influence digestion and absorption of vitamins?

3. Describe the role of vitamin D as a hormone. List the different sources or routes for supplying the body's vitamin D needs. What factors influence the absorption and use of this vitamin? Are any particular groups of older people more likely to have poor vitamin D status? If so, describe the group(s).

4. Make a chart with the following headings: Solubility Medium, Factors Affecting Absorption, Biochemical Test(s), Functional Test(s), RDA, Conditions for Increased/Decreased Vitamin Needs, Health Promotion or Chronic Disease Prevention, and System Affected in Deficiency. Fill in the appropriate headings for each vitamin. Evaluate each vitamin and make a conclusive summary statement for each based on your information.

5. Suppose you were a member of the Food and Nutrition Board reviewing current research on vitamin B-12 in the elderly. What types and categories of research information would you want to have available to use when setting the RDA for vitamin B-12 in older people? Would you recommend changes to the current RDA for older people? Support your decision.

SUGGESTED LEARNING ACTIVITIES

1. Go to the drug store and find two pill vitamin supplements and two milk shake/liquid supplements marketed for the elderly consumer and a common multivitamin marketed to the general public. Compare the levels and types of vitamins in each supplement to the RDA for older people. How do they compare? Include cost as a variable. Based on your investigation, which type of vitamin preparation would you recommend, if any? Justify your decision.
2. Write a lesson plan for a three-part nutrition education program for an audience of older people attending a program at an elder hostel. The title of the lesson plan is "Vitamize your breakfast, lunch, and dinner: How to incorporate more vitamin-rich foods in all of your meals."
3. Construct a composite diagram identifying key vitamins and their role in the prevention and maintenance of bone health. Include associated organ systems and identify age-associated changes in organ function that influence bone health.
4. Construct a list of advantages and disadvantages for the use of (1) plasma or serum levels, (2) serum metabolites, and (3) enzyme activity levels for the evaluation of vitamin status. What recommendations would you make for future research to develop assays appropriate for determining vitamin RDAs and status.
5. Use a computer to access and browse world wide web sites for available information on vitamins and aging. A good starting site is the U.S. Department of Health and Human Services located at www.os.dhhs.gov or the U.S. Department of Agriculture Food and Nutrition Information Center located at www.nalsda.gov/fnic.html.

REFERENCES

1. Allen, L.H., and Casterline, J.: Vitamin B-12 deficiency in elderly individuals: diagnosis and requirements, Am. J. Clin. Nutr. 60:12, 1994.
2. Bendich, A.: The safety of beta carotene, Nutr. Cancer 11:207, 1988.
3. Blanchard, J.: Effects of gender on vitamin C pharmacokinetics in man, J. Am. Coll. Nutr. 10:453, 1991.
4. Blanchard, J., and others: Vitamin C disposition in young and elderly men, Am J. Clin. Nutr. 51:837, 1990.
5. Blanchard, J., Conrad, K.A., and Garry, P.J.: Effects of age and intake on vitamin C disposition in females, Eur. J. Clin. Nutr. 44:447, 1990.
6. Bogden, J.D., and others: Daily micronutrient supplements enhance delayed-hypersensitivity skin test responses in older people, Am. J. Clin. Nutr. 60:437, 1994.
7. Boisvert, W.A., and others: Riboflavin requirement of healthy elderly humans and its relationship to macronutrient composition of the diet, J. Nutr. 123:915, 1993.
8. Bostick, R.M., and others: Reduced risk of colon cancer with high intake of vitamin E: the Iowa women's health study, Cancer Res. 53:4230, 1993.
9. Brady, J.A., Rock, C.L., and Horneffer, M.R.: Thiamin status, diuretic medications, and the management of congestive heart failure, J. Am. Diet. Assoc. 95:541, 1995.
10. Bulux, J., and others: Studies on the application of the relative-dose-response test for assessing vitamin A status in older adults, Am. J. Clin. Nutr. 56:543, 1992.
11. Dawson-Hughes, B.: Calcium and vitamin D metabolism and nutritional status in the elderly: overview. In: Rosenberg, I.H., editor: Nutritional assessment of elderly populations. Measure and function, New York, 1995, Raven Press.
12. DiPalma, J.R., and Thayer, W.S.: Use of niacin as a drug, Annu. Rev. Nutr. 11:169, 1991.
13. Eastell, R., and others: Interrelationship among vitamin D metabolism, true calcium absorption, parathyroid function, and age in women: evidence of an age-related intestinal resistance to 1,25-dihydroxyvitamin D action, J. Bone Mineral Res. 6:125, 1991.
14. Euronut SENECA investigators: Nutritional status: blood vitamins A, E, B-6, B-12, folic acid and carotene, Eur. J. Clin. Nutr. 45:63, 1991.
15. Euronut SENECA investigators: Intake of vitamins and minerals, Eur. J. Clin. Nutr. 45(3):121, 1991.
16. Ferroli, C.E., and Trumbo, P.R.: Bioavailability of vitamin B-6 in young and older men, Am. J. Clin. Nutr. 60:68, 1994.
17. Food and Nutrition Board: Recommended dietary allowances, ed. 10, Washington, DC, 1989, National Academy of Sciences.
18. Freaney, R., McBrinn, Y., and McKenna, M.J.: Secondary hyperparathyroidism in elderly people: combined effect of renal insufficiency and vitamin D deficiency, Am. J. Clin. Nutr. 58:187, 1993.
19. Garry, P.J., and others: Vitamin A intake and plasma retinol levels in healthy elderly men and women, Am. J. Clin. Nutr. 46:989, 1987.

20. Hallfrisch, J., and others: High plasma vitamin C associated with high plasma HDL- and HDL$_2$ cholesterol, Am. J. Clin. Nutr. 60:100, 1994.
21. Hallfrisch, J., Muller, D.C., and Singh, V.N.: Vitamin A and E intakes and plasma concentrations of retinol, beta carotene, and alpha-tocopherol in men and women of the Baltimore longitudinal study of aging, Am. J. Clin. Nutr. 60:176, 1994.
22. Halpner, A.D., and Blumberg, J.B.: Assessment of antioxidant vitamin status in older adults. In: Rosenberg, I.H., editor: Nutritional assessment of elderly populations. Measure and function, New York, 1995, Raven Press.
23. Hodges, S.J., and others: Circulating levels of vitamins K$_1$ and K$_2$ decreased in elderly women with hip fracture, J. Bone Miner. Res. 10:1241, 1993.
24. Holick, M.F.: Environmental factors that influence the cutaneous production of vitamin D, Am. J. Clin. Nutr. 61(Suppl):638S, 1995.
25. Hoppner, K., and Lampi, B.: Folate levels in human liver from autopsies in Canada, Am. J. Clin. Nutr. 33:862, 1980.
26. Jacques, P.F.: Effects of vitamin C on high-density lipoprotein cholesterol and blood pressure, J. Am. Coll. Nutr. 11:139, 1992.
27. Joosten, E., and others: Metabolic evidence that deficiencies of vitamin B-12 (cobalamin), folate, and vitamin B-6 occur commonly in elderly people, Am. J. Clin. Nutr. 58:458, 1993.
28. Kant, A.K., and Block, G.: Dietary vitamin B-6 intake and food sources in the U.S. population: NHANES II, 1976-1980, Am. J. Clin. Nutr. 52:707, 1990.
29. Kiel, D.P.: Vitamin D, calcium, and bone: descriptive epidemiology. In: Rosenberg, I.H., editor: Nutritional assessment of elderly populations. Measure and function, New York, 1995, Raven Press.
30. Krall, E.A., and others: Effect of vitamin D intake on seasonal variations in parathyroid hormone secretion in postmenopausal women, New Engl. J. Med. 321:1777, 1989.
31. Krasinski, S.D., and others: Fundic atrophic gastritis in an elderly population. Effect on hemoglobin and several serum nutritional indicators, J. Am. Geriatr. Soc. 34:800, 1986.
32. Krasinski, S.D., and others: Postprandial plasma retinyl ester response is greater in older subjects compared with younger subjects, J. Clin. Invest. 85:883, 1990.
33. Krasinski, S.D., and others: Relationship of vitamin A and vitamin E intake to fasting plasma retinol, retinol-binding protein, retinyl esters, carotene, α-tocopherol, and cholesterol among elderly people and young adults: increased plasma retinyl esters among vitamin A-supplement users, Am. J. Clin. Nutr. 49:112, 1989.
34. Lee, C.M., and Leklem, J.E.: Differences in vitamin B-6 status indicator responses between young and middle-aged women fed constant diets with two levels of vitamin B-6, Am. J. Clin. Nutr. 42:226, 1985.
35. Lindenbaum, J., and others: Prevalence of cobalamin deficiency in the Framingham elderly population, Am. J. Clin. Nutr. 60:2, 1994.
36. Löwik, M.R.H., and others: Dose-response relationships regarding vitamin B-6 in elderly people: a nationwide nutritional survey (Dutch Nutritional Surveillance System), Am. J. Clin. Nutr. 50:391, 1989.
37. Löwik, M.R., and others: Vitamin C status in elderly women: a comparison between women living in a nursing home and women living independently, J. Am. Diet. Assoc. 93:167, 1993.
38. Maiani, G., and others: Beta carotene serum response in young and elderly females, Eur. J. Clin. Nutr. 43:749, 1986.
39. Manore, M.M., and others: Plasma pyridoxal 5′-phosphate concentration and dietary vitamin B-6 intake in free-living, low-income elderly people, Am. J. Clin. Nutr. 50:339, 1989.
40. Mares-Perlman, J.A., and others: Nutrient supplements contribute to the dietary intake of middle- and older-age adult residents of Beaver Dam, Wis., J. Nutr. 123:176, 1993.
41. McKenna, M.J.: Differences in vitamin D status between countries in young adults and the elderly, Am. J. Med. 93:69, 1992.
42. Meydani, S.N., and others: Vitamin B-6 deficiency impairs interleukin 2 production and lymphocyte proliferation in elderly adults, Am. J. Clin. Nutr. 53:1275, 1991.
43. Meydani, M., and others: Effect of long-term fish oil supplementation on vitamin E status and lipid peroxidation in women, J. Nutr. 121:484, 1991.
44. Meydani, S.N., and others: Assessment of the safety of high-dose, short-term supplementation with vitamin E in healthy older adults, Am. J. Clin. Nutr. 60:704, 1994.
45. Morris, D.L., Kritchevsky, S.B., and Davis, C.E.: Serum carotenoids and coronary heart disease, the lipid research clinics coronary primary prevention trial and follow-up study, J.A.M.A. 272:1439, 1994.
46. Murphy, S.P., Subar, A.F., and Block, G.: Vitamin E intakes and sources in the United States, Am. J. Clin. Nutr. 52:361, 1990.

47. Naurath, H.J., and others: Effects of vitamin B-12, folate, and vitamin B-6 supplements in elderly people with normal serum vitamin concentrations, Lancet 346:85, 1995.

48. Nichols, H.K., and Basu, T.K.: Thiamin status of the elderly: dietary intake and thiamin pyrophosphate response, J. Am. Coll. Nutr. 13:57, 1994.

49. Nieman, D., and others: Dietary status of Seventh-Day Adventist vegetarian and non-vegetarian elderly women, J. Am. Diet. Assoc. 89:1763, 1989.

50. Nilsson-Ehle, H.: Cyanocobalamin absorption in the elderly: results for healthy subjects and for subjects with low serum cobalamin concentration, Clin. Chem. 32:1368, 1986.

51. Nowak, R.: Beta carotene: helpful or harmful?, Science 264:500, 1994.

52. O'Dowd, K.J., and others: Exogenous calciferol (vitamin D) and vitamin D endocrine status among elderly nursing home residents in the New York City area, J. Am. Geriatr. Soc. 41:414, 1993.

53. Oreopoulos, D.G., and others: Renal excretion of ascorbic acid: effect of age and sex, J. Am. Coll. Nutr. 12:537, 1993.

54. O'Rourke, N.P., and others: Thiamine status of healthy and institutionalized elderly subjects: analysis of dietary intake and biochemical indices, Age Ageing 19:325, 1990.

55. Panemangalore, M., and Lee, C.J.: Evaluation of the indices of retinol and *alpha*-tocopherol status in free-living elderly, J. Gerontol. 47:B98, 1992.

56. Pannemans, D.L.E., van den Berg, H., and Westerterp, K.R.: The influence of protein intake on vitamin B-6 metabolism differs in young and elderly humans, J. Nutr. 124:1207, 1994.

57. Posner, B.M., and others: Nutritional risk in New England elders, J. Gerontol. 49:M123, 1994.

58. Ribaya-Mercado, J.D., and others: Vitamin B-6 requirements of elderly men and women, J. Nutr. 121:1062, 1991.

59. Rimm, E.B., and others: Vitamin E consumption and the risk of coronary heart disease in men, New Engl. J. Med. 328:1450, 1993.

60. Rosenberg, I.H., and others: Folate nutrition in the elderly, Am. J. Clin. Nutr. 36(Suppl.):1060, 1982.

61. Rudman, D., and others: Fractures in the men of a veterans administration nursing home: relation to 1,25-dihydroxyvitamin D, J. Am. Coll. Nutr. 8:324, 1989.

62. Russell, R.M., and Suter, P.M.: Vitamin requirements of elderly people: an update, Am. J. Clin. Nutr. 58:4, 1993.

63. Ryan, A.S., Craig, L.D., and Finn, S.C.: Nutrient intakes and dietary patterns of older Americans: a national study, J. Gerontol. 47:M145, 1992.

64. Salamone, L.M., and others: Contributions of vitamin D intake and seasonal sunlight exposure to plasma 25-hydroxy vitamin D concentration in elderly women, Am. J. Clin. Nutr. 58:80, 1993.

65. Saltzman, J.R., and others: Effect of hypochlorhydria due to omeprazole treatment or atrophic gastritis on protein-bound vitamin B-12 absorption, J. Am. Coll. Nutr. 13:584, 1994.

66. Seddon, J.M., and others: Dietary carotenoids, vitamins A, C, and E, and advanced age-related macular degeneration, J.A.M.A. 272:1413, 1994.

67. Selhub, J., and others: Vitamin status and intake as primary determinants of homocysteinemia in an elderly population, J.A.M.A. 270:2693, 1993.

68. Shibata, A., and others: Intake of vegetables, fruits, beta carotene, vitamin C, and vitamin supplements and cancer incidence among the elderly: a prospective study, Br. J. Cancer 66(4):673, 1992.

69. Simon, J.A.: Vitamin C and cardiovascular disease: a review, J. Am. Coll. Nutr. 11:107, 1992.

70. Smidt, L.J., and others: Influence of folate status and polyphenol intake on thiamin status of Irish women, Am. J. Clin. Nutr. 52:1077, 1990.

71. Smidt, L.J., and others: Influence of thiamin supplementation on the health and general well-being of an elderly Irish population with marginal thiamin deficiency, J. Gerontol. 46:M16, 1991.

72. Stampfer, M.J., and others: Vitamin E consumption and the risk of coronary disease in women, New Engl. J. Med. 328:1444, 1993.

73. Stauber, P.M., and others: A longitudinal study of the relationship between vitamin A supplementation and plasma retinol, retinyl esters, and liver enzyme activities in a healthy elderly population, Am. J. Clin. Nutr. 54:878, 1991.

74. Stephensen, C.B., and others: Vitamin A is excreted in the urine during acute infection, Am. J. Clin. Nutr. 60:388, 1994.

75. Toh, S.Y., Thompson, G.W., and Basu, T.K.: Riboflavin status of the elderly: dietary intake and FAD-stimulating effect of erythrocyte glutathione reductase coefficients, Eur. J. Clin. Nutr. 48:654, 1994.

76. Tucker, K.L., Dallal, G.E., and Rush, D.: Dietary patterns of elderly Boston-area residents defined by cluster analysis, J. Am. Diet. Assoc. 92:1487, 1992.

77. Ubbink, J.B., and others: Vitamin requirements for the treatment of hyperhomocysteinemia in humans, J. Nutr. 124:1927, 1994.

78. U.S. Department of Health and Human Services: Dietary intake of vitamins, minerals, and fiber of persons ages 2 months and over in the United States: Third National Health and Nutrition Examination Survey, Phase I, 1988–91, Advance Data from Vital and Health Statistics, Number 258, Nov. 14, 1994, Hyattsville, MD, National Center for Health Statistics.

79. U.S. Department of Health and Human Services: Normal human aging: The Baltimore longitudinal study of aging, NIH Publication No. 84-2450, Washington, DC, 1984, U.S. Government Printing Office.

80. VanderJagt, D.J., Garry, P.J., and Bhagavan, H.N.: Ascorbic acid intake and plasma levels in healthy elderly people, Am. J. Clin. Nutr. 46:290, 1987.

81. Winters, L.R.T., and others: Riboflavin requirements and exercise adaptation in older women, Am. J. Clin. Nutr. 56:526, 1992.

7

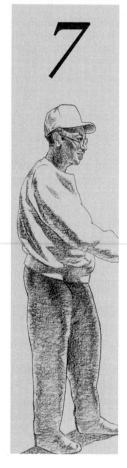

Minerals in Aging

✦✦

Objectives

After studying the chapter, the student should be able to:

✔ *Understand the structural and metabolic functions of the individual essential minerals*

✔ *Identify those minerals of particular concern to older people and the effect of aging on mineral status*

✔ *Describe the nutritional and hormonal factors that regulate calcium balance*

✔ *Outline the dietary, medical, pharmaceutical, and social factors that may influence the mineral status of an older person*

✔ *Estimate an older person's dietary requirement for individual minerals*

✔ *Recognize the need to encourage fluid intake in older people*

Balance techniques, traditionally used to determine mineral requirements, are both costly and tedious, and they demand extraordinary cooperation on the part of subjects. The development of new methods using labeled trace minerals or isotopes has made it possible to measure minute amounts of minerals in tissues and fluids and has sparked renewed interest in both the structural and metabolic roles of these nutrients. The study of minerals is especially important in older people affected by age-related degenerative changes and chronic diseases that involve particular minerals. Bone metabolism, immune function, and regulation of body fluids undergo alterations with advancing age and are influenced by mineral intake and metabolism. The role of macrominerals and trace elements in the prevention of chronic diseases, including cardiovascular disease and cancer, is an active area of research. Currently, we lack sensitive measurements that would allow us to detect marginal mineral status and initiate appropriate intervention before deficiency ensues. This chapter will focus on those minerals that are currently being studied in aging adults.

MACROMINERALS
Calcium

Of the macrominerals, calcium is present in the largest amount. A healthy adult has approximately 1,200 g of body calcium, and about 99% is contained in the skeleton.[1] The remaining 1%, found in cell membranes and extracellular fluids, plays an important role in nerve transmission, muscle contraction, and membrane function. Calcium metabolism has important implications for both nutritional and physical health. Aging is accompanied by a gradual loss of bone mass, which increases the risk of bone fracture.

Control of Calcium Metabolism

Serum total calcium must be maintained very close to 2.5 mmol/l[1] to ensure normal functioning of the heart and nervous system. Serum calcium levels and overall calcium metabolism are controlled by the interaction of several hormones, including parathyroid hormone (PTH), estrogen or testosterone, calcitonin, and the active metabolite of vitamin D [$1,25(OH)_2D$], often referred to as calcitriol. If calcium intake or absorption is inadequate, serum calcium concentrations are maintained at the expense of bone mineral. A slight decrease in serum calcium increases PTH secretion and decreases calcitonin secretion. PTH restores the serum calcium concentration to its former level by (1) stimulating the conversion of $25(OH)D$ to $1,25(OH)_2D$ in the kidneys to promote increased absorption of calcium in the intestine, (2) decreasing renal excretion of calcium by enhancing calcium reabsorption in the renal tubule, and (3) increasing bone resorption and mobilization of bone calcium.[1]

As a consequence of these actions, serum calcium concentration rises slightly above its usual level, resulting in a decrease in secretion of PTH and an increase in secretion of calcitonin. By opposite actions, calcitonin decreases production of $1,25(OH)_2D$ and calcium absorption, increases renal calcium excretion, and decreases bone resorption, thereby bringing about a decrease in serum calcium. The repetition of these events effectively maintains serum calcium concentration within narrow limits. (See chapter 6 for a discussion of vitamin D and PTH.)

Estrogen modulates the effects of PTH and calcitonin by stimulating the synthesis of renal 1-α-hydroxylase, the enzyme necessary to convert $25(OH)D$ to $1,25(OH)_2D$. Estrogen, and probably testosterone, suppress the action of PTH on bone resorption. After estrogen withdrawal, bone becomes increasingly sensitive to PTH, and calcium mobilization is accelerated.[1] The influence of the sex steroid hormones on bone metabolism is more pronounced in women who experience a cessation of estrogen secretion at menopause, compared to men who experience a gradual decline in testosterone secretion at older ages.

Calcium Absorption

Mechanisms of calcium absorption. Calcium is absorbed throughout the small intestine and to a lesser extent in the colon. Calcium is absorbed by both active transport and passive diffusion. At low and moderate intakes, calcium is absorbed by active transport stimulated by $1,25(OH)_2D$, which controls the synthesis of carrier proteins and calcium-dependent ATPase. At high intakes calcium absorption also occurs by passive diffusion. When a person drinks a glass of milk, about 80% of the calcium absorbed crosses the mucosa by active transport, and about 20% is absorbed by passive diffusion.[11]

Decreases in calcium absorption over adulthood in both women and men have been recognized for many years. Calcium absorption in young adults on normal intakes is believed to reach 40% but drops to 25% in older women.[71] The most important factor influencing calcium absorption, however, is calcium intake.[11] Although the total amount of calcium absorbed is directly related to the amount consumed, the proportion absorbed is inversely related to total intake. Dawson-Hughes[11] suggests that the increase in the fraction absorbed compensates in part at a lower intake. It appears that an adjustment period of about two weeks is required to adapt to a different level of intake. Older people may be less able than younger people to increase the percent of calcium absorbed at lower intakes. Individuals with osteoporosis absorb calcium less efficiently than older people who do not have this disease.

Source of dietary calcium. In general calcium is absorbed most efficiently when in a solubilized form, as in milk, or in a highly soluble form, such as the calcium-citrate-malate complex[70] (the form of calcium now added to citrus juices). Calcium is less available when consumed in the form of a relatively insoluble salt, such as calcium carbonate, although it appears that the calcium in calcium carbonate is well absorbed if taken with a meal. The presence of food stimulates more secretion of gastric acid than the supplement alone, and gastric acid enhances the breakdown of insoluble salts. The presence of food also slows gastric emptying and delivers the calcium to the duodenum in smaller amounts, which also may enhance absorption.[70]

The role of gastric acid in calcium absorption becomes important for older people with achlorhydria.[70] When calcium is taken in supplement form under fasting conditions, absorption by achlorhydric subjects is only 4% compared to 23% in normal controls. When calcium carbonate is taken as part of a test meal, the fraction of calcium absorbed by achlorhydric individuals is well within the normal range. Although the particular mechanism that enhances calcium absorption is unknown, components of the meal or the acidity provided by the meal might influence these results. Calcium-food complexes may assist in absorption. Test meals containing carbohydrate from bread or added sugar lower the pH in the intestinal environment. Meals containing acid in the form of orange juice could effectively lower the pH. Pancreatic secretions stimulated by the test meal could contain unknown factors that solubilize calcium salts. An interesting finding was that achlorhydric subjects, when given calcium in a solubilized form, absorbed the mineral at twice the level of normal controls, 45% versus 24%.[70] This may represent an enhanced absorptive response to poor calcium status.

Another practical issue when evaluating calcium absorption in elderly people is the effect of increasing fiber intake. Components of dietary fiber and phytate reduce the bioavailability of many divalent cations, and a high fiber meal can reduce calcium availability by 25%.[70] Studies with achlorhydric subjects and normal controls indicated that calcium absorption fell by more than 5% in both groups given a high fiber meal. Heaney and Weaver[20] looked at the effect of psyllium intake on the absorption of calcium consumed at the same meal by healthy elderly people. This is of particular importance in older people because psyllium is the fiber in many bulk-forming laxatives used to ensure regular bowel movements. When the amount of psyllium present in the recommended dose of a common laxative (Metamucil) was consumed at a breakfast meal that contained 219 mg of calcium in the form of calcium-fortified orange juice, there was no practical difference in the fractional absorption of calcium by the subjects consuming an equivalent amount of neutral fiber, psyllium fiber, or no fiber (absorption among groups varied from 32% to 35%). The phytates or oxalates present in food fiber sources, rather than the fiber itself, may lower the bioavailability of calcium. Absorption of calcium from vegetables high in oxalates, such as spinach, may be as low as 5%.[70]

Calcium Intake

The RDA for calcium for men and women ages 25 and over is 800 mg.[14] Unfortunately, actual intakes of adults of both sexes often fall below this level and decrease with age (fig. 7-1). In the NHANES III study[61] white adults had higher calcium intakes than Mexican American or African American adults, and men had higher intakes than women at all ages. White men ages 30 to 39 had a median daily intake of almost 1,000 mg, 125% of the RDA. By ages 70 to 79 this intake had fallen below 700 mg. The median intake of Mexican American men meets the RDA at younger ages, but by age 80 and over, more than half of this group had a calcium intake below 500 mg. African American men had median calcium intakes of about 500 mg to 600 mg, or 65% to 75% of the RDA. Although white women and Mexican American women are at higher risk of osteoporosis than African American women, over half had calcium intakes below 700 mg at ages 30 to 39, and by age 80 had intakes between 436 mg and 550 mg (below 70% of the RDA). African American women had the lowest calcium intakes, ranging from 62% of the RDA at ages 30 to 39 to 40% of the RDA at ages 80 and over. Discomfort

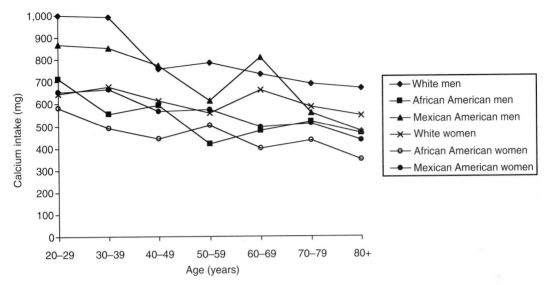

FIG. 7-1   Calcium Intake of Adults by Sex, Age, and Ethnic Group. Calcium intake decreases with age in both men and women, but women consume less calcium than men of similar age and ethnic group; African Americans consume less calcium than white and Mexican American groups.

Data from: U.S. Department of Health and Human Services: Dietary intake of vitamins, minerals, and fiber of persons ages 2 months and over in the United States: Third National Health and Nutrition Examination Survey, Phase I, 1988–91, Advance Data from Vital and Health Statistics, Number 258, Hyattsville, MD, Nov. 14, 1994, National Cancer for Health Statistics.

associated with lactose intolerance or dislike of dairy products may be involved in the poor calcium intakes of older African American adults.

Median calcium intakes were higher in the SENECA study[12] of 2,458 older people in 12 European countries. In the men median dietary intake ranged from 1,323 mg in Greece to 638 mg in Hungary. It would be helpful to explore particular food patterns in different regions of Greece; in women both the highest (1,213 mg) and lowest (521 mg) median intakes were recorded in that country. In none of the 18 European communities represented did median intakes fall below 500 mg.

Income could influence calcium intake. Only 19% and 35% of the older men and women with middle to high income levels who participated in the Boston Nutritional Status Survey were consuming less than 67% of the RDA.[51] In contrast 43% to 44% of the older men and 47% to 54% of the older women from a national sample

fell below two thirds of the RDA for calcium.[50] Centenarians in Georgia[27] consumed nearly 700 mg of calcium per 1,500 kcal. A dietary evaluation of 266 institutionalized older people indicated that availability is an important factor in calcium intake; only 4% to 5% of that group consumed less than 67% of the recommended level.[51] Milk and cheese are significant contributors to the calcium content of the diet. For elderly adults with low (409 mg), moderate (665 mg), or high (1,046 mg) intakes of calcium, milk contributed 38%, 52%, and 64% of the total calcium, respectively.[58] Fluid milk has the added advantage that it is fortified with vitamin D, essential for calcium absorption, to the level of 5 µg per quart.

Calcium supplements are receiving attention as sources of calcium for adults of all ages. Among the Boston elderly,[51] 12% of the men and 18% of the women took calcium supplements that contained 1 mg to 1,607 mg. Median supplement intake was 200 mg in both men and women. In spite of their use of supplements, 25% of the women supplement users were still consuming less than 700 mg of calcium daily.

Over-the-counter and prescription medications can be sources of calcium. In many cases individuals are unaware of the calcium contained in these products, and label information can be incomplete. Although the contribution of medications may be insignificant in people with a high calcium intake from food, it can more than double the apparent intake of individuals who do not consume dairy products regularly.

Calcium Requirement

The calcium requirement for adults over age 25 is likely the most controversial of all the requirements. It has been known for some time that calcium requirements vary over the life cycle. Needs are greater during the periods of rapid growth in childhood and adolescence and during pregnancy and lactation when demand for calcium is high to support fetal development and subsequent milk production.[67] In recent years researchers have proposed that calcium requirements are elevated in postmenopausal women who are estrogen-deficient; however, new data have been interpreted to suggest that even women and men between the ages of 25 and 50 have calcium needs above the current recommendation of 800 mg.[64] Because serum calcium is under strict metabolic control, it does not serve as an indicator of calcium status. Bone mass has been used as the primary measure for evaluation of calcium status, but the wide interindividual variation in bone mineral and the slow turnover of bone tissue can complicate the interpretation of these measurements.[67]

Several approaches have been used to estimate calcium requirements in adults. One approach using epidemiological methods has evaluated the calcium intakes of healthy populations that have experienced a low rate of bone fractures in advanced age. Another approach is determining the level of calcium intake at which the body is in calcium balance, meaning that the total body loss of calcium via all routes of loss does not exceed intake.

Obligatory calcium losses through the urine, feces, and skin have been estimated to be 332 mg

a day for women and 381 mg a day for men.[67] Based on an estimated absorption level of 30%, Weaver[67] has suggested that the calcium requirement is about 1,100 mg a day for older women and 1,270 mg for older men. Balance studies conducted with both men and women support the need for increased calcium intakes. Calcium balance was evaluated in 168 healthy women ages 35 and older who were part of a religious order.[67] These women on self-selected diets were studied over a period of years as they moved through menopause and beyond. It became apparent that premenopausal women or postmenopausal women who were estrogen-repleted required an intake of 990 mg a day to avoid calcium losses. Postmenopausal women who remained estrogen-deprived required 1,500 mg of calcium daily to achieve calcium balance. Spencer and coworkers[55] evaluated calcium requirements in 181 men ages 34 to 71; intakes of 1,200 mg a day brought about calcium balance in 87% of the men studied. On intakes of 800 mg a day, the current RDA, 41% of the men consuming calcium in the form of milk were still losing calcium. Selby[54] evaluated calcium balance in 25 patients with osteoporosis who were following diets representing their usual intakes. Their calcium requirement was 1,480 mg a day, which is similar to the postmenopausal women described earlier who did not have overt bone disease.

On the basis of information now available, the National Institutes of Health (NIH) Consensus Statement has recommended increased calcium intake for all adults age 25 and older (table 7-1).[64] The statement contends that daily intakes of 1,000 mg in young adults will maximize bone retention and bone mass. The decline in estrogen secretion that occurs after the onset of menopause in women results in accelerated bone loss. Increasing calcium intake to 1,500 mg daily may limit bone loss, but it should not be considered a replacement for estrogen.[64] Although bone loss has been less well documented in men, higher calcium intakes are associated with lower rates of hip fracture.

Changes in calcium homeostasis that occur in both men and women ages 65 and over support the need for increased dietary calcium.[11,64] Calcium absorption declines as a result of lower levels of circulating vitamin D metabolites, less

TABLE 7-1 *Optimal Daily Calcium Intakes*

Group	Optimal Intake
Men	
25 to 65 years	1,000 mg
Over 65 years	1,500 mg
Women	
25 to 50 years	1,000 mg
Over 50 years	
Postmenopausal	
Taking estrogen	1,000 mg
Not taking estrogen	1,500 mg
Over 65 years	1,500 mg

Modified from U.S. Department of Health and Human Services: Optimal calcium intake. NIH Consensus Statement, June 6–8; 12(4):1–31, Bethesda, MD, 1994, National Institutes of Health.

efficient conversion of vitamin D to the active form, or resistance of the intestinal mucosa to the action of vitamin D. Continued loss of bone over time can reduce bone mass to the threshold level at which fractures begin to occur.

NIH Consensus Statement and the RDA

The recommendations in the NIH Consensus Statement[64] and the recommendation of the Food and Nutrition Board[14] regarding calcium intakes of adults do not agree. One reviewer[67] pointed to the fact that the current RDAs are based on population averages and provide no margin of safety. Matkovic and Heaney[39] stressed the need to optimize bone mass and proposed the concept of a threshold intake for setting recommended intakes. The **threshold intake** is that intake above which no further increase in calcium retention is observed. The threshold intake for young adults ages 18 to 30 is 957 mg, which is fairly close to the Consensus recommendation of 1,000 mg.

Risks Associated with High Calcium Intake

According to the Food and Nutrition Board,[14] increasing calcium intake to 1,000 mg to 1,500 mg a day is not without risk. The Food and Nutrition Board pointed to the fact that a high calcium intake can increase the risk of urinary stone formation in men with hypercalciuria. A major nutritional issue in both sexes is the potential interference of a high calcium intake with the absorption of iron, zinc, or other divalent cation. Hallberg and others[19] reported that doses of 300 mg to 600 mg of calcium at a meal decreased absorption of both heme and nonheme iron by 50% to 60%. The experts serving on the NIH Consensus Panel[64] considered moderate supplementation raising total daily intake to 1,500 mg to carry limited risk of renal damage or calcium deposits in the soft tissues (milk-alkali syndrome). Intakes of 4 g a day are associated with calcium toxicity, and overuse of antacids containing calcium carbonate can result in milk-alkali syndrome. Individuals with hyperparathyroidism may be at risk if consuming high intakes of calcium. Patients with a history of kidney stones should avoid high levels of calcium supplements. Individuals with total calcium intakes approaching or exceeding 2,000 mg a day are more likely to experience adverse effects and need to be monitored closely. A modest increase in calcium should be safe for most people.[64]

Calcium Relationships with Other Nutrients

Protein intake has been evaluated in respect to urinary calcium loss. Nondairy animal protein decreases renal tubular reabsorption and increases urinary loss of calcium; conversely, plant proteins increase renal tubular absorption and decrease urinary loss. The mechanism for this response appears to be the acid-base status of the diet.[23] Reabsorption of calcium in the kidney tubule is decreased when the kidney must excrete an increased acid load. An evaluation of women from differing geographic regions in China[23] revealed that the women with increased intakes of nondairy animal foods, including fish and eggs, excreted more calcium, regardless of age and calcium intake, than women with a diet based on plant foods. Plant proteins, fruits, and vegetables are alkaline in nature. The sulfur-containing amino acids, methionine and cysteine, found in meat, add significantly to the renal acid load.

Conservation of calcium may be another benefit of the current public health effort to decrease intakes of sodium in the general population. Excessive dietary sodium increases urinary calcium losses.[64] The implications of calcium intake and metabolism for bone mass and the development of osteoporosis will be discussed in chapter 12.

Phosphorus

Phosphorus plays an important role in energy metabolism as a component of high-energy molecules such as adenosine triphosphate. About 85% of body phosphate is found in bone mineral in the ratio of 1 phosphorus to 2 calcium ions.[14] It is generally recommended that calcium and phosphorus be consumed in a ratio of 1:1, but in the presence of adequate calcium, the ratio is considered unimportant. The RDA for phosphorus is 800 mg.[14] Data from the Total Diet Study indicate that dairy products provide 36% of the phosphorus in the food supply; meat, poultry, and fish provide 29%; and grain products provide 13%.[65] Dairy products contain more calcium than phosphorus, whereas meat, poultry, and fish (without bones) contain 15 to 20 times more phosphorus than calcium.[14]

In the NHANES III study[61] median phosphorus intake for all groups ages 65 and over met or exceeded the RDA with the exception of African American and Mexican American women ages 80 and over. Their median intake was about 730 mg. Phosphorus intakes may be underestimated because of incomplete information relating to the amounts of phosphate-containing food additives in processed food. In spite of this, phosphorus intakes still exceed calcium intakes by a considerable margin (see calcium intakes described in fig. 7-1). This disparity between calcium and phosphorus intakes, particularly among older individuals with inadequate calcium intake, could further jeopardize bone health. Phosphorus deficiency, characterized by weakness, pain, and bone mineral loss, has been identified in older individuals with prolonged use of antacids containing aluminum hydroxide.[1] Aluminum hydroxide binds to phosphorus, thus preventing absorption.

Magnesium

Magnesium participates in biochemical and physiologic processes involving energy metabolism, cell membrane permeability, and nerve transmission. About 60% of body magnesium is in the bone.[14] Magnesium requirements are related to body weight and current dietary recommendations are based on the standard of 4.5 mg/kg of body weight.[71]

Magnesium Requirement

At this time little information is available about the magnesium requirement of the elderly. Magnesium absorption in young adults using labeled magnesium was 40% of the test dose.[71] No similar data are available describing absorption in older adults. Recently, attention has been directed toward possible relationships between the incidence of chronic diseases commonly observed in older people and magnesium intakes below recommended levels. These diseases include ischemic heart disease, diabetes mellitus, hypertension, and osteoporosis. Renal handling of magnesium appears to change little with advancing age in the absence of renal disease; however, impaired kidney function can lead to magnesium deficiency or toxicity. Based on the fact that older people with below-recommended levels of intake do not develop overt signs of magnesium deficiency, a recent review suggested that the current RDAs of 350 mg for men and 280 mg for women may be too high.[71]

Magnesium Intake

Magnesium intake is well below the RDA in many older people and decreases with age. In the NHANES III study[61] median intakes for men fell from 299 mg in the 60- to 69-year-old group to 256 mg in the age 80 and over group. Magnesium intakes decreased less in women who had levels of 236 mg to 210 mg over that age range. African American and Mexican American elderly had the lowest intakes, particularly those people above age 79. Median intakes for African American and Mexican American men and women ranged from 55% to 64% of the RDA. The very low intakes of these ethnic elderly may relate to their lower use of milk and dairy products, which provide about

16% of the magnesium in the U.S. food supply.[65] Other food sources of magnesium are nuts, legumes, unmilled grains, bananas, and vegetables. Milk, fruit juices, and meats made the greatest contributions to the magnesium intakes of the economically advantaged older people in the Boston Nutritional Status Survey.[58] Despite an adequate income to purchase food, 43% of the men and 36% of the women in the Boston study consumed less than two-thirds of the RDA.[51] Among institutionalized elderly people, women also had improved intakes relative to men. Only 18% of the institutionalized women as compared to 46% of the institutionalized men fell below two-thirds of the recommended level.[51] Tucker and Rush[58] pointed out that older women consumed proportionately more fruit, fruit juices, and vegetables than older men, which likely contributed to their higher intake. Databases used to calculate the magnesium content of diets are incomplete as to food magnesium content.

Magnesium Plasma Levels and Metabolism

Plasma magnesium levels in healthy individuals are remarkably constant; the site of regulation is the kidneys. About 70% of plasma magnesium is filtered by the kidneys, and on the average, 95% of the filtered magnesium is reabsorbed.[68] The kidneys can adjust the level of reabsorption in response to changes in the plasma magnesium concentration. Magnesium stores in the bone also serve to protect against radical fluctuations in extracellular magnesium levels. Magnesium losses occur when renal tubular reabsorption is impaired as a result of nephritis, particular diuretics, or inappropriate hormone secretion.[32] Diuretics, such as furosemide, decrease magnesium reabsorption. Digoxin enhances magnesium excretion, and magnesium depletion increases sensitivity to digoxin toxicity. In hyperparathyroidism, high urinary calcium levels competitively inhibit the reabsorption of magnesium.[1]

In the Boston study,[68] median serum magnesium levels were identical in both men and women, 0.85 mmol/l, and tended to increase with age. (Normal serum magnesium levels range from 0.65 mmol/l to 1.0 mmol/l.)

Serum levels were similar for both independently living and institutionalized individuals. Those subjects using thiazide diuretics, which increase urinary magnesium excretion, did have lower serum magnesium levels. Gullestad and coworkers[18] evaluated magnesium status in 36 healthy, elderly Norwegians and compared them to 53 healthy, young controls. Subjects were supplemented with a total of 7,500 mg of magnesium over a period of about a month, and then given a magnesium load test which consisted of an infusion of 750 mg over a period of eight hours. The older subjects had an increased retention of magnesium after the magnesium load test, both before and after supplementation. Magnesium retention was lower after supplementation, suggesting that the older subjects had a subclinical deficiency prior to supplementation. A major point for consideration is the fact that serum magnesium levels assessed prior to supplementation were within the normal range, indicating that tissue depletion was coexisting with normal serum levels. Those authors[18] also concluded that overall kidney function improved following magnesium supplementation, based on improved creatinine clearance. Magnesium deficiency does impair kidney function, which returns to normal after magnesium repletion. These elderly subjects did have intakes within the recommended range, indicating a need for further evaluation of factors influencing this requirement.

Magnesium Deficiency and Toxicity

Magnesium deficiency can result from laxative abuse and the loss of large amounts of secretions containing high levels of magnesium from the lower gastrointestinal tract. Chronic alcoholism leads to diminished magnesium intake and absorption and enhances renal excretion. Older individuals with uncontrolled diabetes mellitus are at risk of magnesium deficiency, since excretion is enhanced by the osmotic diuresis induced by high urinary glucose and ketone levels.[32]

Hypermagnesemia is a risk for older people who have impaired kidney function or excessive magnesium intakes. Common magnesium-containing antacids provide 100 mg to 200 mg a dose, and magnesium-containing laxatives can contain as much as 500 mg a dose. Drowsiness, lethargy, loss of coordination and reflexes, and changes in mental function are beginning signs of magnesium toxicity; with increasing severity, cardiac arrhythmias and cardiac arrest can occur.[68]

TRACE ELEMENTS

Iron

Of the trace elements, iron is present in the body in the largest amount. Iron is an important constituent of hemoglobin and myoglobin molecules that transport oxygen and carbon dioxide in the blood and muscle, respectively. Iron is also a component of the cytochrome enzymes that transfer electrons in the metabolism of high-energy molecules.[14] Current evidence indicates a role for iron in immune function and brain function. For many nutrients general status may deteriorate with age as a result of poor intake or chronic disease, but iron status actually improves in women after middle age when menstruation and monthly blood loss ceases. At age 70 and older, women are actually at lower risk of iron deficiency than men.[26] After age 50, the RDA for iron is 10 mg for both sexes.[14]

Iron Absorption

Iron absorption is a complicated and inefficient process in people of all ages. Because there is no established route for the excretion of iron once it has been taken into the body, control is exerted at the point of entry.[14] Iron absorption is influenced by body need, body stores, gastric pH, and foods eaten.

Body need for iron. In a healthy older adult with appropriate iron stores, iron is required to replace obligatory iron losses. Under normal circumstances the major routes of obligatory iron loss are through the desquamation of cells from the skin and gastrointestinal tract. The iron contained in red blood cells is recycled when aged erythrocytes are broken down, and the usual loss of red blood cells in the urine and feces is negligible.[21] Using radiolabeled iron, daily iron losses in young and middle-aged men have been estimated to be 14 μg per kg of body

weight or about 1.1 mg for an 80 kg man.[71] At this time little evidence suggests that iron excretion is higher in older men than younger men. Postmenopausal women have about the same level of iron loss as older men, and about half that of menstruating women with monthly blood loss.[26]

Body stores. Iron stores in a healthy man between the ages of 20 and 50 average about 1,000 mg. In contrast, iron stores in women in this age range are only about 300 mg as a result of menstrual blood loss. After age 50, body iron stores increase proportionately to a greater extent in women than in men. By the age of 70 or 80, men have body iron stores of about 1,200 mg, whereas the postmenopausal women have more than doubled their iron stores, to about 800 mg.[21] As a result, iron deficiency is unlikely in either sex except in the case of pathological blood loss, or extremely low intake or absorption over an extended period of time. Under usual circumstances the percentage of iron absorbed increases as body stores decrease.

Gastric acidity. Decreased secretion of gastric juice by the gastric mucosa affects the absorption of iron in several ways. First, components within the gastric juice bind to iron and enhance its absorption; second, the hydrochloric acid in gastric juice maintains a low pH in the lumen of the stomach, which promotes the reduction of inorganic iron (found in enriched and fortified food products) from the ferric to the ferrous form required for absorption. Antacids that raise pH levels decrease iron uptake.

In light of the importance of gastric acid to iron absorption, Krasinski and coworkers[29] evaluated blood parameters of iron status in normal older people and those with severe, moderate, or mild atrophic gastritis. Serum iron levels and serum ferritin levels did not differ among groups. An increased incidence of anemia was observed in those over age 75 compared to those ages 60 to 74. However, serum vitamin B-12 levels were also lower in the older age group, suggesting that the anemia was related to several factors and not only iron status.

Food source. Heme iron, which constitutes about 40% of the iron found in animal tissues, is more easily absorbed than nonheme iron, which includes the remaining 60% of the iron found in animal tissues and the iron found in egg and plant foods.[14] Absorption of heme iron is not influenced by age or the presence of gastric acid. Absorption of nonheme iron when present as ferric iron is impaired when gastric acid is reduced. The absorption of nonheme iron also can be enhanced or inhibited by other substances in the diet. Ascorbic acid is believed to enhance the absorption of nonheme iron by reducing ferric iron to the more soluble ferrous form and forming soluble complexes with iron ions. This enhanced effect on iron absorption is greatest in people with poor iron status, and when 100 mg to 500 mg of ascorbic acid is consumed at that meal. In those with adequate iron status, ascorbic acid supplementation had little effect on iron absorption. This would suggest that use of ascorbic acid supplements by healthy individuals with appropriate iron stores will not lead to iron overload.[26] However, these observations came from studies of young adults, and similar studies in aging populations are urgently needed. It has been proposed that the addition of heme iron or ascorbic acid can overcome the inhibitory effects of phytates on iron absorption.[26]

Iron absorption and age. Metabolic studies in younger and older healthy men using labeled nonheme iron indicate that age per se does not influence iron absorption.[59] Both age groups absorbed about 8% of the labeled dose fed with a formula diet. Of interest, however, was the magnitude of difference in absorption among the older men. Iron absorption is strongly influenced by body iron stores; thus, percent absorption could be expected to vary among older people with differing iron status. However, the older men in this study were judged to have adequate iron stores based on blood parameters and previous intake. Turnlund and colleagues[59] suggested that the previous iron intake of the men with increased absorption may have included iron that was biologically unavailable, and their iron stores may have been depleted.

Iron stores might also be depleted in older people who have been regular blood donors or experienced pathologic blood loss through injury, bleeding ulcers, or gastrointestinal cancer. Studies with healthy older adults who are regular blood donors[15,16] have established that the regulation of iron absorption, based on body iron stores, remains intact up to age 70 and beyond. An oral iron absorption test that involved administration of 66 mg of ferrous iron under fasting conditions indicated that eight control subjects absorbed 2.5% of the dose as compared to 12 blood donors who absorbed 7.4%.[16] Mean ages of the two groups were 72 to 73 years. Six of the control subjects had little or no change in their body iron stores over a three-year interval. Over that three-year interval the blood donors had each given 13 pints of blood. All subjects had normal gastric acid levels. Based on these findings, Gavin and coworkers[16] suggested that all individuals have a set point for iron stores, and absorption is increased or decreased to maintain or return to that level. In fact, reduced absorption to halt continued increase in iron stores may represent a safety mechanism to prevent iron overload. An observation not discussed in this study was the marked decrease in body iron stores (8.8 mg per kg) among the blood donors, despite their increase in percent absorption. Iron intakes were not reported.

A further evaluation of iron regulation was conducted with 36 healthy volunteers who were 68 years of age and donated blood about every 80 days for three to five years.[15] Iron intake from food averaged 18 mg to 20 mg daily, and several participants were consuming iron supplements providing about 20 mg of iron a day. Decreases in iron stores were similar in both supplemented and unsupplemented men, and mean iron absorption was 4 mg a day. Nonsupplemented women had a greater loss of iron stores than supplemented women, but this could reflect lower iron stores of particular individuals when the study began. Maximal iron absorption among the women was a bit lower than among the men, reaching 3.6 mg a day. The most interesting finding from this study was the relationship between total iron intake and percent absorption (fig. 7-2). The subjects consuming 18 mg of iron daily absorbed about 20% of the iron consumed; those with intakes of 38 mg

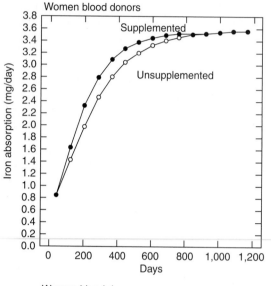

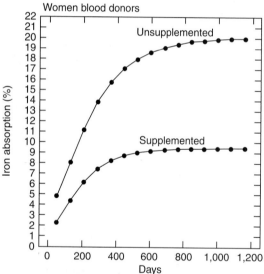

FIG. 7-2 Iron Intake and Iron Absorption in Healthy Elderly Blood Donors. Women with iron intakes of 18 mg a day from dietary sources absorbed about the same total amount of iron (3.6 mg/day) as those with intakes of 38 mg a day, which included a 20-mg supplement. The percent of iron absorbed was about double in the unsupplemented women, allowing them to absorb a greater proportion of their lower intake.

Garry, P.J., Koehler, K., and Simon, T.L.: Iron stores and iron absorption: effects of repeated blood donations, Am. J. Clin. Nutr. 62:611, 1995. (Used with permission.) © American Society for Clinical Nutrition.

transport oxygen. When iron is absorbed, it enters the portal vein bound to the carrier protein transferrin. At that point it may be transported to the bone marrow for incorporation into an erythrocyte or to the liver where it is stored. In an adult with adequate iron status, about one-third of the available transferrin is saturated with iron, and this measurement serves as an indicator of iron status. In an individual who is iron deficient, the synthesis of transferrin increases as a physiologic response to increase the amount of iron carried across the mucosal cell and into the body.[21]

Body iron stores can be estimated on the basis of the plasma ferritin level. Plasma ferritin iron is in direct equilibrium with storage iron and, according to Herbert,[21] the plasma ferritin level (in nanograms per milliliter), when multiplied by 10, will indicate the milligrams of iron stored. If plasma or serum ferritin falls to 20 ng/ml, it means that iron stores have dropped to 200 mg. If iron depletion continues, erythropoiesis is impaired and anemia will ensue. Protein-energy malnutrition, infection, inflammation, defective erythropoiesis, or chronic blood loss can result in iron-deficiency anemia and disordered iron metabolism (see chapter 12). Based on average absorption levels, the current RDA of 10 mg[14] will provide sufficient iron to replace normal losses.

Dietary Iron and Biochemical Parameters

Iron intake and biochemical parameters of iron status are influenced by age, sex, income,

absorbed about 10%. There does appear to be a lag time after body iron stores begin to decrease before a commensurate increase in absorption is initiated. Eventually, absorption increases to replace iron losses that continue to occur; however, the initial level of iron stores is not reached unless blood loss is interrupted.

Iron Requirements and Metabolism

The major physiologic role of iron within the hemoglobin molecule in the red blood cell is to and dietary pattern. Among 686 noninstitutionalized people in Boston[51] who ranged in age from 60 to 98 years, none of the men and only 3% of the women consumed less than two-thirds of the RDA; however, these individuals came from areas with a median annual income of $21,600. In contrast, 12.5% of the men and 17% of the women ages 65 to 74 from a national survey[50] representing all income levels had less than 67% of the RDA for iron. As an indication of how age may influence iron intake, the number of women who were deficient in dietary iron rose from 17% to 23% above age 74, but fell from 12.5% to 7% in the men of that age.[50] Puerto Rican women ages 60 to 74, interviewed in the Hispanic Health and Nutrition Examination Survey,[63] had a mean intake of only 7.8 mg of iron. Institutionalized older people who have their meals provided may be less likely to have poor intakes. The Boston Nutritional Status Survey[51] included 266 institutionalized subjects, and all of the men and 95% of the women were consuming at least two-thirds of the recommended level of iron.

Iron intake is generally related to energy intake; thus, older people with diets low in kilocalories are also likely to be low in iron. It appears, however, that older people may compensate for a lower energy intake by deliberately choosing foods high in nutrient density, including iron. Although the average American diet contains about 6 mg of iron per 1,000 kcal, participants in the Georgia Centenarian Study[27] had intakes of about 7 mg per 1,000 kcal, and the diets of healthy Arizona women[66] ages 75 and over contained 8 mg per 1,000 kcal.

Income can be a significant factor in iron intake. This could be expected since protein foods high in iron tend to be costly. In the NHANES II study,[33] older people who were eligible for food stamps but were not participating in the program had a mean iron intake of only 6.8 mg. Eating less meat can influence total iron intake and the bioavailability of all iron consumed. In a New Mexico survey[28] iron intakes from meat, fish, or poultry dropped from 2.7 mg to 1.9 mg between women ages 75 or younger and women ages 76 or older. Intakes in men of similar ages dropped from 3.4 mg to 3.0 mg. Nevertheless, older vegetarian women

in California[42] who consumed no meat had higher iron intakes than their nonvegetarian counterparts; 4% of the vegetarian women versus 7% of the nonvegetarian women consumed less than the RDA for iron.

Biochemical parameters indicate that many older people maintain appropriate iron status into advanced age. Among 69 independently living older adults in Arizona,[38] with a mean age of 80, only two individuals had erythrocyte counts below 3.5 trillion/liter, and only one woman and one man had hemoglobin concentrations indicative of deficiency (less than 12 g/dl for women and less than 14 g/dl for men). Ten of the subjects (14%) had low serum iron and transferrin saturation levels, but no one had a serum ferritin level below 20 ng/ml. Only one person consumed less than 67% of the RDA, but 22% of the subjects took supplements. An evaluation of health conscious older people in Paris[48] who ranged in age from 70 to 89 indicated that iron status was generally satisfactory, but some problems were detected. Mean levels of plasma iron, total iron-binding capacity, serum ferritin, and erythrocyte ferritin fell within normal ranges for both men and women. At the same time, iron deficiency was identified in 8.8% of the group. Iron status in these elderly people was similar to the young control subjects, except for the serum and erythrocyte ferritin levels which increased with age.

Iron status does differ in well-nourished versus poorly nourished older people. Elderly African Americans tend to have lower dietary iron levels than white elderly people of the same sex.[61] Among 186 very-low-income elderly African Americans in Washington, D.C.,[37] 48% of the men and 33% of the women had hemoglobin levels below established standards, and 23% had serum ferritin levels below 20 ng/ml. Forty-one percent of this group consumed less than the RDA for iron, and their level of intake was directly related to biochemical status. In addition to low intakes, these individuals also may have been consuming iron sources with low bioavailability. Their low body weight coupled with poor iron status suggested low food intake overall.

A comparison by Löwik and coworkers[35] of older omnivores and older vegetarians in the Netherlands suggests that heme iron plays an important role in maintaining appropriate iron status. All subjects in the Dutch study were at least age 65; the 44 vegetarians refrained from eating meat, fish, or poultry and had followed this practice for most of their adult lives. The vegetarians tended to have fewer erythrocytes, decreased transferrin saturation, and significantly lower serum ferritin levels compared to the omnivores. The vegetarians also were older, which may have contributed to these findings; however, the low serum ferritin levels suggest that, over time, iron absorption had been diminished.

Practical Aspects of Iron Intake

Many older people, even those on limited incomes, obtain a portion of their iron from animal foods. For low-income elderly people in Arizona,[66] 21% of their dietary iron was provided by flesh foods. Nonetheless, cereals are a popular food of older people at all income levels. How well the iron salts added to enriched and fortified cereal products are absorbed by older people with some degree of hypochlorhydria requires further study.

There is the potential for hemochromatosis in older people with excessive iron intakes or absorption. Manore and coworkers[38] reported a median iron intake of 27 mg among their supplement users age 75 and over. In Boston elderly people serum ferritin levels (and likely liver iron stores) were directly related to alcohol ingestion.[25] Serum ferritin levels increased dramatically with intakes of 15 g or more of alcohol a day. In the high alcohol users, one-fourth of the men had serum ferritin levels above 256 µg/L and one-fourth of the women had levels above 203 µg/L. Jacques and Russell[25] noted that alcohol may enhance iron absorption. Iron overload should be suspected when serum ferritin levels reach 300 µg/L.

Selenium

Selenium is a cofactor for glutathione peroxidase, an enzyme that, in concert with vitamin E, plays an important role in antioxidant function. Selenium deficiency in humans results in a degenerative disease of the myocardium that was identified in young people in areas of China where the soil is lacking in selenium. The RDA

for selenium, established in 1989, is 55 µg for women and 70 µg for men.[14]

Selenium Intake and Biochemical Levels

Little is known about the usual daily intake of selenium in the aging population. Based on the selenium content of analyzed food composites typical of the American diet, the intake of the average adult is estimated to be 108 µg per day;[14] however, the selenium content of individual food items is largely undetermined. In older British men and women[6] selenium intakes were 54 µg a day among those in good health who had a varied diet, and 38 µg a day among those in poor health who were housebound and dependent on others to bring their food. It does appear that older people can absorb selenium contained in food or in a yeast product. Apparent absorption from food was 57% of intake among the British elderly, regardless of health status. A study carried out with elderly people in Denmark[30] indicated that supplements of inorganic selenium can be absorbed and bring about a 30% increase in the levels of selenium-dependent glutathione peroxidase in both plasma and erythrocytes. No increase in enzyme levels occurred in the elderly control subjects.

The progressive decline in serum selenium levels and erythrocyte glutathione reductase levels after age 80 leads to serious questions about antioxidant function in advanced age.[30,36,43] At the same time the concentration of lipid peroxidation products in erythrocytes is about the same in young adults with higher plasma and erythrocyte selenium as in older adults with lower plasma and erythrocyte selenium, if compared on the basis of erythrocyte polyunsaturated fatty acids.[43] Serum selenium and serum glutathione reductase activity are lower and serum lipid peroxidation levels are higher in patients with chronic renal failure, especially those on hemodialysis.[34] Loughrey and coworkers[34] pointed out that selenium intake is likely to be low in patients on protein-restricted diets.

The major sources of dietary selenium are seafood (especially canned tuna) and liver, with lesser amounts in other meats, eggs, and grain products,[63] although the selenium content of grains is related to the selenium content of the soil in which they were grown. Because intake of grain products tends to be lower when kilocalories are reduced, the age-related decline in serum selenium levels observed in some older people could be, in part, the result of decreased food intake.

Requirement for Selenium

Current research has pointed to a possible involvement of selenium in immune function and in the development of atherosclerosis and cancer. The relationship between selenium status and cardiovascular disease or cancer is not consistent and may be influenced by vitamin E status.[71] Daily supplements of selenium at levels about two times the RDA increased the lymphocyte proliferation responses in older adults.[71] Further work is required to determine the long-term advantages of such supplementation. Buchman and coworkers[5] emphasized the need to monitor serum selenium levels in patients on tube feedings. Several of their patients required intakes of 100 µg to 200 µg of selenium daily to maintain appropriate serum selenium because of excessive urinary losses.

Zinc

Zinc is a cofactor for enzymes involved in DNA and protein synthesis and is essential for cell growth and repair. Because we lack sensitive indicators of zinc status, the evaluation of zinc nutriture among older people and the estimation of a daily requirement are uncertain.

Zinc Absorption and Metabolism

Controlled studies in older adults have produced mixed results about the effect of age on zinc absorption. Zinc absorption measured using stable isotopes was only 17% to 21% in older subjects as compared to 31% to 39% in younger subjects. When fed zinc-restricted diets, however, those older adults did retain the ability to increase the percentage of zinc absorbed.[71] Other food constituents present in the meal influence zinc absorption in adults of all ages. Couzy and coworkers[9] fed labeled zinc as part of a low- or high-availability test meal to eight older men ages 70 to 83 and nine younger men ages 24 to 40. The percent absorption

from the high-availability meal was 35% to 39% in the two groups with no significant differences. Absorption was lower, ranging from 20% to 23%, for both the younger men and the older men when given the low-availability meal containing phytates.

The differences in findings among studies could reflect differences in zinc status among the older people evaluated. Plasma zinc levels, currently used as a measure of zinc status, lack sensitivity in identifying marginal status. Endogenous losses of zinc are lower in older adults; thus, lower absorption could be a response to a lower requirement.[71] Older men have a reduced amount of lean body mass, lower exercise levels, and lower ejaculation frequency, which could lower the requirement. A current gap in the literature is information regarding zinc absorption in older women. In older people in poor health, chronic negative nitrogen balance contributes to endogenous zinc loss.[6]

The effect of added calcium in a meal on zinc bioavailability remains controversial. In postmenopausal women increased calcium (about 470 mg) consumed as 400 ml of fluid milk or as a calcium supplement did not reduce zinc absorption or retention on a diet supplying 16 mg of zinc.[72] It is important to note, however, that this diet supplied a liberal level of zinc (the RDA for women is 12 mg), well above average intakes. Effects may differ on diets marginal in zinc. This will continue to be an important issue as older women are encouraged to increase their intakes of calcium to maintain bone health.

Zinc Intake and Biochemical Parameters

Zinc intake often falls below the RDA of 15 mg for men and 12 mg for women. Median intakes of people age 60 and over, estimated from dietary records obtained in the NHANES II study,[65] ranged from 5.6 mg to 9.4 mg. Age, sex, ethnic group, and income influence dietary zinc. Zinc intakes declined from 12.9 mg a day in the men ages 60 to 69 to 10.8 mg in those ages 80 and over in a population of economically advantaged Boston elderly.[51] Comparable intakes among the women in that study were 10.6 mg and 10 mg. In a nationwide study including all income levels,[50] 50% of both the men and women over age 74 consumed less than two-thirds of the RDA for zinc. African American and Mexican American elderly are particularly vulnerable to zinc deficiency. Median intakes measured in the NHANES III study[61] ranged from 7 mg to 8.7 mg among the men, and from 5.2 mg to 6.9 mg among the women. When comparing these values to their respective RDAs of 15 mg and 12 mg, it is apparent that about half of older African American and Mexican American elderly are consuming no more than 50% of the RDA. Zinc intake of patients in a long-term care facility based on chemical analysis of the diet was found to be 5.5 mg.[52]

Dietary zinc is influenced by total energy intake and increases proportionately as total kilocalories increase. Older men with energy intakes of 1,800 kcal consume about 10.6 mg of zinc. Older women consuming about 1,300 kcal take in about 7.2 mg of zinc (60% of the RDA).[53] Those with low energy intakes can compensate by selecting foods rich in zinc. In the Boston Nutritional Status Survey 26% of the dietary zinc was contributed by meat and 16% was contributed by dairy products.[58] But the most common source of zinc in the American diet is beef, a relatively expensive item in the food budget. Legumes and whole-grain products are rich in zinc, although it is present in a less bioavailable form. Diets emphasizing highly processed breads and cereals and poultry will be limited in zinc.[57] Older vegetarian women in California[42] who avoided meat, fish, and poultry had mean zinc intakes of only 6.2 mg.

In light of the relatively low zinc intakes of many older people, zinc deficiency, defined on the basis of serum zinc, is not as common as one would expect. In the Boston study[69] low serum zinc levels (below 11 μmol/L) were few in number, despite zinc intakes well below the RDA. On the other hand, 30% of elderly living in a New Jersey community[4] had low serum zinc levels. Older Dutch vegetarians[35] had significantly lower serum zinc levels than omnivores similar in age (fig. 7-3). Older people who avoid flesh foods, regardless of reason, may be at greater risk of poor zinc status based on the reduced bioavailability associated with other food sources of zinc.[24]

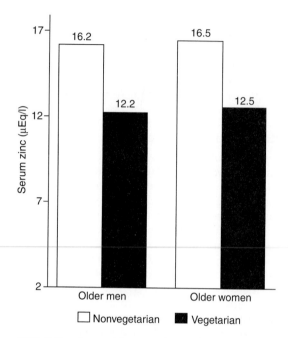

FIG. 7-3　Serum Zinc Levels in Older Vegetarians and Omnivores. Vegetarian men and women ages 65 and over have lower serum zinc levels than omnivores of the same sex, age, and geographic region.

Data from Löwik, M.R.H., and others: Long-term effects of a vegetarian diet on the nutritional status of elderly people (Dutch Nutrition Surveillance System), J. Am. Coll. Nutr. 9:18 and 600, 1990.

Suspicions that marginal zinc status is widespread among the elderly population cannot be confirmed or refuted because definitive indicators of zinc status are lacking. Bales and coworkers[3] fed healthy older volunteers with normal plasma zinc a low zinc diet (about 4 mg) for 15 days and then a high zinc diet (about 28 mg) for six days. Plasma zinc and erythrocyte metallothionein levels (metallothionein is a zinc protein complex) were unchanged throughout the study, suggesting that the period of depletion and repletion was too short to bring about observable changes. Plasma levels of the zinc-dependent enzyme 5-nucleotidase did fall sharply and rise rapidly through the depletion and repletion phases and may hold promise as an indicator of zinc status. Among the healthy New Jersey subjects described earlier,[4] 12 months of daily supplementation with 15 mg of zinc failed to raise their serum zinc levels below 11 μmol/L to the normal range. The relationship between zinc intake and zinc status, especially as related to plasma zinc levels, requires further study.

Zinc Status and Metabolic Function

Zinc plays a key role in several important functions of particular concern in older people. Wound healing, taste acuity, and immune function are altered in classic zinc deficiency. Alternatively, there is no convincing evidence that zinc supplementation above recommended levels will reverse age-related changes in these functions. Wound-healing is improved in malnourished elderly patients who are given physiologic levels of zinc; wound-healing is not improved in older people whose zinc status was adequate prior to supplementation.[53]

An area of current research is the effect of zinc supplementation on immune function. A well-controlled study carried out with community living older people between the ages of 60 and 89[4] indicated that zinc supplements of 100 mg a day exerted a transient improvement in natural killer cell function, but depressed delayed hypersensitivity immune function. Individuals receiving 15 mg of zinc per day showed some increase in delayed hypersensitivity immune function if their baseline measures had indicated marginal deficiency. These researchers concluded that older people should avoid supplements containing high levels of zinc.

Zinc supplements in excess have been associated with other deleterious effects in addition to the observed effect on immune function. Supplements providing 50 mg to 75 mg a day lower HDL-cholesterol levels in younger people and may have a similar effect in older people.[71] In insulin-dependent diabetics given a daily supplement of 50 mg of zinc,[10] glucose control worsened and glycosylated hemoglobin levels increased. Older people should be cautioned against self-medication with zinc.

Copper

Copper is a component of several important proteins and enzymes and is essential for erythropoiesis. The Food and Nutrition Board recommends 1.5 mg to 3 mg a day as an estimated safe and adequate daily dietary intake for adults (ESADDI). Current data suggest that average intakes fall below this amount, with men averaging 1.2 mg and women 0.9 mg a day.[14]

Poor copper status is more likely the result of low intake rather than poor absorption or retention. August and coworkers[2] studied young and elderly men and women given natural food diets containing about 3 mg of copper. Absorption levels were 60% in the younger subjects and 53% in the older ones. Moreover, the older individuals increased their rate of absorption to 67% when given a diet low in copper (about 0.5 mg). Healthy British elderly people[6] on self-selected diets were able to maintain copper balance on intakes of 1.28 mg.

It is of interest that older vegetarian women in California[42] had significantly higher copper intakes than older nonvegetarian women (1.42 mg versus 0.99 mg a day). Copper intakes of older New Jersey men and women[4] ranged from 1.05 mg to 1.38 mg a day, respectively. Organ meats, nuts, seeds, and legumes are good sources of copper.

Milne and Neilsen[41] observed 12 postmenopausal women fed a low copper diet for four months and called for a reevaluation of copper status in humans. In those women no changes in plasma copper, ceruloplasmin, or cholesterol levels were observed in spite of copper depletion. In contrast, platelet cytochrome C oxidase and erythrocyte glutathione oxidase levels responded dramatically to copper depletion with a rapid fall as depletion progressed and a slow increase when copper intake was increased. Intakes above 2 mg daily were necessary to restore copper status to optimum levels. Animal studies[73] suggest that high intakes of iron can depress copper absorption. In view of the widespread use of iron supplements by elderly people for whom copper intake may be marginal, attention to the evaluation of sensitive indicators of copper status is warranted.

Manganese

Manganese is a component of several mitochondrial metalloenzymes and is found in most edible plants; thus, deficiency among people with access to plant foods is unknown. The ESADDI for adults is 2 mg to 5 mg.[14] Gibson and coworkers[17] determined the manganese intakes of 90 noninstitutionalized Canadian women ranging in age from 58 to 89 years. Those researchers chemically analyzed 24-hour duplicate diet composites collected by the subjects. Median manganese intake was 3.5 mg, although there were intakes as low as 1.6 mg and as high as 11 mg. Because of the limited database describing the manganese content of common foods, it was surprising that the mean manganese intake as determined by chemical analysis (3.8 mg) was about the same as the intakes calculated from the food records for that day (3.9 mg).

The manganese intakes of these Canadian women[17] are about twofold higher than those of older vegetarian women[42] and threefold higher than those of older nonvegetarian women[42] studied in California. The vegetarian women had a mean intake of 2.18 mg, barely adequate under current standards, and the nonvegetarian women had a mean intake of 1.25 mg, considerably below the recommended range of 2 to 5 mg. Whole-grain bread and cereal products, the best sources of manganese, tend to be consumed in low amounts by some older women, although fruits and vegetables also contribute manganese to the diet. The higher intakes of the Canadian women[17] may have been due in part to their high consumption of tea; median intake was 1.5 cups, or 360 ml a day. Tea is high in manganese, containing approximately 1.1 mg per 500 ml. Excessive iron intakes can interfere with manganese absorption.

Chromium

Chromium is essential for maintaining normal glucose and lipid metabolism; it facilitates the interaction of insulin with the receptor site on the cell membrane.[14] Based on this relationship with insulin, chromium status has been associated with glucose tolerance. Because tissue chromium concentrations decline with increasing age and parallel the gradual deterioration in glucose tolerance that often occurs in later adulthood, the chromium status of older people as related to impaired glucose tolerance and the onset of diabetes mellitus has been a topic of interest. Unfortunately, this relationship is still unclear.

Chromium Absorption

Chromium absorption is low in all age groups. In 22 apparently healthy older people on self-selected diets, mean absorption appeared to be 2% to 3% of dietary intake.[6] Mean daily intakes were 30 µg in men and 20 µg in women. Despite their low intakes, 20 of the 22 participants were in chromium balance. Diets very high in fiber contribute to chromium losses in older people.

Chromium Intake

The ESADDI for chromium is 50 µg to 200 µg per day.[14] Because data on the chromium content of foods are scarce, evaluation of dietary intake requires chemical analyses of food composites. Older Canadian women[17] had chromium intakes ranging from 21 µg to 274 µg per day with a mean of 96 µg; nevertheless, 22% of the women consumed less than 50 µg and 7% consumed more than 200 µg. The women in the latter group were consuming high amounts of tea reported to be a good source of chromium. Other food sources include brewer's yeast, liver, potatoes, oysters, whole-grain bread and cereal products, cheese, and chicken. The milling of grain products results in the loss of almost 90% of the chromium. Based on available studies of chromium intake in adults of all ages, an individual would need to consume about 3,000 kcal a day to obtain the suggested intake of 50 µg.[71] In the NHANES III study,[62] median energy intakes for people ages 60 to 69 were about 1,900 kcal in men and about 1,500 kcal in women. Median intakes fell to 1,700 kcal and 1,300 kcal, respectively, in people over age 79. Based on this finding, the majority of older people will not be able to obtain the suggested level of chromium from food alone. Wood and coworkers,[71] in their extensive review of mineral requirements for the elderly, urged that the chromium recommendation be reconsidered in the next revision of the RDAs.

Chromium Status, Glucose Tolerance, and Lipid Metabolism

The relationship between chromium status and glucose metabolism in older people remains unclear. Although some researchers have observed an improvement in glucose tolerance following chromium supplementation in the range of 200 μg a day, this is not always the case.[71] The inconsistency in observations likely relates to the individuals being studied. Elderly people who are deficient in chromium may demonstrate an improvement in glucose tolerance as chromium status improves, whereas those with appropriate levels of body chromium may not. Whether or not chromium supplements exert a pharmacological effect on glucose metabolism has not been established. Chromium may play a role in lipid metabolism as chromium supplements of 250 μg a day reduced very low density lipoprotein (VLDL) cholesterol and increased HDL cholesterol in healthy older subjects.[71] Further studies with well-nourished older people that include young control subjects are required to answer these questions.

Fluoride

Fluoride is not classified as an essential element, although it does support optimum mineral crystallization in bones and teeth. Epidemiologic comparisons of people living in areas with high or low levels of naturally occurring fluoride in the soil or drinking water point to a positive effect of fluoride in maintaining bone density and decreasing dental caries. Large bone crystals that develop in the presence of fluoride are less susceptible to resorption than smaller crystals. The potential toxicity of fluoride, however, has limited its use in treating bone disorders (see chapter 12). The ESADDI for fluoride is 1.5 mg to 4 mg per day.[14] Fluoridation of public drinking water is recommended when natural fluoride levels are low.

WATER AND ELECTROLYTES

Water and the principal electrolytes (potassium, sodium, and chloride) are supplied to the body through the diet. Water balance and electrolyte concentrations in body fluids and tissues can be altered through disordered control mechanisms or chronic disease.

Potassium

Potassium is the principal intracellular cation, and about 98% of body potassium is in the cell.[14] Plasma potassium is carefully controlled, since fluctuations affect the transmission of nerve impulses, the control of blood pressure, and the contraction of muscles, including the heart.

Potassium Absorption and Metabolism

Potassium is well absorbed at a level of 90% or more,[14] and there is no evidence to suggest less than adequate absorption at older ages. The kidneys regulate potassium concentration in the extracellular fluid. The kidneys can both reabsorb and secrete potassium ions and are capable of reabsorbing up to 95% of the potassium in the glomerular filtrate. If this degree of potassium reabsorption were continuous, toxic and eventually lethal levels of potassium would accumulate.

The reabsorption and secretion of potassium ions is controlled by two different feedback systems: 1) a rise in potassium levels in the extracellular fluid triggers an increase in tubular potassium secretion, and 2) an increase in aldosterone secretion indirectly increases potassium excretion, because the reabsorption of a sodium ion in the renal distal tubule results in the secretion of a potassium ion. Both low-sodium concentrations and high-potassium concentrations in the extracellular fluid stimulate the secretion of aldosterone by the adrenal cortex which initiates increased sodium reabsorption and potassium excretion by the kidneys. Age-related changes in kidney function and use of certain drugs can alter potassium balance in older adults.[32]

Serum potassium levels are closely maintained between 3.5 mmol/l and 5 mmol/l.[40] Replacing daily fecal and renal losses of potassium requires an intake of 1,600 mg to 2,000 mg (40 to 50 mmol). On low intakes of only 800 mg (20 mmol), metabolic equilibrium is maintained at the expense of body stores, and potassium plasma levels may fall below 4 mmol/l.[14] Because increased levels of dietary potassium are believed to be beneficial in controlling blood pressure, the Committee on Diet and Health convened by the National Research Council[56] recommended five or more servings a day of vegetables and fruits, especially green and yellow vegetables and citrus fruits, which will provide about 3,500 mg (90 mmol) of potassium.

Potassium Intake

Potassium intake varies widely, depending on an individual's food habits. The richest sources of dietary potassium are fruits and vegetables, and individuals who consume large amounts of these foods may have intakes from 8,000 mg to 11,000 mg a day.[14] Conversely, potassium in-takes among older people can be rather low. In the NHANES III study,[61] median potassium intakes of men and women ages 60 to 69 were 2,861 mg and 2,422 mg, respectively. Median intakes decreased to 2,456 mg and 2,129 mg in those ages 80 and older. Potassium intake is particularly low among older African American and Mexican American women whose median intakes ranged from 1,585 mg to 1,888 mg. Education and possibly income influence the use of potassium-rich foods: older women with at least one year of college consumed about 500 mg more potassium a day than women from the same community who had 12 years or less of school.[22] All of these women lived alone. Overall, the women consumed on the average 19 servings of fruits a week and 21 servings of vegetables.

The centenarians living in the community who participated in the Georgia study[27] had 16 servings of fruit a week and 23 servings of vegetables. Vegetables eaten each week included six servings of green and yellow vegetables, three servings of tomatoes, and one serving of carrots. In the American diet fruits and vegetables contribute 38% of the potassium, and dairy foods contribute 21%.[65] Older people should be encouraged to have at least five servings a day from the fruit and vegetable group. Increased use of dairy foods would add both calcium and potassium to the diet.

Potassium Deficiency and Toxicity

Hypokalemia. Hypokalemia is defined as a decreased level of potassium in the blood, falling below 3.5 mmol/l. It can result from inadequate potassium intake, but the most common cause is the use of loop diuretics such as furosemide or thiazide diuretics. About 20% of patients receiving thiazide diuretics develop hypokalemia.[40] Potassium depletion can occur in older people with severely compromised kidney function for whom potassium losses may exceed 20 mmol (800 mg) a day. Hypersecretion of aldosterone, increasing renal reabsorption of sodium at the expense of potassium, will lead to excessive potassium excretion. Potassium can be lost in large amounts through the chronic use of laxatives or bouts of diarrhea. Vomiting not only reduces food intake but also results in the loss of gastric acid. This loss of gastric acid and hydrogen ions can produce a metabolic alkalosis that causes potassium to move from the extracellular fluids into the cell, thus seriously reducing serum potassium levels. In diabetic acidosis, potassium moves out of the cell and into the extracellular fluid and is subsequently lost in the urine.[40] Magnesium depletion can lead to hypokalemia.[32] Low potassium intake will exacerbate the potassium depletion associated with any of these conditions.

Serum potassium levels below 3.5 mmol/l can affect several organ systems. Changes in the resting membrane potential and excitability of nerves and muscles can lead to cardiac arrhythmias, deterioration in glucose tolerance, disorientation and confusion, decreased motility of the gastrointestinal tract, inability of the kidney to concentrate urine, and muscle weakness and cramps.[32] Susceptibility to digoxin intoxication increases in potassium deficiency.[40] Also, potassium appears to have a protective effect in reducing the hypertensive action of sodium. Unfortunately, hypokalemia can go unnoticed, since many of these clinical signs tend to be associated with aging and older patients in general.

The relative prevalence of hypokalemia and the advisability of potassium-sparing diuretics or potassium supplementation of older people on loop or thiazide diuretics remains unsettled.[32] The major argument for using potassium supplements is to prevent losses in total body potassium. Follow-up studies of diuretic users over several years, however, revealed no changes in total body potassium. Moreover, when potassium supplements were provided to patients who were losing body potassium, they had no effect. Lindeman and Beck[32] were convinced that foods rich in potassium can prevent a potassium deficiency in people using thiazide or loop diuretics. When low serum potassium levels are accompanied by a metabolic alkalosis, potassium chloride is the appropriate supplement, since chloride is also required to correct the problem.

Hyperkalemia. Hyperkalemia, or an elevated level of potassium in the blood, is characterized by a serum potassium level greater than 5 mmol/l. Usually, total body potassium is normal but its distribution between the intracellular and extracellular compartments is abnormal.[40] Hyperkalemia is most commonly associated with impaired kidney function with decreased urinary excretion of potassium. Inappropriate use of potassium supplements, use of potassium-sparing diuretics such as triamterene that cause retention of potassium, or use of other potassium-containing drugs such as penicillin can contribute to this condition. Metabolic or respiratory acidosis, especially diabetic ketoacidosis, results in a small shift in potassium from the cells into the blood and a marked elevation in serum potassium.[40]

Reduced secretion of aldosterone leading to enhanced reabsorption of potassium occurs in older people and results in higher potassium retention. Older individuals with both compromised kidney function and reduced secretion of aldosterone are more susceptible to hyperkalemia when given potassium supplements than are younger people. In the Boston Collaborative Drug Surveillance Program, overseeing 16,000 patients, fewer than 1% of the 1,404 patients under age 50 developed hyperkalemia as compared to about 6% of those over 50.[32] Early symptoms of hyperkalemia are muscle weakness and apprehension; however, cardiac arrhythmias and cardiac arrest can occur with little prior warning. Older individuals taking potassium supplements or using potassium-sparing diuretics require regular monitoring of their serum potassium levels.

Sodium

Sodium intakes of all age groups are receiving increasing attention based on the fact that diets high in sodium are associated in some individuals with elevated blood pressure.[14] Although sensitivity to sodium-induced hypertension is genetically related, we have no way to identify these individuals; thus, it is appropriate for all adults to use some discretion in limiting their sodium intake since it carries no risk for the general population.[14]

Sodium Homeostasis and Requirement

Sodium is the principal cation in the extracellular fluid and is important in the regulation of extracellular fluid volume. Excessive sodium retention increases fluid retention with a possible rise in blood pressure and edema. Sodium excretion is controlled primarily by the renin-angiotensin-aldosterone system.[44] This system, which is activated in response to either a drop in blood pressure or decreased sodium concentration in the filtrate in the renal tubule, stimulates the renal tubule to increase sodium reabsorption. The kidneys can reabsorb as much as 99% of the sodium in the glomerular filtrate.[14] When dietary sodium levels are high, aldosterone secretion is low, and more sodium is excreted. When sodium intake is low, aldosterone secretion rises and sodium excretion can be reduced to almost zero.

Older individuals appear to be less able to adapt to changes in sodium intake and to conserve sodium when necessary. Both circulating renin and aldosterone levels are decreased by 30% to 50% in older people, and this may influence both the time sequence and the degree of response to a change in sodium level. Because secretion of aldosterone can be increased with administration of adrenal-stimulating hormones, the reduced aldosterone secretion in response to a lower sodium intake likely relates to a defect in renin secretion or metabolism and not the adrenal gland.[44]

Sodium conservation and loss is also controlled by the atrial natriuretic peptide. This hormone, secreted by the heart, acts to decrease water and sodium reabsorption in the kidneys, counteracting the action of the renin-angiotensin-aldosterone system. Both basal blood levels of atrial natriuretic peptide and blood levels after stimulation of the volume receptors are increased in older people.[40] Based on the older person's impaired ability to respond to major changes in sodium levels, it is judicious to avoid either extreme sodium restriction or administration of a sodium load.

Obligatory sodium losses are estimated to be 5 mmol (115 mg) a day.[14] The safe minimum daily intake established by the Food and Nutrition Board is 500 mg. The Committee on Diet and Health recommends that all people limit their sodium intake to 2,400 mg, or 6,000 mg of salt.[56] Sodium chloride, or table salt, is 40% sodium by weight, and 1 teaspoon of salt (5 g) contains 2,000 mg of sodium.

Sodium Intake

Estimates of sodium intake in the general population range from 4 g to 5.8 g (10 g to 14.5 g of sodium chloride).[14] In the United States a major source of sodium is sodium chloride, or table salt. A British study[56] concluded that only 10% of dietary sodium was naturally present in food, and only 15% came from salt added at home, either in cooking or at the table; 75% came from salt or other sodium-containing additives used in food processing and manufacturing. This finding has important implications for elderly people who, because of physical disability or living situation, are dependent on preprepared food items. Also, food items fairly popular among older age groups—grain products, including bread, rolls, and crackers, and processed meats such as hot dogs and luncheon meats—were the two highest contributors of dietary sodium in the general population evaluated in the NHANES II study.[56]

Because individuals find it difficult to estimate the amount of salt they add in cooking and at the table, most surveys report sodium intake based on food composition tables, the amount of table salt in standard recipes for mixed dishes, and information on sodium content of processed foods provided by food manufacturers. Sodium intakes do decrease with age, which may relate to dietary advice given to older people being treated for cardiovascular disease, hypertension, or diabetes mellitus. In the NHANES III study,[61] median sodium intakes were 4,126 mg in men ages 20 to 29 and only 3,140 mg and 2,278 mg at ages 60 to 69 and 80 and older, respectively. Women appear to consume less sodium at all ages with intakes of 2,759 mg at ages 20 to 29, and 2,379 mg and 2,172 mg at ages 60 to 69 and 80 and older.

Older African American men consume lower levels of sodium than older white men.[61] African American men ages 60 to 69 had median sodium intakes of 2,490 mg which dropped to 1,739 mg at older ages. Older Mexican American men had sodium intakes about midway between the older African American men and the older white men. Older African American and Mexican American women consumed about 300 mg less of sodium per day than their white counterparts. In all of these populations it is likely that true sodium intake, which includes salt added at the table, sodium in drinking water, and sodium in medications, is actually higher. In general, older women appear more likely than older men to fall within the recommended level of 2,400 mg.

Sodium Depletion and Retention

Hyponatremia. Hyponatremia, a below-normal concentration of sodium in the blood, is more likely to occur in older people than in younger people. A serum sodium concentration below normal can result from an excessive loss of sodium through the kidney, retention of water in excess of retained sodium, or a combination of both.[32] For the most part older kidneys retain the ability to conserve sodium and maintain serum sodium concentrations in the normal range. But excessive amounts of diuretics can lead to depleted volumes of both sodium and water. Depleted fluid volume stimulates the secretion of antidiuretic hormone (ADH) and the subsequent reabsorption of water in the renal tubule to restore fluid volume to normal. If sodium loss continues as water is being replaced, hyponatremia ensues.[32] Older adults appear to become increasingly sensitive to serum osmolality and may secrete increased and inappropriate levels of ADH, leading to water retention and dilution of the sodium concentration in extracellular fluids.[44] Chronically ill older people who are taking a number of prescription drugs have a higher prevalence of hyponatremia. Hyperglycemia, causing a shift of water from the intracellular space to dilute the glucose-related hyperosmolality, leads to hyponatremia. Vomiting and chronic diarrhea cause abnormal sodium loss. Muscle cramps, mental impairment, confusion, and seizures resulting from fluid retention and pressure in the brain are the major symptoms of serious hyponatremia. Extremely low serum sodium levels can result in sudden death.[32]

Hypernatremia. An increase in serum sodium concentration is more likely related to insufficient intake of fluids than excessive water loss.[40] Hypernatremia is most common in frail, chronically ill older people who are unable to drink without help. An increase in serum sodium concentration is a powerful stimulator of the thirst mechanism, so older people with access to water are less likely to develop serious hypernatremia. A derangement in central nervous system function can blunt the thirst mechanism.[45] Continued vomiting or diarrhea causes significant loss of body water, as does an extremely elevated body temperature with excessive sweating. Among hospitalized elderly people, hypernatremia is associated with pneumonia and fever, highly concentrated nutritional supplements following surgery, and glycosuria in poorly controlled diabetes.[32] Age-related changes in the ability of the kidneys to conserve water contributes to this condition. Hypernatremia is characterized by thirst and confusion in the early stages, progressing to delirium and coma as water moves from the brain cells into the vascular space.

Fluid Balance in the Older Adult

Water is the most abundant constituent in the human body. It accounts for about 60% of body weight in young adults and decreases to about 50% in older adults (see chapter 5). Because the body cannot store water, fluid must be replaced daily. Normal daily body water turnover is estimated to be 4% of body weight.[47] Fluid replacement may be especially critical for the older adult in whom total available body water is reduced. It was believed that the loss of body water over adult life was related to the loss of body muscle, high in water content; however, a longitudinal study[47] of healthy adults between the ages of 70 and 81 found the body water lost over that period came from the extracellular fluid compartment. Reiff[47] suggested that the decline in body water involves not only the loss of cells but also some decline in water content in existing cells as a result of changes in cell proteins and osmotic relationships.

Fluid intake. Fluid is supplied to the body in the form of water and other liquids, in foods, and as water of oxidation. In younger people the thirst mechanism tends to ensure an adequate fluid intake, but, as noted earlier, a diminished sensitivity to dehydration reduces fluid intake in older adults. The physically impaired or seriously ill individual who cannot drink without help is particularly vulnerable to low fluid intake. Those subject to incontinence may consciously restrict fluid intake to avoid embarrassment.

Among older adults participating in the National Food Consumption Survey,[60] intakes of liquids differed according to age and sex. Nonalcoholic liquid intake calculated from coffee, tea, soda, fluid milk, juices, and fruit drinks totalled 3.9 cups and 3.5 cups in the men and women ages 65 to 74, respectively. Liquid intake fell to 3.6 cups in the men ages 75 and over and to 3.3 cups in the women of that age. However, these values do not include the plain water consumed by these older people. Also, other foods and the water derived from the complete oxidation of carbohydrates, fats, and proteins contribute to fluid intake. Fruits and vegetables, for example, contain 85% to 95% water by weight.[14] The water of oxidation supplied by a 2,000 kcal diet is about 250 ml.[14] Unfortunately, current and accurate data regarding the fluid intake of older people are generally not available from nutrition surveys. Fluid intake is an important consideration in the nutritional well-being of older people, but it has not been evaluated on a routine basis.

Fluid requirement. The water requirement of an adult is influenced by many factors. About half of the fluid to be replaced each day is lost through the lungs and skin (insensible water loss). These losses are increased in environments with high ambient temperatures or dry air, in physical exercise, or when body temperature is increased as in febrile illness. Loss of fluid in the feces is limited under normal conditions but escalates dramatically in diarrhea. The water required to handle the solute load excreted through the kidneys varies according to diet composition. The breakdown products of protein metabolism, primarily urea but also sulfates and phosphates, are a major factor in the amount of water required for urine formation.

The Food and Nutrition Board[14] recommends 1 ml of water per kilocalorie as a general guideline for water consumption; others suggest a minimum intake of 1,500 ml a day. Because water intoxication is less likely to occur, the specified requirement often is increased to 1.5 ml/kcal to allow for individual variations in activity level, insensible water loss, and urinary solute load. Older adults are more vulnerable to dehydration as a result of less efficient kidney function, drugs that increase water loss, and reduced thirst sensation. On this basis they should be encouraged to raise their fluid intake to about 2,000 ml daily[7] unless this is contraindicated by particular cardiac or renal conditions necessitating fluid restriction.

Regulation of fluid balance. Water and sodium homeostasis are interrelated and require a balance between intake and output. Intake is controlled by the thirst mechanism and the appetite for sodium. The excretion of both water and sodium is handled by the kidneys. Alterations in both the thirst mechanism and the kidneys' ability to conserve water predispose older adults to problems in fluid balance.

Excretion of water by the kidneys is controlled by ADH (also known as vasopressin) secreted by the posterior lobe of the pituitary gland. ADH is secreted in response to increased osmolality of the extracellular fluid acting on osmoreceptors in the hypothalamus and decreased blood volume and blood pressure acting on receptors in the major arteries. An immediate action of ADH is to conserve water by increasing water reabsorption in the renal tubule. Under normal circumstances this leads to an increase in urine solute concentration and a decrease in urine flow. However, aging kidneys cannot concentrate solute and conserve water to the extent possible at younger ages. Consequently, an older person requires a larger amount of water than a younger person to excrete the same solute load. In some older people osmoreceptor sensitivity appears to be enhanced and ADH secretion increased above the levels in younger adults.[44] Increased ADH secretion in response

to osmotic stimuli or other factors increases the risk of hyponatremia, especially in the case of high fluid intake; this reaction is sometimes referred to as the syndrome of inappropriate secretion of antidiuretic hormone.[40] At the same time, some older people have low levels of ADH despite higher levels of plasma osmolality, suggesting that they have established a different set point for body fluid and electrolyte concentration.[13]

Impaired thirst. A physiologic change that significantly influences fluid homeostasis in older people is altered thirst. Medical textbooks over the years have pointed out that older patients do not ask for fluids.[49] Research studies with healthy older men (ages 67 to 75) and healthy young controls (ages 20 to 31) have confirmed a blunting of the thirst mechanism.[49] After 24 hours of water deprivation, resulting in about a 2% loss in body weight in both groups, the older subjects still experienced little thirst, whereas the younger subjects were extremely thirsty.

A major concern was the response of the older men when unlimited amounts of water were made available to them. The older individuals consumed only 3.4 ml per kg of body weight, whereas the younger subjects consumed 8.5 ml per kg of body weight (fig. 7-4).[49] In other words, the younger men consumed the amount of fluid required to raise their plasma volume to predeprivation levels. The older subjects did not replace the water they had lost in spite of a significant increase in plasma sodium concentration, which normally stimulates thirst. The young men had very little increase in plasma sodium yet experienced strong thirst. Older people are less able to measure serum osmolality and appropriate fluid replacement levels, leading to chronic dehydration in even healthy elderly.

Several physiologic and hormonal systems could contribute to changes in thirst and fluid regulation.[46] First, the osmoreceptors that respond to dehydration in the cell, and the baroreceptors that respond to changes in plasma volume may be less sensitive. The renin-angiotensin-aldosterone activity decreases with age, and angiotensin II is thought to be a strong

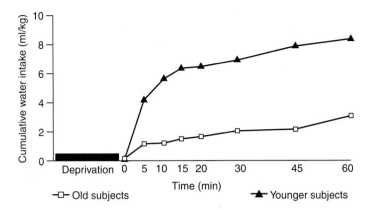

FIG. 7-4   Cumulative Water Intake of Younger and Older Men Following Water Deprivation. Because the thirst mechanism is impaired in older adults, older men as compared to younger men do not consume enough water to replace body losses following a period of water deprivation.

Adapted with permission from Phillips, P.A., and others: Reduced thirst after water deprivation in healthy elderly men, New Engl. J. Med. 311:753, 1984. © 1984 Massachusetts Medical Society. All rights reserved.

stimulant of thirst. The age-related increase in level of atrial natriuretic peptide contributes to diminished thirst, since this peptide not only inhibits renin but also directly inhibits thirst. Decreased sensations of thirst may also involve changes in the brain and hypothalamus which control the translation of these messages. Fluid consumption that stimulates the pharyngeal receptors in the mouth causes an immediate fall in plasma ADH in young men even though the water consumed has not been absorbed yet into the vascular system. This response does not occur in elderly men.[46] As mentioned in chapter 4, taste sensitivity is also altered in advanced age, suggesting a disruption in the nerve pathways from the oral cavity to the brain. The disordered thirst response also has serious implications for temperature regulation and the ability to handle heat stress. Sweating, a usual means of lowering body temperature, also is less effective in older people.

Dehydration in the older adult. The older person's inability to recognize the need for fluid, coupled with limited access to water in some situations, increases the risk of serious dehydration with significant consequences.

Body water is a diluent for medications, and a dehydrated individual is more vulnerable to drug toxicity. Temperature regulation is less efficient with a decreased level of body water to act as a thermal buffer. Consequently, older people living in hot, humid conditions are more susceptible to heat stroke.

Physical signs of dehydration include dry tongue, flushing, reduced turgor of the skin, and, as the condition increases in severity, confusion or delirium. Serum sodium and blood urea nitrogen levels usually are elevated. Among 339 nursing home residents,[31] 103 were determined to be dehydrated based on elevated serum sodium and an elevated ratio of blood urea nitrogen to creatinine. Dehydrated patients were most likely to be women, over age 85, and bedridden with several chronic conditions requiring various medications. Use of laxatives was a risk factor for severe dehydration. Those needing assistance with feeding or drinking were 11 times more likely to be dehydrated than those able to feed themselves. This suggests a need for a dietary prescription for fluids among those needing constant care, whether institutionalized or at home.

❖ ❖ ❖

CASE STUDY

Mr. J is a 68-year-old retired man who lives with his wife who prepares all of their meals. He has a history of high blood pressure. Mr. J had a stroke several months ago and is recovering well, but currently has minimal use of his arms. His diet is fairly well balanced but approximately 30% of his energy intake is coming from animal protein foods. He is not on medication for his blood pressure nor has he been checking it as instructed by his doctor. He makes no attempt to avoid salt or sodium in his diet although before his stroke he was able to lower his blood pressure by reducing his sodium intake.

1. Could his stroke have been related to his history of high blood pressure? Defend your answer.
2. What additional information related to food and mineral intake and fluid balance would you want to have before counseling Mr. J? Would it be important to assess his current medications? Why?
3. Is his protein intake appropriate? How could his protein intake influence his high blood pressure? Would you recommend a change in his protein intake? If so, what recommendation would you give?
4. Are there any risks associated with a severe reduction in dietary sodium? Explain.
5. Outline the teaching program you would use for Mr. J. Include in your outline behavioral changes you would recommend, foods to avoid with appropriate substitutes, and foods to include. Explain why you are making specific recommendations.

Dehydration has been reported in older individuals receiving tube feedings high in protein (1 g per kg of body wt). Chernoff[8] recommends a fluid intake of 30 ml per kg of body weight or a fluid level that is 125% of the volume of the formula for patients given this level of protein. When dehydration has been reported in patients receiving tube feedings, total fluid intake was about 2 l per day and the onset of dehydration was gradual. To rehydrate older individuals with chronic dehydration, 600 ml to 1,200 ml of fluid to replace insensible water loss will be needed.[8] When a patient has been vomiting or having diarrhea, it may be necessary to provide 2.5 l to 4 l of fluid to replace the water lost.

The prevalence of dehydration among older people at home is unknown, although the finding that laxatives predispose chronically ill older people to dehydration emphasizes the need to educate healthy older people about appropriate amounts of fluid. Reduced fluid intake exacerbates a constipation problem and puts a greater burden on the kidneys, particularly among those with high intakes of protein and electrolytes. Individuals who have problems with mobility may consciously restrict their fluid intake to avoid frequent trips to the bathroom, particularly if they must ask for help or climb stairs. Food records and diet histories used in nutrition counseling should include water intake as well as intakes of other fluids.

Summary

The roles of the essential minerals in maintaining the health and well-being of older people are receiving increasing attention. The macrominerals (e.g., calcium, phosphorus, magnesium) are vital for maintaining the structural integrity of the bones as well as a number of metabolic functions. The dietary requirements for the macrominerals are controversial. The NIH Consensus Statement recommends a calcium intake above the current RDA for all adults. Recent evidence suggests that the RDA for magnesium may be too high. The absorption and metabolism of most minerals are unchanged as a consequence of increasing age, although zinc and calcium are absorbed less well in older adults. For calcium this change is likely related to hormonal influences and estrogen withdrawal at menopause. For calcium and many of the trace minerals, intakes fall below even two-thirds of the RDA in many older groups. Common medications taken by older people, such as antacids and laxatives, may increase intake or increase excretion of some minerals, enhancing risk of deficiency or toxicity. Because sensitive measurements of mineral status are not currently available, marginal deficiencies are difficult to identify. Likewise, the effects on the health of older persons of mineral supplements in excess of requirements are uncertain.

Water and electrolyte balance in aged individuals, who are ill or in good health, requires continual attention. Impaired thirst and the kidneys' decreased ability to conserve water increase the risk of dehydration and potentially dangerous alterations in electrolyte levels. Although the institutionalized older person who cannot drink without help is especially vulnerable to low fluid intake, older people who live in areas with high ambient temperatures, who exercise regularly, who use laxatives, or who consume large amounts of protein also need to be advised about appropriate fluid intake.

REVIEW QUESTIONS

1. Why is there a renewed interest in the role of minerals in the health of elderly people? What is the difference between a macromineral and a trace mineral? Which minerals are associated with immune status, hypertension, bone metabolism, glucose tolerance, and cardiovascular disease?
2. What hormones are involved in the control of calcium balance? What role does each hormone play in maintaining normal serum calcium? Are serum calcium levels an accurate reflection of bone density?
3. How does aging influence calcium status? Is the effect different in men and women? Explain. Does dietary intake of protein and sodium influence calcium balance? Describe.
4. How can laxative intake, alcohol intake, and prescription medications for hypertension and congestive heart failure influence mineral status? If kidney function is impaired, which minerals are more likely to rise to higher levels? How do vegetarian diets influence mineral status?
5. What factors contribute to lower total body water in older people? Why is this a serious situation? What is the water requirement for the elderly? What situations predispose the older person to dehydration?

SUGGESTED LEARNING ACTIVITIES

1. Go to your local drug store and examine the labels of available over-the-counter laxatives and antacids. Prepare a report that includes for each medication any mineral that is a component or an ingredient. Identify any potential effect of each drug on the absorption, metabolism, or excretion of one or more minerals.
2. Review NHANES III dietary intake data. Prepare a report that (1) identifies each mineral consumed at a level of less than 70% or more than 125% of the RDA by older people, (2) describes potential functional or metabolic effects of intakes at the current level by older people, and (3) suggests dietary changes that will allow for dietary mineral intake within 10% of the RDA.
3. Prepare a short answer to each of the following questions that you have received from elderly people through the local "Dial-A-Dietitian" service in your community:
   a. "I read that zinc supplements will strengthen my immune system and make my food taste better. Should I start taking a supplement of zinc?"
   b. "Will drinking tea with my meals cause poor absorption of the minerals in my foods?"
   c. "I just started going through menopause. Should I start taking a calcium supplement to protect my bones?"
4. Prepare a one-page handout to be used at a senior center on choosing preprepared foods for the older person who has hypertension and is concerned about sodium intake.

REFERENCES

1. Arnaud, C.D., and Sanchez, S.D.: Calcium and phosphorus. In: Brown, M.L., editor: Present knowledge in nutrition, ed. 6, Washington, DC, 1990, International Life Sciences Institute, Nutrition Foundation.
2. August, D., Janghorbani, M., and Young, V.R.: Determination of zinc and copper absorption at three dietary Zn-Cu ratios by using stable isotope methods in young adult and elderly subjects, Am. J. Clin. Nutr. 50:1457, 1989.
3. Bales, C.W., and others: Marginal zinc deficiency in older adults: responsiveness of zinc status indicators, J. Am. Coll. Nutr. 5:455, 1994.
4. Bogden, J.D., and others: Daily micronutrient supplements enhance delayed-hypersensitivity skin test responses in older people, Am. J. Clin. Nutr. 60:437, 1994.

5. Buchman, A.L., Moukarzel, A., and Ament, M.E.: Selenium renal homeostasis is impaired in patients receiving long-term total parenteral nutrition, J. Parent. Enter. Nutr. 18:231, 1994.

6. Bunker, V.W., and Clayton, B.E.: Research review: studies in the nutrition of elderly people with particular reference to essential trace elements, Age Ageing 18:422, 1989.

7. Carter, W.J.: Macronutrient requirements for elderly persons. In: Chernoff, R., editor: Geriatric nutrition: the health professional's handbook, Gaithersburg, MD, 1991, Aspen Publishers.

8. Chernoff, R.: Thirst and fluid requirements, Nutr. Rev. 52(8II):S3, 1994.

9. Couzy, F., and others: Zinc absorption in healthy elderly humans and the effect of diet, Am. J. Clin. Nutr. 58:690, 1993.

10. Cunningham, J.J., and others: Hyperzincuria in individuals with insulin-dependent diabetes mellitus: concurrent zinc status and the effect of high-dose zinc supplementation, Metab. 43(12):1558, 1994.

11. Dawson-Hughes, B.: Calcium and vitamin D metabolism and nutritional status in the elderly: overview. In: Rosenberg, I.H., editor: Nutritional assessment of elderly populations. Measure and function, New York, 1995, Raven Press.

12. Euronut SENECA investigators: Intake of vitamins and minerals, Euro. J. Clin. Nutr. 45(suppl. 3):121, 1991.

13. Faull, C.M., Holmes, C., and Baylis, P.H.: Water balance in elderly people: is there a deficiency of vasopressin?, Age Ageing 22:114, 1993.

14. Food and Nutrition Board: Recommended dietary allowances, ed. 10, Washington, DC, 1989, National Academy of Sciences.

15. Garry, P.J., Koehler, K.M., and Simon, T.L.: Iron stores and iron absorption: effects of repeated blood donations, Am. J. Clin. Nutr. 62(3):611, 1995.

16. Gavin, M.W., McCarthy, D.M., and Garry, P.J.: Evidence that iron stores regulate iron absorption—a setpoint theory, Am. J. Clin. Nutr. 59:1376, 1994.

17. Gibson, R.S., Macdonald, A.C., and Martinez, O.B.: Dietary chromium and manganese intakes of a selected sample of Canadian elderly women, Hum. Nutr. Appl. Nutr. 39A:43, 1985.

18. Gullestad, L., and others: Magnesium status in healthy free-living elderly Norwegians, J. Am. Coll. Nutr. 13(1):45, 1994.

19. Hallberg, L., and others: Calcium: effect of different amounts on nonheme- and heme-iron absorption in humans, Am. J. Clin. Nutr. 53:112, 1991.

20. Heaney, R.P., and Weaver, C.M.: Effect of psyllium on absorption of co-ingested calcium, J. Am. Geriatr. Soc. 43:261, 1995.

21. Herbert, V.: Nutritional anemias in the elderly. In: Prinsley, D.M., and Sandstead, H.H., editors: Nutrition and aging, New York, 1990, Alan R. Liss.

22. Holcomb, C.A.: Positive influence of age and education on food consumption and nutrient intakes of older women living alone, J. Am. Diet. Assoc. 95:1381, 1995.

23. Hu, J.F., and others: Dietary intakes and urinary excretion of calcium and acids: a cross-sectional study of women in China, Am. J. Clin. Nutr. 58:398, 1993.

24. Hunt, J.R., and others: High- versus low-meat diets: effects on zinc absorption, iron status, and calcium, copper, iron, magnesium, manganese, nitrogen, phosphorus, and zinc balance in postmenopausal women, Am. J. Clin. Nutr. 62(3):621, 1995.

25. Jacques, P.F., and Russell, R.M.: Alcohol. In: Hartz, S.C., Russell, R.M., and Rosenberg, L.H., editors: Nutrition in the elderly. The Boston nutritional status survey, London, 1992, Smith-Gordon and Company.

26. Johnson, M.A., and others: Iron nutriture in elderly individuals, FASEB J. 8:609, 1994.

27. Johnson, M.A., and others: Nutritional patterns of centenarians, Inter. J. Aging Hum. Develop. 34:57, 1992.

28. Koehler, K.M., Hunt, W.C., and Garry, P.J.: Meat, poultry, and fish consumption and nutrient intake in the healthy elderly, J. Am. Diet. Assoc. 92:325, 1992.

29. Krasinski, S.D., and others: Fundic atrophic gastritis in an elderly population: effect on hemoglobin and several serum nutritional indicators, J. Am. Geriatr. Soc. 34:800, 1986.

30. Lassen, K.O., and Horder, M.: Selenium status and the effect of organic and inorganic selenium supplementation in a group of elderly people in Denmark, Scand. J. Clin. Lab. Invest. 54:585, 1994.

31. Lavizzo-Mourey, R., Johnson, J., and Stolley, P.: Risk factors for dehydration among elderly nursing home residents, J. Am. Geriatr. Soc. 36:213, 1988.

32. Lindeman, R.D., and Beck, A.A.: Mineral requirements. In: Chernoff, R., editor: Geriatric nutrition: the health professional's handbook, Gaithersburg, MD, 1991, Aspen Publishers.

33. Lopez, L.M., and Habicht, J.P.: Food stamps and the iron status of the U.S. elderly poor, J. Am. Diet. Assoc. 87:598, 1987.

34. Loughrey, C.M., and others: Oxidative stress in haemodialysis, Q. J. Med. 87:679, 1994.
35. Löwik, M.R.H., and others: Long-term effects of a vegetarian diet on the nutritional status of elderly people (Dutch Nutrition Surveillance System), J. Am. Coll. Nutr. 9:600, 1990.
36. Löwik, M.R.H., and others: Marginal nutritional status among institutionalized elderly women as compared to those living more independently (Dutch Nutrition Surveillance System), J. Am. Coll. Nutr. 11(6):673, 1992.
37. Macarthy, P.O., Johnson, A.A., and Walters, C.S.: Iron nutritional status of selected elderly black persons in Washington, D.C., J. Nutr. Elderly 6(2):3, 1986.
38. Manore, M.M., Vaughan, L.A., and Carroll, S.S.: Iron status in free-living, low-income very elderly, Nutr. Rep. Inter. 39:1, 1989.
39. Matkovic, V., and Heaney, R.P.: Calcium balance during human growth: evidence for threshold behavior, Am. J. Clin. Nutr. 55:992, 1992.
40. Miller, M.: Water and electrolyte disorders. In: Abrams, W.B., Beers, M.H., and Berkow, R., editors: Merck manual of geriatrics, Whitehouse Station, NJ, 1995, Merck Research Laboratories.
41. Milne, D.B., and Nielsen, F.H.: Effects of a diet low in copper on copper-status indicators in postmenopausal women, Am. J. Clin. Nutr. 63:358, 1996.
42. Nieman, D.C., and others: Dietary status of Seventh-Day Adventist vegetarian and nonvegetarian elderly women, J. Am. Diet. Assoc. 89:1763, 1989.
43. Oliviero, O., and others: Selenium status, fatty acids, vitamins A and E, and aging: the Nove Study, Am. J. Clin. Nutr. 60:510, 1994.
44. Pfeil, L.A., Katz, P.R., and Davis, P.J.: Water metabolism. In: Morley, J. E., Glick, Z., and Rubenstein, L.Z., editors: Geriatric nutrition. A comprehensive review, ed. 2, New York, 1995, Raven Press.
45. Phillips, P.A., and others: Reduced osmotic thirst in healthy elderly men, Am. J. Physiol. 261:R166, 1991.
46. Phillips, P.A., Johnston, C.I., and Gray, L.: Disturbed fluid and electrolyte homeostasis following dehydration in elderly people, Age Ageing 22:26, 1993.
47. Reiff, T.R.: Body composition with special reference to water. In: Horwitz, A., and others, editors: Nutrition in the elderly, New York, 1989, Oxford University Press.
48. Research Group on Aging: Extensive laboratory assessment of nutritional status in fit, health-conscious, elderly people living in the Paris area, J. Am. Coll. Nutr. 13(6):646, 1994.
49. Rolls, B.J.: Regulation of food and fluid intake in the elderly, Ann. N.Y. Acad. Sci. 561:217, 1989.
50. Ryan, A.S., Craig, L.D., and Finn, S.C.: Nutrient intakes and dietary patterns of older Americans: a national study, J. Gerontol. 47:M145, 1992.
51. Sahyoun, N.: Nutrient intake by the NSS elderly population. In: Hartz, S.C., Russell, R.M., and Rosenberg, L.H., editors: Nutrition in the elderly. The Boston nutritional status survey, London, 1992, Smith-Gordon and Company.
52. Sandstead, H.: Is zinc deficiency a public health problem?, Nutrition 11:87, 1995.
53. Sandstead, H., and others: Zinc nutriture in the elderly in relation to taste acuity, immune response, and wound healing, Am. J. Clin. Nutr. 36:1046, 1982.
54. Selby, P.L.: Calcium requirement—a reappraisal of the methods used in its determination and their application to patients with osteoporosis, Am. J. Clin. Nutr. 60:944, 1994.
55. Spencer, H., and others: Calcium requirement in humans, Clin. Orthop. 184:270, 1984.
56. Thomas, P.R.: Improving America's diet and health. From recommendations to action, Washington, DC, 1991, National Academy Press.
57. Tucker, K.: Micronutrient status and aging, Nutr. Rev. 53(9II):S9, 1995.
58. Tucker, K., and Rush, D.: Food choices of the elderly. In: Hartz, S.C., Russell, R.M., and Rosenberg, L.H., editors: Nutrition in the elderly, The Boston nutritional status survey, London, 1992, Smith-Gordon and Company.
59. Turnlund, J.R., Reager, R.D., and Costa, F.: Iron and copper absorption in young and elderly men, Nutr. Res. 8:333, 1988.
60. U.S. Department of Agriculture: Food intakes: individuals in 48 states, year 1977–78, Nationwide Food Consumption Survey 1977–78, Report No. I-1, Washington, DC, 1983, U.S. Government Printing Office.
61. U.S. Department of Health and Human Services: Dietary intake of vitamins, minerals, and fiber of persons ages 2 months and over in the United States: Third national health and nutrition examination survey, Phase I, 1988–91, Advance Data from Vital and Health Statistics, Number 258, Nov. 14, 1994, Hyattsville, MD, National Center for Health Statistics.

62. U.S. Department of Health and Human Services: Energy and macronutrient intakes of persons ages 2 months and over in the United States: Third national health and nutrition examination survey, Phase I, 1988–91, Advance Data from Vital and Health Statistics, Number 255, Oct. 24, 1994, Hyattsville, MD, National Center for Health Statistics.

63. U.S. Department of Health and Human Services: Nutrition monitoring in the United States. Chartbook I: Selected findings from the national nutrition monitoring and related research program, DHHS Publication No. (PHS) 93-1255-2, Hyattsville, MD, 1993, U.S. Public Health Service.

64. U.S. Department of Health and Human Services: Optimal calcium intake. NIH Consensus Statement, June 6–8; 12(4):1–31, Bethesda, MD, 1994, National Institutes of Health.

65. U.S. Department of Health and Human Services, U.S. Department of Agriculture: Nutrition monitoring in the United States. An update report on nutrition monitoring, DHHS Publication No. (PHS) 89-1255, Washington, DC, 1989, U.S. Government Printing Office.

66. Vaughan, L.A., and Manore, M.M.: Dietary patterns and nutritional status of low income, free-living elderly, Food Nutr. News 60(5):1, Nov.–Dec., 1988.

67. Weaver, C.M.: Age-related calcium requirements due to changes in absorption and utilization, J. Nutr. 124:1418S, 1994.

68. Wood, R.J.: Magnesium. In: Hartz, S.C., Russell, R.M., and Rosenberg, L.H., editors: Nutrition in the elderly. The Boston nutritional status survey, London, 1992, Smith-Gordon and Company.

69. Wood, R.J.: Zinc. In: Hartz, S.C., Russell, R.M., and Rosenberg, L.H., editors: Nutrition in the elderly. The Boston nutritional status survey, London, 1992, Smith-Gordon and Company.

70. Wood, R.J., and Serfaty-Lacrosniere, C.: Gastric acidity, atrophic gastritis, and calcium absorption, Nutr. Rev. 50(2):33, 1992.

71. Wood, R.J., Suter, P.M., and Russell, R.M.: Mineral requirements of elderly people, Am. J. Clin. Nutr. 62:493, 1995.

72. Wood, R.J., and Zheng, J.J.: Milk consumption and zinc retention in postmenopausal women, J. Nutr. 120:398, 1990.

73. Yu, S., West, C.E., and Beynen, A.C.: Increasing intakes of iron reduce status, absorption, and biliary excretion of copper in rats, Br. J. Nutr. 71:887, 1994.

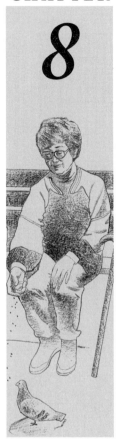

8

Food Selection Patterns in Older People

++

Objectives

After studying the chapter, the student should be able to:

✔ *Recognize how the aging process influences food selection*

✔ *Identify current trends in food patterns among older Americans*

✔ *Understand the psychologic, physiologic, sociologic, and economic factors influencing food selection by the elderly*

✔ *Identify the effects of income, race, and ethnicity on food choices in the elderly*

✔ *Describe appropriate methods of feeding and nutrition support for the functionally impaired and chronically ill elderly*

INTRODUCTION

Many aspects of our lives change as we grow older. We retire from full-time employment, creating time for new interests, social activities, and recreation. We may develop health problems that require changes in our dietary pattern or lifestyle. We may move to a retirement community that offers a wide variety of social and educational opportunities. Our food choices and resources adapt in response to changes in leisure time, income, health status, and personal needs. In this chapter we will explore the factors that influence food selection in older adults.

FOOD SELECTION AS A CONTINUUM

What Influences Food Selection?

Food has nutritional significance, but also important social and emotional significance. Angulo[1] observed that not only do we eat to live, we eat to achieve health, to derive pleasure, and to express our cultural and ethnic heritage. Our selection, preparation, and consumption of food is shaped by psychological and social values. Food becomes more than a tangible substance; food is placed into such categories as

❖

INFLUENCES ON FOOD CHOICES

- Psychologic factors
  Social activity
  Self-esteem
  Nutrition knowledge
  Perceived health benefit
  Loneliness
  Bereavement
  Symbolism of food
  Mental awareness
  Food aversion
  Food faddism
- Physiologic factors
  Appetite
  Taste acuity
  Olfactory acuity
  Dental status
  Prescribed diets
  Chronic disease

Food intolerance
Health status
Physical status (based on activities of daily
  living [ADLs] and instrumental activities
  of daily living [IADLs])
Physical exercise
Use of drugs (prescribed and over-the-counter)
- Socioeconomic factors
  Age
  Gender
  Income
  Cooking facilities
  Daily schedule
  Retirement/leisure time
  Education
  Distance to food store
  Availability of transportation
  Availability of familiar foods

---

healthy or providing comfort. Such food meanings appear to translate into action. McIntosh and coworkers[36] found that elderly people who assigned a health value to foods and compared "health foods" to "regular foods" actually had higher vitamin intakes than those who did not hold health food beliefs. In an older person food patterns reflect lifelong attitudes and habits influenced by the changing environment. To better understand the influence of lifestyle, health, and economic status on the food choices of older adults, individual factors have been identified and evaluated. Examples of these factors are listed in the box.

Although each factor influencing food behavior may be viewed individually, all act in combination. The older woman who enjoys food preparation and prides herself on "cooking from scratch" will face a dilemma as worsening arthritis makes it more difficult to shop for and prepare food. Her possible alternatives are using the motorized carts available in many larger supermarkets, using more preprepared items requiring little cooking, relying on home-delivered meals, or relocating to a retirement community that offers meal service. In the case of a couple,

the husband may be able to take over some food responsibilities when his spouse becomes disabled. Helping older people solve their food problems often involves seeking alternatives and doing things differently from their usual practice.

Changes in Lifelong Food Patterns

Throughout the life cycle, human behavior, including nutrition behavior, constantly undergoes transition, adaptation, and change. In the later years family size changes as children leave home and establish their own households. With a change in family size, food patterns also change. For example, the couple now living by themselves may go out to eat more frequently. In contrast, recent social and economic changes are resulting in single parents with children returning to their family home; grandparents are sometimes becoming responsible for the care and feeding of their grandchildren.

A loss in income at retirement or at the death of a spouse poses the need for a change in food buying habits if less money is now available for food. Retirement may open up opportunities for more socialization involving food, such as taking part in a congregate meal program or regularly meeting other retirees or friends for breakfast at a fast food restaurant. Increasing social interaction can result in more snacking and a higher overall food intake or a higher intake of particular foods.

For many older people, food intake is more a continuation of their previous habits than a change in their pattern. Schlettwein-Gsell[64] pointed out that both physical and social factors contribute to the persistence of dietary patterns into old age. Changes in gastrointestinal function may lessen one's ability to adapt to new foods. For elderly people at home, familiar meal patterns provide a structure for the day. Some older people select new foods for health reasons,[30] although little information is available describing the relationship between self-perceived health and dietary intake. Older women who perceived their health as good chose foods needed for roughage, foods that were easy to prepare, and foods that they enjoyed eating.[64] In reality the food selection patterns of older people reflect many attitudes and wants.

The diet of the older person also reflects the current food supply. Their survival points to their ability to select a reasonably adequate diet from the foods available over a period of time. Sometimes, changes in food intake are detrimental to nutritional status, but this is not always the case. When older individuals consume very limited types or amounts of food, it is usually the result of very extenuating circumstances; such situations will be discussed later in this chapter. For most older people, positive aspects of the diet can be a foundation for any improvement that may be required.

AGE AND FOOD INTAKE
Level of Food Intake

Normal aging brings about a decrease in both the energy requirement and the amount of food consumed (fig. 8-1).[18,32] Food records collected in the Third National Health and Nutrition Examination Survey (NHANES III) indicated that men lower their food intake to a greater extent than women, and black and Mexican American elderly lower their food intake to a greater

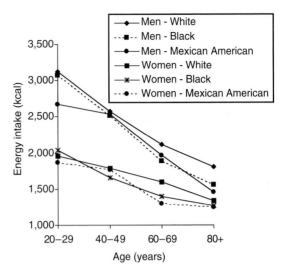

FIG. 8-1   Changes in Energy Intake Over Adulthood. Energy intake declines to a greater extent in men and in black and Mexican American women.

Data from Life Sciences Research Office, Federation of American Societies for Experimental Biology: Third Report on Nutrition Monitoring in the United States, Vol. I and II, Washington, DC, December 1995, U.S. Government Printing Office.

extent than white elderly.[32] In men, energy intake fell from a mean of 3,025 kcal at ages 20 to 29 to 1,776 kcal at age 80 and older. In women, energy intake dropped from 1,957 kcal to 1,329 kcal over this age range. In general, blacks and Mexican Americans have lower energy intakes than their white counterparts at all ages.

The most recent evaluation of food records gathered from the Baltimore Longitudinal Study of Aging (BLSA) between 1960 and 1987 indicated changing trends in energy intake among the older subjects.[22] In the 1960s older men had lower energy intakes than younger men, but this was not true in the 1970s and 1980s. The older men maintained a protein intake of about 15% to 16% of total energy, but kilocalories obtained from fat declined from 42% to 34%. Kilocalories supplied by carbohydrate increased from 39% to 44%. These findings imply that both older and younger individuals are reducing their intake of fat and adopting more healthful dietary practices. However, the men participating in the BLSA tend to be well educated and economically advantaged and are not representative of the general population. The NHANES III study,[32] in contrast with the BLSA, reported little change in the contribution of particular macronutrients to total energy intake over adulthood.

The Georgia Centenarian Study[25] indicates that centenarians who are able to remain in the community do not reduce their food intake to any extent after age 60. The mean energy intake of the centenarians was 1,581 kcal as compared to the 1,605 kcal consumed by individuals ages 60 to 69 from the same geographic area. Georgia subjects ages 80 to 89 had an energy intake of 1,423 kcal. In the NHANES III study,[32] the mean energy intake for all subjects age 80 and older was 1,484 kcal.

Patterns of Food Intake

Older people continue to select many of the same foods as younger people, despite a decrease in energy intake. The Continuing Survey of Food Intake of Individuals (CSFII) conducted by the U.S. Department of Agriculture[32] reported the percentages of younger and older adults consuming particular food items at least once over a three-day record period. About the same proportion of men and women age 20 and older and age 70 and older used bread or yeast rolls (91% to 95%); however, over 80% of the older people had cereal, compared to 64% of the younger group. The older participants also were more likely to have cake, cookies, or pastry.

The group age 70 and older reported about the same use of vegetables as the group age 20 and older, although some differences existed. Older people were more likely to use dark green and deep yellow vegetables than younger people. Older women reported less use of lettuce and more use of green beans. Older men were more likely to use corn, green peas, and lima beans. Older people continue to eat fruit. As compared to younger groups, older people use more citrus fruits and juices, dried fruits, bananas, melons and berries, and more fruit mixtures, including canned fruits. Their higher use of bananas and citrus fruit may relate to the

high potassium content of these foods and the importance of potassium intake in older people using diuretic drugs. More older women consumed at least five servings of fruits and vegetables a day as compared to young and middle aged women.

Older people use milk products to about the same extent as younger people but are more likely to choose low fat milks and milk desserts. Use of meat, poultry, and fish varied little between younger and older groups. About 52% of older men and 43% of older women had frankfurters, sausage, or luncheon meat at least once over the three-day record period. Of foods from the meat group only beef was higher for the older men (53% used beef) and poultry for the older women (52% used poultry), as compared to their younger counterparts.

Some older adults decrease their energy intake by consuming less of all the foods normally eaten rather than selectively reducing intake. The detrimental effect of this practice on diet quality was apparent in two groups of women[18] whose mean ages were 72 and 81 and whose energy intakes were 2,074 and 1,674 kcal, respectively. Protein intake decreased from 53 to 48 gm, calcium from 924 to 760 mg, and iron from 11.3 to 8 mg. In the Georgia Centenarian Study,[25] protein intake was 66 g in the 60- to 69-year-olds, 58 g in the 80- to 89-year-olds, and 52 g in those age 100 and older.

Selecting protein and dairy foods lower in fat allows a reduction in energy intake, if needed, yet ensures adequate amounts of the B complex vitamins, iron, magnesium, calcium, and zinc. Whole-grain products add valuable vitamins and trace minerals to the diet. Foods that contain primarily simple carbohydrates and fat (e.g., sweet baked items, soft drinks, crackers, and alcoholic beverages) should be the first items to be deleted from the diet when energy intake must be reduced. Food preparation methods that add additional kilocalories in the form of fat or rich sauces should be avoided.

Older people, as compared to younger people, do seem to use their kilocalories more wisely and choose foods higher in nutrient density.[27] Food records available from the NHANES II study[27] were analyzed for the use of foods from six basic food groups: meat, dairy, grain, fruit, vegetable, and other (fats, sweets, and alcohol). People above age 65 consumed only 19% of their total energy from the fats, sweets, and alcohol group, whereas the 19- to 34-year-olds consumed 32% of their kilocalories from this group.

Food patterns also differ among the older and younger segments of the over-60 population. Fischer and coworkers[19] found that people age 60 to 70 ate more high-fiber breads, pasta, and rice and more fresh and frozen vegetables than those age 75 to 85. The older group used fewer low-fat milk products and more high-fat cheeses, pastries, pies, and cakes, compared to the 60 to 70 age group.

The influence of educational level and health beliefs on the food selection patterns of the very old warrants further investigation. Fischer and coworkers[19] found that the older seniors, age 75 to 85, believed that an improved diet would result in improved health, although they tended to select less nutritious foods. It may be that health professionals who encourage dietary changes in the young-old do not make the same effort toward nutrition education in the old-old. Those in the oldest age group may lack information on food content. The food choices of the old-old also are more likely to be influenced by changes in economic status as health expenditures rise and by increases in functional disability.

Health Considerations

Medical advice or the belief that a particular food is good or bad for health can lead to changes in food preparation and consumption in the older population.[12] In the Georgia Centenarian Study[20] 83% of those age 60 to 69, 56% of those age 80 to 89, and 32% of those age 100 and older reported trying to avoid high-cholesterol foods. In a recent Gallup Survey,[76] 77% of older Americans indicated that they are eating a healthier diet now than they did three years ago. For many this involved selecting more low-calorie, sugar-free, and reduced-fat foods.

Older people are becoming increasingly interested in food components other than fat that may influence health. A study of older people in

Wales[77] reported that 7% of the men and 10% of the women age 65 to 74 had changed their diet for health reasons. Specific changes included eating more fish and fiber and eating less meat, salt, fats, and sugar. Moreover, these older people indicated a desire for more information on food labels. These findings support the idea that nutrition education can be effective in helping older people modify their food patterns. Such modifications could be significant for health, since research has demonstrated that improved nutrition helps offset the development of chronic diseases such as coronary heart disease, cancer, and osteoporosis.

The relationship between food choices and perceived health outcome appears to be somewhat complex in older age groups. Although health considerations are a factor in food selection, the converse is also true: the dietary choices made seem to influence health perception.[49] In a study of nearly 1,100 New England residents over age 70,[49] a change in diet as a result of illness was positively related to perceived health. Apparently, the action of making a dietary change was associated with an increased sense of physical well-being. This response from taking a positive step toward improving one's health might also apply to other positive behavior changes such as increasing physical activity or stopping smoking.

Food intake records collected from older people between 1977 and 1987 by the U.S. Department of Agriculture indicate a trend toward changes in food patterns.[48] Fewer people used high-fat cuts of beef and pork in 1987 as in 1977, although there was little change in the use of frankfurters and luncheon meats. About 30% selected low-fat dairy items in 1977 whereas 44% had moved from high-fat to lower-fat dairy items by 1987. Lower-fat meat, poultry, and fish increased in use over the 10-year period, and more than 15% of those interviewed changed from white bread to whole grain, high fiber bread.

The impact of these changes on actual nutrient intake, however, was modest. Despite these trends toward selection of food items higher in fiber and lower in fat, use of high-fat desserts such as pastries or butter or margarine did not decrease to any extent. Nor did use of important fiber and micronutrient sources, such as fruits, vegetables, cereals, or legumes, increase. High-fat desserts remained the single major source of energy in both surveys. Based on these findings, Popkin and coworkers[48] raised concerns regarding the type and effectiveness of current health messages. Emphasis is now placed on food items to be avoided rather than on food items and meal patterns that support optimum nutrition and health. Practical advice to be used in meal planning that emphasizes greater use of fruits, vegetables, legumes, whole-grain breads and cereals, and lower-fat dairy foods might have a greater influence on overall nutrient intake.

Ethnic Food Patterns

As the older population increases in number, so will it increase in diversity.[69] Of the total elderly in 1990, 87% were white, 8% were black, about 3% were Hispanic, and the remaining 2% were American Indian, Eskimo, or Asian and Pacific Islanders. By the year 2010, African Americans will make up 10% and Hispanics 6% of the population age 65 and older. Older African Americans will number almost 4 million and older Hispanics 2.5 million.[69] Heart disease, diabetes, severe high blood pressure, and cancer are more prevalent among African Americans than whites, and all of these conditions are influenced by dietary intake and preventive health care.[16] Heart disease is less prevalent among Hispanics than among African American or white populations, but diabetes is especially high among Mexican Americans. Overweight is also common among Mexican Americans, especially among Mexican American women. Heart disease is lower among Asians and Pacific Islanders, but cancer incidence is higher.[72]

Very limited information is available describing the food habits of elderly African Americans, Hispanics, or Asians. It will be important in the years ahead for health professionals to characterize the food patterns of these groups and suggest culturally appropriate interventions if needed.[16] It does appear that ethnic and racial origin continue to exert an influence on food patterns into advanced age.

Hispanic elderly. A survey of 254 low-income Mexican American and white elderly in Texas[2] indicated that ethnic background is more important than socioeconomic status in predicting dietary patterns in older adults. The Mexican Americans consumed flour tortillas, legumes, poultry, eggs, and organ meats more frequently than the non-Hispanics of similar age. The Mexican Americans were more likely to cook with saturated fats and had a higher sugar intake. Major limitations in the diet of the older Mexican Americans were their low use of dairy foods and fruits and vegetables rich in beta carotene and vitamin C. These patterns are reflected in a recent NHANES III report[32] indicating low intakes of vitamin A and magnesium in this group (fig. 8-2).

Asian elderly. Tong[70] examined the food habits of 62 elderly Vietnamese who had lived in the United States for 15 years. Based on a 24-hour dietary recall record, it was evident that many ethnic foods were still part of the meal pattern. Breakfast consisted of the traditional pho (beef soup with rice noodles, bean sprouts, and fresh herbs), and both lunch and dinner usually consisted of a stir-fried item and rice. Typical American foods such as hamburgers, pancakes, and pizza were not well liked. Only 5% of this group used milk or cheese regularly.

A study of 45 elderly Chinese women in California[9] revealed that 95% still consumed mainly Chinese staple foods, including rice, noodles, and dumplings at lunch and dinner. Breakfast varied between American breakfast items—bread, rolls, pastries, hot cereal, cookies, and crackers—and traditional Chinese foods. There was no association between the length of time lived in the United States and their use of American foods. A problem for older ethnic groups may be the availability of ethnic food items. Buying them may require transportation to a particular market. These items may also be high in cost.

Among Chinese elderly, Korean elderly, and Japanese elderly residing in a senior apartment complex in Chicago,[28] some serious nutrient deficiencies were identified. Over half of the Chinese and Korean women had low energy intakes and were taking in less than 67% of the

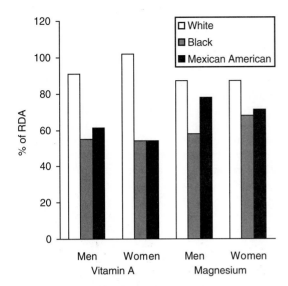

FIG. 8-2 Differences in Nutrient Intake Among Elderly of Different Race and Ethnic Groups. Black and Mexican American elderly people have low intakes of vitamin A and magnesium as compared to white elderly. Black and Mexican American elderly may be eating fewer portions of dark green and deep yellow vegetables; lower use of milk products among black and Mexican American elderly may contribute to their lower magnesium intakes.

Data from Life Sciences Research Office, Federation of American Societies for Experimental Biology: Third Report on Nutrition Monitoring in the United States, Vol. I and II, Washington, DC, December 1995, U.S. Government Printing Office.

recommended level of calcium. In the Korean women protein, vitamins A and C, and riboflavin were problem nutrients. The Chinese, Korean, and Japanese men and the Japanese women tended to have better diets. Underweight was more prevalent than overweight in these older people. Although the study did not report intakes of specific foods, Kim and coworkers[28] commented that these elderly Asian Americans had not adopted American food patterns, but continued to prefer their ethnic foods.

African American elderly. Older African Americans are more likely to be at nutritional risk than older white people. In a survey of 109 elderly African Americans in Louisiana,[23] more than 87% had less than 67% of the RDA for riboflavin, iron, and thiamin, and almost half had low intakes of calcium and vitamin C. In contrast only 2% were low in vitamin A and 6% in protein. Among old-old African Americans ranging from 74 to 96 years and living in an urban senior housing complex,[4] relative body weight ranged from 90 to 247. Nearly half were taking vitamin supplements. Intakes of fat and cholesterol were low in this group, falling in the range of the American Heart Association Step I diet; however, the low intake of fat could be related to low food intake overall. Older blacks in the Georgia Centenarian Study[25] were less likely to eat breakfast than older whites and had a diet higher in sweets and fat but lower in fruits and eggs. Johnson and coworkers[25] pointed out that eggs are an economical source of protein and avoidance of eggs may not be necessarily desirable for older people at risk for malnutrition. Older African Americans living in public housing in Massachusetts reported eating a variety of foods.[10] Most preferred refined grains to whole grains, but rice, grits, macaroni, and cornbread were popular foods. White potatoes, sweet potatoes, cabbage, collard or mustard greens, and tomatoes were consumed regularly by older Kansas blacks.[24] Chicken, eggs, cheese, and ground beef were the protein foods used most frequently by the Kansas elderly. African American elderly may be changing their traditional pattern of using dark green and deep yellow vegetables, resulting in lower intakes of vitamin A (fig. 8-2).

It is important to understand and respect the cultural food patterns of older people belonging to various ethnic or racial groups. Recognizing the need to preserve traditional values is important in the development of programs that are appropriate for meeting the social and health needs of individual groups.

PSYCHOSOCIAL ASPECTS OF FOOD SELECTION

Eating is an important psychosocial activity. It is a symbol of prestige, friendship, and reward.[6] Good food, well prepared, conveys the message that an individual is important and that someone cares about his or her well-being.[47] Feelings of worthlessness or rejection can cause a loss of interest in food and subsequent low food intake. Changes in food patterns challenge the cultural and personal values embodied in these patterns. As children, many older people were taught that protein builds muscle and is important for growth and health,[6] and this belief is likely reflected in the fact that older people who have control over their food intake tend to eat the recommended (or even higher) level of protein. As people age they must continually give up parts of their lives: their job or profession, their home, their spouse or peers who die.[6] Food may be one of the few things left that they can control. Food can provide comfort and pleasure when other sources of enjoyment have been lost. Stressful events, including losing a spouse, moving to a new location or long-term care facility, experiencing a change in health status, not having an adequate income to meet medical or living expenses, or losing old friends, have been associated with poor nutrient intake.[46]

Level of Social Interaction

Throughout life eating is a social activity. Typical examples are birthday parties, wedding receptions, or sharing a pizza. Losing a spouse or friend results in a loss of eating companions for the older adult, who may now be eating alone for the first time in his or her life. Loneliness contributes to malnutrition in some older people.

Walker and Beauchene[78] evaluated the effect of loneliness on dietary adequacy in 61 independently living older people ranging in age from 60 to 94. They found that loneliness was related to number of social contacts; those who had more social contacts were less lonely. The average number of social contacts over the three-day reporting period was 17.7, with a range of 3 to 48. A surprising finding, however, was that the length of time spent in contact with others was not related to the degree of loneliness. This implies that even a short telephone call or visit to bring a home-delivered meal may add to an older individual's psychological or emotional well-being. Neither age nor physical health influenced the degree of loneliness, although the older black people interviewed had higher loneliness scores than the older white people. Loneliness, in turn, was significantly related to overall dietary adequacy; the greater the degree of loneliness, the lower the intake of protein, iron, riboflavin, niacin, ascorbic acid, and phosphorus.

Within the context of social interaction or isolation, Troll[71] maintains that it is important to differentiate between isolation and desolation. Isolates are those who are relatively content living alone and may have done so most of their lives. The desolates, on the other hand, live alone but experience a high degree of loneliness. Physical isolation may be far less important than the frequency of communication or exchange of messages. An individual who lives with other people but is ignored is far more lonely than the person who lives alone but has a daily telephone conversation with a friend or child.

A study of 145 older people receiving home care services[46] indicated that most (81%) had social contact at least once a week with relatives, neighbors, friends, or acquaintances, but more than half (51%) reported feeling lonely much of the time. In fact the more frequent their social contacts with others, the greater their loneliness. Despite these feelings, the number of social contacts or degree of social isolation was not a predictor of dietary intake. Nevertheless, those older people who reported having friends had a higher energy intake. These findings have importance for the increasing number of elders who are homebound and need help with activities of daily living (see chapter 1). The home care provider serves as a social contact and could provide emotional support to an isolated individual. Also, the home care provider is in a unique position to watch for signs of malnutrition and to initiate corrective action before health status is threatened.

Changing Household Roles

Just as advancing age leads to changes in personal roles, so it can bring about changes in household roles. Although the woman in a two-person household may take primary responsibility for meal planning and food preparation in the early and middle stages of the family life cycle, in retirement, the husband's involvement in food decisions may increase. In 82 retired

Iowa couples,[61] not only did retired husbands participate to a greater extent in food-related decisions, but their level of participation also had nutritional implications. The greater the husband's involvement in both meal planning and actual food purchasing, the better the diet. Women who expressed dissatisfaction with their traditional role showed little interest in food-related activities. This finding has important implications for nutrition education. Although food programs are often directed toward women, leaders should make an effort to involve men who may strongly influence food decisions within a retired family.

Food Preferences

Food preferences are molded by our ethnic, cultural, and religious backgrounds. Older people, like most people, prefer foods associated with pleasant experiences or related to their home or place of origin. Preferred foods may have been given as special treats or served on holidays or special occasions. For lonely older people, food cravings may arise from their need for emotional gratification.[64] Age-appropriate expectations can sometimes influence food selection, although these are more likely to be the expectations of younger individuals as to what "older people should eat" rather than the expectations of older people themselves.

MENTAL STATUS AND FOOD INTAKE

Mental disorders in an older adult can result in confusion, irritability, acute depression, or, in extreme situations, true dementia. Causes of dementia include **senile dementia of the Alzheimer type (SDAT)**, multi-infarct dementia arising from a stroke or other cerebrovascular incident, or dementia associated with excessive long-term alcohol intake. An estimated 15% of those over age 65 have dementia of some form and degree.[7] Whatever the cause, dementia is likely to pose nutritional problems. Those with severe organic brain disease or SDAT may forget to eat or may be unable to differentiate between breakfast, lunch, and dinner. If they are unable to prepare food, meals may consist

totally of bread and jam or prepackaged foods, limiting nutrient intake both quantitatively and qualitatively. (The biological aspects of dementia will be discussed in chapter 13.)

Stages of Dementia and Nutritional Implications

SDAT is a progressive neurologic disease in which the older individual becomes increasingly unable to function, both mentally and physically. Complications associated with SDAT can include behavioral symptoms (e.g., hostility, extreme agitation, or uncooperativeness), psychiatric problems (e.g., depression, anxiety, or paranoia), and metabolic disturbances (e.g., dehydration, infection, or drug toxicity).[7]

The development of SDAT usually is divided into three stages, although Butler[7] emphasizes that there is tremendous variability among individual patients. The initial stage is characterized by recent memory loss, the inability to retain new information, and problems in judgment. Difficulties in shopping and preparing and storing food are likely. Impaired memory and judgment can lead to such nutrition complications as forgetting to eat or eating the same meal twice. SDAT patients have difficulty recognizing and detecting odors. This olfactory malfunction often appears as a greater preference for sweet and salty foods.[43]

In the intermediate stage of dementia, increased agitation becomes evident. Energy requirements may escalate by as much as 600 kcal a day.[33] Patients seldom consume sufficient kilocalories to meet these increased energy needs and often begin to lose weight. In this stage individuals may require some assistance with eating, such as cutting food into bite-size pieces or spreading margarine or butter on bread.

During the final stage of SDAT, the patient may be unable to swallow and may require tube feeding. Some patients simply refuse to open their mouths or swallow when spoon fed, whereas others become compulsive eaters or try to consume inedible objects.[43] Dementia is a leading cause of weight loss in the elderly.[19] Memory loss, disorientation, impaired judgment, apathy, apraxia, combative feeding behavior, and appetite disturbances are factors identified with the weight loss occurring in demented patients.

Nutrient Intake in Dementia

Nutritional supplements are very important in meeting the needs of patients with advanced SDAT. In two reports[33,68] describing the food intake of SDAT patients in long-term care facilities, mean energy intakes were 1,532[33] and 1,558 kcal,[68] although individual intakes ranged from 995 to 2,120 kcal. Nutritional supplements, such as fortified beverages and puddings, provided 29% of total kilocalories and 41% of total protein in the patients studied by Suski and Nielson.[68] Without nutritional supplements the daily intake of their 19 nonambulatory SDAT patients was deficient in kilocalories and all nutrients but vitamin C and iron. Among the 13 elderly SDAT patients studied by Litchford and Wakefield,[33] calcium and niacin fell below 25% of the recommended dietary allowances (RDA) when supplements were not included. In SDAT patients classified as wanderers, daily energy intake even with supplements fell 600 kcal below their energy expenditure; in those who were sedentary, intake fell only 200 kcal below their energy expenditure.[33] Continual pacing, a characteristic of some SDAT patients, can increase energy needs by more than 1,600 kcal a day.[54] Changes in energy metabolism also may occur among sedentary SDAT patients. Five sedentary SDAT patients were found to have a mean weight loss of 4.5 kg in six months despite an energy intake of 37 kcal per kg of body weight.[53] (See chapter 5 for energy recommendations.)

Feeding Patients with Dementia

When feeding patients with dementia, it may help to offer fewer choices and small portion sizes with between-meal snacks as needed. Distractions such as a television or ringing telephone should be avoided as much as possible. Food temperatures need to be checked because patients may not be sensitive to burning their mouths. Also, food consistency may need to be modified and tough or crispy foods excluded. Pureed foods may be necessary to prevent choking. (See chapter 12 for guidelines on feeding individuals with swallowing disorders.)

Providing major nutrient sources at the noon meal when cognitive and attentive abilities are at their peak may optimize nutrient intake.[68]

Long-term care facilities should implement procedures to quantify the amount of food eaten on a regular basis. Notations regarding the amount of food on the tray that was actually eaten are influenced by individual perceptions of staff members.[57] Staff who consume lower amounts of food themselves may consider food intake "good" when only half of the food offered to the patient is actually eaten.

Areas for Further Research

In a clinical situation the older patient with dementia should be weighed regularly, since weight loss can be significant. It also appears that nonambulatory patients are more likely to lose weight than ambulatory patients. Whether ambulatory patients receive food from visitors or other sources requires further study. Likewise, the effect of other medical complications associated with dementia bears further investigation. Infection and dehydration are not uncommon in patients with SDAT. Drugs used to control the behavioral problems associated with the disease can affect liver function and blood pressure and cause urinary retention.[7] Metabolic complications rather than food intake alone may be a significant factor in the nutrient deficiencies and weight loss associated with dementia.

PHYSIOLOGIC ASPECTS OF FOOD SELECTION

The physical changes that occur as a result of normal aging and degenerative disease influence food habits. Loss of appetite or diminished taste sensitivity makes eating less pleasurable. A physical disability that restricts food shopping and meal preparation limits food choices. Because physiologic changes affect both psychologic outlook and level of social activity, it sometimes is difficult to identify the true cause of any observed change in food pattern.

Sensory Aspects of Food Selection

Appetite. Research indicates that food intake regulation is impaired in healthy elderly people and may contribute to lower food intake. Such factors as diminished taste, prescription drugs, and poor dental status, all issues of concern in older people, also adversely affect appetite. Nevertheless, in the Georgia Centenarian Study[25] only 4% to 5% of those older adults ranging in age from 60 to over 100 reported that a physical condition interfered with their appetite. Among older Canadians receiving home care services,[46] men were more likely than women to report having a good appetite; overall, 64% reported good appetite.

Older people with health problems are more likely to have poor appetites. Anorexia is a common side effect of many prescription drugs such as digoxin, which causes nausea and anorexia. Appetite may be affected by psychological factors. Individuals who are depressed are more likely to have low energy intake.[43]

Taste acuity. Older people sometimes have loss of taste or distorted taste perception. As described in chapter 4, the sense of taste is controlled by the number and functional capacity of the taste buds on the tongue and pharynx and the integrity of the nerve supply to this region. Schiffman[62] concluded that many older adults do have elevated taste thresholds to the basic modalities of sweet, salty, sour, and bitter. This means that a taste must be present in a test solution at a higher concentration to be detected by an older person. On the other hand, Zallen and others[82] contend that actual taste does not diminish when concentrations of the taste stimuli fall within the normal continuum found in food. When their older subjects were presented with various salt concentrations in the form of mashed potatoes and chicken broth, their taste acuity did not differ from the younger subjects. For older people with extensive loss of taste, the addition of flavor enhancers may increase their food intake and improve their nutritional status. Older people living in a retirement home ate more food when it was flavor enhanced and demonstrated improved function as measured by an increased hand grip strength.[63]

Some older individuals have distorted taste. Although an intense degree of sweetness becomes unpleasant for most younger people, this is not true for many older people. This may explain why some older people crave items high in sugar. Wearing dentures or poor dental hygiene can leave a residual taste in the mouth that overpowers other taste. Certain prescription drugs cause an interfering taste. Nutritional status may influence taste; however, poor zinc status has not been shown to be a primary cause of decreased taste in older people (see chapter 7).

Olfactory function. Changes in the ability to detect or identify odors vary among individuals and particular odors.[62] Medical conditions such as diabetes, liver disease, or renal disease, drugs such as antihypertensive agents, and smoking can exert a greater effect on olfactory function than age itself. In a study of 80 older women living in the community[15] who had a high level of personal function (their mean age was 76), nearly half had olfactory dysfunction. Although reduced ability to smell did not result in poor nutrient intake, it was associated with less interest in cooking, eating a less wide variety of foods, lower use of fruits and vegetables with a sour or bitter taste such as citrus fruits, a higher intake of sweets, and a fat intake pattern with greater cardiovascular risk (a higher intake of saturated fat and lower ratio of polyunsaturated to saturated fat). Greater attention to color, texture, and flavor fortification of foods for older people may help to overcome olfactory losses and enhance food enjoyment.

Dental Problems and Food Selection

In general, dental health in the United States has improved. Americans are seeing a dentist more regularly for preventive dental care, they are reducing dental caries through self-care, and they are keeping their teeth longer. Regardless, dental problems are frequent in the older population.[35] Data obtained from a national survey (table 8-1) indicate a large unmet need for dental care. Most older people are not covered by dental insurance and may not be able to afford dental services to repair cavities, treat gum disease, or prepare dentures. Serious periodontal disease and decayed teeth are painful and can cause people to avoid certain foods. Foods that are very hot or very cold can aggravate oral pain, as can very crisp or fibrous foods that require significant biting force. Despite its importance, oral health is sometimes neglected in long-term care facilities.

TABLE 8-1 *Oral Health Status of Older Adults*

Condition	Occurrence (%)
Edentulous	41
Need for denture replacement or repair	27
Root caries	57
Periodontal weakening (loosening of teeth)	95
No dental visit in past two years	44
Perceived need for dental care	36

Adapted from Martin, W.: Oral health in the elderly. In: Chernoff, R., editor: Geriatric nutrition: the health professional's handbook, Gaithersburg, MD, 1991, Aspen Publishers.

Use of dentures increases with age.[44] In the Boston Nutritional Status Survey[44] 54% of the men ages 60 to 69 wore partial or full dentures as compared to 100% of those age 90 or older. In the women the use of dentures increased from 61% to 79% over this age range. Although loss of teeth and a lack of dentures or ill-fitting dentures can interfere with chewing and decrease the pleasure associated with eating, the influence of dental status on nutrient intake is controversial. In the Boston Nutritional Status Survey[44] individuals wearing partial or complete dentures had lower energy, protein, and niacin intakes and higher carbohydrate intake. However, denture use increased with age which also is a factor in energy intake. Individuals who are edentulous tend to avoid meat and cheese which are difficult to chew, and this influences both protein and niacin intakes. In the Boston study denture wearers were taking more medications and were more likely to have been hospitalized recently. In an evaluation of over 1,600 elderly Chinese living in Hong Kong,[81] 45% of the women and 37% of the men reported problems with chewing; however, there were no differences in the frequency of eating vegetables, fruits, or meat. Nevertheless, recent weight loss of more than 2 kg, general poor health, and depression were associated with chewing problems.

Providing nutrient sources requiring only limited chewing is important for those with poor dental status. Dairy products, eggs, ground meat, well-cooked chicken and fish, and legumes are good sources of high-quality protein. Fruit juices, cooked green and yellow vegetables, and potatoes can provide folate and vitamins A, C, and B-6. Many fresh fruits, including apples, melons, or bananas, can be eaten by those who are partially or completely edentulous if the fruit is ripe, peeled, and cut into small pieces. Pureed foods should be considered only when all other possibilities have been exhausted.

Physical Disability and Food Selection

Prevalence of physical disability. A significant number of older people living in the community have some limitation in activity that can affect both food shopping and meal preparation. Functional limitations or difficulty in performing personal care tasks or home management tasks increase with age.[69] Only 9% of people between the ages of 65 and 69 have difficulty with Activities of Daily Living (ADLs) or Instrumental Activities of Daily Living (IADLs), but this increases to 45% by age 85 (see chapter 1 for review of ADLs and IADLs). Data from the National Health Interview Survey[69] indicated that relatively few (4%) people age 85 and older who live in the community need help with eating. On the other hand, 26% need help preparing meals, and 37% need help with shopping. Minority elderly are more likely to need help with everyday activities than white elderly. In those age 65 and older, 15% of whites, 23% of blacks, and 19% of Hispanics need help with at least one ADL or IADL. Arthritis, a common cause of functional limitation and disability, is reported by over half of all older people living in the community.[69] If the older person has limited vision or movement, he or she may not be able to shop for groceries; consequently, all food supplies must be delivered. Preparing vegetables can be difficult for someone whose hands are crippled with arthritis. Moving about the kitchen requires special effort for a person who must grasp a cane or walker for support. Poor eyesight can interfere with reading a nutrition label or package directions for food preparation or seeing the numbers on an oven temperature dial.

Nutrient intake and physical disability. Unfortunately, there has been little nutritional evaluation of people with physical disabilities who live at home. In a study of about 2,200 frail elderly in New York state,[56] the very-low-income people with reduced mobility had the highest nutritional risk. Those who were home-bound and lived alone indicated an unmet need for help with food preparation and reported more days without eating. About half of those with both financial problems and restricted mobility had days with nothing to eat. One measure of diet quality is the frequency of use of green or yellow vegetables. Those who needed help with meal preparation consumed green and yellow vegetables infrequently.

Energy intake and protein intake were evaluated in 145 older Canadians receiving home care services.[46] In that group 38% of the men and 15% of the women reported that functional limitations interfered with meal preparation. Sixty-nine percent of the men and 26% of the women never prepared their own meals but depended on relatives and neighbors for assistance. A new and significant finding in this study was the effect of good or poor vision on dietary intake. A mean difference of nearly 6 g of protein a day separated the individuals with good vision from those with poor vision; this difference was independent of other medical conditions. An estimated one in five older people has a vision problem.

Physical disability that compromises food intake could increase the occurrence of acute illness and hospitalization. Mowé and coworkers[40] evaluated dietary habits and nutritional status in a group of older people recently admitted to the hospital from their own home and a group of older people from the same geographical area and similar financial, educational, and social status who were living at home. The hospitalized group had lower hemoglobin and serum albumin and ascorbic acid. The mean BMI was 22 for those in the hospital but the mean BMI was 24 to 25 in those at home. The poor nutritional status in the hospital group as compared to the group at home suggests that food intake was less

than adequate prior to hospital admission. The hospital group also reported having more difficulties in obtaining and preparing food prior to hospitalization.

In a follow-up of 17,065 people age 70 years and over interviewed in the National Center for Health Statistics Longitudinal Study of Aging,[73] the need for assistance with meal preparation was related to mortality. After six years 76% of those who could not prepare their own meals had died; only 24% were still alive. Individuals who can no longer prepare meals may have a serious illness that contributes to an early death; however, a person dependent on others for food also may have a lower nutrient intake that contributes to a decline in immune function or increase in cardiovascular or cancer risk.

Food items that can be heated in a microwave oven offer an alternative for older people with limited movement. Individually portioned packages, although more expensive, eliminate the problem of having to deal with leftovers. Nutrition education should focus on the selection of preprepared foods that contain limited amounts of sodium and fat and generous amounts of protein, vitamins, minerals, and fiber. Food technologists must continue efforts to develop food items high in nutritional quality that require little preparation.

Prescribed Diets and Food Selection

Diabetes mellitus, cardiovascular disease, kidney disease, or other chronic diseases often include a dietary prescription as part of their management. Older individuals following a prescribed diet may be restricted in sodium, fat, cholesterol, protein, carbohydrate, or energy. In the Georgia Centenarian Study,[25] 17% of those 100 years of age or older were following a "low-salt" diet, and 4% were following a low-cholesterol diet. Of the participants age 60 to 69, 15% and 18%, respectively, were on "low-salt" or low-cholesterol diets. The study did not indicate whether these special diets were prescribed by a physician. Race may be a factor in the adoption of low-sodium diets, since 25% of the older black participants in the Georgia study were following "low-salt" diets, as compared to only 11% of the older white participants.

TABLE 8-2   *Sources of Special Diets*
*Followed by Older Adults**

Diet	Prescribed by a Professional	Self-Prescribed
Low sodium	85%	14%
Low fat, low cholesterol	81%	19%
Diabetic	91%	8%
Low calorie	64%	35%
High fiber	53%	44%

*Percentages may not add up to 100%; not all sources represented.
Data from Lee, C.J., and others: Impact of special diets on the nutrient intakes of southern rural elderly, J. Am. Diet. Assoc. 93(2):186, 1993.

A nutrition survey of nearly 3,300 men and women ranging in age from 65 to 106 years who lived in 11 southern states[31] reported that 44% were following a special diet. The most common diet was a low-fat/low-cholesterol diet, followed by a diabetic diet and a high-fiber diet. The lowest energy intake (63% of the RDA) occurred in the people following a diabetic diet and the highest energy intake (70% of the RDA) occurred in those following the high-fiber diet. Energy intake was the same (67% of the RDA) among the people on the low-fat/low-cholesterol diet or no diet. Fat made up 33% of total energy in all of the diets described above and 35% of total energy for the people following no particular diet.

Further study is needed on the sources of the diets being followed by older people. In the survey of southern elderly[31] many older people had self-prescribed their special diet (table 8-2). There was no indication as to where they obtained their information or the appropriateness of the food choices they were making. It is important to follow up on an older person who has been placed on a special diet. Although the plan may be tentative or designed for short-term treatment, the individual may continue to follow the diet for months or even years, even when it is no longer appropriate.

Prescribed diets have a positive influence on nutrient intake if foods high in kilocalories and low in nutrient density are limited or omitted. Yet, omitting favorite foods or severely limiting the use of salt can reduce the pleasure associated with eating. It is important to take an individual approach in developing a diet for an older person, recognizing the need to consider favorite foods from the lifelong pattern. Including the patient in the decision-making process promotes development of a diet that will be accepted and followed.

SOCIOLOGIC ASPECTS OF FOOD SELECTION

Social Characteristics of the Aging Population

Marital status, living arrangements, and education differ within the aging population according to age, gender, and race or ethnic group.[69] Between the ages of 65 and 74, older people are likely to be married and living with their spouse. After age 84, a greater proportion of older people live alone or with other relatives. Older men usually live with their spouses as compared to older women who often live alone.[69]

Marital Status

At age 65 and older, 74% of men are married and living with their spouse as compared to only 40% of women. Although most older men remain married until they die, most older women are widowed. In fact elderly women are three times more likely to be widowed than elderly men. Because women have a longer life expectancy, they tend to outlive their husbands. Differences in marital status become even more pronounced with increasing age. By age 85, 80% of all women are widowed, whereas 47% of all men are still married. At all ages over 64, black women are less likely to be married than white women.[69]

Educational Level

In the population age 65 and older, fewer people have completed high school than is true for the population age 25 to 64. In general, 55% of community living older people completed high school as compared to 82% of other adults, but only one-fourth of elderly blacks completed high school. Nearly 30 of every 100 elderly people completed up to eighth grade or less. Years of schooling are lowest among elderly people age 85 and older.[69] The limited formal education of the oldest-old suggests the need for more visual methods of nutrition education, such as videos or demonstrations.

Living Arrangements

Most older people (95%) live in the community with their spouse, with other family members, with nonrelatives, or alone; only 5% of older people are institutionalized.[69] As women age, it becomes increasingly likely that they will live alone. The most recent census indicated that 42% of all older women live alone and 57% of older women above age 84 live alone. Older women also are more likely than older men to live with a relative other than a spouse. This may relate to elderly widowed women going to live with a child. Older black and Hispanic women more often live in households with three or more people as living arrangements involving extended families, including adult children and grandchildren, are more common in these groups. Fewer older men than older women live alone, but the greatest proportion living alone (30%) are white men age 85 and older. Women who live alone seem to fare better than men who live alone. Women who live alone typically have social contacts and diets similar to those of married couples.[69]

Household Size and Food Selection

Household size and nutrient intake. It is true that a person eating alone may be less motivated to prepare an adequate meal, but many other factors, including age, sex, economic situation, health status, and number of social contacts with family or friends, also influence food intake in those who live alone. Davis and coworkers[13] evaluated the influence of household size on dietary quality in the 4,402 adults age 55 and over who participated in the National Food Consumption Survey (NFCS). Older men living alone were more likely to have poorer diets than older women living alone, and

the proportion of single men with poor quality diets increased with age. Fourteen percent of the single men ages 55 to 64 had poor diets, but this nearly doubled to 25% among those age 75 and older. The pattern for single women was less consistent: 22% of those in the youngest age group (ages 55 to 64) had poor diets, compared with 16% and 21% in the groups ages 65 to 74 and 75 and over, respectively. In this evaluation a poor diet was defined as one with an intake below 67% of the RDA for at least five of the nine nutrients evaluated. These nutrients included vitamins A, C, B-6, and B-12, thiamin, riboflavin, iron, calcium, and magnesium.

As described in table 8-3, poverty status, a lower weekly food expenditure, and poor health contributed to poor quality diets.[13] However, the variable that was most important was the energy intake. Individuals eating alone did not make poorer food choices, they just consumed less food overall. Older people living alone are more likely to skip meals and consume a higher proportion of their total kilocalories away from home. Meals consumed away from home could include congregate meals obtained at senior centers. Skipping meals may be an indication that food resources are inadequate.

Living alone is not consistently related to poorer quality diets in older people. Posner and coworkers[50] considered the fact that social isolation or loneliness rather than living alone might be a key factor; individuals living in one-person households may participate actively in clubs or churches or other groups and have a high level of social interaction. In 1,156 New England elderly over age 69,[50] lower nutrient intake was related to less education (eight years of schooling or less) and not to living alone. In fact, those living alone had a diet lower in fat and saturated fat. About 20% of both groups (living alone and not living alone) had low intakes of protein and vitamin C, about 40% had low intakes of vitamin A, and about 75% were low in several nutrients. In that study individuals living alone were more likely to be female and age 85 or older; socially isolated individuals were more likely to be male.

Among 539 Dutch elderly[80] nutritional status evaluated on the basis of blood analyses did not

TABLE 8-3   *Factors Related to Dietary Quality in Older People*

Quality of Diet	Men		Women	
	High	Low	High	Low
Energy intake (kcal)	2,136	1,222	1,593	934
Money spent for food (per week)	$19.42	$16.09	$19.02	$15.70
Poor health (% of group)	29	51	32	45
Income below poverty level (% of group)	9	15	15	26

Adapted from Davis, M.A., and others: Living arrangements and dietary quality of older U.S. adults, J. Am. Diet. Assoc. 90:1667, 1990.

differ by household size. Total plasma carotenoids were lower in those living alone, although total fruit and vegetable consumption was similar in all households. Those living alone did tend to prepare their meat, potatoes, and vegetables for two or more days at a time. Reheating vegetables could decrease the vitamin content but preparing food ahead does ensure the availability of an appropriate meal for reheating on days when physical illness precludes extensive meal preparation. If there is no one else in the house and no neighbor or relative close by, the older person who is sick and forced to remain in bed may have nothing to eat or drink. This can lead to dehydration and, over a period of time, malnutrition.

Household size and cooking facilities. People who continue to live in their own home usually have adequate facilities for food storage and preparation, including a working stove, oven, and refrigerator. The type and size of an appliance affect its use. Older people may hesitate to heat their conventional oven for one item such as a baked potato. The ease, convenience, and lower utility cost of a microwave oven or small toaster oven make it an acceptable alternative. An older refrigerator or an apartment-size refrigerator with a small freezer compartment is a problem for someone who shops or has groceries delivered only infrequently. Food storage and preparation facilities can be less than adequate in senior housing apartments that have little counter space, limited cabinet space, and a small refrigerator.

Individuals who rent a room and have no access to kitchen facilities are forced to eat in restaurants or elsewhere. They may heat some foods on a hotplate in their room or use a heating coil for hot water for soup or beverages. These people are likely to be at or below the poverty level and, consequently, at high risk for poor nutrition. This group includes the hidden elderly who reside in rundown hotels in deteriorating inner city neighborhoods. These individuals need access to government-funded nutrition programs, including congregate or home-delivered meals and food stamps. Participation in these programs has been shown to reduce the nutritional risk of such older people (see chapter 14 for further discussion of meal programs).

Food Selection in Men and Women

Older men consume more kilocalories than older women but have diets lower in nutrient quality.[13] Older men are more likely than older women to skip meals[59] and have higher intakes of alcohol.[50] In a study of New England elderly, a greater proportion of men than women were in need of dental care, and poor dental status may influence food choices in this group.[50] Marital status affects nutrient intake to a greater extent in older men than women. Single older men tend to have poorer diets than single older women. Davis and coworkers[13] found that in the United States, single men age 75 or older were at the highest risk for diets low in important nutrients. The current generation of older men is less accustomed to food preparation and, if widowed, may have diets lacking in variety. Older men are more likely to have inadequate dietary levels of vitamins A and C which could relate to lower use of fruits and vegetables. Overall, men are more likely to reach adequate intakes of most nutrients because generally they consume more food.

Food Shopping Patterns

Food shopping can be a recreational or leisure time activity for the healthy older person with available transportation; conversely, it can be a difficult problem for the physically disadvantaged. Physical limitations, lack of transportation, and the changing locations of supermarkets present obstacles in food shopping for older people. In an older Canadian population receiving home care,[46] 41% of the men and 63% of the women were unable to food shop. In a national survey[69] 15% of those ages 75 to 84 and 37% of those above age 84 needed help with food shopping.

For many older people with a high level of physical function, shopping is an important social activity. In rural America, more than 51% of the elderly go to the grocery store at least twice a week, and they usually spend at least half an hour there.[65] With the changing face of today's supermarket, older people actually may increase the time they spend shopping. Today's convenience-conscious consumer wants everything under one roof, from a traditional supermarket to a pharmacy, post office, bank, in-store restaurant, and caterer. It is predicted that home-delivery, order-ahead service, and drive-through grocery pick-up will become available in the future. Supermarkets are responding to the growing elderly population with such services as benches to rest on, small-size packages, and help in handling groceries and carts.

Although the young-old may look forward to shopping, the old-old or frail elderly find food shopping somewhat difficult. Reported problems include lifting heavy items, difficulty in reaching or stooping for items on high or low shelves, and failing eyesight, which affects the ability to read labels or find an item on the shelf. Dependence on a cane or walker interferes with pushing a market basket, although many supermarkets now provide motorized carts for shoppers who need them.

Transportation to a food store is a problem for older people who no longer drive. In rural areas, if a store is within walking distance, it usually is a general store with a limited variety of items and package sizes, and prices tend to be higher. Urban elderly have similar problems, since inner city supermarkets are closing because of poor profit margins and the growth of suburban malls. Independently owned grocery markets are often replaced by self-service convenience stores with higher prices and less selection.

Walking to the store and carrying heavy bags home is difficult for those who must use a cane. In northern locations, sidewalks covered with ice and snow may preclude walking for several days at a time. Research evaluating the influence of shopping patterns on the nutritional adequacy of the diet is not currently available. Helping older people with shopping might be encouraged for those seeking worthwhile volunteer activities.

Lifestyle and Food Selection

Daily meal pattern. Because the daily schedule is more flexible after retirement, older people sometimes move away from the traditional pattern of three meals a day. Breakfast, however, is a popular meal with older people and in a national study[59] only 8% of the men and 4% of the women age 65 to 74 skipped breakfast. More men above age 75 (11%) skipped breakfast, but few of the women above age 75 (2%) skipped breakfast. Breakfast has a major impact on overall dietary quality in older age. In the CSFII,[32] breakfast contributed about 25% of the total energy, 25% to 29% of the vitamin A, about 30% of the vitamin C, 28% of the vitamin B-6, 31% of the calcium, and 29% of the magnesium in the diets of people age 70 and older. Use of a fortified ready-to-eat cereal likely contributed to these intakes.

It is interesting that the centenarians interviewed in Georgia[25] were more likely to regularly eat breakfast than were the participants ages 60 to 69. Also, the white elderly people were more likely to eat breakfast than the black elderly people. Lunch is the meal most likely to be skipped by older people. In a national study[59] about 30% of the older men and 21% of the older women skipped lunch.

Snacking patterns. Americans have been moving away from the traditional three meals a day to a grazing pattern, with an increase in mini meals and snacks. A concern in the case of younger people has been the nutritional quality of those snacks, which in some instances provide primarily kilocalories and fat. Murphy and others[41] found in older age groups that while snacking increased energy intake, it did not decrease the overall quality of the diet. This suggests that foods of reasonable nutrient density were being selected as snacks. In the CSFII,[32] nearly 80% of the participants age 60 and older had at least one snack over the reporting period. Ryan and coworkers[59] found that 35% of the men and 40% of the women above age 74 snacked. Snacking patterns may reflect ethnic patterns. Vietnamese elderly[70] snacked very infrequently. Those who reported snacking chose fruit, cake, cookies, soup with crackers, tea, or coffee. For older Chinese women in California,[9] fresh fruit was a common snack.

Promoting appropriate snacks could be of particular importance to older people for whom television watching or evening snacking is frequent. In a national study of older people[11] salty items such as pretzels or crackers, followed by ice cream, were the most popular evening snack. Fruit was the most popular morning snack. In the CSFII,[32] snacks provided about 10% of total energy, about 5% of the vitamin A, 7% of the vitamin B-6, 10% of the calcium, and 9% of the magnesium in the diets of people age 60 and older. It would appear that milk-based snacks are a frequent choice in this age group. Snack choices such as fruit, a low-fat dairy food, or a whole-grain bread or cereal will improve the nutrient intake of older adults.

Food away from home. Eating away from home has been increasing in the general population, and older adults are also part of this trend. The NFCS[32] found that 33% of people age 20 and older had a meal or snack away from home at least once during a three-day record period. Twenty percent of the men and women ages 60 to 69 had lunch or brunch away from home, but this fell to 14% in the group age 70 and older.

Older men were more likely to have breakfast away from home than older women. Fast food restaurants are attracting the older market. In 1989, McDonald's restaurants did 30% of their business with people over age 50.[65] Over half of older people surveyed in Texas and New Jersey frequented fast food restaurants.[39] Reasons given for eating at fast food outlets were not having to cook and the availability of economical food choices. Meals away from home also may include congregate meal programs or social potluck dinners at senior centers or other locations.

Trends in Social Patterns

Socioeconomic status influences both social participation and nutrition in older people. For example, the 50- to 64-year-old group spends about 14% more money on food than do younger groups.[65] Individuals between 40 and 60 years of age spend a greater proportion of their discretionary income on "catered experiences," such as travel tours and culinary events. As the older population becomes more diverse, it will be increasingly important to evaluate the influence of social contact on food intake in all groups. For the older adult who travels extensively, social contacts may be primarily short-term acquaintances, whereas for the older adult in poor health who seldom leaves home, visits or calls from family members may be the usual source of social interaction. For elderly people whose children have moved to different geographic locations, neighbors or workers from social agencies may be the only visitors. Each of these groups has different social patterns and expectations and different levels of accessibility to food. Another area for study is the food pattern of older widowed versus older single people. The single person who is accustomed to eating alone may be less vulnerable to nutritional inadequacy in later years than the individual for whom eating alone is a new experience.

FAILURE TO THRIVE: A MULTIFACETED PROBLEM
Food Intake and Failure to Thrive

Failure to thrive was first described in the pediatric literature in the late 1800s.[17] In children the characteristics associated with the failure to thrive include poor growth, poor appetite, apathy and the appearance of unhappiness, and lack of movement or activity. In infants these feelings of hopelessness and helplessness are believed to contribute to cachexia, repeated infections, and death.[5] Failure to thrive has recently been identified in older adults, although the symptoms are somewhat different. Whereas children exhibit a failure to grow and develop normally, the elderly experience a failure to maintain, with a loss of body weight, functional capacity, and cognitive and social skills.[17] The failure to thrive concept in adults involves several key elements:

1. A decline in biologic, psychologic, and social function. Any chronic disease can result in failure to thrive but heart failure, cancer, uncontrolled diabetes, or chronic obstructive pulmonary disease are most common. Dementia leading to social withdrawal or social isolation is associated with failure to thrive. Depression is an important component of this syndrome. Egbert[17] emphasized that deterioration must occur in all three areas of function for a true diagnosis of failure to thrive.
2. Loss of weight or undernutrition. A major characteristic of failure to thrive is reduced food intake, which can be both a cause or a result of this condition. Medications associated with many chronic diseases induce lower food intake and nausea, anorexia, distorted taste, or confusion. In some older people depression and isolation cause a lack of interest in eating. Failing eyesight interferes with food shopping and meal preparation. For the older person whose income is below the poverty level and who is taking several expensive prescription drugs, there may be little money left to purchase a sufficient amount of nutritious food.
3. No immediate explanation for the condition observed.

Failure to thrive is not a consequence of normal aging but instead results from a combination of aging changes that predispose older people to a downhill spiral involving chronic disease, weight loss, and malnutrition. Malnutrition may be an initial and critical factor in failure to thrive, leading to depression, mental changes, and further deterioration in physical or mental status.

Failure to thrive is not always recognized by health professionals, thus delaying intervention and resulting in unnecessary hospitalization or loss of independence. Loss of weight or change in mental function may be considered the result of old age, negating further investigation of possible underlying causes. Symptoms of disease are sometimes altered in the older person; for example, a serious infection is usually accompanied by fever in a young adult, but fever may be absent in an older adult. A review of 82 elderly patients diagnosed with failure to thrive[3] indicated that 81% had problems with at least two ADLs, 70% had trouble walking, 55% had anorexia, 45% were incontinent or had severe chronic pain, and 56% had impaired mental status. Although only 5% of these individuals were admitted to the hospital from institutional settings, 30% were discharged to such settings.

Intervention strategies for older people with failure to thrive include:[17]

- Use a team approach. A physician, nutritionist or dietitian, and social worker should be included. A psychologist or psychiatrist is needed if dementia or mental illness is identified. A speech pathologist can assist with swallowing disorders.
- Emphasize nutrition intervention. Undernutrition can be both a cause and an effect of failure to thrive, and in most cases nutrient intake can be improved. Dietary, anthropometric, and biochemical assessment is essential for a complete diagnosis of the condition (see chapter 11).
- Focus on factors that can be improved. For individuals with long-term chronic disease, difficulty in walking or swallowing, or physical pain, the condition may not be treatable. On the other hand, providing appropriate meals through use of home-delivered meals or homemaker services, reducing social isolation by regular visits from family or other social support people, and reconsidering the medications prescribed to reduce anorexia may be feasible interventions. Performing surgery for cataracts or providing needed glasses to improve vision

or fitting the edentulous patient with dentures can improve social involvement and eating behavior.

Control of Food Intake and Body Image

Despite the fact that weight loss is common among elderly people, the specific biologic or psychologic factors involved are poorly understood. A study of 35 healthy older and younger normal weight men[55] suggested that the metabolic signals that regulate food intake in younger people and prevent weight loss do not act the same way in older people. While younger men actively compensate with increased food intake following several weeks of underfeeding, older men do not. Older animals become increasingly sensitive to cholecystokinin, the gastrointestinal hormone believed to promote satiety as food moves through the gastrointestinal tract.[38] Morley and Silver[38] suggest that the early satiety associated with anorexia in some elderly people may be caused by increased signals from this hormone.

Inappropriate attitudes toward eating and body image may be involved in weight loss among the elderly. Hall and Driscoll[21] reported the case studies of two women ages 64 and 61 who weighed 33.5 kg (height = 1.69 m), and 37.5 kg (height = 1.71 m), respectively, and met the diagnostic criteria for anorexia nervosa. Both wished to avoid fatness, used laxatives to prevent weight gain, and died within five years of cachexia. Others have reported a distorted body image and inappropriate self-control around food among undernourished older men.[37] One patient, age 74, whose weight for height was 76% of the average indicated that he was preoccupied with a desire to be thinner.

Restrained eating appears to be more prevalent in older white women than older black women. Among 404 older women whose mean age was 73,[67] overweight African American women were only half as likely to feel guilty after overeating or to go on a diet as overweight white women. More than twice as many overweight African American women were satisfied with their weight as compared to overweight white women. The inappropriate attention to thinness that is growing within younger populations appears to be influencing older groups as well. Of particular concern is the preoccupation with reduced food intake among elderly people who are already underweight. It would be interesting to evaluate body image and restrained eating among older people with failure to thrive.

ECONOMIC ASPECTS OF FOOD SELECTION
Aging and Economic Status

In general the economic status of older people has improved measurably in the last 25 years; however, all groups have not shared equally in these gains.[69] The economic picture for older people can be uncertain as life expectancy increases along with ever-growing health care expenditures. For the most part people age 65 and older have less cash income than people under age 65. This decrease in cash income is related to retirement, when people become dependent on Social Security or other pensions. Social Security payments, which are based on one's income when working, are the principal source of income for most older Americans. Since 1975 Social Security benefits have increased annually according to the increase in the Consumer Price Index the previous year, but income still may be inadequate or uncertain for the older adult. The death of her husband is critical for an older woman who depended on his pension and is eligible for no or very low Social Security or pension benefits of her own. Health problems resulting in continuing medical costs that are not covered by Medicare or private health insurance can deplete the older person's savings, creating financial anxiety. Costly prescription drugs can divert money from the food budget. Older adults are more likely than younger adults to fall below the poverty level and are less able through marriage or employment to increase their income above this level.

Age, marital status, education level, ethnic group, and former occupation all influence income in later life.[69] Based on 1990 dollars the median income for elderly men was $14,183, but for elderly women it was only $8,044. Older

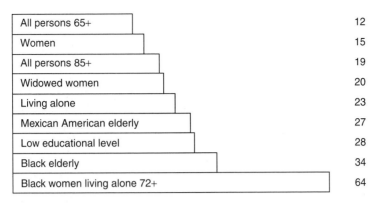

All persons 65+	12
Women	15
All persons 85+	19
Widowed women	20
Living alone	23
Mexican American elderly	27
Low educational level	28
Black elderly	34
Black women living alone 72+	64

Data for persons age 65+ unless noted otherwise

FIG. 8-3   Percentage of Typical Groups with Incomes Below the Poverty Level. Age, sex, race, and marital status influence poverty status in older people. Elderly women living alone who belong to minority groups are at highest risk of being poor.

Data from U.S. Senate Special Committee on Aging: Aging America. Trends and projections (annotated), Serial No. 101-J, Washington, DC, 1990, U.S. Government Printing Office.

married couples had a median income of $20,996 whereas older women living alone had a median income of only $7,863. Among the elderly, advancing age increases the risk of being poor. While only 8% of people ages 65 to 69 are poor, 17% of those ages 80 to 84 are poor. Black and Hispanic elderly have lower incomes than white elderly. Blacks and Hispanics are more likely to have lower incomes as younger adults and therefore receive lower Social Security or pension benefits.[69] As shown in figure 8-3, individuals having several of these characteristics have an even greater chance of being poor.[75] Now that more women have entered the workforce and are establishing Social Security or pension accounts in their own right, the prevalence of poverty among older women is likely to decline in future decades.

Older people spend a larger proportion of their income on food, utilities, and health care than younger people do.[75] Conversely, younger households spend proportionately more on clothing, transportation, and entertainment. Both groups spend about the same amount on housing. Out-of-pocket costs for health care are the greatest threat to the economic security of the older person. Out-of-pocket costs for health

care use 9% of the income of those ages 65 to 74 and 15% of the income of those above age 74, compared to only 4% of the income of younger adults.

Food Expenditures in Older Households

Older households spend a greater proportion of their total income on food than younger households. In 1990, the average proportion of income spent for food across all households was about 12%;[29] in contrast retired households included in a 1986–87 survey spent about 20% of their income for food.[58] As income level rises, a decreasing proportion of income is spent for food.[29] Households with an income of about $6,000 spent 42% of their money for food, whereas those with an income of $14,000 spent only 22% for food.[29] Although retired married couples, retired single men, and retired single women spend about the same proportion of their income (20%) for food, this represents very different amounts in actual dollars.[58] A survey of 1,597 retired households[58] revealed that married couples spent $3,683 for food a year, single men spent $2,381, and single women spent $1,779.

A major trend across all U.S. households is an increasing amount of money being spent for food eaten away from home. Kinsey[29] noted that while median household income rose by 21% since 1960, expenditures for food away from home rose by 183%; in 1990, 37% of the food dollar was spent for food away from home. Across all retired households food away from home used about 5% of the food dollar;[58] retired single men and retired married couples eat away from home more frequently than retired single women. Retired married couples and single men also spend more money for alcohol than retired single women. Money spent for food continues to decline with advancing age regardless of retirement. The average annual expenditure for food per person (in 1984 dollars) by older Americans ages 55 to 64 was $3,602, compared to $1,865 by those age 75 or older.[65]

Level of Income and Nutritional Adequacy

Several studies suggest a relationship between income and nutrient intake.[41,51] Posner and coworkers[51] found 53 homebound, low-income older people to be at nutritional risk. Depending on the particular dietary component (kilocalories, protein, vitamin A, vitamin C, thiamin, riboflavin, niacin, iron, or calcium), 40% to 80% of these older people did not meet the RDA. The decline in the nutritional quality of the diet with decreasing income was not the result of poor food choices, but of the limited amount of food available.

Murphy and coworkers[41] analyzed the factors influencing dietary adequacy in people over age 64 and found the significant predictor to be money spent for food. People with better quality diets spent on the average $3.33 to $3.60 more for food a week. Money spent for food was significantly related to total energy intake. Individuals ages 65 to 84 with better quality diets had higher incomes than those with poorer quality diets. Surprisingly, income was not a factor in the dietary quality of those age 85 or older. In a study of community living people age 70 or older in New England,[49] lack of money for food, eating fewer than two meals a day, and eating few fruits and vegetables were the strongest predictors of inadequate nutrient intake. Eating fewer meals as an indicator of inadequate nutrient intake is consistent with the finding among the low-income homebound elderly[51] described earlier who reported a lack of available food. Fruits and vegetables, usually popular foods among the elderly, also tend to be relatively expensive and would be less available on a low food budget.

It is difficult to separate the effects of income, education, and ethnic group on food intake. Individuals with less than a high school education are more likely to have low intakes of protein, vitamins A and C, thiamin, and calcium than those who have at least a high school education.[50] Older people with less education are likely to have lower incomes but also may have limited reading ability and less opportunity to learn about good food choices.

Level of income and poverty status influence food consumption but not all nutrients are affected in the same way (fig. 8-4). In the CSFII[32] mean protein intake among people over age 60 ranged from 109% to 110% of the RDA, despite incomes that were less than 30% above the poverty level; protein intakes increased to 124% to 130% of the RDA in older women and men with incomes more than 3.5 times the poverty level. It appears that older people value protein and make an effort to obtain this nutrient regardless of income. While protein intake was adequate in the lowest income group, zinc intake was well below the recommended level. This suggests that milk, poultry, or highly processed prepared foods that tend to be low in zinc rather than meat or whole-grain breads and cereals that are good sources of zinc are the major food sources of protein. Zinc intake met only 65% of the RDA for the older men and 67% of the RDA for the older women with the lowest income; the older men with the highest income increased their intake of zinc to 98% of the RDA, but the older women with the highest income still fell way below with intakes of only 81% of the RDA.

Despite the relatively high cost of some fruits and vegetables, particularly in the winter months, the men and women with the lowest incomes met at least 100% of the RDA for vitamin A, and

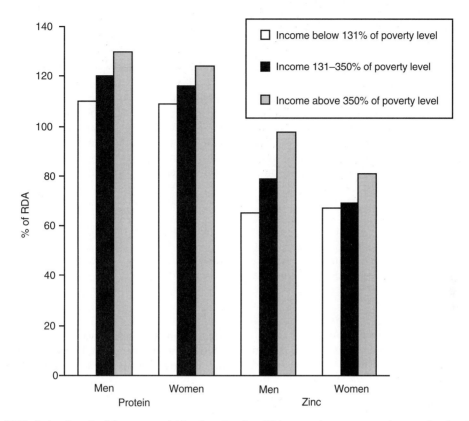

FIG. 8-4   Level of Income and Nutrient Intake. Older people consume adequate levels of protein regardless of income level; in contrast, zinc intakes are below recommended levels in low-income elderly and climb as income level rises.

Data from Life Sciences Research Office, Federation of American Societies for Experimental Biology: Third Report on Nutrition Monitoring in the United States, Vol. I and II, Washington, DC, December 1995, U.S. Government Printing Office.

intakes rose to 150% of the RDA as income increased.[32] Vitamin B-6 was eaten at a level of only 81% to 84% of the RDA in the lowest income group, but exceeded the recommended level in the highest income group. Manore and coworkers[34] pointed out that breakfast cereals and bananas are major sources of vitamin B-6 in the diets of older people. Seasonal availability and cost appeared to influence the use of bananas among low-income Arizona elderly, and cost was related to lower intakes of meat, poultry, and fish. Over 85% of an older population studied in Norway[79] believed that a proper meal ought to include vegetables and potatoes, but about 20%

of that group indicated that cost limited their use of vegetables. Canned vegetables are often less expensive than fresh or frozen vegetables but many types have added sodium. (The influence of poverty status on all major nutrients will be discussed in chapter 9.)

Use of Food Stamps

Food assistance programs like the food stamp program that increase buying power can improve the quality of the diet. Unfortunately, eligible older people are less likely to participate in the food stamp program than eligible younger people; national estimates indicate that only 22% of poor elderly receive food stamps.[74] Black and Hispanic elderly are about twice as likely to participate in the food stamp program as white elderly. A survey of nearly 1,700 low-income elderly[45] revealed that only 25% participated in the food stamp program. Among those who indicated they had been without food for more than three days in a row in the last month, only 32% were receiving food stamps. Older people may be less informed about food stamps, may lack transportation to the appropriate office, or may choose not to apply because of pride.

Efforts to ease these problems have included processing food stamp applications by mail or telephone and giving application materials to outreach workers at senior centers and congregate meal sites. These methods also eliminate the embarrassment of having to appear at the local family assistance or welfare office. Although several areas are testing giving cash payments rather than food stamps, it has been shown that food stamps are two to seven times more effective than cash income in increasing food purchases.[66] Health and social service professionals working with elderly who are eligible to receive food stamps need to encourage and facilitate the application process and ongoing participation.

Community Meal Programs for the Poor

A national survey[45] found participation in soup kitchen and food pantry programs to be low among older adults, despite the fact that three-fourths had incomes below the poverty level. Of those who indicated they did not have enough money to buy food, 76% never used a soup kitchen, and 83% never used a food pantry. Identification of individuals using food pantries in New York state[8] indicated that only 9% of urban users were age 60 or older as compared to 28% of rural users. The low utilization of soup kitchens and food pantries by impoverished older people is largely unexplained. Pride, lack of transportation, or fear of personal harm in the neighborhood where the program is located may deter participation by needy older people.

NUTRITION FOR OLDER PEOPLE WITH SPECIAL NEEDS

Helping the Functionally Impaired

Older people who are seriously ill or recovering from illness are sometimes unable to feed themselves. This can be temporary with self-feeding resuming as strength is regained. In the case of a stroke, organic brain syndrome, or chronic neuromuscular disease such as Parkinson's disease or myasthenia gravis, some degree of paralysis or loss of coordination can be permanent and prohibit the usual motions involved in self-feeding. Data from the National Health Interview Survey[69] indicate that 4% of people age 85 or older living in the community need help with eating. Among physically impaired older people receiving home health services,[14] nearly 14% needed help with eating.

Problems in meal preparation and self-feeding can be caused by weakness in the hand and arm muscles, making it difficult to lift utensils such as a bowl, cup, or spoon. Partial paralysis can limit range of motion or make it difficult to flex the fingers and hand to grasp a plate or fork. If the affected muscle group has an adequate blood and nerve supply, weakened muscles often can be strengthened by appropriate exercises. If, however, the neuromuscular weakness resulted from wasting of the muscle tissue or denervation of the muscle because of brain damage or one of the diseases noted above, it is less likely that normal function can be restored. Changes in muscle fibers may cause a permanent change in the joint so that the arm remains bent at the elbow and cannot be extended.

Utensils for Special Needs

Various devices have been developed to assist individuals with some degree of functional loss. Sometimes only a slight modification of existing utensils will facilitate food handling. Special aids often are available from local hospital supply companies or by mail order. (See selected resources in appendix D.)

Cups. Lightweight plastic cups are easier to handle than glass or china. A cup with a partial lid or small opening (plastic travel cup) will prevent spills for those with abrupt movements and poor coordination. Sports drink containers, with their wide base, plastic composition, and fitted lid and straw, are also good alternatives. A stretch-knit coaster slipped onto the bottom of a glass or an adhesive-backed bathtub safety tread attached around the sides provides a non-slippery surface for grasping.

Forks and spoons. Utensils with extra-thick bamboo or plastic handles are easier to grasp if flexing the fingers is difficult. An inexpensive solution is placing a foam curler over the handle of a standard utensil, since the foam surface increases the friction and aids in holding. For those unable to grasp, a cuff with a pocket holding a standard utensil can be slipped over the hand to facilitate self-feeding. A swivel spoon or spoon with an extra long handle is helpful when motion is limited.

Plates and bowls. A suction device to prevent a dish or bowl from moving will assist the older person attempting to self-feed with the use of only one hand. A plate with a broad edge to push food against when filling a spoon or fork will help those with limited motor skills. Because self-feeding can require considerable time for one who is slowly regaining skills, a plastic dish with a lower compartment filled with hot water is necessary to keep food at a palatable temperature.

When the older individual with some functional loss returns home, meal preparation must also be resumed. Use of a microwave oven can facilitate the transition, since it requires little dexterity of movement and can heat or reheat food in short periods of time. The major difficulty associated with preprepared microwavable foods can be opening or preparing the package for placement in the microwave oven. Many packages require use of a scissors and hand strength for cutting through a cardboard covering.

Regaining Self-Feeding Skills

Types of food for self-feeding. Relearning feeding skills can be a long and difficult process. Careful selection and preparation of the foods offered and a positive approach will facilitate progress and encourage effort. If chewing or swallowing is also a problem, a soft diet rather than a pureed diet is not only more palatable but

also requires less skill in eating. Avoid cutting foods into many small pieces; fewer motions are required to eat fewer medium-sized pieces. Finger foods are ideal because they require less effort and energy to eat. Ideas for making difficult items into finger foods include putting ground meat or sandwich filling in a pita pocket, serving an egg hard-cooked and peeled, or cutting raw fruits and vegetables into strips, flowerets, or quarters. An easy-to-eat meal might include a pita sandwich, soup served in a mug, apple slices (peeled and cored), and a carton of milk with a straw.

Environment for self-feeding. Attention and praise provide incentive for continuing what may be a painful and frustrating activity. Having the individuals in a self-feeding program sit at a table facing each other promotes both social interaction and mutual support as patients become helpful to each other. Reducing the general noise level so that patients can converse with staff and each other contributes to a positive meal environment. Sensitizing staff to avoid negative outbursts, such as when a self-feeding patient accidentally spills food, is essential for a rehabilitation program to succeed.

Feeding the Chronically Ill

Many factors contribute to feeding difficulties and subsequent malnutrition in a frail chronically ill elderly adult. The older person may actively resist feeding, may have difficulty chewing and swallowing, or may have altered appetite and taste because of medications he or she is taking. Preserving the dignity of the individual who has to be fed influences general receptivity to the food offered. The emotional empathy between the individual performing the feeding and the patient is critical to successful feeding and continuing nutritional intake. A sensitive and patient attitude on the part of the caregiver will encourage food intake in a frail older person for whom food mastication and swallowing require concentrated effort. Sanders and coworkers[60] emphasized the need to allow sufficient time for feeding. In that report one-third of caregivers fed an entire meal in 5 to 10 minutes. The following guidelines are important when feeding the older adult:[52]

The position of the person: The individual should be sitting upright with hips at a 90-degree angle. Never feed a person in a supine position, because this increases the danger of choking and food aspiration.

The presentation of the food: Only small amounts of food should be offered at a time; forcing food into the mouth too rapidly increases the fear of choking and the danger of food aspiration. Straws that supply liquid more rapidly than it can be swallowed should not be used. Infant rice cereal is a relatively inexpensive and effective thickener for thin liquids that are difficult to handle. Commercial thickeners are also available.

The nutrient density of the food: Items rich in energy, protein, vitamins, and minerals should be emphasized since the older person may tire quickly and consume only limited amounts of food. (See chapter 12 for ideas on fortifying foods with powdered protein supplements.)

A Team Approach

Evaluating any loss in function and planning appropriate therapy to help the patient achieve the highest level of independence possible requires a cooperative effort of the nurse, physician, nutrition professional, occupational therapist, and physical therapist. Successful feeding of patients who cannot feed themselves requires attention to the type of food to be offered and the appropriate feeding techniques. The rehabilitation necessary to help a patient relearn self-feeding skills demands careful planning and supervision. The dietary intake of patients with feeding problems must be monitored carefully and adjustments made as necessary.

DIETARY PATTERNS: IMPLICATIONS FOR NUTRITION EDUCATION

Older people generally have a varied diet that includes foods from all major food groups. Most older people regularly consume protein foods (meat, fish, poultry, and eggs); more than 94% of the men and 88% of the women over age 64 participating in a national survey had at least one serving a day of these foods.[32] Among the 2,650 older people interviewed in the NHANES I Epidemiologic Follow-Up Study (NHEFS),[42] white participants had an average of 1.6 servings a day from the protein group but black participants had only 1.2 servings. In the CSFII,[32] men age 70 and over averaged 7 oz. of food a day from the meat group and women averaged 5 oz.

Breads and cereals are popular foods with older people and are consumed daily. In the CSFII,[32] 51% of those age 70 and older had a ready-to-eat cereal at least once during the record-keeping period; 61% had a sweet baked product. The NHEFS population[42] consumed 2.5 servings of grains, bread, or cereal each day. Current recommendations suggest at least six servings each day.

Use of milk products is lower than recommended in older men and women. Although over 80% report using milk, average total intake represents less than one cup of milk a day or less than 300 mg of calcium.[32] The elderly white people in the NHEFS study[42] averaged 1.6 servings a day from the dairy group, but the elderly black people averaged only 1.2 servings. The recommended level is at least two servings a day.

Fruits and vegetables were eaten in the recommended amounts by the NHEFS subjects.[42] They had 2.7 servings of fruit each day and 3.2 servings of vegetables to meet their total of Five A Day; however, use of vegetables was lower among black elderly. On the average all of the participants had one serving a day of a citrus fruit, but the daily intake of vegetables supplying vitamin A precursor carotenoids was only about a half serving. Limited use of dark green and deep yellow vegetables was also observed in the older CSFII participants.[32] Less than 20% had a dark green or deep yellow vegetable, although about 30% had tomatoes during the record-keeping period.

Regardless of limited budgets, older people appear to regularly consume foods from the meat group. These items, coupled with increased servings of enriched or whole-grain bread and cereal, should provide adequate iron, although iron absorption may be compromised in some older people. Encouraging use of whole-grain products would add important minerals such as zinc, magnesium, and chromium to the diet.

❖ ❖ ❖

CASE STUDY

Mrs. W just had her 85th birthday and lives alone. At a recent checkup, her doctor found that she has lost a significant amount of weight and seems to be confused as to the day of the week and recent events. Her husband of 65 years died in the past year. She has two children and five grandchildren, but they live more than 100 miles away. Her current medications include digoxin and an antihypertensive agent.

1. Based on the available information, what factors might have contributed to her weight loss? Explain.

2. Do you have enough information to determine whether or not Mrs. W is suffering from failure to thrive? If not, what additional information is needed?

3. How could her medications affect her appetite and food choices?

4. What dietary information would you need her to provide to assess her current status? What nutrition and dietary recommendations might you offer her?

5. Would psychosocial recommendations and referrals be appropriate? If so, describe.

Frankfurters and luncheon meats were used by nearly half of the older people participating in the CSFII;[32] protein foods lower in sodium or fat that provide more quality protein for less cost, such as lean meat, eggs, and legumes, should be encouraged.

Incorporating dairy products into the daily meal pattern is essential for intakes of calcium and riboflavin to be adequate. These foods also contribute vitamin A, protein, and magnesium, and fluid milk provides added vitamin D. The role of grain products in a healthy diet must continue to be a priority in nutrition education. Also, many older people are not consuming adequate amounts of dark green or deep yellow vegetables. This may relate to cost or problems in the preparation of fresh vegetables. Frozen or canned vegetables are a good alternative to fresh, particularly in the winter months.

Dietary diversity based on the number of food groups included in the daily diet has been associated with reduced mortality risk.[26] The five food groups evaluated included: dairy, meat, grain, fruit, and vegetable. Participants in the NHEFS study[26] who consumed foods from only two groups had a 50% greater risk of death after seven years than individuals consuming foods from three or more groups. Of all age groups evaluated, those age 65 and older had the most diverse diets. About 41% of the older men and women ate foods from five food groups, and about 35% ate foods from four

groups. It appears that older people recognize the importance of all food groups, providing a sound basis for further nutrition education.

Summary

Adaptation to changes in lifestyle, health, and economic status can bring about changes in eating patterns. Increasing age and decreasing energy requirements result in consumption of less food and can lead to nutritional inadequacy. Older people do change their food patterns according to general food trends and product availability and so can be receptive to nutrition education.

Social activity and social contact are positively related to the nutritional quality of the diet. Depression, loneliness, and diminished feelings of self-worth can lead to disinterest in food. Mental disorders in the older adult, including dementia, can influence nutritional requirements as well as food behaviors, and dietary and behavioral interventions are often indicated. Patients with organic brain syndrome who cannot feed themselves often show weight loss and should be monitored closely. Efforts at rehabilitating patients with loss of motor skills or partial paralysis should include self-feeding.

Changes in taste and smell, loss of teeth, and physical disability can adversely affect nutrient intake. A person who is homebound and dependent on others for food delivery or a functionally impaired older person who cannot move about easily in the home to carry on meal preparation is forced to depend on preprepared food items and can have limited intake of fresh fruits and vegetables and dairy products. Drugs or prescribed diets used to treat chronic diseases that are common in older people can result in diminished appetite or problems in food selection. Snacking can either add to or detract from the quality of the diet, and nutrition education should emphasize healthy, nutrient-dense snack choices.

Failure to thrive, traditionally related to pediatric populations, has recently been identified in older adults. In the elderly, failure to thrive is a failure to maintain, with a loss of body weight, functional capacity, and cognitive and social skills. Intervention includes use of a team approach, emphasis on nutrition intervention, and a focus on factors that can be modified to improve food intake and social interaction.

Older people generally have a varied diet that includes food from all major food groups. Most older people regularly consume meats, fish, and poultry, breads and cereals, and fruits and vegetables. Use of milk products is lower than recommended in many older men and women. Older people with a low income are likely to have diets poorer in nutritional quality than older people with higher incomes. Food stamps can make a significant contribution to the food availability and nutritional quality of the diets of older recipients. Unfortunately, eligible older people are less likely to participate in the food stamp program than eligible younger people. Older people should be encouraged to participate in food assistance programs and helped in identifying such opportunities in their community.

REVIEW QUESTIONS

1. How does aging alter energy and nutrient intake? Does race or ethnic group or very old age influence energy intake in older people? What is the Baltimore Longitudinal Study of Aging, and what information about nutrition and aging is the study providing?
2. How do changes in roles within the family structure influence eating patterns? Does social interaction positively or negatively influence eating patterns in the elderly? What does "age-appropriate expectations" mean when it comes to food selection?
3. What are the three stages of dementia? How are food choices and nutrient intake affected at each stage? What dietary modifications may be required at each stage of dementia? What general guidelines should be considered when feeding patients with dementia?
4. Do taste and smell change as people age? What effect might these sensory changes have on food selection? What dental problems are common in older people and how do they influence food intake? How does arthritis influence food choices and eating habits?
5. What is failure to thrive in the elderly? What key elements are involved in failure to thrive? Is failure to thrive a normal consequence of aging? What intervention strategies are appropriate for older people with failure to thrive?

SUGGESTED LEARNING ACTIVITIES

1. Go to the frozen food section of your grocery store and prepare a list of all frozen meals that would be acceptable meeting the following criteria: no more than 800 mg of sodium and no more than 30% of the kilocalories from fat. Prepare a handout for use in an education class for older people.
2. Prepare a handout describing risk factors for nutritional inadequacies to be used by community groups working with older people. Include physiologic, psychologic, sociologic, and economic risk factors.
3. Develop a resource list of food assistance programs in your community that are available to older people, listing what assistance is provided and eligibility requirements. Include the name, address, and telephone number of a contact person for each program who could help an older person who wished to participate. Make your list available to activity leaders in senior centers and directors of congregate meal sites and home-delivered meals programs.
4. Prepare a recipe booklet with feeding hints for caregivers of persons with senile dementia of the Alzheimer type.
5. Interview an older relative about the foods eaten, household composition, meal times, and foods served for special holiday or religious meals when he or she was a young adult. Have his or her food patterns changed since that time, and, if so, how have they changed? Prepare an oral report for your class on your findings, and point out the differences and similarities between your older person's food pattern as a young adult and your food pattern.

REFERENCES

1. Angulo, J.F.: Foodways, ideology, and aging: a developmental dilemma, Am. Behavioral Scient. 32(1):41, 1988.
2. Bartholomew, A.M., and others: Food frequency intakes and sociodemographic factors of elderly Mexican Americans and non-Hispanic whites, J. Am. Diet. Assoc. 90:1693, 1990.
3. Berkman, B., Foster, L.W.S., and Campion, E.: Failure to thrive: paradigm for the frail elder, Gerontologist 29:654, 1989.
4. Bernard, M.A., Anderson, C., and Forgey, M.: Health and nutritional status of old-old African Americans, J. Nutr. Elderly 14(2/3):55, 1995.
5. Braun, J.V., Wykle, M.H., and Cowling, W.R.: Failure to thrive in older persons: a concept derived, J. Gerontol. 28(6):809, 1988.
6. Briley, M.E.: Food preferences of the elderly, Nutr. Rev. 52(8):S21, 1994.
7. Butler, R.N.: Senile dementia of the Alzheimer type. In: Abrams, W.B., Beers, M.H., and Berkow, R., editors: Merck manual of geriatrics, ed. 2., Whitehouse Station, NJ, 1995, Merck Research Laboratories.
8. Clancy, K.L., and Bowering, J.: The need for emergency food: poverty problems and policy responses, J. Nutr. Ed. 24:12S, 1992.
9. Chau, P., and others: Dietary habits, health beliefs, and food practices of elderly Chinese women, J. Am. Diet. Assoc. 90:1667, 1990.
10. Cohen, N.L., and Ralston, P.A.: Factors affecting dietary quality of elderly blacks, final report, Washington, DC, 1992, AARP Andrus Foundation.
11. Cross, A.T., Babicz, D., and Cushman, L.F.: Snacking habits of senior Americans, J. Nutr. Elderly 14(2/3):27, 1995.
12. Davies, L.: Nutrition education of the elderly. In: Prinsley, D.M., and Sandstead, H.H., editors: Nutrition and aging, New York, 1990, Alan R. Liss.
13. Davis, M.A., and others: Living arrangements and dietary quality of older U.S. adults, J. Am. Diet. Assoc. 90:1667, 1990.
14. Dey, A.N.: Characteristics of elderly men and women discharged from home health services: United States, 1991–92, Advance Data, No. 259, Vital and Health Statistics, U.S. Department of Health and Human Services, 1995, Hyattsville, MD.
15. Duffy, V.B., Backstrand, J.R., and Ferris, A.M.: Olfactory dysfunction and related nutritional risk in free-living, elderly women, J. Am. Diet. Assoc. 95:879, 1995.
16. Dwyer, J.: Nutritional problems of elderly minorities, Nutr. Rev. 52(8):S24, 1994.
17. Egbert, A.M.: The dwindles: failure to thrive in older patients, Nutr. Rev. 54(No. 1, Part II):S25, 1996.
18. Exton-Smith, A.N., and Stanton, B.R.: Report on an investigation into the dietary of elderly women living alone, London, 1965, King Edward's Hospital Fund for London.
19. Fischer, C.A., and others: Nutrition knowledge, attitudes, and practices of older and younger elderly in rural areas, J. Am. Diet. Assoc. 91:1398, 1991.
20. Fischer, J.G., and others: Dairy product intake of the oldest-old, J. Am. Diet. Assoc. 95(8):918, 1995.
21. Hall, P., and Driscoll, R.: Anorexia in the elderly—an annotation, Intl. J. Eating Disorders 14(4):497, 1993.
22. Hallfrisch, J., and others: Continuing diet trends in men: the Baltimore Longitudinal Study of Aging (1961–1987), J. Gerontol. 45:M186, 1990.
23. Hollingsworth, D.S., and Hart, W.D.: Effects of gender, ethnicity, and place of residence on nutrient intake among elderly residents of southwestern Louisiana, J. Nutr. Elderly 10(4):51, 1991.
24. Jerome, N.W.: Dietary intake and nutritional status in older U.S. blacks: an overview. In: Jackson, J.S., editor: The black American elderly, New York, 1988, Springer Publishing Co.
25. Johnson, M.A., and others: Nutritional patterns of centenarians, Inter. J. Aging Hum. Develop. 34(1):57, 1992.
26. Kant, A.K., and others: Dietary diversity and subsequent mortality in the First National Health and Nutrition Examination Survey Epidemiologic Follow-up Study, Am. J. Clin. Nutr. 57:434, 1993.
27. Kant, A.K., and Schatzkin, A.: Consumption of energy-dense, nutrient-poor foods by the U.S. population: effect on nutrient profiles, J. Am. Coll. Nutr. 13(3):285, 1994.
28. Kim, K.K., and others: Nutritional status of Chinese-, Korean-, and Japanese-American elderly, J. Am. Diet. Assoc. 93:1416, 1993.
29. Kinsey, J.D.: Food and families' socioeconomic status, J. Nutr. 124:1878S, 1994.
30. Krondl, M., and others: Food use and perceived food meanings of the elderly, J. Am. Diet. Assoc. 80:523, 1982.
31. Lee, C.J., and others: Impact of special diets on the nutrient intakes of southern rural elderly, J. Am. Diet. Assoc. 93(2):186, 1993.

32. Life Sciences Research Office, Federation of American Societies for Experimental Biology: Third Report on Nutrition Monitoring in the United States, Vol. I and II, Washington, DC, December 1995, U.S. Government Printing Office.

33. Litchford, M.D., and Wakefield, L.M.: Nutrient intakes and energy expenditures of residents with senile dementia of the Alzheimer's type, J. Am. Diet. Assoc. 87:211, 1987.

34. Manore, M.M., Vaughan, L.A., and Lehman, W.R.: Contribution of various food groups to dietary vitamin B-6 intake in free-living, low-income elderly persons, J. Am. Diet. Assoc. 90:830, 1990.

35. Martin, W.: Oral health in the elderly. In: Chernoff, R., editor: Geriatric nutrition: the health professional's handbook, Gaithersburg, MD, 1991, Aspen Publishers.

36. McIntosh, W.A., and others: The relationship between beliefs about nutrition and dietary practices of the elderly, J. Am. Diet. Assoc. 90:671, 1990.

37. Miller, D.K., and others: Abnormal eating attitudes and body image in older undernourished individuals, J. Am. Geriatr. Soc. 39:462, 1991.

38. Morley, J.E., and Silver, A.J.: Anorexia in the elderly, Neurobiol. Aging 9(1):9, 1988.

39. Morris, J., Schneider, D., and Macey, S.M.: A survey of older Americans to determine frequency and motivations for eating fast food, J. Nutr. Elderly 15(1):1, 1995.

40. Mowé, M., Bohmer, T., and Kindt, E.: Reduced nutritional status in an elderly population (> 70 y) is probable before disease and possibly contributes to the development of disease, Am. J. Clin. Nutr. 59:317, 1994.

41. Murphy, S.P., and others: Factors influencing the dietary adequacy and energy intake of older Americans, J. Nutr. Ed. 22:284, 1990.

42. Murphy, S.P., Everett, D.F., and Dresser, C.M.: Food group consumption reported by the elderly during the NHANES I Epidemiologic Follow-up Study, J. Nutr. Ed. 21:214, 1989.

43. Nutrition Screening Initiative: Nutrition interventions manual for professionals caring for older Americans, Washington, DC, 1992, Nutrition Screening Initiative.

44. Papas, A.S.: Oral health. In: Hartz, S.C., Russell, R.M., and Rosenberg, I.H., editors: Nutrition in the elderly. The Boston Nutritional Status Survey, London, 1992, Smith Gordon and Company.

45. Parker, S.L.: A national survey of nutritional risk among the elderly, J. Nutr. Ed. 24:23S, 1992.

46. Payette, H., and others: Predictors of dietary intake in a functionally dependent elderly population in the community, Am. J. Public Health, 85:677, 1995.

47. Peters, G.R., and Rappoport, L.: Aging and the psychosocial problematics of food, Am. Behavioral Scient. 32:31, 1988.

48. Popkin, B.M., Haines, P.S., and Patterson, R.E.: Dietary changes in older Americans, 1977–1987, Am. J. Clin. Nutr. 55:823, 1992.

49. Posner, B.M., and others: Nutrition and health risks in the elderly: the nutrition screening initiative, Am. J. Public Health 83:972, 1993.

50. Posner, B.M., and others: Nutritional risk in New England elders, J. Gerontol. 49(3):M123, 1994.

51. Posner, B.M., Smigelski, C.G., and Krachenfels, M.M.: Dietary characteristics and nutrient intake in an urban homebound population, J. Am. Diet. Assoc. 87:452, 1987.

52. Practical solutions to eating problems of the elderly, J. Am. Diet. Assoc. 91:1417, 1991.

53. Renvall, M.J., and others: Body composition of patients with Alzheimer's disease, J. Am. Diet. Assoc. 93:47, 1993.

54. Rheaume, Y., Riley, M.E., and Volcier, L.: Meeting nutritional needs of Alzheimer patients who pace constantly, J. Nutr. Elderly 7:43, 1987.

55. Roberts, S.B., and others: Control of food intake in older men, J.A.M.A. 272:1601, 1994.

56. Roe, D.A.: In-home nutritional assessment of inner-city elderly, J. Nutr. 120:1538, 1990.

57. Rouse, J.H., and Gilster, S.D.: An improved method of documenting and evaluating nutritional intake of persons with Alzheimer's disease, J. Nutr. Elderly 14(1):45, 1994.

58. Rubin, R.M., and Nieswindomy, M.: Expenditure patterns of retired and nonretired persons, Monthly Labor Rev. 117(4):10, 1994.

59. Ryan, A.S., Craig, L.D., and Finn, S.C.: Nutrient intakes and dietary patterns of older Americans: a national study, J. Gerontol. 47(5):M145, 1992.

60. Sanders, H.N., Hoffman, S.B., and Lund, C.A.: Feeding strategy for dependent eaters, J. Am. Diet. Assoc. 92:1389, 1992.

61. Schafer, R.B., and Keith, P.M.: Social-psychological factors in the dietary quality of married and single elderly, J. Am. Diet. Assoc. 81:30, 1982.

62. Schiffman, S.: Changes in taste and smell: drug interactions and food preferences, Nutr. Rev. 52(8):S11, 1994.

63. Schiffman, S.S., and Warwick, Z.S.: Effect of flavor enhancement on nutritional status: food intake, biochemical indices, and anthropometric measures, Phys. Behav. 53:395, 1993.

64. Schlettwein-Gsell, D: Nutrition and the quality of life: a measure for the outcome of nutritional intervention, Am. J. Clin Nutr. 55:1263S, 1992.
65. Senauer, B.H., Asp, E., and Kinsey, J.: Food trends and the changing consumer, St. Paul, MN, 1991, Eagen Press.
66. Splett, P.L.: Federal food assistance programs, Nutr. Today 29(2):6, 1994.
67. Stevens, J., Kumanyika, S.K., and Keil, J.E.: Attitudes toward body size and dieting: differences between elderly black and white women, Am. J. Public Health 84:1322, 1994.
68. Suski, N.S., and Nielson, C.C.: Factors affecting food intake of women with Alzheimer's type dementia in long-term care, J. Am. Diet. Assoc. 89:1770, 1989.
69. Taeuber, C.: Sixty-five plus in America, Curr. Pop. Rep., Spec. Studies, P23-178, Washington, DC, August 1992, U.S. Bureau of the Census.
70. Tong, A.: Eating habits of elderly Vietnamese in the United States, J. Nutr. Elderly 10:35, 1991.
71. Troll, L.E.: Eating and aging, J. Am. Diet. Assoc. 59:456, 1971.
72. U.S. Department of Health and Human Services: Healthy people 2000: National health promotion and disease prevention objectives, DHHS Publication No. (PHS) 91-50213, Washington, DC, 1991, U.S. Government Printing Office.
73. U.S. Department of Health and Human Services: Trends in the health of older Americans: United States, 1994, Vital and Health Statistics, Series 3, No. 30, DHHS Publication No. (PHS) 95-1414, Hyattsville, MD, April 1995, National Center for Health Statistics.
74. U.S. General Accounting Office: Elderly Americans. Health, housing, and nutrition gaps between the poor and nonpoor, Report to the Chairman, Select Committee on Aging, House of Representatives, GAO/PEMD-92-29, Washington, DC, 1992, U.S. Government Printing Office.
75. U.S. Senate Special Committee on Aging: Aging America. Trends and projections (annotated), Serial No. 101-J, Washington, DC, 1990, U.S. Government Printing Office.
76. Use of light products growing fastest among older Americans, Calorie Control Commentary 16(2):6, 1994.
77. Vetter, N.J., and others: The relationship between dietary habits and beliefs in elderly people compared with younger people, J. Nutr. Elderly 9(4):3, 1990.
78. Walker, D., and Beauchene, R.E.: The relationship of loneliness, social isolation, and physical health to dietary adequacy of independently living elderly, J. Am. Diet. Assoc. 91:300, 1991.
79. Wandel, M: Dietary intake of fruits and vegetables in Norway: influence of life phase and socioeconomic factors, Intl. J. Food Sci. Nutr. 46:291, 1995.
80. Westenbrink, S., and others: Effect of household size on nutritional patterns among the Dutch elderly, J. Am. Diet. Assoc. 89:793, 1989.
81. Woo, J., and others: Chewing difficulties and nutritional status in the elderly, Nutr. Res. 14(11):1649, 1994.
82. Zallen, E.M., Hooks, L.B., and O'Brien, K.: Salt taste preferences and perceptions of elderly and young adults, J. Am. Diet. Assoc. 90:947, 1990.

9 *Nutritional Status of Older Adults*

Marie Fanelli Kuczmarski

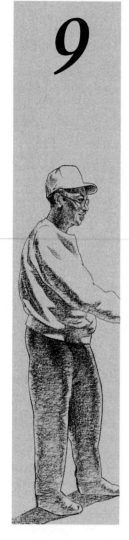

+++

Objectives

After studying the chapter, the student should be able to:

✔ *List the national nutrition surveys that provide information on older people, the government agencies that carry out these surveys, and the specific types of data collected*

✔ *Understand the difference between nutritional status and dietary status and recognize the factors that contribute to nutritional status*

✔ *Understand the physical and biochemical markers used to assess nutritional status in older people*

✔ *Recognize the differences in nutritional status between institutionalized older people and those living in the community*

✔ *Apply the information gained from national nutrition surveys to the nutritional care of older people*

INTRODUCTION

Nutritional status encompasses anthropometric, biochemical, clinical, dietary, and socioeconomic factors. Although the term "nutritional status" sometimes is used interchangeably with "dietary status," these terms do have different connotations. Dietary status is a more limited term that refers to intake of foods, beverages (both nonalcoholic and alcoholic), and nutrients, including supplements.

The data on food intake and dietary status representative of noninstitutionalized older adults in the United States presented in this chapter are derived from the 1989–91 and 1994–96 Continuing Survey of Food Intakes by Individuals (CSFII), conducted by the U.S. Department of

Agriculture. Data on nutritional and dietary status are derived from the Third National Health and Nutrition Examination Survey (NHANES III), 1988–94, conducted by the U.S. Department of Health and Human Services. NHANES III was designed as a six-year survey and completed in three-year phases (1988–91 and 1991–94). The most recent information on food intake of selected American Indian populations is also included in this chapter. These data were obtained from the Strong Heart Dietary Survey, conducted by the U.S. Department of Health and Human Services between 1989 and 1991.

This chapter presents selected data from national and smaller local surveys to provide a descriptive picture of the dietary and nutritional status of noninstitutionalized older Americans. Where possible, survey findings are stratified by age, race or ethnic group, gender, and income level. Even though older adults typically are defined as individuals age 65 or older, data for people over age 50 also are presented for comparison.

OVERVIEW OF U.S. GOVERNMENT SURVEYS
Continuing Survey of Food Intake by Individuals (CSFII)

CSFII, 1989–91, was designed to provide a probability sample representative of individuals in households in the 48 conterminous states. The survey was composed of two separate samples: households with incomes at any level and households with incomes less than or equal to 130% of the poverty threshold (low-income sample). Information on food consumed by individuals both at home and away from home was collected by trained interviewers for three consecutive days using a 24-hour recall and a two-day food record. Dietary data were collected on all days of the week, beginning in April and continuing through March of the next year. About 20% of the total sample, or 2,340 people age 60 or older, satisfactorily completed both the dietary recall and food record.[11]

The CSFII, 1994–96, was designed to provide a probability sample representative of noninstitu-

tionalized individuals in all 50 states. Food intake information was collected through in-person interviews for two nonconsecutive days. Low-income and elderly populations were oversampled. The survey had no upper age limit, and the age range for older adults interviewed in 1994 was 65 to 97 years. There were 736 individuals 65 years of age and older who satisfactorily completed the dietary recalls, and they comprised about 13% of the total 1994 sample.

Third National Health and Nutrition Examination Survey (NHANES III)

NHANES III used probability sampling to select a representative sample of the civilian population living in households from all 50 states. Due to the structure of the NHANES III sample design, unbiased estimates of nutritional status and health can be independently produced from both phase 1 and 2. This survey collected information on nutritional and health status through interviews and direct physical examinations. Food intake data were gathered with a 24-hour dietary recall and questions relating to eating habits, food insecurity, and nutrition-related practices. Physical examinations included anthropometric measurements, hematologic and biochemical assessments, bone density measurements, and dental examinations.[16]

Trained interviewers administered the 24-hour recall using an automated interactive dietary interview and coding system. This recall contained information on specific food items and beverages consumed by the respondent from midnight to midnight preceding the interview. The interviews were scheduled on all days of the week. For phase 1, the highest proportion of recalls were for Wednesday (19%), Thursday (17%), and Friday (26%). Therefore, phase 1 intake data reflect weekday food consumption.

Unlike NHANES II, there was no upper age limit. Non-Hispanic blacks, Mexican Americans, and adults ages 60 years and older were oversampled to provide reliable statistics for these population groups. The sample included 4,369 people 60 years of age and older, or 21.5% of the total NHANES III phase 1 sample. Of those older adults selected, 3,468 (79%) were interviewed, and 2,920 (67%) had a physical examination.

Strong Heart Dietary Survey

Because of sampling designs, the national nutrition surveys do not consistently include American Indians living on reservations. The Strong Heart Dietary Survey, conducted by the Indian Health Service of the U.S. Public Health Service and the Centers for Disease Control and Prevention, collected food intake data from American Indians residing in South Dakota, Arizona, and Oklahoma, who ranged in age from 45 to 74. A 24-hour recall and a quantitative food frequency questionnaire were used to collect food intake information. The data collection and data analysis methods were the same as those used for NHANES III, 1988–91. Data were analyzed for two age groupings, 45 to 59 years and 60 to 74 years.[11]

DIETARY INTAKE

Dietary intake data can be used to describe the actual foods eaten, eating patterns, and the level of energy and nutrients consumed. That data aids in the development of nutritional interventions and educational programs and for policy-making decisions.

Food Intakes

The 1989–91 CSFII data have been used to describe the use of food groups and selected food items in the diets of older men and women. Table 9-1 provides the percentage of older adults by two age groups (60 to 69 and 70+ years) who reported consuming particular items during the three days when dietary data were collected.[12] Almost all the older adults interviewed consumed yeast breads; approximately half used ready-to-eat cereals and dessert items (cakes, cookies, pastries, and pies); and about 20% ate rice. Pasta was the item with the least reported use. Among men and women ages 60 to 69 and 70 and over using grain products, the percentages were similar for all items with the exception of ready-to-eat cereals and dessert items. The use of these products was slightly higher for the 70 and over age group.

In the vegetable category, about 3 in 10 people age 60 and over consumed dark green and deep yellow vegetables during the three dietary interview days.[12] Between 46% and 61% of all older adults consumed tomatoes and lettuce. More men 70 years and over used tomatoes, and fewer men and women of that age used lettuce, compared to men and women 60 to 69 years of age. The reported use of specific fruits in descending order was citrus fruits, bananas, apples, melons or berries, and dried fruits.[12] There were no marked age or sex differences in percentages of older adults using citrus fruits or melons or berries. More men age 70 or over reported using bananas, apples, and dried fruits, compared to men 60 to 69 years of age (table 9-1). The Five A Day for Better Health Survey, conducted in 1991 by the U.S. Department of Health and Human Services, found that for both men and women, the proportion of adults consuming five or more servings of fruits and vegetables a day was greatest for people 60 and older.[11] Nineteen percent of older men and 34% of older women consumed five or more fruits and vegetables daily. Approximately half of the older age group consumed between 2.5 and 5 servings of fruits and vegetables daily.

Among dairy products, use of cheese generally outranked fluid milks.[12] Cheese is used less by men and women 70 and older versus the 60- to 69-year-old men and women (table 9-1). Of the fluid milks, low-fat milk was the type consumed by the greatest proportion of older adults interviewed. The percentage of older men and women using beef, pork, poultry, fish, eggs, and legumes was not dramatically different by age group. However, a notable gender difference arose when ranking these items by use. For older men, beef and eggs were reported with the greatest frequency, while poultry was used the most frequently by older women.

Although dietary patterns, such as core food listings, derived from the most recent CSFII or NHANES III have not been published, reports of the dietary patterns of the oldest-old (85+ years) and centenarians are available. The Georgia Centenarian Study, initiated in 1988, is providing food intake data on sexagenarians, octogenarians, and centenarians. Compared to the sexagenarians included in the study, the centenarians were more likely to consume a more varied

TABLE 9-1   *Percentage of Older Adults Who Reported Use of Selected Food Groups*

	Men		Women	
Age, Years n	60–69 461 %	70+ 426 %	60–69 666 %	70+ 787 %
Grain products				
Yeast breads	94.5	91.2	91.2	94.8
Ready-to-eat cereals	45.5	50.9	47.0	51.6
Rice	19.2	20.5	17.7	19.2
Pasta	11.0	14.0	13.9	10.0
Cakes, cookies, pastries, pies	59.6	64.0	58.9	62.4
Vegetables				
Dark green	27.9	28.2	29.0	30.2
Deep yellow	30.5	33.2	35.1	37.0
Tomatoes	54.2	61.4	55.3	50.8
Lettuce	57.9	51.0	58.4	45.5
Fruits				
Citrus	51.1	50.2	53.7	55.3
Dried	9.2	14.8	11.0	10.7
Apples	23.8	30.3	29.1	25.9
Bananas	34.8	43.5	36.9	41.8
Melons/berries	19.6	23.4	20.9	23.1
Dairy products				
Whole milk	26.1	29.2	26.5	28.5
Lowfat milk	37.9	41.2	38.1	43.3
Skim milk	19.9	17.3	16.5	17.1
Yogurt	1.3	6.7	7.6	5.9
Cheese	47.5	39.7	51.9	45.3
Protein foods				
Beef	51.4	53.4	45.5	42.7
Pork	45.4	41.9	38.1	37.4
Poultry	49.0	49.0	52.0	51.7
Fish	36.3	27.0	31.9	30.7
Eggs	47.7	48.0	35.8	39.1
Legumes	31.6	32.0	26.4	22.6

From Life Sciences Research Office, Federation of American Societies for Experimental Biology: Third report on nutrition monitoring in the United States, Vol. 2, Washington, DC, 1995, U.S. Government Printing Office.

diet that included breakfast.[7] Their frequency of consumption of whole milk, biscuits, and coffee was more than that of either the sexagenarians or octogenarians, while their use of bran cereal and fruit was less than that of the octogenarians. In addition, the centenarians and octogenarians consumed chicken less frequently than the sexagenarians. The women in this study tended to consume "healthier" diets than the men. The men consumed more bacon and sausage, while the women consumed more fruit, especially fresh fruit. This higher fruit consumption may have contributed to the higher intakes of dietary fiber of the women compared to the men.

Fischer and associates[4] reported that the participants in the Georgia Centenarian Study who lived alone consumed dairy products more frequently than those participants living with others. They attributed this difference to the ease of preparation and consumption of dairy products relative to other food items. They also found that women consumed more yogurt and cottage cheese compared to men and that the black participants consumed more whole milk and less low-fat (2%) milk compared to the white participants.

Holcomb[6] completed a survey of dietary habits of healthy older women who lived alone. These women resided in both urban and rural areas in Kansas. The findings of this study revealed that the weekly reported consumption of fruits, vegetables, meats, and dairy products of the oldest-old (85+ years) was similar or even superior to that of women ages 65 to 74 years or 75 to 84 years. The weekly frequency of fruit and vegetable consumption for the entire study population was 18.8 and 21.3, respectively. The women also consumed a variety of fruits and vegetables; five different fruits and seven different vegetables were eaten during the reported week. There were no significant differences in frequency of weekly food consumption between urban and rural residents. These data suggest that living alone does not necessarily mean that an older adult is at risk for poor nutrition.

Energy and Nutrient Intakes

Mean energy and selected nutrient intakes that differed for men and women, ages 50 to 64

and 65 and over, interviewed in the 1994 CSFII are presented in tables 9-2 and 9-3. These data were derived from one-day dietary recalls and do not include nutrient intakes from supplements. The mean energy intake of both sexes ages 50 to 64 was significantly higher than that of the men and women ages 65 and older. The decline in reported mean energy intake across age groups was generally accompanied by a decrease in mean nutrient intakes. Mean intakes of protein, total fat, and saturated, monounsaturated, and polyunsaturated fats were significantly lower in diets consumed by the older age group compared to those 50 to 64 years of age. On the other hand, mean intakes of vitamin A and carotene were significantly higher for the men 65 and older, compared to the younger men.

For both men and women ages 65 years and older, energy intakes were considerably less than the 1989 Recommended Dietary Allowances (RDA).[17] Fat provided 32% of the total energy for women and 34% of the total energy for men, levels which exceed the recommendation of less than 30% of total energy from fat. Saturated fat provided 11% of the energy for both sexes. Within each gender, individuals age 65 and older had mean intakes of dietary fiber, calcium, zinc, copper, magnesium, and vitamin B-6 that were below recommended levels, while their mean sodium intakes exceeded the recommended upper limit of 2,400 mg a day.[15,17]

Median intakes of energy and 26 nutrients by men and women according to age and race or ethnic group are presented in tables 9-4 and 9-5.[12] These data were obtained from 24-hour dietary recalls collected during phase 1 of NHANES III. As was the case with the CSFII data, dietary supplements are not included in the calculations. Median values, which are presented in bold type in both tables, indicate an intake less than the RDA or recommended level established by an alternate criterion. It should be noted that the numbers of non-Hispanic black and Mexican American men and Mexican American women ages 80 and over are small; in fact, they are less than the minimum number recommended for estimating a reliable national statistic for this subgroup.

TABLE 9-2 Mean (± SEM)* Nutrient Intakes of Older Men†

Age (years)	50–64 (N = 395)		65+ (N = 371)	
	Mean	(± SEM)	Mean	(± SEM)
Food energy (kcal)	2,148	(55.0)	1,928	(46.0)
Protein (g)	85.5	(2.9)	76.1	(1.8)
Total fat (g)	83.6	(2.7)	71.8	(2.0)
Saturated fat (g)	26.9	(1.0)	23.9	(0.8)
Monounsaturated fat (g)	32.5	(1.1)	27.4	(0.8)
Polyunsaturated fat (g)	17.7	(0.7)	14.6	(0.5)
Cholesterol (mg)	309	(16.0)	269	(10.0)
Sodium (mg)	3,702	(113.0)	3,324	(98.0)
Niacin (mg)	26.1	(0.9)	23.2	(0.7)
Vitamin A (RE)	1,060	(64.0)	1,502	(105.0)
Carotene (RE)	521	(42.0)	693	(58.0)

*SEM = Standard error of the mean
†Means for the two age groups are significantly different (p < .05)
From Continuing Survey of Food Intakes by Individuals, U.S. Department of Agriculture, 1994.

TABLE 9-3 Mean (± SEM)* Nutrient Intakes of Older Women†

Age (years)	50–64 (N = 410)		65+ (N = 365)	
	Mean	(± SEM)	Mean	(± SEM)
Food energy (kcal)	1,546	(28.0)	1,408	(32.0)
Protein (g)	62.1	(1.5)	58.2	(1.2)
Total fat (g)	59.2	(1.5)	49.9	(1.7)
Saturated fat (g)	19.3	(0.5)	16.5	(0.7)
Monounsaturated fat (g)	22.2	(0.6)	18.7	(0.6)
Polyunsaturated fat (g)	13.1	(0.5)	10.6	(0.4)
Vitamin E (TE)	7.2	(0.3)	6.2	(0.2)

*SEM = Standard error of the mean
†Means for the two age groups are significantly different (p < .05)
From Continuing Survey of Food Intakes by Individuals, U.S. Department of Agriculture, 1994.

As might be anticipated, median energy intakes of both men and women declined with each subsequent age group. Median energy intakes of men were consistently higher than those of women of similar age and race or ethnic group. Within each ethnic group, median nutrient intakes, with the exception of vitamin A and carotene, generally decreased with increasing age.

White older men and women tended to have higher intakes for approximately half of the nutrients listed in tables 9-4 and 9-5. There

TABLE 9-4   *Median Energy and Nutrient Intakes of Older Men*

Age, Years n	White Men			Black Men			Mexican American Men		
	60–69 247	70–79 285	80+ 250	60–69 141	70–79 93	80+ 21*	60–69 152	70–79 60	80+ 19*
Energy (kcal)	1,932	1,813	1,725	1,630	1,346	1,394	1,805	1,480	1,464
Protein (g)	79	70	65	67	60	56	74	64	60
Carbohydrate (g)	239	223	211	196	173	147	227	190	136
Dietary Fiber (g)	15.31	14.73	15.07	12.25	10.31	6.73	18.15	16.84	13.12
Fat (g)	71	66	64	59	50	50	62	52	52
SFA[1] (g)	24	23	22	20	18	17	19	16	19
MFA[2] (g)	26	25	24	22	19	18	23	19	20
PUFA[3] (g)	14	12	11	11	10	8	12	10	8
Cholesterol (mg)	232	217	190	280	225	276	296	244	235
Calcium (mg)	734	688	671	480	516	467	810	558	476
Iron (mg)	14.71	13.24	13.27	10.59	9.78	8.66	13.50	11.52	11.69
Sodium (mg)	3,205	2,987	2,767	2,490	2,422	1,739	2,828	2,712	2,429
Potassium (mg)	2,924	2,760	2,505	2,093	1,961	1,766	2,629	2,406	2,073
Zinc (mg)	11.52	10.34	9.06	8.77	7.84	7.04	8.71	8.13	7.74
Magnesium (mg)	306	282	263	205	198	173	273	244	216
Vitamin A (RE)	914	916	851	551	543	455	613	583	395
Carotene (RE)	245	217	203	109	199	96	243	310	170
Vitamin E (TE)	7.49	6.50	6.49	5.43	4.86	3.77	6.60	5.30	4.60
Vitamin C (mg)	82	86	82	58	72	83	79	67	31
Thiamin (mg)	1.66	1.61	1.50	1.30	1.19	1.10	1.45	1.33	1.35
Riboflavin (mg)	2.04	1.90	1.78	1.54	1.42	1.46	1.68	1.53	1.48
Vitamin B-6 (mg)	1.83	1.71	1.75	1.33	1.20	1.38	1.47	1.28	1.14
Folate (ug)	302	268	261	218	187	170	268	197	234
Vitamin B-12 (ug)	4.51	4.00	3.89	3.43	3.30	2.50	3.57	2.49	2.47

[1]Saturated fatty acids; [2]Monounsaturated fatty acids; [3]Polyunsaturated fatty acids.
* All values in this column represent a small sample size and may be potentially unreliable.
From Life Sciences Research Office, Federation of American Societies for Experimental Biology: Third report on nutrition monitoring in the United States, Vol. 2, Washington, DC, 1995, U.S. Government Printing Office.

TABLE 9-5 *Median Energy and Nutrient Intakes of Older Women*

	White Women			Black Women			Mexican American Women		
Age, Years	60–69	70–79	80+	60–69	70–79	80+	60–69	70–79	80+
n	246	253	251	148	93	35	153	51	23*
Energy (kcal)	1,510	1,380	1,294	1,405	1,326	1,199	1,306	1,057	1,264
Protein (g)	60	55	49	51	57	45	53	45	41
Carbohydrate (g)	185	180	173	180	154	161	165	148	140
Dietary Fiber (g)	13.44	12.92	11.70	11.04	11.02	9.96	11.72	11.22	6.91
Fat (g)	55	50	44	45	50	42	44	32	48
SFA[1] (g)	18	16	15	14	15	13	13	11	14
MFA[2] (g)	20	17	17	17	17	17	15	11	17
PUFA[3] (g)	11	10	9	9	10	7	8	7	8
Cholesterol (mg)	162	154	134	151	215	125	178	220	196
Calcium (mg)	660	586	544	399	436	347	494	511	436
Iron (mg)	10.68	10.26	9.57	9.29	9.89	9.15	8.66	8.32	6.78
Sodium (mg)	2,427	2,246	2,182	2,090	1,894	1,854	1,801	1,812	2,008
Potassium (mg)	2,495	2,221	2,146	1,850	1,777	1,585	1,888	1,607	1,678
Zinc (mg)	7.71	7.18	6.59	6.93	6.37	5.92	6.80	6.42	5.26
Magnesium (mg)	245	226	211	189	193	174	200	169	154
Vitamin A (RE)	816	903	754	431	710	451	435	577	480
Carotene (RE)	275	312	226	190	255	129	224	198	146
Vitamin E (TE)	6.31	5.74	5.43	4.48	5.02	3.79	4.21	4.09	4.71
Vitamin C (mg)	89	78	87	86	76	60	64	58	50
Thiamin (mg)	1.26	1.19	1.15	1.06	1.03	1.16	0.95	0.93	0.90
Riboflavin (mg)	1.57	1.41	1.41	1.12	1.32	1.19	1.17	1.27	1.22
Vitamin B-6 (mg)	1.44	1.38	1.37	1.16	1.23	0.98	1.13	0.98	0.91
Folate (ug)	229	236	205	174	185	174	173	147	150
Vitamin B-12 (ug)	3.01	2.64	2.60	2.19	2.55	2.12	2.37	2.23	1.63

[1]Saturated fatty acids; [2]Monounsaturated fatty acids; [3]Polyunsaturated fatty acids.
*All values in this column represent a small sample size and may be potentially unreliable.
From Life Sciences Research Office, Federation of American Societies for Experimental Biology: Third report on nutrition monitoring in the United States, Vol. 2, Washington, DC, 1995, U.S. Government Printing Office.

were no notable differences in the proportion of energy contributed by the macronutrients among ethnic groups. Protein contributed approximately 16% of energy intake among all groups surveyed. The percent of energy contributed by total fat was 32% for Mexican American older adults, 33% for white and black women, and 34% for white and black men. Carbohydrates contributed the remaining 48% to 53% of energy.

In general, median intakes of energy, calcium, zinc, magnesium, vitamin A, vitamin E, and vitamin B-6 were less than the RDA.[17] Median dietary fiber intake was less than the range of 20 to 30 g recommended by the National Cancer Institute (NCI).[15] Median iron intakes were less than 10 mg for black men 70 and older, and for all the women, with the exception of white women between 60 and 79.[17] Only the white men and women met or exceeded the RDA for folate.[17]

Recently, the U.S. Public Health Service completed a dietary survey of American Indians in various regions to gain information that would be helpful in developing disease prevention programs. Mean nutrient intakes for American Indians residing in Arizona, Oklahoma, and South Dakota were similar to median intakes reported for the older age groups in NHANES III. As shown in table 9-6, mean energy intakes were below RDA values for American Indian men and women, ages 60 to 74.[11] Mean intakes of total fat as a percentage of energy were consistently above 30% of total kilocalories, and mean intakes of dietary fiber were below the recommended intake of 20 to 30 g a day for healthy adults.[15] Mean cholesterol intakes for American Indian men and women residing in Arizona were far above 300 mg a day, but this was not the case in South Dakota or Oklahoma. Mean vitamin A intakes were below the RDA for only the American Indian men residing in Arizona, and mean iron intakes were slightly below the RDA value for only the American Indian women residing in Oklahoma.[17]

Quartiles of energy and nutrient intakes by income level, using data from CSFII, are presented in tables 9-7 and 9-8. Income was categorized as either less than 130% or 130% or more of the federal poverty income guideline. The difference in energy intakes between the 25th and 75th percentiles was approximately twofold for men and women 50 and older. For older women, regardless of income status, energy intakes at the 25th percentile were less than 1,200 kcal. At this energy level, it is difficult to obtain adequate amounts of essential nutrients without supplementation. Of the nutrients presented in tables 9-7 and 9-8, intakes of iron and vitamins A and C appear to be related to income.

Vitamin and Mineral Supplements

For the most accurate dietary assessment, intakes from vitamin and mineral supplements should be added to the nutrient intakes from food. The median daily intake for vitamins from supplements was between 100% and 300% of the RDA and, for minerals, from 15% to 270% of the RDA.[14] These findings indicate that vitamin and mineral supplements are commonly used by older Americans, and that intakes from supplements can exceed 100% of the RDA. Therefore, it seems prudent to use information on supplement use when evaluating the adequacy of diets of older adults.

ANTHROPOMETRIC EVALUATION

Several body measurements were performed by trained health technicians in NHANES III. The height and weight data obtained were used to calculate body mass index (BMI) or the ratio of weight (kg) to height squared (m²). BMI was similar for the men ages 60 to 69 and 70 to 79 who had mean BMI levels of 26.9 and 26.5, respectively. BMI fell sharply to 24.7 in the men age 80 and over. This pattern was also observed in the women for whom the BMI was 27.3, 26.7, and 24.6 at ages 60 to 69, 70 to 79, and 80 and over, respectively.[10]

Estimates of the prevalence of overweight use BMI. A BMI equal to or greater than 27.8 was used to define overweight for men and a BMI equal to or greater than 27.3 was used for

TABLE 9-6   *Mean One-Day Nutrient Intakes of Selected Groups of American Indians (60–74 years)*

	State of Residence			RDA Value or Criterion for Comparison
	Arizona	Oklahoma	South Dakota	
Energy (kcal)				
Men	1,621	1,567	1,594	2,300
Women	1,476	1,204	1,469	1,900
Fat (% kcal)				
Men	36	36	36	30*
Women	34	36	36	30*
Cholesterol (mg)				
Men	447	288	240	300*
Women	361	190	269	300*
Dietary fiber (g)				
Men	16	13	12	20–30†
Women	17	11	12	20–30†
Vitamin A (RE)				
Men	886	1,068	1,003	1,000
Women	954	833	1,119	800
Beta carotene (RE)				
Men	265	434	413	None
Women	389	343	484	None
Vitamin C (mg)				
Men	79	101	75	60
Women	122	101	89	60
Iron (mg)				
Men	17	11	11	10
Women	15	9	10	10

*Recommendations by the Expert Panel on Detection, Evaluation and Treatment of High Blood Cholesterol in Adults (Adult Treatment Panel II), 1993.

†Recommendations by National Cancer Institute, 1987.

From Life Sciences Research Office, Federation of American Societies for Experimental Biology: Third report on nutrition monitoring in the United States, Vol. 1, Washington, DC, 1995, U.S. Government Printing Office.

TABLE 9-7   Dietary Intakes of Energy and Selected Nutrients of Older Men by Poverty Status

	25th Percentile		50th Percentile		75th Percentile	
	< 130%	≥ 130%	< 130%	≥ 130%	< 130%	≥ 130%
Men 50–64 years **(n = 349)**						
Food energy (kcal)	1,270	1,630	1,700	2,127	2,288	2,693
Protein (g)	53.1	61.3	70.9	84.3	91.7	108.9
Total fat (g)	40.0	48.5	61.1	79.5	84.8	116.6
Vitamin C (mg)	32	37	83	78	198	129
Vitamin A (RE)	430	593	1,126	1,382	1,958	2,393
Calcium (mg)	373	427	590	640	812	962
Iron (mg)	8.8	10.4	11.5	14.3	17.5	19.2
Sodium (mg)	1,907	2,466	3,138	3,594	4,131	4,811
Cholesterol (mg)	136	146	250	243	441	441
Men 65+ years **(n = 308)**						
Food energy (kcal)	1,255	1,368	1,582	1,831	2,115	2,508
Protein (g)	43.6	54.5	74.6	70.8	90.8	94.8
Total fat (g)	38.1	42.4	63.7	65.7	90.6	94.3
Vitamin C (mg)	33	42	66	78	130	130
Vitamin A (RE)	697	814	1,276	1,504	2,410	3,725
Calcium (mg)	344	392	552	710	1,032	1,006
Iron (mg)	7.9	9.8	13.2	15.1	20.3	21.3
Sodium (mg)	2,039	2,296	3,136	3,059	4,338	4,116
Cholesterol (mg)	107	121	219	205	418	326

From Continuing Survey of Food Intakes by Individuals, U.S. Department of Agriculture, 1994.

women. These values are the gender-specific 85th percentile values of BMI for the men and women ages 20 to 29 years who were examined in NHANES II; these standards were chosen using a statistical approach. The 20-to-29 age group was selected as a reference standard because these individuals are considered to be relatively lean, and increases in body weight that are observed with advancing age generally reflect an increased accumulation of fat. These cutoff points represent approximately 124% and 120% of desirable weight for men and women, respectively, and the mid-point of the range of weights for a medium frame in the 1983 Metropolitan Height and Weight tables, after appropriate adjustments for clothing and shoes.[10]

Between NHANES II and NHANES III, phase 1, the prevalence of overweight increased 14% (from 26.8% to 40.9%) for men 60 to 74 years of age, and 4% (from 37.3% to 41.3%) for women 60 to 74.[10] As shown in figures 9-1 and 9-2, within sex and race and ethnic groups, the proportion of individuals overweight decreased as age increased.[12] Among both race and ethnic groups, prevalence of overweight varied by sex. The highest overweight prevalence among women was found in older blacks, ages 60 to 69, and among men, the highest overweight prevalence was found in Mexican Americans, ages 60 to 69.[12]

The Dietary Guidelines Advisory Committee recommended the use of a BMI of 25 to define

TABLE 9-8   *Dietary Intakes of Energy and Selected Nutrients for Older Women by Poverty Status*

	25th Percentile		50th Percentile		75th Percentile	
	< 130%	≥ 130%	< 130%	≥ 130%	< 130%	≥ 130%
Women 50–64 years **(n = 352)**						
Food energy (kcal)	1,011	1,125	1,367	1,506	1,976	1,880
Protein (g)	38.2	44.0	53.5	59.4	72.8	79.2
Total fat (g)	34.3	35.0	52.7	57.1	74.1	78.0
Vitamin C (mg)	22	33	44	66	88	127
Vitamin A (RE)	339	533	692	1,113	1,543	2,437
Calcium (mg)	268	334	437	535	715	772
Iron (mg)	6.5	7.8	8.7	10.5	11.3	14.2
Sodium (mg)	1,570	1,812	2,563	2,535	3,040	3,362
Cholesterol (mg)	85	96	162	166	300	264
Women 65+ years **(n = 290)**						
Food energy (kcal)	1,000	1,101	1,133	1,446	1,505	1,762
Protein (g)	37.1	44.0	50.6	56.6	63.5	77.6
Total fat (g)	24.2	34.5	40.6	47.6	52.1	65.7
Vitamin C (mg)	24	42	49	85	113	137
Vitamin A (RE)	485	757	956	1,357	1,800	3,144
Calcium (mg)	348	347	491	507	770	771
Iron (mg)	6.5	8.3	9.0	11.1	12.5	15.4
Sodium (mg)	1,446	1,836	2,090	2,361	2,936	3,328
Cholesterol (mg)	99	109	146	154	261	261

From Continuing Survey of Food Intakes by Individuals, U.S. Department of Agriculture, 1994.

the upper boundary of healthy weight.[2] This recommendation was based on data from recent studies which demonstrated that mortality increased significantly above a BMI of 25. Using this criterion with the NHANES III data, the prevalence of overweight would be 65% for men ages 60 to 79 years, 47% for men age 80 and older, 58% for women ages 60–79 years, and 50% for women age 80 and older.

CLINICAL ASSESSMENTS

Hypertension

In the NHANES III, six readings of systolic and diastolic blood pressure were obtained during the physician's examination, and the results were averaged. If mean systolic pressure was 140 mm Hg or higher and/or average diastolic pressure was 90 mm Hg or higher, or if the person reported taking antihypertensive medications, the individual was classified as hypertensive. More than half of those age 60 or older were hypertensive (figs. 9-3 and 9-4).[12] The prevalence of hypertension generally increased with age. Within race and ethnic groups, black older men and women had the highest prevalence.[12]

Bone Density

The NHANES III, phase 1, provided the first quantitative estimates of total femur bone mineral density on a nationally representative sample of older women. The total femur density

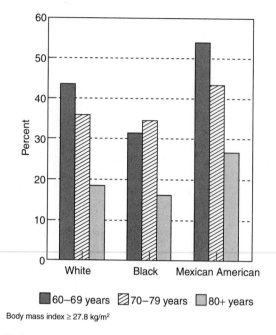

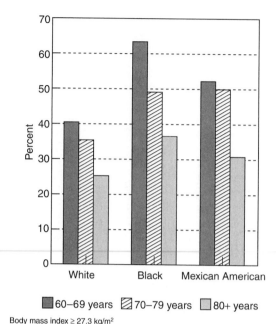

■ 60–69 years ▨ 70–79 years ▢ 80+ years

Body mass index ≥ 27.8 kg/m²

FIG. 9-1 Percent of Overweight Older American Men. Overweight is more frequent among men ages 60 to 79 than men ages 80 or older; Mexican American men are more likely to be overweight than white or black men.

Life Sciences Research Office, Federation of American Societies for Experimental Biology: Third report on nutrition monitoring in the United States, Vol. 2. Washington, DC, 1995, U.S. Government Printing Office.

■ 60–69 years ▨ 70–79 years ▢ 80+ years

Body mass index ≥ 27.3 kg/m²

FIG. 9-2 Percent of Overweight Older American Women. Women ages 60 to 79 are more likely to be overweight than women age 80 and older; black women tend to have a higher prevalence of overweight than white or Mexican American women.

Life Sciences Research Office, Federation of American Societies for Experimental Biology: Third report on nutrition monitoring in the United States, Vol. 2, Washington, DC, 1995, U.S. Government Printing Office.

included measurements of the femur neck, trochanter, and intertrochanter. Looker and associates[13] published prevalence estimates of femoral osteopenia and osteoporosis for white women by decade starting at age 50 (fig. 9-5). Femoral osteopenia and osteoporosis were defined using the criteria proposed by the World Health Organization. Osteopenia was defined as a total bone mineral density between 1 and 2.5 standard deviations below the average for adult women and osteoporosis was defined as greater than 2.5 standard deviations below the group mean. The research used white women, ages 20 to 29 years, as its reference group.[13]

As described in Figure 9-5, 35% or more of the white women, age 50 or older, had osteopenia.[12] The prevalence of osteopenia peaked in women ages 70 to 79 years. The prevalence of osteoporosis increased steadily with each succeeding decade—from 6% in women 50 to 59 to 52% in women ages 80 and over.

BIOCHEMICAL MEASUREMENTS
Serum Cholesterol

A high blood cholesterol level (≥ 240 mg/dl), especially a high level of low density lipoproteins (LDL) (≥ 160 mg/dl) increases risk for coronary

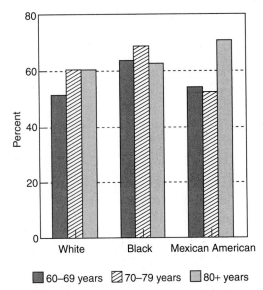

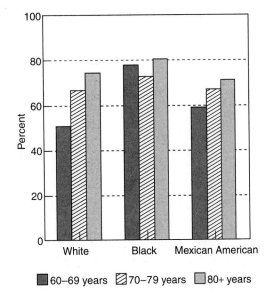

Systolic pressure ≥140 mm Hg and/or diastolic pressure ≥90 mm Hg or taking antihypertensive drugs

Systolic pressure ≥140 mm Hg and/or diastolic pressure ≥90 mm Hg or taking antihypertensive drugs

FIG. 9-3   Percent of Older American Men with Hypertension. Hypertension is less prevalent in white men ages 60 to 69 and Mexican American men ages 60 to 79 than in black men of similar age.

Life Sciences Research Office, Federation of American Societies for Experimental Biology: Third report on nutrition monitoring in the United States, Vol. 2, Washington, DC, 1995, U.S. Government Printing Office.

FIG. 9-4   Percent of Older American Women with Hypertension. Within race and ethnic groups, women ages 80 and older and black women of all ages are most likely to have hypertension.

Life Sciences Research Office, Federation of American Societies for Experimental Biology: Third report on nutrition monitoring in the United States, Vol. 2, Washington, DC, 1995, U.S. Government Printing Office.

heart disease.[3] Low levels of high density lipoproteins (HDL) (< 35 mg/dl) appear to increase risk for coronary heart disease, whereas high levels of HDL decrease risk.[3] Between NHANES II and NHANES III, phase 1, the prevalence of high serum cholesterol levels decreased from 33.1% to 28.6% for men 60 to 74 and from 53.6% to 42.5% for women of that age range.[12] NHANES III, phase 1, data indicate that the prevalence of high serum total cholesterol is lower in individuals age 75 and older— 19.9% for men and 39.2% for women compared to older adults of the same sex ages 60 to 74 years.[12] Changes in mean LDL and HDL cholesterol levels also occurred between NHANES II and NHANES III, phase 1. LDL cholesterol

decreased 7% in men and 13% in women ages 65 to 74.[9] HDL cholesterol dropped 1% in men, but it increased 3% in women ages 65 to 74.[9]

Older white and black women had higher prevalences of elevated LDL cholesterol than their male counterparts (fig. 9-6).[12] By gender, Mexican American men and black women, ages 60 to 69, had the highest prevalence. In contrast, older men were more likely to have low HDL cholesterol compared to older women, regardless of race or ethnic group (fig. 9-7).[12] Applying the Adult Treatment Panel II guidelines to phase 1 NHANES III participants, approximately 50% of all men and women, 65 years of age and older, would be candidates for dietary intervention.[3,23]

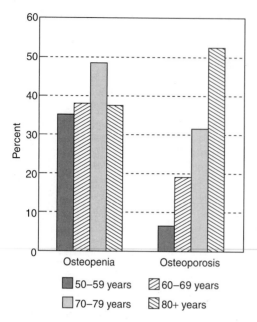

FIG. 9-5   Percent of White Women with Bone Disorders. Women ages 70 to 79 are most likely to have osteopenia; at ages 80 and older, osteoporosis is the most common bone disorder.

Looker, A.C., and others: Prevalence of low femoral bone density in older U.S. women from NHANES III, J. Bone Mineral Res. 10:797, 1995.

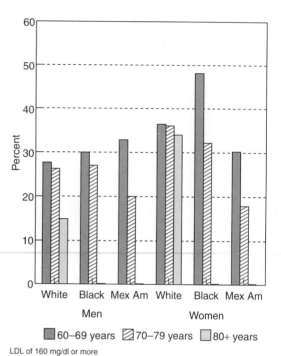

LDL of 160 mg/dl or more

FIG. 9-6   Percent of Older American Adults with High Serum Low Density Lipoprotein (LDL). Serum LDL levels decline with age among all race, sex, and ethnic groups; white and black women have the highest LDL levels.

Life Sciences Research Office, Federation of American Societies for Experimental Biology: Third report on nutrition monitoring in the United States, Vol. 2, Washington, DC, 1995, U.S. Government Printing Office.

Older adults with very low serum total cholesterol (< 160 mg/dl) are a mix of individuals with either minimal or high risk for mortality. It is possible that individuals with low serum cholesterol may represent a group of "survivors." On the other hand, low serum cholesterol has been associated with increased cancer risk, morbidity, and mortality. A study of non-institutionalized, ambulatory older people compared the health and two-year mortality rates of rural elderly with serum cholesterol levels below 150 mg/dl to controls, matched for age and sex, with serum cholesterol levels between 200 and 240 mg/dl.[8] Eligible participants were without a diagnosis of cancer within the five years preceding the study. Approximately 3% of the study sample (n = 3,874) had low serum cholesterol values. After two years, 13% of the low cholesterol group had died compared to 7% of the control group. Although there was no statistically significant relationship between cholesterol level and specific cause of death, the investigators suggest that a low serum cholesterol may be a warning sign of early subclinical disease or asymptomatic condition. The findings stress the importance of regular medical checkups. Among institutionalized older adults, a low serum cholesterol level is an indicator of protein-energy malnutrition (see chapter 12).[22]

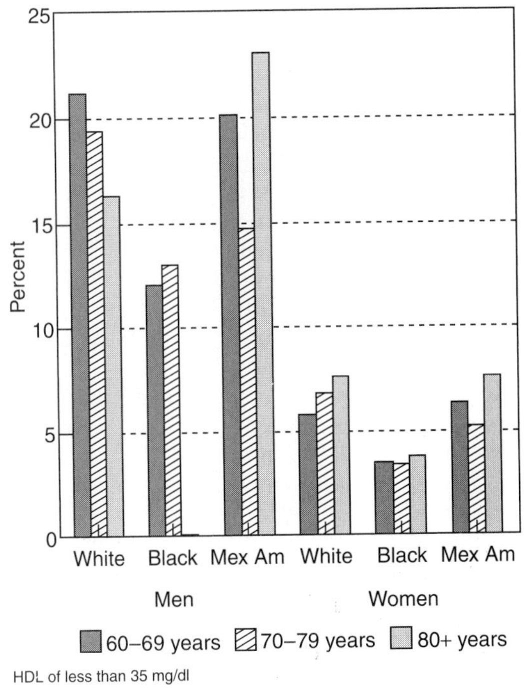

25
20
15
10
5
0
Percent
White
Black
Mex Am
White
Black
Mex Am
Men
Women
60–69 years
70–79 years
80+ years
HDL of less than 35 mg/dl

FIG. 9-7 Percent of Older American Adults with Low Serum High Density Lipoproteins (HDL). Men are more likely to have low serum HDL levels; white and Mexican American elderly have lower HDL levels than black elderly.

Life Sciences Research Office, Federation of American Societies for Experimental Biology: Third report on nutrition monitoring in the United States, Vol. 2, Washington, DC, 1995, U.S. Government Printing Office.

HEALTH AND NUTRITIONAL STATUS OF OLDER ADULTS OVER THE CONTINUUM OF CARE

Health Status

Respondent-assessed health is one of the simplest and most informative measures of health. It is strongly associated with life satisfaction, mortality, and objective health status measures such as physical examinations and physicians' ratings.[24,26,27] Health status varies with race and ethnicity among older adults.[24] Compared with white elderly, Hispanic elderly, and Asian Pacific Islanders, a greater percentage (43%) of black older adults rate their health as fair or poor.[24] The smallest proportion of respondents age 65 and older in national surveys who reported fair or poor health status were Asian Pacific Islanders. The Asian Pacific Islanders were also less likely to report limitations of activities compared to all other race and ethnic groups (23% of Asian Pacific Islanders have any activity limitation as compared with 37% of white, 40% of Hispanic, and 46% of black elderly).[24]

Our knowledge of the health status of minority elderly is generally limited to comparisons between blacks and whites. Among these two racial groups, self-assessed health varied by age. A greater proportion of adults above age 74 living in the community rated their health as fair or poor compared to adults ages 65 to 74.[26] Among blacks, the percentage increased from about 15% for people 65 to 74 years old, to 23% for people ages 75 and older; among whites, the increase was from 7% to 10% for the same age groupings. Black people, 70 and older, were twice as likely to be limited in performing personal care activities such as eating, dressing, and getting around the home as white people of similar age.[26]

Data from national surveys were used to compare respondent-assessed health of people age 65 and older based on metropolitan versus nonmetropolitan residence.[27] From 1990 census data, people age 65 and older comprise 12% of the metropolitan population and 15% of the nonmetropolitan population. (A metropolitan area is defined as a county or counties containing a place or urbanized area of ≥ 50,000 people and a total population of ≥ 100,000 people; a nonmetropolitan area consists of counties outside a metropolitan area.) In 1990 approximately 27% of the metropolitan elderly and 30% of the nonmetropolitan elderly assessed their health as fair or poor.[27] Of all groups, blacks in nonmetropolitan areas were the most likely to rate their health as fair or poor. About 56% of black older adults in nonmetropolitan areas rated their health as fair or poor compared to 43% of blacks in metropolitan areas. These nonmetropolitan black elderly were more likely to have higher risk for mortality and lower life satisfaction compared to those in metropolitan areas. Although there were differences in self-perceived health, there were no significant differences in the percentage of older adults consuming a diet low in fat and high in dietary fiber by metropolitan versus non-metropolitan residence.[27]

Nutritional Status

Optimal nutritional status is essential for promoting health and ensuring quality of life. Access to food and healthful, well-balanced meals are important for maintaining independence, avoiding premature nursing home placements, and using expensive health care services. Compared to malnourished individuals, individuals with good nutritional status have reduced incidence of hospitalization and, if hospitalized, have reduced stays and fewer major complications.

Malnutrition is defined as a nutritional deficit, excess, or imbalance. Overweight and underweight are examples of malnutrition. Among noninstitutionalized older Americans and older adults in other developed nations, overweight is prevalent and the prevalence is increasing.[10] Underweight is also a problem that exists among the free-living older adult population; however, prevalence estimates are lower than for overweight. Posner and coworkers[21] reported that 12% to 24% of older New England adults, 70 years of age and older, were underweight, defined as a BMI less than 22 kg/m². Among the institutionalized elderly, the prevalence of underweight has been reported to be approximately 50%.[21]

Malnutrition is a potential, although not necessary, consequence of food insecurity. **Food insecurity,** also known as food insufficiency, exists whenever the availability of nutritionally adequate and safe foods or the ability to acquire acceptable foods in socially acceptable ways is limited. Results from a mail survey conducted in 1992 by the Urban Institute indicated that between 2.5 million (8%) and 4.9 million (16%) of older adults age 65 and older suffer from food insecurity and hunger.[1] The highest levels of food insecurity were found among older Hispanic adults, older adults with incomes below the poverty index, and older adults with serious health problems that interfere with eating or result in changes in eating patterns.[1]

Deficient energy intakes appear to be a main contributor to the development of malnutrition in older adults. Data from national and international surveys and localized U.S. surveys of older adults indicate that dietary intakes of free-living older adults are limited in energy.[12,18,19,21] Low energy intakes result in intakes of essential nutrients that are less than recommended. Calcium, iron, zinc, and magnesium are usually limited in the diets of older adults, especially older women. The prevalence of undernutrition in free-living older adult populations has been reported to be between 5% and 8%.[5]

Health care administrators estimate that 2 in 5 of older adults receiving home care assistance are malnourished.[20] The prevalence of low-energy and nutrient intakes in functionally dependent elderly populations has been reported to be considerably higher than for healthy, independent elderly populations.[19] Van der Weilen and associates[28] reported that sedentary older adults living in or awaiting admission to a nursing home had significantly lower intakes of water-soluble vitamins, namely thiamin, riboflavin, vitamin B-6 and vitamin C, compared to independently living, physically active older adults. These researchers only examined water-soluble vitamin intakes. Payette and Gray-Donald[19] completed a cross-sectional study of functionally dependent elderly who receive home care services and assessed overall diet quality. More than half their subjects consumed diets that provided less than recommended levels of energy, protein, calcium, zinc, magnesium, folate, and vitamins A, D, and E. In fact, for 2 in 10 men and 3 in 10 women, the diet was not adequate to provide two-thirds of the recommended amounts of more than four essential nutrients.[19] The results from these studies clearly demonstrate that functionally dependent older adults are at a higher risk for developing malnutrition compared to independent older adults.

Perceived prevalence of protein-energy malnutrition by U.S. gerontological nurses, physicians, and health care administrators was assessed in a national telephone survey in 1993.[20] Nurses and physicians perceived that one in four of their patients was not receiving proper nutrient intake and that one in two hospital patients was

❖ ❖ ❖

CASE STUDY

You were recently hired as the nutritionist for a nursing home on an American Indian reservation in Arizona. The residents are all over 70 years old and are functionally dependent.

1. Based on currently available national survey data, what percentage of the residents are likely to be malnourished? Which specific micronutrients are likely to be consumed at suboptimal levels?

2. Based on currently available survey data of American Indians in Arizona, what foods should be consumed in lower amounts? What foods should be consumed in higher amounts? What culturally appropriate foods would you suggest to correct existing nutrient deficiencies?

3. What chronic diseases are the residents at risk of having or developing based on their dietary intake? Explain.

4. How will you determine whether the dietary status of the residents in your nursing home is similar to the older Americans represented in the national surveys?

5. Which anthropometric, biochemical, and clinical indicators of nutritional status will you measure routinely?

---

malnourished.[20] They also perceived that 2 in 5 of older adults residing in nursing homes were malnourished.[20] These subjective estimates are close to prevalence estimates from published studies. In hospitals and nursing homes the prevalence of malnutrition is higher—32% to 50% in acutely hospitalized patients and 23% to 85% in nursing home residents.[25] The high prevalence of protein-energy malnutrition in nursing homes may reflect the transfer of malnourished patients from acute care hospitals to long-term care facilities following an acute illness.

Nutritional deficiencies are common in nursing home populations. Energy intakes for older women in nursing care facilities generally range from 1,300 kcal to 1,500 kcal, while for noninstitutionalized women, energy intake has been reported to be approximately 1,600 kcal.[18] Oakland and Speer[18] conducted a study of 26 women over the age of 95 years who resided in long-term care facilities. All the women were on a liberalized, geriatric diet plan, with many selecting their own meals. The mean energy intake of these women was 1,710 kcal, a level higher than previous reports. Yet, protein, calcium, iron, zinc, and vitamin A were the nutrients most commonly consumed at less than recommended amounts.[18] In addition to these nutrients, low dietary intakes of folate, thiamin, riboflavin, and vitamins B-6, C, and D have been reported for nursing home populations.[22] Subnormal blood values have also been found for these micronutrients. Nursing home residents are frequently underweight and have substandard adipose mass.[22] These populations clearly need extra nutritional care.

In institutionalized older adult populations, the incidence of infection and the mortality rate have been shown to be higher in malnourished patients than in patients judged to be adequately nourished. The annual mortality rate in the nursing home population is 10% to 40%.[22] In general, among the institutionalized population, the individuals most likely to die soon have low serum albumin, low serum cholesterol, a small triceps skinfold, low BMI, and low hemoglobin and hematocrit.[22]

Summary

Populations at greater risk of nutritional problems include minority groups, individuals with an income below the poverty index, sedentary older adults awaiting admission to a nursing home, and institutionalized older adults. Malnutrition is more prevalent among the institutionalized population as compared with community-dwelling older adult populations. Malnutrition adversely affects not only the length but also the quality of life. The challenge to nutritionists, dietitians, and other health professionals is to improve or maintain the nutritional health of all older Americans, thereby improving their quality of life.

REVIEW QUESTIONS

1. Why are data from national surveys useful to the study of the nutritional status of older people? How do the surveys differ in their data collection methods, and what do they reveal about the nutritional status of older people?
2. How is the quality of a diet assessed? What is the dietary quality of older people in the United States? Are there any differences in the quality of diets consumed by older people of different races, ethnic background, or socioeconomic status? Which nutrients are consumed in insufficient quantities by older people?
3. What is the prevalence of hypertension in the older population? Among the elderly, which group has the highest incidence of hypertension? How does the prevalence of osteoporosis change as women age? What biochemical measures provide an indication of risk of coronary heart disease? Which groups are at greatest risk of coronary heart disease based on biochemical measures?
4. What are the benefits of optimal nutritional status in older Americans? What is food insecurity? What are the causes of food insecurity among the elderly?
5. Does nutritional status differ between institutionalized and noninstitutionalized older people? If so, in what ways?

SUGGESTED LEARNING ACTIVITIES

1. Visit your library, and find statistics on how many Hispanic older people live in your community. Find information on the food patterns of Hispanics and identify the foods most commonly eaten. Relate the typical food pattern to the national survey data on nutrient intakes of Hispanics. Identify ethnic foods that could provide the nutrients that are consumed at below optimum levels. Plan a three-day diet for an older Hispanic person, using preferred cultural foods.
2. Instruct an older person on keeping a three-day food diary. Obtain the diary after it has been completed and analyze it for nutrient content, using a computer dietary analysis program. Compare your results to data found in NHANES III. Schedule a time to talk with the older person about his or her diet and provide recommendations if needed.
3. Plan a 20-minute program on vitamin and mineral supplements for an audience of older adults. Develop a survey instrument of vitamin and mineral use, and distribute the survey after your program. Stratify the results by age group, sex, and race. Compare your findings to those found in the national surveys.
4. Telephone a nursing home in your community, and obtain the number of the consulting dietitian. Set up an appointment with the dietitian, and interview her on the nature of her work at the nursing home, the nutritional status of the residents, and the methods used to monitor nutritional status.

REFERENCES

1. Burt, M.R.: Hunger among the elderly: local and national comparisons, 1993, Washington, DC, 1993, Urban Institute.
2. Dietary Guidelines Advisory Committee: Report of the dietary guidelines committee on the dietary guidelines for Americans, Washington, DC, 1995, U.S. Department of Agriculture.
3. Expert Panel on Detection, Evaluation, and Treatment of High Blood Cholesterol in Adults: Summary of the second report of the National Cholesterol Education Program (NCEP) Expert Panel on Detection, Evaluation, and Treatment of High Blood Cholesterol in Adults, J. Am. Med. Assoc. 269:3015, 1993.
4. Fischer, J.G., and others: Dairy product intake of the oldest old, J. Am. Diet. Assoc. 95:918, 1995.
5. Guigoz, Y., and others: Mini nutritional assessment: a practical assessment tool for grading the nutritional state of elderly patients. In: The mini nutritional assessment: MNA, Facts and Research in Gerontology (Supplement No 2), Paris, 1994, Serdi Publishing Co.
6. Holcomb, C.M.: Positive influence of age and education on food consumption and nutrient intakes of older women living alone, J. Am. Diet. Assoc. 95:1381, 1995.
7. Houston, D.K., and others: Individual foods and food group patterns of the oldest-old, J. Nutr. Elderly 13:5, 1994.
8. Ives, D.G., and others: Morbidity and mortality in rural community-dwelling elderly with low total serum cholesterol, J. Gerontology 48:M103, 1993.
9. Johnson, C.L., and others: Declining serum total cholesterol levels among U.S. adults, J. Am. Med. Assoc. 269:3002, 1993.
10. Kuczmarski, R.J., and others: Increasing prevalence of overweight among U.S. adults, J. Am. Med. Assoc. 272:205, 1994.
11. Life Sciences Research Office, Federation of American Societies for Experimental Biology: Third report on nutrition monitoring in the

United States, Vol. 1, Washington, DC, 1995, U.S. Government Printing Office.

12. Life Sciences Research Office, Federation of American Societies for Experimental Biology: Third report on nutrition monitoring in the United States, Vol. 2, Washington, DC, 1995, U.S. Government Printing Office.

13. Looker, A.C., and others: Prevalence of low femoral bone density in older U.S. women from NHANES III, J. Bone Mineral Res. 10:797, 1995.

14. Moss, A.J.: Uses of vitamin and mineral supplements in the United States: current users, types of products, and nutrients, Vital and Health Statistics, Advance Data, No. 174, Hyattsville, MD, 1989, National Center for Health Statistics.

15. National Cancer Institute: Diet, nutrition & cancer prevention: a guide to food choices. Publication No. 87-2878, Bethesda, MD, 1987, National Institutes of Health.

16. National Center for Health Statistics: National health and nutrition examination survey III data collection forms, Hyattsville, MD, 1991, U.S. Department of Health and Human Services.

17. National Research Council: Recommended dietary allowances, ed. 10, Washington, DC, 1989, National Academy Press.

18. Oakland, M.J., and Speer, M.G.: Dietetic research in long-term care facilities: nutrient intake and nutritional status indicators in the oldest old. Top. Clin. Nutr. 8:26, 1993.

19. Payette, H., and Gray-Donald, K.: Risk of malnutrition in an elderly population receiving home care services. In: The mini nutritional assessment: MNA, Facts and Research in Gerontology (Supplement No. 2), Paris, 1994, Serdi Publishing Co.

20. Peter D. Hart Research Associates, Inc.: National survey on nutrition screening and treatment for the elderly, Washington, DC, 1993, Peter D. Hart Research Associates.

21. Posner, B.M., and others: Nutritional risk in New England elders, J. Gerontology 49:M123, 1994.

22. Rudman D., and Feller, A.G.: Protein-calorie undernutrition in the nursing home, J. Am. Geriatr. Soc. 37:173, 1989.

23. Sempos, C.T., and others: Prevalence of high blood cholesterol among U.S. adults, J. Am. Med. Assoc. 269:3009, 1993.

24. Tanjasiri, S.P., and others: Picture imperfect: hidden problems among Asian Pacific Islander elderly, Gerontologist 35:753, 1995.

25. Thomas, D.R.: Outcome from protein-energy malnutrition in nursing home residents. In: The mini nutritional assessment: MNA, Facts and Research in Gerontology (Supplement No. 2), Paris, 1994, Serdi Publishing Co.

26. U.S. Department of Health and Human Services: Trends in the health of older Americans: United States, 1994. Vital and Health Statistics, Series 3, No. 30, DHHS Publication No. (PHS) 95-1414, Hyattsville, MD, 1995, National Center for Health Statistics.

27. Van Nostrand, J.F., and others: Health. In: Common beliefs about the rural elderly: what do national data tell us?, Vital and Health Statistics, Series 3, No. 28, DHHS Publication No. (PHS) 93-1412, Hyattsville, MD, 1993, National Center for Health Statistics.

28. Van der Weilen, R.P.J., and others: Dietary intakes of energy and water-soluble vitamins in different categories of aging, J. Gerontology 51A:B100, 1996.

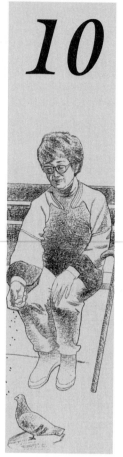

10

Drugs and Nutritional Considerations in the Aging Adult

+++

Objectives

After studying the chapter, the student should be able to:

✔ *Recognize the reasons why older people take 25% of all prescription medications*

✔ *Define polypharmacy and list factors that contribute to polypharmacy in the elderly*

✔ *Identify reasons for heavy drug use in long-term care populations*

✔ *List the age-related changes in drug metabolism*

✔ *Recognize the most common drug-nutrient interactions in the elderly*

INTRODUCTION

As a group, the elderly are the primary consumers of prescribed drugs. The actual use of nonprescription drugs by the elderly is unknown, but estimates put use by older people at seven times the amount used by the general adult population.[39] By the year 2050, it is projected that older adults will make up 25% of the population and will continue to be the largest users of drugs.[51] Today, older adults comprise about 12% of the population, yet they take 25% of all prescription medications.[4]

Physicians today have approximately 10,000 drugs available for use in diagnosis or treatment.[19] Based on a survey of the Pharmaceutical Manufacturers Association, 221 drugs were in some stage of clinical development to treat 23 diseases commonly affecting the older adult.[61] This fact, coupled with a widespread assumption that there is a pill for every malady, makes the older population particularly vulnerable to the undesirable consequences that can occur with drug therapy.

There is a fine line between the therapeutic and detrimental effects of many drugs. The consequences of doing nothing must be compared with the potential benefits of an intervention tempered by the adverse effects that frequently accompany drug use. Different approaches should also be considered because the primary goal of improving the quality of life for an older person may be accomplished without drug therapy.[76]

DRUG USE BY THE ELDERLY

Basis for Use

The prevalence of symptoms and diseases increases with age, and life expectancy has been extended. Elderly people commonly have several health problems. More than 80% of elderly individuals have one or more chronic diseases.[60] Consequently, drugs are prescribed by the physician or self-prescribed by the older individual to resolve or manage chronic conditions. Older adults frequently report several vague and nonspecific symptoms, posing difficulties for the physician attempting to diagnose correctly and prescribe appropriate treatment. Some symptoms are so common among the older age group that diagnostic significance is lost. Several drugs may be prescribed for treatment, making it even more difficult to establish an accurate diagnosis. The adverse side effects resulting from use of medications may not be ascribed to the proper culprit. It is more likely that new drugs will be prescribed to treat symptoms attributed to a new disease state, exacerbation of an existing condition, or simply the aging process.[48]

Self-prescription of medications can also pose problems for the elderly. Over-the-counter (OTC) drugs may relieve an individual's symptoms, and the older adult may hesitate to seek medical attention in a timely manner—especially if health care seems unaffordable. Elderly people may self-medicate with former prescriptions, with drugs borrowed from others, or with nonprescription preparations. Nonprescription drugs frequently are viewed as harmless, because a physician's prescription is not required. However, many OTC drugs have active ingredients that would require a prescription if taken in greater amounts. Older adults may neglect to tell their physician about OTC drugs they are taking, believing that these drugs present no risk.

Neither the use of prescription drugs nor self-medication by older adults is expected to decline, because sophisticated diagnostic techniques have enabled physicians to identify more diseases amenable to drug treatment. The pattern of drug use among ambulatory elderly, as assessed through population-based household surveys, underscores this premise.

Currently, even though the number of new drugs approved by the U.S. Food and Drug Administration (FDA) is increasing, research on drug therapy in the elderly is limited.[16,22,28,77] Drug studies typically are conducted on large populations without specific attention to the elderly.[16] A physician is likely to prescribe drugs for the elderly according to guidelines based on use by healthy young adults. Most studies fail to identify which conditions are the result of normal aging and which are caused by multiple diseases and multiple drug regimens.[33] Difficulties in research design and administration and the cost of longitudinal studies on drugs and the elderly exacerbate the problem of limited research. Efforts are being made to encourage representation of the elderly in drug trials.[21] A 1989 FDA guideline on the testing of drugs in older adults states "there is no good basis for the exclusion of patients on the basis of advanced age alone, or because of the presence of any concomitant illness or medication, unless there is reason to believe that the concomitant illness or medication will endanger the patient or lead to confusion in interpreting the results of the study."[21]

An increase in the use of drugs to treat the elderly also means an increase in cost. Drug costs are expected to continue to rise.

Polypharmacy in the Elderly

Factors contributing to polypharmacy. As the number of older adults increases, in concert with a growing number of drugs to treat and prevent their related health problems, the concern of polypharmacy is becoming acute. **Polypharmacy** is the use of several medications, either prescribed or OTC, at the same time by an individual.[42] Polypharmacy may be related to a host of symptoms, including weakness, unsteadiness, confusion, anorexia, incontinence, and immobility.[39] Some authors use the term "polypharmacy" to describe only excessive and unnecessary use of medications without regard to a specific number of drugs.[37,61] A number of features associated with polypharmacy and the elderly are described below:

- Use of medications without a defined need or condition
- Use of duplicate medications
- Concurrent use of interacting medications
- Use of contraindicated medication
- Use of inappropriate doses of a medication
- Use of drugs to treat adverse drug reactions
- Improvement following discontinuation of medications

This pattern of taking medications can have several causes.[37,43] An older person may improperly use drugs which have been appropriately prescribed by the physician, or the individual may select from formerly prescribed drugs that have been stored or even hoarded for future need. The older person seeking information regarding nutritional supplements may heed advice from clerks in health food stores or from television commercials. The physician may be inappropriately prescribing medications, partly because the suitability of drug therapy for the elderly can be difficult to predict. Elderly individuals frequently are seen in several clinics, and they may fail to inform each physician of drugs they are taking. Compounding the problem with prescribed medications, some older people may be self-prescribing OTC drugs and may neglect to tell the physician about these substances.

Other factors contribute to polypharmacy among the elderly.[12,20] Unintentional errors in drug use may be attributed to unclear directions. Instructions may be given when the patient is particularly anxious or in physical discomfort. Also, just when the elderly need more time to learn about the medicines they will be taking, they actually receive less. Errors can occur when instructions are delivered hastily, particularly when medical jargon is used. Elderly people whose hearing is impaired may not fully comprehend verbal instructions about the medicines prescribed. Many elderly people have impaired sight and are also vulnerable to problems associated with packaging and labeling. A person with arthritis may have difficulty opening childproof drug containers, and special instructions may be written in print too small to be read clearly and understood.

Polypharmacy in the elderly occurs in community-living, hospitalized, and long-term care populations.

Drug use among community-living elderly. One 10-year, cross-sectional study indicated that the average number of drugs used increased significantly among the 4,509 older people living in the community who were surveyed.[61] The number of prescription and nonprescription medications increased by 0.52 and 0.21 per person, respectively, from 1978–79 to 1987–88. The four most common categories of therapeutic drugs reported (as a percentage of all drugs used for the 1978–79 period) were antihypertensives, analgesic-antipyretics, antirheumatics, and cathartics; by 1987–88 the most common categories were antihypertensives, analgesic-antipyretics, anticoagulants, and antirheumatics. An overall decline in all drug categories was attributed to the availability of new classes of drugs and the effects of aging on the population. For example, new anticoagulant therapies gained in popularity during this 10-year period. The participants in this study were typically white, upper middle class, retired volunteers, healthy enough to attend all screening visits and thus not representative of all older people in the country.

The Iowa 65+ Rural Health Study involved 3,467 older people living in rural areas.[28] The three most common types of prescription drugs used were cardiovascular agents, central nervous system agents, and analgesics; the three most commonly used OTC drugs were analgesics, vitamin and mineral supplements, and laxatives. Not surprisingly, average prescription and overall drug use increased significantly with age; OTC drug use remained relatively unchanged. Conversely, the number of individuals reporting no drug use declined with increasing age. When the participants were asked about the purpose of each medication they took, 10% of the responses were either inappropriate or showed that the person did not know the purpose of the medication.[58]

Opdycke and associates[47] reported on 70 individuals, ages 61 to 94, who participated in the Focused Drug Therapy Review Program conducted by the University of Michigan College of Pharmacy and Institute of Gerontology. Pharmacists were surveyed to identify medication-related education problems in this group of elderly. The most common problem was inadequate understanding of the purpose of medications, followed by noncompliance, inappropriate use of medications, and inadequate communication with health professionals.

In an investigation of drug use in a group of relatively healthy and functional individuals ages 76 to 96, most of the 61 subjects could name their medications and identify their use.[16] Also, drug use was not excessive. Almost half of the OTC drugs were vitamin and mineral supplements. However, problems can be traced to inappropriate drug prescriptions for older people. In an investigation of 416 successive hospital admissions of elderly people, 73% of adverse drug reactions identified on admission were attributed to unnecessary drugs, potential drug-drug interactions, and drug contraindications.[40]

Drug use among hospitalized elderly. Gosney and Tallis[25] examined drug orders for 573 elderly patients on admission to the hospital and daily thereafter through discharge or death, to establish how often contraindicated and interacting drugs were prescribed. On admission, patients reported using an average of about two drugs. During hospitalization they were taking about six drugs, and on discharge about three or four. The drugs most commonly prescribed (in descending order) were antibiotics (70% of all patients), analgesics (65%), diuretics (51%), hypnotics or sedatives (36%), potassium salts (24%), digoxin (16%), and antacids (15%). Of the 6,160 prescriptions analyzed, 200 drugs were contraindicated or had the potential for adverse reactions. The study did not consider OTC drugs or dosage errors. The authors concluded that 66% of the contraindicated prescriptions were avoidable.

Beers and associates[6] studied the effect of hospitalization on medications used by the elderly after discharge. They reviewed the medical and pharmacologic records of 197 patients, age 65 or older, who were admitted to a large Veterans Administration Hospital. On admission these individuals were taking 4.5 drugs each, with a range of none to 16 drugs. On discharge, little change was seen in the average number of drugs taken per person (4.8; range, none to 12). Most subjects (71%) had at least one admission drug deleted before discharge. The 29% of admission drugs not continued at discharge were replaced with a similar type of drug. Patients who were taking an above-average number of drugs on admission were discharged with fewer drugs. Although the overall number of drugs before and after hospitalization did not change significantly, the type of drugs prescribed did change. At discharge the use of narcotic analgesics, laxatives, and antibiotics had increased. The findings support the thesis that polypharmacy may be influenced by hospitalization.

Drug use in long-term care patients. Approximately 5% of those age 65 or older in this country are institutionalized. Two recent review articles on multiple drug use in nursing home residents[37,43] noted that although the elderly in long-term care facilities suffer from the same maladies as their community-dwelling counterparts, nursing home residents are among the heaviest users of drugs. Intensive drug use in this setting may be quite appropriate to optimize medical and functional status.[3] Nursing home placement frequently involves a person with altered mental status, for whom required medications result in altered central nervous system (CNS) function. Nursing home residents are most likely to be recipients of excessive psychotherapeutic drugs, and the need for chronic use of these drugs has been questioned. Depression, anxiety, insomnia, and agitation are symptoms frequently seen in the nursing home, and drugs may be indiscriminately prescribed to control them. Although changes in staffing patterns and a commitment to promote interaction between health care personnel and the nursing home resident could lessen the need for psychotherapeutic drugs, medications are likely to be used because they are easy to prescribe and quickly satisfy both resident and caregiver.

Beers and associates[7] monitored 12 intermediate-care facilities in Massachusetts for one month.

Approximately 40% of all drugs prescribed in those nursing homes were to be given "as needed," or **pro re nata** (PRN) (on average, three drugs per resident). Geriatric residents received an average of almost six drugs given at least once; about 50% of these drugs were prescribed PRN. PRN drugs are primarily sedatives, hypnotics, analgesics, and laxatives.

In another study which looked at the quality of drug prescriptions for residents in 12 nursing homes, 14% of the residents were prescribed over 10 drugs.[5] Physicians wrote orders for an average of seven drugs per resident. An expert panel evaluating the appropriateness of those drug orders concluded that 0.52 drugs per resident were prescribed inappropriately.

Patrick and coworkers[49] compared drug prescription patterns of 21 nursing homes with a **gerontological nurse practitioner** (GNP) and 21 without a GNP. The GNP is a nurse with advanced education who, in most states, can prescribe medications. The drug records of 210 elderly residents were selected for review. Significantly fewer drugs and doses of drugs were prescribed in the nursing homes with GNPs. Residents of these nursing homes were prescribed an average of about eight drugs. Residents of nursing homes without GNPs were given an average of 10 drugs. A similar finding was noted regarding OTC drugs. Annually, projected drug costs were $120,192 for nursing homes with a GNP and $156,828 for the facilities without a GNP.

In summary, the use of medications prescribed by physicians is increasing, along with OTC preparations which are self-prescribed by elderly people. While those living at home are known to take a significant number of drugs, elderly long-term care residents receive even more. With this increase in drug use comes the likelihood of inappropriate and/or excessive drug use and adverse drug reactions.

Adverse Drug Reactions

An **adverse drug reaction** (ADR) is defined as any drug-induced undesirable or unwanted consequence that necessitates treatment, a decrease in dosage or cessation of a drug, and/or selection of an alternate drug or treatment.[12] ADRs in the elderly are related to (1) the increasing number of

drugs they take, (2) the diminished functional capacity of organs involved in drug absorption, distribution, and elimination, and (3) noncompliance with medication regimens.[24] Whether aging itself is an independent risk factor for ADRs is unclear, but older people are definitely at increased risk.[14,28,49,61] The most important reason for the development of ADRs, however, is polypharmacy, with an exponential increase in the incidence of ADRs with the number of drugs taken.

Drug-induced iatrogenic health problems are a major concern for the elderly, although the frequency of ADRs in the elderly is unknown.[41] It has been estimated that 10% to 15% of hospital admissions of older people are the result of ADRs.[76] The figure may reach 31% when the definition is broadened to a "drug-related problem." Within six months of discharge from the hospital, approximately 22% to 36% of elderly individuals are readmitted.[9] Bero and coworkers[9] observed that 24% of the 706 elderly individuals they followed were readmitted because of ADRs.

Drugs frequently implicated in ADRs among the elderly are those used to treat high blood pressure, congestive heart failure, cardiac arrhythmias, lung disease, arthritis, and blood clots.[41] Most of these drugs have a narrow **therapeutic index,** which means there is only a slight difference between therapeutic and toxic doses.[51] Thus, dose-related toxicity is a heightened concern, and concentrations of these drugs in the body should be aggressively monitored. The possibilities for adverse reactions may be underscored when a brand-name drug is substituted with a generic drug, not unlikely when one considers the cost savings of most generic versions. Legally the total bioavailability of a generic drug may not vary by more or less than 20% of the brand-name drug. However, this percentage can represent a substantial difference in a drug with a narrow therapeutic range.

A number of factors make the aged particularly vulnerable to the iatrogenic illness caused by ADRs. Just as increasing drug use is correlated with increasing age, reactions are more likely to occur in the very young and the very old.[12] Women are more likely than men to have

ADRs. People being treated with several drugs are at greater risk of adverse drug reactions. Reactions are also associated with certain diseases, such as those of the gastrointestinal tract, liver, and kidney. Undesirable drug effects increase with the severity of the disease and as a result of age-related changes in tissue responsiveness to drugs.[24,38] Compensatory mechanisms seen in the young that buffer the body against troublesome side effects are not as effective in the elderly. The elderly may present with different symptoms than the younger population as a result of an ADR.

AGE-RELATED CHANGES IN DRUG METABOLISM

Increasing intolerance to drugs is a characteristic identified with increasing age and relates to the diminished functional capacity of many body organs.[24] Under normal conditions a drug is absorbed from the gastrointestinal tract into the bloodstream and is distributed to various body compartments. Some drugs may be further broken down into intermediate compounds for excretion in the urine, but certain drugs may also be eliminated through bile, feces, sweat, and saliva. Differences in drug distribution and response to drugs in older people can be attributed to age-related changes in pharmacokinetics and pharmacodynamics.[19]

Pharmacokinetics

Pharmacokinetics refers to how the body absorbs, distributes, metabolizes, and excretes a drug and its metabolites. The most commonly prescribed route of drug administration is the oral route, or through the mouth. Drug absorption depends on two factors: the rate of absorption and the extent of absorption.

Drug absorption. With advancing age, gastric pH increases as the secretion of gastric acid decreases (see chapter 4).[69] Drugs designed to dissolve in an acid environment may dissolve poorly as pH rises and therefore may not be absorbed as well.[12] In the elderly, splanchnic (hepatic) blood flow is reduced 40% to 45%, which may delay drug absorption. The number

of mucosal cells and cell types change as a person ages, resulting in some loss of absorptive surface and a decrease in the amount of an administered drug that enters the systemic circulation. In contrast, the longer intestinal transit time reported in some elderly subjects may actually enhance absorption because of increased exposure of the mucosal surface to the drug.

Nevertheless, there appears to be a lack of conclusive evidence that drug absorption is significantly affected in the elderly; that is, it is unlikely that drugs are less bioavailable in the healthy elderly than in the healthy young.[48]

Drug distribution. Changes in body composition that occur with normal aging can affect drug disposition, depending on the chemical nature of the drug. However, an age-related effect on drug distribution is difficult to differentiate from a change caused by chronic disease. The percentage of body water decreases by 10% to 15% between 20 years and 40 years of age.[66] Lean body mass and skeletal muscle decrease with age, and body fat increases. These changes are more marked in women than men. In men, body fat increases from 18% to 35%. In women, body fat increases from 33% to 48%.

The blood levels of drugs that are distributed primarily in body water and those distributed in lean body tissues will increase as the total body water and muscle compartments decrease in size. Also, water-soluble drugs may not be adequately distributed because of the decline in the relative amount of body water. Conversely, highly lipid-soluble drugs may be stored in adipose tissue, thus prolonging or possibly increasing their effects.[12]

Changes in blood flow associated with aging may be another cause of altered pharmacokinetics. Cardiac output is reduced, and overall circulation becomes sluggish, favoring the brain, heart, and kidney.[66] Drug arrival at target receptors is delayed, and drug release from storage tissues is impaired. The glomerular filtration rate declines, as does renal blood flow; consequently, the rate at which a drug or its by-products is excreted decreases. Blood concentrations of flow-dependent drugs rise. A reduction in blood flow to the gastrointestinal tract may decrease the rate of absorption of drugs. Decreased blood flow to the liver and kidney, major sites for drug metabolism and elimination, contributes to a decrease in the removal of drugs from the body. Thus, as blood flow is decreased, a higher plasma concentration of water-soluble drugs may be noted.

Changes in drug binding to plasma proteins, red blood cells, and other body tissues can also affect drug distribution. Some older people have lower plasma albumin levels, with less albumin available for drug binding. The result is an increase in unbound or free drug available for pharmacologic action. A small reduction in the plasma protein available for drug binding could mean a twofold or threefold increase in the concentration of the free, and hence active, drug available.[69] For example, warfarin, an anticoagulant, is a protein-bound drug whose action is enhanced when albumin is decreased. Thus the potential for serious bleeding is heightened. Small reductions in serum albumin in the healthy aged do not appear to be clinically significant, based on epidemiological studies.[13] However, in an older adult with a chronic disease or for an individual taking several drugs simultaneously, the incidence of adverse drug reactions is likely to increase when plasma albumin levels are below optimum.

Drug metabolism. After the drug has been distributed to body tissues, it is removed from the body through metabolism and excretion. The site of metabolism for most drugs is the liver.[48] Age-related changes in hepatic-drug metabolism are difficult to separate from other factors that can influence the ability of the liver to process drugs. These other factors include chronic diseases, environmental factors such as tobacco or alcohol intake, multiple drug use, and possibly genetic factors.[41,78] The liver's capacity to metabolize drugs is reduced with advancing age due to decreases in hepatic mass and blood flow. The liver loses 35% of its weight between early adulthood and late old age.[77] Disintegration of hepatocytes is evident; thus a reduction in the liver's capacity to metabolize drugs may be related to the number of functioning liver cells. A slower metabolic rate suggests that a drug remains in the body longer, increasing the risk of drug toxicity.

Drug excretion. Drugs may be eliminated via the liver through the bile and into the feces. However, the predominant route of drug elimination is through the kidney into the urine. Changes in drug elimination occur in concert with age-related alterations in kidney function.

The best documentation of altered pharmacokinetics in aging is the decreased rate of drug elimination by the kidneys.[43] The glomerular filtration rate may diminish by as much as 50% between the ages of 20 and 90. Renal blood flow declines 1.9% a year after age 30. The body's ability to concentrate urine declines, particularly with water deprivation, and renal sodium conservation is also retarded with age. The overall effect of diminished renal function is less efficient drug clearance, leading to higher circulating blood levels of a drug.[12] Slow renal excretion, drug accumulation, and the potential for toxicity resulting from renal changes are aggravated by dehydration, congestive heart failure, renal disease, hypotension, and diabetes.[11,20]

Pharmacodynamics

Pharmacodynamics refers to the effect of a drug on a target organ.[12,44,49] Studies on pharmacodynamics in the elderly are more limited than those on pharmacokinetics.

Receptor sites in a target organ may be altered by a change in number, function, or sensitivity with increasing age.[27] For example, receptor sensitivity usually increases, which explains the high incidence of toxic drug reactions in this age group. However, decreased receptor sensitivity also may develop, resulting in a reduced therapeutic response to a drug. In that case a larger dose is required to achieve the desired therapeutic response, which puts the elderly person at risk of drug toxicity. Age-related differences in responsiveness vary with the drug studied, emphasizing the need for caution in prescribing medications according to guidelines based on research using young, healthy adults. Metoclopramide (used in treatment of nausea and vomiting), warfarin (an anticoagulant), and benzodiazepines (used to treat seizures) are drugs which have age-related pharmacodynamic changes.[48] Because there is such a wide variation in the elderly population, from the 65-year-old active adult to the frail 100-year-old, merely recommending a blanket dosage reduction for any elderly person is not realistic.

DRUG-NUTRIENT INTERACTIONS

Drugs can influence the nutritional status of an individual by exerting physiologic and biochemical actions that alter patterns of absorption, utilization, and excretion of nutrients. Conversely, profound changes in drug metabolism and efficacy can be brought about by changes in a person's diet. Drug-nutrient interactions are significantly more problematic in the elderly, particularly the frail elderly and those on marginal diets who are already at increased nutritional risk.[66] Nutritional risk increases with chronic and multiple drug use. The symptoms of a nutrient deficiency resulting from drug-nutrient interactions may be more severe than those resulting from a dietary deficiency.[50] For example, animals receiving an antithiamine drug had greater brain deterioration than those who received thiamine-deficient diets. Unfortunately, drug-induced nutritional side effects are often subtle in manifestation and slow to be identified. Frequently, they escape detection.

Drug Effects on Nutrition

Short-term drug use is unlikely to have a significant impact on nutritional status. However, chronic use of some drugs may have a substantial effect and may exacerbate existing dietary deficiencies.[78] Drugs can interfere with nutritional status through their effect on food intake, nutrient absorption, metabolism, and excretion.

Drugs and food intake. Drug-induced changes in appetite or the senses of taste or smell may influence the dietary intake of an older person. The adverse gastrointestinal side effects of a drug may also influence food intake. For example, many antineoplastic drugs cause anorexia and nausea or vomiting when food is consumed, thus reducing food intake.[50] Cardiac glycosides also cause anorexia accompanied by nausea.[11] Nausea, vomiting, and diarrhea are common side effects of several antihypertensive drugs, such as hydralazine and diazoxide, and suppress the appetite.

Not all effects on appetite are negative. Psychotropic medications used to treat anxiety and depression can stimulate the appetite and may result in weight gain.[50] Another **hyperphagic drug,** a medication which increases appetite, is tolbutamide, an oral diabetic agent.

Although some drugs may be classified as hypophagic or hyperphagic, the effect on appetite is influenced by individual factors.[11] For example, an improvement in appetite frequently accompanies an improvement in mood in older people, whose rate of drug metabolism is slowed. However, the typical improvement in mood and psychologic function and subsequent increase in food intake associated with psychotropic agents in younger patients is not seen in most older patients. To the contrary, these drugs may cause drowsiness and disinterest in food. Although amitriptyline hydrochloride is a hyperphagic drug in younger people, the result in older people may be behavioral agitation, which interferes with eating.

Drugs and nutrient absorption. The effect of drugs on nutrient absorption is the most common and clinically significant type of drug-nutrient interaction because most drugs are taken by mouth.[65,74] Drug-induced changes in absorption and utilization appear to have a more significant influence on micronutrients than macronutrients.[78]

Drugs can interact with nutrients in several ways to compromise nutrient absorption.[50] For example, the environment of the gastrointestinal lumen may be affected by changes in the composition of bacterial flora. Laxatives may change gastrointestinal transit time, resulting in loss of calcium and potassium. Generalized malabsorption can occur with the change in gastrointestinal motility associated with anticholinergic drugs. Antacids may cause a change in gastrointestinal pH, leading to a thiamin deficiency. Nutrient bioavailability may be decreased through inactivation of bile salts, impairing the formation of micelles required for the absorption of fat.[11] For example, cholestyramine disrupts the formation of micelles and prevents the reabsorption of bile salts, thus decreasing absorption of the fat-soluble vitamins.[55] Cholestyramine also binds to intrinsic factor, preventing uptake of vitamin B-12, as does paraaminosalicylic acid. Some medications form insoluble precipitates or chelate with a nutrient and impair absorption. The classic example of the latter type of drug-nutrient interaction is the interaction between tetracycline and various minerals, including calcium and magnesium; chelates are formed and absorption of these nutrients is decreased.

Certain drugs may damage the intestinal mucosa and destroy villi and microvilli, leading to the loss of brush border enzymes and intestinal transport systems.[73] Colchicine, an anti-inflammatory drug used in the treatment of gout, can damage the intestinal mucosa resulting in decreased absorption of fat, vitamin B-12, carotene, sodium, and potassium; it also can inhibit the intestinal enzyme lactase, with a reduced breakdown of lactose. Enzyme inactivation is a possible mechanism of neomycin, an antibiotic, and clofibrate, a lipid-lowering drug, resulting in decreased carbohydrate absorption.[59] Some drugs may produce a physical barrier to absorption. Laxatives containing emollients, such as mineral oil or phenolphthalein, dissolve fat and fat-soluble vitamins. The nutrients are then excreted in the feces.

Blumberg and Suter[11] have identified secondary mechanisms which can interfere with nutrient absorption. Digestion of food may be affected by drug-related changes on gastric or intestinal secretions, pancreatic exocrine function, or hepatic bile secretion. For example, cimetidine, an H_2-receptor antagonist used to decrease gastric acid secretion and treat peptic ulcers can induce vitamin B-12 deficiency. Release of vitamin B-12 from its protein-bound form is decreased when gastric acid is not present in normal amounts, and less of the free vitamin is available for association with intrinsic factor and absorption.

The effect of a drug on one nutrient may have secondary consequences for yet another. For example, absorption of calcium may be impaired by a vitamin D deficiency induced as a result of the antitubercular drug, isoniazid, which inhibits the hydroxylation of vitamin D.

Drug absorption is favored when drugs are in a dilute solution.[75] The greater volume and relative hypotonicity of the dilute solution results in a more rapid gastric emptying and greater exposure to the intestinal surface area. Unfortunately, many elderly persons, especially those with incontinence, tend to limit their fluid intake to as little as possible. Drugs are more efficiently absorbed when taken with generous amounts of water or other liquids with no pharmacologic function. Elderly people should be advised not to take medications with carbonated beverages, acidic fruit or vegetable juices, or caffeinated beverages.

Drugs and nutrient metabolism. Drugs may affect nutrient status by altering the intermediary metabolism of a nutrient or by promoting catabolism of a nutrient.[50] In some instances this action may be a deliberate and desired therapeutic effect. Oral anticoagulants such as warfarin act as vitamin K antagonists to depress blood-clotting mechanisms. Similarly, the therapeutic advantage of methotrexate is to antagonize the metabolism of folic acid, which is necessary for DNA and amino acid metabolism, making the drug useful as an antineoplastic agent.

Drugs may increase the rate of metabolism of certain vitamins by enhancing the production of catabolic enzymes or inhibiting controlling enzymes. Although the anticonvulsant phenytoin is believed to interfere with folate absorption, the folate depletion observed may also relate to enhanced activation and destruction of folate.[54] Conversely, supplements with folate may precipitate a seizure, increasing the required dosage of the drug to control convulsions. In addition to its antifolate action, phenytoin increases the metabolic inactivation of vitamin D by inducing vitamin D-degrading enzymes.[59]

Isoniazid, a drug used in the treatment of tuberculosis, can interfere with the hydroxylation of vitamin D and ultimately result in impaired calcium absorption.

Drugs and nutrient excretion. Drugs may affect nutrient status through hyperexcretion accomplished by replacing nutrients on carrier protein binding sites, by chelation, or by disturbances in renal excretion.[50] Aspirin enhances the plasma clearance of folic acid by competing for the vitamin's binding sites. A zinc deficiency is possible in those receiving long-term administration of penicillamine. This anti-inflammatory drug, used in the treatment of rheumatoid arthritis, chelates with zinc and copper, resulting in increased urinary excretion of these minerals.

The desired effect of diuretics, which is decreased reabsorption of sodium, generally is accompanied by hyperexcretion of potassium, magnesium, and zinc, particularly with long-term administration.[50] Increased renal excretion of thiamin is also an effect of furosemide, a loop diuretic. The cardiovascular abnormalities associated with thiamin deficiency are important considerations when these diuretics are prescribed for older people with chronic congestive heart failure.

Effect of Food on Drugs

Just as drugs may affect nutrient status, so may food and dietary patterns affect the activity of a drug. Foods or specific components in food can decrease the effectiveness or increase the hazards of drug therapy. Diet can influence drug activity in one of several ways. First, dietary constituents may affect absorption of the drug. Through enzyme induction or inhibition, a food may alter drug metabolism. Foods may also cause hyperexcretion of a drug as a consequence of excessive acidification or alkalization of the urine. For example, urinary acidification will increase the excretion of diazepam, an antianxiety tranquilizer. Pharmacologically active substances in foods may alter the effect of a particular drug administered at the same time the food is eaten.

Food and drug absorption. Drug absorption may be enhanced, reduced, delayed, or unaffected by concomitant food intake, by particular foods, or by specific nutrient or nonnutrient constituents of the diet. Food may have a clinically significant effect on a drug when the impact on drug absorption is substantial and the drug has a narrow therapeutic range.[50] Nutrients that enhance drug absorption may result in life-threatening drug intoxication. Conversely, concurrent administration of nutrients that reduce absorption of a drug with a narrow therapeutic range may minimize the drug's efficacy.

Food may affect drug absorption by altering the rate of gastric emptying and drug dissolution. Absorption is likely to be most efficient when a drug has sufficient time to dissolve in the stomach and then empties quickly into the intestine, or it can dissolve rapidly in the proximal small intestine. The rate of diffusion of drugs to mucosal absorptive sites and subsequent drug absorption is reduced by hot foods, heavy meals, and highly viscous solutions. Solid meals, particularly those with a high fat content, tend to slow the stomach emptying rate by activating receptors in the duodenum. Conversely, light, liquid meals activate stretch receptors in the stomach, thereby speeding up the emptying rate. A drug may be barred access to the mucosal surface of the small intestine by foods that act as mechanical barriers. The bioavailability of a drug may be markedly compromised by chelation with specific food components and nutrient supplements.

Food and drug metabolism. Drugs are metabolized by mucosal enzymes and by microflora in the intestines. Although a change in the diet may affect mucosal enzyme secretion, the microbial population in the gastrointestinal tract, and the overall rate of drug metabolism, studies with older populations are limited. After a drug has been absorbed, its therapeutic effect is influenced by how quickly the drug is extracted from the bloodstream. Dietary components (carbohydrates, proteins, and fats) regulate splanchnic blood flow and the rate of hepatic extraction and thus may alter the therapeutic efficacy of drugs. For example, the short-term postprandial effect of a protein-rich meal (more than 20% of kilocalories) is an increase over fasting levels in splanchnic blood flow.[50] A high-fat meal (more than 50% of kilocalories) also enhances the rate of hepatic perfusion. A meal with more than 70% of kilocalories from carbohydrate has little or no effect.

A change in the diet may alter the composition of microflora and influence the intestinal metabolism of drugs. Manipulating sources of dietary fiber may affect the gut microflora and intestinal transit time.

Food and drug excretion. Changes in dietary patterns can result in changes in urinary pH. For example, fruits such as prunes, plums, rhubarb, and cranberries contain large amounts of quinic acid, which, instead of being completely oxidized in the body, is converted to hippuric acid. Hippuric acid is eliminated through the urine and increases urinary acidity and decreases urinary pH. Diet-induced alkalization or acidification of the urine may change the excretion rates of certain drugs and influence the therapeutic effect.

Drugs may be classified as either weak acids or weak bases.[50] In an acid urine, renal tubule excretion of weak acids is slowed, and their effective concentration in the blood is prolonged. Conversely, excretion of drugs that are weak bases is increased in a decreasing urinary pH, and their effective concentration is lessened. Quinidine is an antiarrhythmic agent classified as a weak base. Reabsorption in the kidney tubule is enhanced in an alkaline urine, which results from a large intake of fruit juices (more than 1 l a day); in that case, the plasma concentration of the drug is increased.[59]

Pharmacologically active foods. A number of foods contain **pharmacologically active substances,** or substances that exert drug-like actions or alter drug action in the body. The classic example of this type of food-drug interaction occurs between foods that contain tyramine or other high pressor amines and monoamine oxidase (MAO) inhibitors.[15] MAO inhibitors are prescribed as antidepressants, and although experience with these drugs in the elderly is limited, attention is warranted. Foods and beverages containing tyramine stimulate the release of norepinephrine from storage sites within neurons. Normally, monoamine oxidase inactivates dietary tyramine, and excessive norepinephrine release is prevented. The tyramine-MAO inhibitor interaction may result in severe headaches and acute hypertensive attacks, which can be fatal. Restricted foods are foods which are spoiled, decayed, fermented, overripe, old, or aged. Examples of excluded items include aged cheeses (bleu, Swiss, and cheddar), aged or smoked meats (herring, sausage, and corned beef), sour cream, and ripe bananas and avocados. Red wines are prohibited although other forms of alcohol may be consumed in moderation. Broad bean pods and fava beans are restricted foods. MAO inhibitors are not recommended for the elderly because of the possibility of interactions with other drugs that may be prescribed[10] and because it is difficult to ensure that restricted foods will not be consumed.

Licorice imported from European countries contains a substance, glycyrrhizic acid, which has pharmacologic action. The active ingredient has mineralocorticoid activity. When this licorice is consumed in excessive amounts by people taking antihypertensive drugs, hypokalemia, sodium retention, and edema may result.

NUTRITIONAL CONSIDERATIONS OF PRESCRIPTION DRUGS

A significant number of drugs pose particular risk for the elderly. A few of the most frequently prescribed drugs have been selected for elaboration. Table 10-1 offers some examples of the possible drug-nutrient interactions of chronic drugs commonly used by the elderly.

Drug Management of Cardiovascular Disease

Digitalis glycosides. The digitalis glycosides increase myocardial contractility. In the failing heart, such as in congestive heart failure, these drugs increase overall cardiac efficiency. The drugs also are used in the treatment of certain cardiac arrhythmias, including atrial fibrillation and atrial tachycardia.

Digoxin, the most commonly used digitalis glycoside, has a narrow therapeutic range, which increases the likelihood of digitalis toxicity.[51] Absorption of the drug can be delayed by the presence of food in the gastrointestinal tract or by delayed gastric emptying. In these cases more of the drug is likely to be metabolized, leaving less of the unchanged drug available for absorption.[11] The result is an erratic therapeutic response. Because the distribution of digoxin is closely related to lean body mass, the elderly require lower-than-normal doses. Furthermore, because renal function and renal clearance are reduced in the elderly, the serum concentration of digoxin is often elevated.[43] Digitalis intoxication commonly occurs in as many as 30% of those taking this drug. Digoxin may also increase urinary excretion of magnesium and

Text continued on p. 243.

TABLE 10-1 *Drug-Nutrient Interactions Possible with Prescription Drugs Commonly Used by the Elderly*

Type of Drug*	Mechanism/Risk of Interference	Nutritional Considerations
Antiarrhythmic drug		
Quinidine *Quinalan***	Vitamin K deficiency if given with anticoagulants.	With high intake of fruit or juices: quinidine toxicity.
Anticoagulant		
Warfarin *Coumadin Panwarfin*	Antagonism of anticoagulant effects by vitamin K. Fatty foods may reduce absorption.	Large amounts of vitamin K-containing foods (cabbage, green peas, turnip greens, broccoli) should be avoided.
Anticonvulsants		
Phenytoin *Dilantin*	Impaired nutrient metabolism and utilization: vitamin B-12 and folate deficiencies. Increases inactivation of 25-OH-vitamin D: osteomalacia (long-term use).	Should be taken with food or immediately after meals to minimize gastric irritation. Folic acid supplement may be prescribed (limit 1 mg/day).
Primidone *Mysoline*	Impaired nutrient metabolism and utilization: folate deficiency; neurologic complications. May interfere with bone mineralization via interruption of vitamin K-dependent bone proteins.	Supplementation with vitamin K may be considered.
Antidepressants		
Imipramine *Tofranil*	Possible induction of riboflavin deficiency; interferes with assessment of riboflavin status. Acidifies urine. Causes gastric discomfort; constipation.	Should be administered with or immediately after food to reduce gastric irritation. May require increase in dietary fiber and fluid to overcome drug-induced constipation.
Phenelzine *Nardil*	Monoamine oxidase (MAO) antidepressant: concomitant intake of tyramine foods can precipitate sudden hypertensive crisis. Can cause GI distress, dry mouth, and appetite changes.	Foods and beverages high in tyramine and other pressor amines should be avoided. Body weight should be checked and any unusual changes reported. Sugarless candy or gum may help stimulate salivary flow.

Continued.

*Drug classes are included in the Glossary.
**Brand names indicated in *italics*.

239

TABLE 10-1 *Drug-Nutrient Interactions Possible with Prescription Drugs Commonly Used by the Elderly—cont'd*

Type of Drug*	Mechanism/Risk of Interference	Nutritional Considerations
Antigout drug		
Colchicine *Novocolchine*	Damage to intestinal mucosa: decreased absorption of vitamin B-12, carotene, fat, cholesterol, lactose, D-xylose. Long-term administration leads to megaloblastic anemia.	To reduce gastric irritation, should be taken with water immediately before or after meals. Encourage adequate fluid intake.
Antihypertensive drug		
Hydralazine *Apresoline*	Administration with food: increased drug bioavailability. Vitamin B-6 deficiency: risk vitamin B-6 deficiency causing neuritis.	Medication should be taken with food. Diet restricted in kilocalories and sodium may be warranted. Supplementation with vitamin B-6 may be considered.
Angiotensin converting enzyme inhibitors *Capoten* *Vasotec* *Monopril*	Reduces potassium excretion. Food *may* decrease absorption.	Avoid potassium supplements. Dietary counseling depends on drug taken: *Capoten* should not be taken with food; *Vasotec* should be taken with food; *Monopril* may be taken without regard to food.
Beta-adrenergic blocking agents *Inderal* *Lopressor*	May cause hypoglycemia in insulin-dependent patients but mask tachycardia, a warning sign. Food can enhance bioavailability.	Should be taken with food. However, once a food/drug pattern is established, consistency with that pattern is important.
Anti-infective drugs		
Isoniazid *INH, Isotamine*	Altered nutrient excretion and vitamin B-6 antagonist: vitamin B-6 deficiency; pellagra secondary to vitamin B-6 deficiency. Interferes with vitamin D metabolism: risk of osteomalacia. Food decreases drug absorption.	Supplementation with vitamin B-6, niacin, and vitamin D may be considered. Risk of osteomalacia is greatest in homebound or institutionalized elderly who do not drink milk. Should be taken on an empty stomach with water.
Sulfadiazine (a sulfonamide) *Microsulfon*	Impaired **folic acid** absorption. Anorexia. Administration with food alters GI motility and transit time: decreased drug absorption rate.	Foods rich in **folic acid** should be encouraged. Supplementation with folic acid may be considered. To minimize gastric irritation, drug should be taken with food or after meals. Adequate fluid intake should be encouraged.

Drug	Effect	Dietary recommendation
Tetracycline *Achromycin* *Panmycin*	Impaired nutrient metabolism and utilization. Interferes with vitamin K intestinal synthesis. Milk, dairy products, and iron supplements decrease drug absorption.	Supplementation with riboflavin, ascorbic acid, and calcium may be considered. Should be taken on an empty stomach with water. No milk, dairy products, or iron-containing foods should be taken within three hours of drug administration. Adequate fluids should be encouraged.
Anti-inflammatory drug Penicillamine *Cuprimine*	Appetite suppression: weight loss.	Supplementation with multivitamin and mineral pill may be advised because the drug can increase need for vitamin B-6 and zinc. Should not be administered with iron **or** other mineral supplements. Should be taken one hour before or three hours after meals. Adequate fluid intake is necessary.
Antiparkinsonian drug Levodopa *Dopar* *Larvodopa*	Vitamin B-6 causes accelerated conversion of levodopa to dopamine: decreased dopamine penetration of blood-brain barrier. May reverse antiparkinsonian effect. High protein diets interfere with drug transport to the CNS.	Intakes of vitamin B-6 in diet and supplements should be restricted. Foods high in protein should be limited.
Cardiac stimulant Digoxin *Lanoxin*	Anorexia and nausea: weight loss. Low potassium intake: digoxin toxicity. Bran cereal: slows drug absorption. Vitamin E: hypercalcemia and arrhythmias.	Well-balanced meals and adequate potassium intake should be encouraged. High-sodium foods should be avoided. Bran should be avoided in the meal that accompanies or follows drug administration. Should be taken with meals. However, once a food/drug pattern is established, consistency with that pattern is important.

Continued.

241

TABLE 10-1 **Drug-Nutrient Interactions Possible with Prescription Drugs Commonly Used by the Elderly—cont'd**

Type of Drug*	Mechanism/Risk of Interference	Nutritional Considerations
Diuretics		
Furosemide *Lasix*	Enhances excretion of sodium, chloride, potassium, magnesium, calcium, and water.	High-sodium foods should be restricted. Foods rich in potassium, calcium, and magnesium should be encouraged.
Spironolactone *Aldactone*	Enhances excretion of sodium, chloride, and water. Reduces excretion of potassium. Food enhances absorption.	Potassium supplements should not be used, nor should a salt substitute. Take with food or milk to lessen gastric irritation.
Thiazides *Hydrodiuril*	Enhances excretion of sodium, potassium, magnesium, and water.	High-sodium foods should be restricted. Foods rich in potassium and magnesium should be encouraged.
Lipid-lowering drug		
Cholestyramine *Questran*	Interferes with bile acid activity: vitamins A, D, E, K, B-12 and folate deficiencies. Depletes iron stores.	Supplementation is recommended with vitamin A, D, K (if hypoprothrombinemia occurs) and folic acid for those with reduced serum or red cell **folic acid**). Low-cholesterol diet is indicated. A high-bulk diet and increased fluid intake should be encouraged as tolerated.
Tranquilizers		
Chlorpromazine *Thorazine*	Increases appetite. Possible inducement of riboflavin deficiency; fiber interferes with assessment of riboflavin status. May result in constipation, fecal impaction; sore mouth and gums.	May require increase in dietary fiber and fluid to overcome drug-induced constipation. **Sore** mouth may be relieved by rinsing mouth or frequent sips of water. Sugarless candy or gum may also help stimulate salivary flow.
Analgesics		
Nonsteroidal anti-inflammatory drugs	**Renal** clearance decreases with age. Can cause sodium and fluid retention. Some foods may contribute to adverse gastrointestinal problems.	Increased risk of gastric and duodenal ulcer. May exacerbate hypertension or congestive heart failure. Administering immediately after eating is desirable. Limit citrus fruit and juices, alcohol, and caffeine.

calcium.[33] The drug's effects may be potentiated by concurrent administration of calcium or vitamin D supplements.

The clinical manifestations of digitalis toxicity include anorexia, nausea, vomiting, diarrhea, headaches, confusion, delirium, and diet- or drug-induced changes in plasma electrolytes. High doses of the drug may lead to digitalis cachexia. Gastrointestinal disturbances may also affect food intake, resulting in compromised nutritional status. Because many of the symptoms associated with digitalis toxicity are similar to those associated with conditions for which the drug is prescribed (e.g., nausea and vomiting attributable to heart failure or arrhythmias), it is important to know the elderly person's dietary habits.

Antiarrhythmic drugs. Antiarrhythmic drugs are used to treat irregularities in the rate and rhythm of heart contractions, disturbances that pose the risk of cardiac failure. Quinidine, an antiarrhythmic agent, has a narrow therapeutic index.[43,49] An increased elimination **half-life,** the time required for elimination of one-half of the drug, and decreased renal clearance are also characteristic of quinidine in the elderly. Because of altered pharmacokinetics in the elderly, elimination of the drug is prolonged. Thus, older people are at an increased risk of toxic effects, including **cinchonism,** a cluster of adverse effects characterized by gastrointestinal distress, headache, tinnitus, dizziness, blurred vision, and mild tremors.[59] Cinchonism occurrence is more commonly associated with low body weight. An older adult taking quinidine should be cautioned to avoid consumption of large amounts of citrus fruit juices (more than 1 l a day) because these juices increase urinary pH. Renal clearance of the drug is reduced in an alkaline urine, and therefore serum concentration of the drug is increased.

Anticoagulants. Anticoagulant therapy is intended to prevent the development of intravascular thromboses that can block the passage of blood and lead to a stroke or heart attack. The hypoprothrombinemic effect of oral anticoagulants may be enhanced by drugs that decrease vitamin K levels, such as antibiotics.[33] Older people who drink herbal teas containing naturally

occurring coumarin should also be counseled that the anticoagulant action of their medication may be increased. Alcohol inhibits the metabolism of anticoagulant drugs. Conversely, a decreased anticoagulant effect may be observed in those who currently consume large quantities of green tea and foods high in vitamin K, such as green leafy vegetables, liver, cheese, egg yolks, tomatoes, meats, and cereal. It is essential to know the older individual's dietary habits to provide appropriate counseling.

Antihypertensive drugs. Drug therapy for hypertension aims to reduce elevated arterial blood pressure. Antihypertensive agents exert their effects through numerous mechanisms and on many sites in the body. Drugs used in the management of hypertension include adrenergic inhibitors, vasodilators, angiotensin converting enzyme inhibitors, and diuretics.

Adrenergic inhibitors. Beta-adrenergic blocking agents reduce or block myocardial stimulation, vasodilation, and bronchodilation.[73,75] Ventricular and myocardial contractility are decreased. In response to a slowed heart rate, blood pressure is reduced. The bioavailability of these drugs is enhanced in the presence of food because of food-related increases in splanchnic blood flow.[53] Because renal clearance rates are reduced in the elderly and almost all beta-blockers are excreted by the kidney, drug excretion may be retarded. The risk of prolonged retention is also significant in elderly people with hypoalbuminemia.[55] Having less albumin to bind the drug means that more of the medication can diffuse into nervous tissue and give rise to side effects in the central nervous system.

Vasodilators. Hydralazine is a nondiuretic antihypertensive vasodilator whose primary effect is dilation of the blood vessels, particularly the arterioles.[59] In response to the vasodilation, blood pressure drops. The bioavailability of hydralazine is enhanced in the presence of food. The peripheral neuropathy that occurs in some individuals taking hydralazine is related to its antipyridoxine effect, because the drug combines with pyridoxine coenzymes, making them unavailable.[14] Thus the patient has an increased need for vitamin B-6, and supplementation (25 mg a day) may be prescribed to counter this side effect.[53] Older patients should be cautioned against taking vitamin B-6 in amounts above that found in a daily multivitamin pill unless advised to do so by their physician.[56] High dosages of vitamin B-6 can be toxic and lead to neuropathy and muscle weakness.

Angiotensin converting enzyme (ACE) inhibitors. ACE inhibitors lower blood pressure by blocking enzymes which act to constrict blood vessels and cause sodium and fluid retention. Some ACE inhibitors are used in combination with other drugs to manage certain types of heart failure by increasing the heart's ability to pump blood. These drugs also reduce potassium excretion by the kidneys and can cause hyperkalemia.[48] Because of the increased risk of hyperkalemia, older people being treated with ACE inhibitors should not take potassium supplements.

Diuretics. Retention of excess fluid by the body results primarily from excess sodium retention. The effectiveness of a diuretic is related to its ability to bring about excretion of excess sodium, which is accomplished by reducing the reabsorption of sodium ions in the renal tubules. Older people using diuretics need ongoing medical supervision as they are more susceptible to fluid and electrolyte disorders than are younger people.

The several types of diuretics differ in their particular action on the kidney tubule and the reabsorption of minerals and electrolytes. Loop diuretics, such as furosemide and ethacrynic acid, decrease sodium and chloride absorption in the ascending loop of Henle.[53] It is important to carefully monitor electrolyte levels in these patients, because low blood levels of sodium, potassium, magnesium, and calcium are possible side effects. Although the older person should be counseled to avoid foods high in sodium and avoid indiscriminate use of OTC medications, a very restrictive sodium diet (less than 1.5 gm of sodium a day) is not appropriate. Conversely, a strong argument for a mild sodium restriction in these situations is that potassium loss is directly proportional to sodium excretion, which increases with dietary intake.[72] Wilber[72] suggests limiting sodium intake to 75 mEq per day, accomplished by eliminating highly salted, preprepared foods from the diet and by not adding salt at the table. This approach enhances the effectiveness of the oral diuretic and may eliminate the need for potassium supplements or the relatively expensive potassium-sparing diuretic combinations. To compensate for the increased urinary excretion of calcium, which can speed up the development of osteoporosis, an older patient should be encouraged to drink milk each day.[55]

Thiazide diuretics decrease sodium reabsorption in the distal kidney tubules and can lead to fluid and electrolyte imbalances. The risk of significant magnesium and potassium loss is increased with thiazide diuretics. Conversely, calcium retention has been observed, and elevated blood levels of calcium may occur with prolonged thiazide therapy.[55,78] The potential for hyperglycemia is heightened for older people with diabetes.

Not all diuretics increase the risk of potassium loss. Potassium-sparing diuretics conserve potassium by reducing distal tubular secretion of potassium in conjunction with sodium reabsorption. The principal use of potassium-sparing drugs is in combination with other diuretics. If potassium-sparing drugs are used alone, significant hyperkalemia can result. For an elderly person taking potassium-sparing drugs, potassium supplements or salt substitutes will exacerbate the risk of hyperkalemia.

Lipid-lowering drugs. The National Cholesterol Education Program/Adult Treatment Program[20] supports the use of lipid-lowering medications as adjunctive therapy to dietary changes, but does not approve the use of these drugs as a substitute for such changes.

Cholestyramine is an effective plasma cholesterol-lowering drug that combines with bile acids in the intestine. Bile acid reabsorption is prevented, and the excretion of bile acids in the feces is increased. Bile acid sequestrants such as cholestyramine should be used cautiously in the elderly, because gastrointestinal discomfort, severe constipation, and nutrient malabsorption are likely.[59] Long-term therapy with bile acid sequestrants, including colestipol, has been shown to depress the absorption of fat-soluble vitamins, folate, and vitamin B-12 by inhibiting absorption or decreasing the availability of bile acids.[53] Nutrition counseling should encourage a liberal intake of dietary fiber to counter the constipating effects of cholestyramine.

In pharmaceutical doses, niacin may be prescribed to decrease serum lipids by decreasing very low density lipoproteins (VLDL) and low density lipoproteins (LDL).[66] However, the use of niacin as a lipid-lowering drug is limited by the adverse effects of flushing and itching. In addition, any ulcers present may be aggravated, and vomiting, diarrhea, and dyspepsia may result. Liver function may be impaired with increasing serum transaminase activity, and jaundice has been reported. Niacin in the form of nicotinamide (rather than as nicotinic acid) does not produce flushing. Since tolerance frequently develops after a few weeks, increasing dosage gradually may minimize the flushing reaction.

Niacin is available without a prescription and has become a well-known therapeutic agent. Its popularity has been enhanced by numerous lay articles and books. However, because of the potential for hepatotoxicity and other side effects and aggravation of other chronic conditions such as diabetes mellitus, active peptic ulcer disease, and acute gout, older people should be cautioned against self-medicating with niacin.

Pulmonary Drugs

A number of changes occur in the lungs with increasing age, including a 50% increase in residual lung volume between early adulthood and age 70.[74] A decrease in vital capacity is the result of reduced elasticity of the chest wall. Weaker respiratory muscles, impaired ciliary action, and a less effective cough further predispose an older person to a variety of pulmonary diseases and disorders. Pulmonary conditions commonly seen in the elderly include pneumonia, chronic obstructive pulmonary disease (COPD), pulmonary embolism, and tuberculosis.

Bronchodilators. Bronchodilators relax and expand the bronchioles, the small airways that lead to the air sacs where oxygen and carbon dioxide are exchanged. Theophylline is a xanthine-derivative bronchodilator used to treat COPD in the elderly.[55] The presence of food has little effect on theophylline availability, although absorption of the drug may be somewhat slower when food is present than when the stomach is empty. However, variations in food components can affect the drug's efficacy. A high-protein, low-carbohydrate diet may decrease the effect of the drug by increasing its metabolism and clearance through the kidney. Conversely, a high-carbohydrate, low-protein diet slows theophylline metabolism and predisposes the individual to undesirable side effects such as dizziness, flushing, and headache.[55] A high-fat intake potentiates the risk of dizziness by promoting rapid absorption of the drug. Taking theophylline with beverages containing caffeine may result in an increased incidence of adverse effects. Elimination of the drug is enhanced by the high polycyclic carbon content of charcoal-broiled foods.[73]

Antitubercular agents. Isoniazid, a vitamin B-6 antagonist, can produce clinical symptoms of vitamin deficiency by inhibiting pyridoxal kinase.[78] As many as 40% of those taking the drug may develop vitamin B-6 deficiency. The adverse effect is increased in those with concurrent intake of other antitubercular agents, in individuals with low vitamin B-6 intakes, and in those not given supplementation. Vitamin B-6 supplementation of 25 mg a day is recommended.[55] Isoniazid inhibits the enzyme which breaks down histamine, allowing elevation of histamine levels in the blood. The high histamine content of foods such as sardines, skipjack, tuna, sauerkraut juice, and yeast extract predisposes the individual taking isoniazid to severe headaches, low blood pressure, itching, chills, palpitations, and loose stools.[59]

Gastrointestinal Disease

H₂-receptor antagonist. Long-term administration of cimetidine coupled with a high-fiber diet may result in the formation of gastric phytobezoars, or hard balls of fiber.[45] A diet low in cellulose may need to be considered for the elderly person receiving long-term therapy with cimetidine or for those with chewing problems. Antacids may impair oral absorption of H₂-blockers if administered concurrently.[10] Cimetidine can induce vitamin B-12 depletion by impairing its absorption, particularly in vegans who take the drug for a prolonged time (greater than one year).

Psychotherapeutic Drugs

The use of psychotherapeutic medications, now the third most commonly prescribed type of drug, is increasing among the elderly.[48] Unfortunately, evidence indicates that these drugs are being misused in this segment of the population. One aspect of the problem may be an improper diagnosis of mental disorders, but also these drugs are being prescribed as a panacea for the problems of daily living, to quiet an individual in an institution or even within the family. Psychotherapeutic drugs such as sedatives or antidepressants frequently are prescribed for the elderly to control disruptive behavior. Older people are especially sensitive to the intended pharmacologic effects and the undesirable adverse effects of psychotherapeutic drugs.

Tranquilizers. The side effects of many tranquilizers may include nausea and vomiting, which may cause loss of appetite and lead to malnutrition. However, phenothiazine antipsychotic drugs, which include chlorpromazine, may actually stimulate the appetite to the point that the older individual with free access to food may grossly overeat.[55] Obesity then becomes a concern. Chlorpromazine may also induce riboflavin depletion.[56] Researchers conducting animal studies observed interaction between this drug and the metabolism of riboflavin, which has a similar chemical structure.[78]

Antidepressants. The reported incidence of depression in the elderly is approximately 10%. Tricyclic antidepressants (amitriptyline and imipramine) are frequently prescribed for the elderly and are accompanied by potentially serious side effects, such as cardiac dysrhythmias, hypotension, and anticholinergic effects.[15,34,49] Consequently, constipation may be a severe problem and the importance of incorporating an adequate amount of fiber to the diet should be stressed. These drugs are also known to alter riboflavin metabolism and induce riboflavin depletion.[56]

Enhanced appetite may be observed in some elderly people taking tricyclic antidepressants, and this may lead to weight gain.[59] This improved appetite may be due to an improved mental state or an improved taste perception.

Dry mouth is a possible side effect with tricyclic antidepressants. To cope with the problem, the individual should avoid drinking high-calorie beverages; rather, low-calorie beverages, sugarless gum or candy, or ice should be selected. A new class of drugs, selective serotonin reuptake inhibitors, has comparable antidepressant actions with fewer anticholinergic adverse effects.[15]

Drug therapy in Alzheimer's disease. Senile dementia of the Alzheimer type (SDAT) is the most common type of dementia in the United States and the number of cases is increasing.[14] Treatment is primarily supportive, although drug therapy for those with secondary behavioral disturbances, such as depression, hallucinations, agitation, and wandering, has been helpful in some cases.[15] Currently between 10 and 20 drugs are undergoing the clinical trials required before gaining final approval from the FDA. The drugs used in the treatment of SDAT are divided into two broad categories: drugs directed at improving abnormal behavior and those directed at improving cognitive function.

Numerous drugs are available to treat behavioral problems, although none is specific for SDAT; these drugs may be useful in dementia of any origin. Neuroleptics are the most widely prescribed drugs to treat abnormal behavior, although their mode of action in controlling psychotic behavior has not been established. No one drug within this category has been shown to have greater effectiveness than another. Chlorpromazine, once a favorite, has largely been replaced by thioridazine hydrochloride, because the latter is less likely to cause such adverse symptoms as immobility, rigidity, restlessness, and tremors.[17] Other side effects associated with neuroleptic drugs include seizures, inappropriate secretion of antidiuretic hormone, jaundice, and weight gain.[14] Sedatives or minor tranquilizers are indicated for use in short-term treatment of anxiety or in less severe cases, but they may increase the risk of falling. The exact mechanism of effectiveness of drugs such as propranolol and carbamazepine (used to treat agitation and violent behavior) is unknown and the role of these drugs is largely undefined.

More recent drug development has centered on attempts to improve cognitive function in

SDAT patients. Because SDAT is recognized as a deficiency of acetylcholine in neural tissues, researchers have sought ways to increase brain levels of acetylcholine. Because the enzyme cholinesterase degrades acetylcholine, drugs that inhibit the enzyme's action could potentially increase acetylcholine levels. A second category of drugs, nootropic drugs, is also used to improve cognitive function. Although the way in which these drugs affect memory is unknown, nootropic drugs act to improve nerve cell function. The third subcategory of drugs to improve cognitive function are the calcium channel blockers, which act on the vascular system. In addition to their vasodilating properties, these drugs have the ability to block calcium entry into injured or hypoxic brain neurons, which may be a key to their effectiveness.

At best drugs may slow the progression of SDAT; none has yet been discovered that will reverse the course of this disease. Multiple drug therapies may be the best line of treatment for SDAT, a disease characterized by multiple defects.

Antiparkinsonian Drugs

Drug treatment of Parkinson's disease is directed toward augmenting dopamine activity or reducing acetylcholine activity. Clinical manifestations of this incurable disease include bradykinesia, rigidity, and tremors. Difficulties with mastication and swallowing also may be observed.

Levodopa, an antiparkinsonian agent, has a structure similar to that of amino acids and therefore competes with amino acids for absorption sites in the small intestine.[56] If the drug is taken concurrently with a high-protein diet, its bioavailability may be significantly compromised. The suggested protein intake of individuals taking levodopa is 0.5 g per kg body weight, which should be adequate if protein foods of high biological value are stressed. Eating protein foods later in the day is another strategy to suggest. Older individuals taking levodopa should avoid multivitamin supplements containing pyridoxine (vitamin B-6) because this vitamin enhances the peripheral conversion of levodopa to dopamine, and the drug's effects will be reduced.

Antineoplastic Drugs

Whether the elderly as a group are less likely to receive vigorous, potentially beneficial chemotherapy treatment for cancer has received considerable attention.[57] In a comparison of toxicity from chemotherapy in individuals under age 70 and those age 70 or older, no significant difference was observed between the two groups in important predictors of outcome, including functional status, weight loss, and previous therapy.[8] Toxicity was similar for both groups, with the exception of hematologic toxicity causing changes in the blood-forming tissues in the bone marrow. A significantly greater number of elderly adults experienced hematologic toxicity. Red blood cell production may be affected, accompanied by anemia, leukopenia, and thrombocytopenia. An increase in toxicity with age may be associated with the presence of age-related physiologic decline in specific organ systems such as reduced renal function.

Essentially all neoplastic agents cause nausea and vomiting, resulting in a reduced food intake, fluid and electrolyte imbalance, and weight loss. The effects of the drugs on the gastrointestinal tract may induce anorexia. Antineoplastic drugs, particularly methotrexate, cause malabsorption through desquamation of intestinal epithelial cells, and malabsorption may continue after chemotherapy has been discontinued. Inflammation of the mucous membrane lining the mouth, throat, and esophagus, stomatitis, and glossitis may cause discomfort with eating. If a person tries to eat when the drug is causing side effects, an aversion to those foods eaten may result from an association between the food item and the unpleasant side effects experienced.[54] It is unlikely that a change in appetite associated with the drug alone will induce a nutritional deficiency.[55]

Prescription Analgesics

Individuals age 65 or older are the greatest users of analgesics. Narcotic analgesics include natural pain relievers (opium, codeine, and morphine) and synthetic narcotics (opioids).[33] A prescription is required. Nonnarcotic analgesics are sold without a prescription and will be discussed later. Both narcotic and nonnarcotic drugs are used to treat pain. Narcotics are typically prescribed for moderate to severe pain and act primarily on the central nervous system.

NUTRITIONAL CONSIDERATIONS OF OVER-THE-COUNTER DRUGS

The use of nonprescription medication is high among elderly people, although reports vary as to its extent. Almost one-third of drug expenditures by the elderly goes to OTC drugs.[41] Further, use of nonprescription drugs among the elderly is expected to continue to increase in concert with the expansion of home health care, the fastest growing segment of the health care market.[34] The most frequently used OTC drugs are analgesics, cough and cold preparations, vitamin supplements, antacids, and laxatives. Use of nonprescription medicine is more likely with advancing age, particularly among women. However, elderly adults are not likely to discuss the use of OTC drugs with a physician, and the physician is not likely to ask about their use.

Unfortunately, indiscriminate use of these therapeutically valuable drugs can lead to unexpected consequences. The elderly are particularly at risk for the hazards associated with nonprescription drugs for several reasons. Additive effects and interactions with prescribed drugs can develop in people undergoing complex drug regimens. In self-prescribing OTC drugs, the elderly person may not correctly diagnose the condition, select an appropriate drug, and follow directions.

In this era of increasing self-care, more prescription drugs are being changed to nonprescription status, increasing the potential for further adverse effects. For example, in 1995 cimetidine (Tagamet HC) became available as an OTC drug. Users of drugs are generally reimbursed for prescription medications but not for OTC drugs, thus making the prescription-to-OTC switch desirable for the government and health care plans.[62] The trend is likely to continue.

Table 10-2 offers some nutritional considerations for OTC drugs commonly used by the elderly.

Nonprescription Analgesics

Nonnarcotic analgesics are used to treat mild to moderate pain and act on the peripheral nervous system at the receptor sites for pain.[33] Most analgesics have an antipyretic effect and may be prescribed to reduce elevated body temperature. The most commonly used and oldest analgesic in the United States is aspirin (acetylsalicylic acid). This drug also has an anti-inflammatory effect, making it useful to treat the symptoms of inflammatory conditions (e.g., rheumatoid arthritis and osteoarthritis). Because aspirin produces an inhibitory effect on platelet aggregation or clotting, it is also prescribed to reduce the risk of heart attack or stroke.

Aspirin is classified among the nonsteroidal anti-inflammatory drugs (NSAIDs), valuable as pain relievers. NSAIDs inhibit the synthesis of prostaglandins which accumulate at injured tissue sites, resulting in inflammation and pain. NSAIDs are not without side effects. For example, common side effects of aspirin include gastric distress, dyspepsia, and nausea.[35] Salicylate toxicity can occur at high doses or with prolonged use, particularly with the older adult chronic aspirin user who tends to have less serum protein to bind salicylate and also is less able to excrete it.[59] Symptoms of salicylate toxicity include confusion, irritability, tinnitus, impaired hearing or vision, nausea, vomiting, and diarrhea. Because of aspirin's antipyretic action, subnormal body temperatures can occur. Gastritis, ulceration of the gastric mucosa, and hemorrhaging are harmful side effects experienced by the elderly who, because of inadequate diets and poor nutritional status, are less able to compensate for even small blood loss. Iron-deficiency anemia may be induced. Folic acid deficiency and macrocytic anemia are associated with chronic aspirin therapy, particularly in those with a marginal intake of the vitamin. Vitamin C depletion has also been observed.

Other NSAIDs are now available without prescription, including ibuprofen and naproxen sodium, which have stronger analgesic and significant antipyretic effects than aspirin with fewer gastrointestinal side effects.[33] The presence of food may delay or reduce the absorption rate of these drugs.[70] However, the rate of

TABLE 10-2 *Nutritional Considerations with Over-the-Counter Drugs Commonly Used by the Elderly*

Type of Drug		Nutritional Considerations
Analgesics		
Aspirin	*Anacin,* * *Bayer, Bufferin, Ecotrin, Excedrin*	Chronic ingestion may be associated with depressed plasma ascorbic acid and folate levels; supplementation may be indicated. May cause iron-deficiency anemia as a result of GI blood loss. Some brands may contain appreciable amounts of sodium.
Acetaminophen	*Datril, Panadol, Tylenol*	Coadministration with a high-carbohydrate meal may significantly retard absorption. Individuals with poor nutrition or who have ingested alcohol over prolonged periods are prone to liver disease, and drug may cause anorexia, nausea, vomiting, dyspepsia, constipation, or diarrhea. May increase urinary loss of ascorbic acid.
Ibuprofen Naproxen sodium	*Advil, Motrin, Nuprin Aleve*	Can cause gastric distress. Should be taken with food, at meal times, or with plenty of fluids. Avoid alcohol. May cause iron-deficiency anemia as a result of GI bleeding.
Antacids		
Aluminum hydroxide	*Amphojel*	Large doses for prolonged periods along with a diet low in phosphorus and protein can lead to a phosphorus-deficiency syndrome; the elderly person in poor nutritional status is at high risk. Vitamin A and thiamin deficiencies can occur as a result of reduced absorption. Constipation occurs commonly, and intestinal obstruction has been reported.
Magnesium hydroxide	*Milk of Magnesia*	Excessive dosage can cause nausea, abdominal cramps, diarrhea, alkalization of urine, and dehydration. Magnesium toxicity can develop in those with kidney failure. May decrease absorption of vitamin A, phosphorus, and calcium; inactivates thiamin.

*Brand name indicated in italics.

Continued.

TABLE 10-2   *Nutritional Considerations with Over-the-Counter Drugs Commonly Used by the Elderly—cont'd*

Type of Drug		Nutritional Considerations
Antidiarrheal drugs	*Lomotil, Kaopectate*	May cause nausea, vomiting, abdominal discomfort, constipation, and fecal impaction. Caffeine beverages and alcohol should be avoided, since both increase peristalsis. Prolonged use may interfere with intestinal absorption of nutrients and promote constipation.
Antiemetics	*Dramamine, Bonine*	May cause dry mouth, nose, and throat, epigastric distress, and constipation.
Antihistamines Diphenhydramine Chlorpheniramine maleate	*Benedryl* *Chlor-Trimeton*	GI side effects may be lessened by administration of drug with meals or milk. Dry mouth may be relieved by sugarless candy or gum or rinses with water. Elderly people are especially likely to experience dizziness, sedation, and hypotension.
Cold preparations Dextromethorphan	*Robitussin DM, Sucrets*	Fluid intake should be increased to 2 to 3 l daily to help thin and mobilize respiratory secretions, but the elderly should be monitored closely to avoid fluid overload.
Laxatives Bulk-forming	*Metamucil, Mitrolan*	Adequate fluid intake must be maintained; fecal impaction can occur if intake by mouth is insufficient. Can decrease appetite through abdominal fullness. Products contain varying amounts of sugar and salt. Electrolyte imbalance is possible with chronic use.
Fecal softeners Stimulants	*Colace* *Bisacolax, Correctol,* *Dulcolax, Ex-Lax*	Adequate fluid intake must be maintained. Abuse can cause electrolyte imbalance, including potassium depletion; malabsorption, with weight loss, can also occur. Frequent use may result in laxative dependence.

hospitalization of the elderly due to bleeding ulcers is at least twice that of the general population, and this may be related to the fact that the elderly use more than 50% of all NSAIDs consumed. Therefore, these drugs should be given with food to prevent gastrointestinal irritation. Older people should be advised that consuming alcohol with ibuprofen may increase the risk of gastrointestinal bleeding.

Acetaminophen, second only to aspirin in popularity, is a para-aminophenol derivative which possesses analgesic and antipyretic action and has a wide therapeutic index.[48] It is a commonly used aspirin substitute, although not an NSAID. For the older adult with degenerative joint disease, acetaminophen often provides satisfactory pain relief with several advantages over NSAID therapy.[3] A lower incidence of gastrointestinal upset and bleeding has been observed as well as fewer reports of hypersensitivity reactions. However, unlike aspirin, acetaminophen has no significant anti-inflammatory activity. The major concern is that a massive overdose of acetaminophen can induce hepatotoxicity. Liver damage is also possible with long-term use in alcoholics and those with impaired liver function.

Antacids

Antacids are frequently used to treat upper gastrointestinal disorders, ranging from mild indigestion and heartburn to peptic ulcer. Appropriate antacid therapy should be selected cautiously, because indiscriminate use of many widely available and easily obtainable preparations result in serious, harmful effects. This is particularly important for elderly people with altered bowel habits, severe organ-system disease, or renal impairment.[23]

With antacid therapy, the absorption of acidic drugs may be increased and the absorption of basic drugs decreased. If possible, other drugs should not be taken within one to two hours of antacid ingestion. By delaying gastric emptying, antacids delay the absorption of a number of drugs. The elimination of other drugs is influenced by the effect of antacids in raising urinary pH.

Some antacids contain significant amounts of sugar. The sodium content of antacids should also be explored, especially for older people who have been advised to restrict sodium in their diets because of hypertension, edema, or congestive heart failure. Antacids containing more than 5 mEq of sodium per dose carry a precautionary warning on the label, but sodium bicarbonate and effervescent forms of antacids are exempt from this rule.[23]

Antacids with calcium ions may induce a rebound hyperacidity in the stomach.[33] Milk-alkali syndrome is a possible complication associated with high doses of calcium-containing antacids over several years. The condition is exacerbated with the concurrent intake of milk products. Symptoms include metabolic alkalosis, hypercalcemia, vomiting, confusion, headache, calcium crystals in the urine, and renal insufficiency. More acute problems have been observed with calcium-containing antacids at lower doses. Constipation and fecal impaction may be promoted.

Aluminum-containing antacids may be constipating and may result in intestinal obstruction, particularly in the bedridden individual. This type of antacid has also been implicated in the dementia observed in elderly uremic patients. High levels of aluminum have been identified upon autopsy in brain specimens of patients with dementia.[23] Brain alterations were similar to those seen in Alzheimer's disease. A toxicity of aluminum has been proposed but not confirmed. Phosphate depletion is likely, since aluminum antacids bind phosphate ions in the intestine and accelerated elimination of the nonabsorbable phosphates follows. Symptoms of phosphate depletion include anorexia, muscle weakness, impaired reflexes, depression, and osteomalacia.

Aluminum hydroxide is sometimes paired with magnesium hydroxide to reduce the occurrence of constipation associated with aluminum-containing antacids and the diarrhea frequently associated with magnesium-containing antacids. Antacids containing magnesium can cause profound diarrhea, leading to dehydration and significant losses of vitamins and electrolytes, particularly potassium. Magnesium toxicity, characterized by nausea, vomiting, impaired reflexes, hypotension, and respiratory depression, can develop in people with impaired renal function.[56]

Antacid preparations containing sodium carbonate are appropriate for short-term use only because of the potential for sodium overload, which is significantly enhanced during prolonged treatment. Milk-alkali syndrome and rebound hypersecretion of gastric acid similar to that noted with calcium preparations are also possible. With use of antacids the pH of the jejunum may be sufficiently raised to decrease the absorption of folic acid.

Laxatives

A laxative is an agent that facilitates evacuation of the bowel. It has been estimated that 90% of the elderly who are laxative dependent or laxative abusers are women.[23] Laxative use among the elderly is similar to the use of analgesics, and use of both drugs continues to be high. Laxatives can be classified by their respective mechanisms of action.

Stimulant laxatives increase the frequency and intensity of muscle contractions in the intestine, which may produce excessive catharsis, leading to the development of fluid and electrolyte disturbances. The intensity of the response to these drugs is directly proportional to the dose. Side effects may include intestinal cramps, increased secretion of mucus, and excessively fluid evacuations. Castor oil is an example of a stimulant laxative, and it should be used cautiously by the elderly because of its potential for dehydration. Prolonged use of stimulant laxatives can result in the cathartic syndrome, impaired motility, dilated colon, exacerbated constipation, and laxative dependency.[3] Severe malabsorption, with steatorrhea, protein-losing enteropathy,[11] and decreased absorption of glucose, calcium, potassium, and vitamin D, have been observed.

Saline or osmotic cathartics should also be used with caution in the elderly because of potential side effects. These drugs mechanically stimulate peristalsis and alter stool consistency by increasing water retention in the intestinal lumen. The older individual should be encouraged to drink sufficient water to prevent dehydration.

Emollient laxatives soften the fecal mass by reducing surface tension of interfacing liquids in bowel contents.[74] Fluid accumulation in the bowel is promoted. Stool softeners are relatively safe and recommended for conditions in which hard or dry stool might prove painful or when straining is undesirable, such as in elderly people with heart disease. Potassium deficiency, associated with gastrointestinal losses and lack of potassium reabsorption in the colon, has been observed with some stool softeners.[59]

Bulk-producing laxatives are cellulose derivatives that swell in intestinal fluid and stimulate peristalsis by retaining water in the stool. The size of the stool is increased, and transit time is decreased. These laxatives are the preferred type for short-term treatment of most types of mild constipation. However, they should be administered with and followed by large amounts of water. Bulk-forming laxatives are contraindicated for individuals prone to intestinal ulcers or disabling adhesions, because of the danger of impaction.[23]

The preferred measures for maintaining a soft, formed stool and regular bowel habits are a sufficient fluid intake and a well-balanced diet rich in high-fiber foods. Important sources of dietary fiber include whole-grain cereals and breads, fruits and vegetables, and nuts. Cereals are preferable sources of fiber because they are high in soluble fiber, which has proved to be more effective in producing fecal bulk. Bran has been shown to be particularly effective in decreasing constipation and maintaining bowel function. Adding high-fiber foods to the diet should be done slowly to prevent flatulence and abdominal cramps. Excessive fiber intake can interfere with the absorption of minerals and may lead to intestinal obstruction.

ALCOHOL USE IN OLDER PEOPLE

Alcohol is one of the most pervasive drugs in our society. Its use or abuse places the elderly at risk for a variety of adverse and life-threatening effects, including liver disease, gastritis, peptic ulcer disease, heart muscle disorder, malnutrition, and changes in mental status.[18]

Until recently, use and abuse of alcohol by the elderly did not receive a great deal of attention. This may have been partly due to an attitude that abusers would "mature out" of their habits.[71] Also, symptoms associated with a problem drinker (tremors, impaired memory, disturbed sleep patterns, peripheral neuropathy, unsteady gait, depression) may be mistakenly identified as common problems of aging.[19] However, as the population as a whole ages, current interest in the use of alcohol by older age groups is heightened.

Use of Alcohol

Sulsky and associates[64] observed that alcohol consumption decreased with age among 611 noninstitutionalized, nonalcoholic elderly people ages 60 to 95. Men were more likely to drink than women, and men also were more likely to consume large quantities of alcohol than women. In a random sample of 241 British elderly, 76 (32%) identified themselves as drinkers, and 161 (68%) identified themselves as nondrinkers.[31] As with other community studies, men were more likely to drink than women.

One estimate puts the number of adults over the age of 65 with a drinking problem at 10%, based on hospital and treatment facility admissions.[67] Another investigation concluded that alcohol-related hospitalizations for this population were comparable to those for myocardial infarctions, the number one cause of death among older Americans.[1] Figures for the latter study were based on data from 1989 Medicare claims.

Although a significant number of older people appear to consume alcoholic beverages regularly, the number of alcohol abusers is not clear. Widner and Zeichner[71] purport that a significant number go undetected and that drinking behavior may be underreported by as much as 50%. Analysis from the 1988 National Health Interview Survey indicates that 50% of men age 65 or older identified themselves as abstainers, as did 74% of women age 65 or older.[19] Twenty-six percent of men and 16% of women were light drinkers (1 to 13 drinks per month). Moderate drinkers (4 to 13 drinks weekly) included 15% of the men and 7% of the women. Nine percent of the men and 3% of the women in this age group were considered heavy drinkers (on average, two or more drinks daily). One must keep in mind when interviewing the older adult and when interpreting the number of drinks consumed that problems related to alcohol in this population are likely to develop at relatively low levels of consumption.

Although elderly alcohol abusers cannot be described as a homogenous group based on behavioral characteristics, they do fall into two classes: the early-onset and the late-onset problem drinker.[70] The early-onset problem drinker has a long history of heavy alcohol consumption beginning before age 40. The support network of family and friends is less likely to be as strong as that of the late-onset problem drinker whose history of heavy drinking began after age 40. Early-onset drinkers are likely to be unmarried and male. Typically they have fewer alcohol-related physical problems and appear more responsive to treatment. Late-onset problem drinkers account for as many as 40% of all elderly problem drinkers, and onset seems to be related to a stressful event. They also are likely to be depressed and using a variety of drugs.

Underreporting of true alcohol consumption by the elderly may be associated with their isolation from an active support network that typically would recognize and report alcohol-related problems.[71] On the other hand, family members may hesitate to report the older person's drinking problem in an attempt to protect the dignity of the individual. Many of the physical complaints (musculoskeletal pain, insomnia, depression) and complications (falls and liver disease) of heavy drinking are masked as common complaints associated with aging.[70]

Nutritional Aspects

Tolerance to alcohol decreases and adverse side effects increase with age.[70] Elevated blood alcohol levels in the older person following a typical drink are likely due to decreased hepatic blood flow, body water content, and lean body mass. The risk of nutritional deficiency arising from use of other drugs is markedly increased by excessive use of alcohol or when prior alcoholism has depleted nutrient stores. Enzyme induction is enhanced with chronic alcohol use which enhances a drug's metabolism.[65] The result may be the necessity of greater drug dosage to achieve the desired effect. Moreover, alcohol interacts with some drugs to exacerbate negative effects. Both alcohol and aspirin irritate the gastric mucosa and can lead to gastrointestinal bleeding. When both drugs are combined, the anticoagulant effect of aspirin can result in serious hemorrhage.[33]

A high alcohol intake decreases potassium levels. This presents a serious danger to the cardiac patient taking digoxin, since both cardiac arrhythmias and digoxin toxicity can result. The insulin-dependent diabetic may become hypoglycemic following high alcohol intake, since alcohol interferes with gluconeogenesis.[55] The non-insulin-dependent diabetic taking an oral antidiabetic drug such as tolbutamide may experience hyperglycemia, because alcohol can shorten the drug's period of action.[55] Chlorpropamide, another oral antidiabetic agent, can result in a chlorpropamide-alcohol flush reaction in some non-insulin-dependent diabetics when the drug is mixed with alcohol in beverages, foods, or other drugs.

Thiamin deficiency. Alcohol interferes with thiamin absorption. At the low concentrations in which it is normally found in the intestine, thiamin is absorbed against a concentration gradient by an active transport mechanism requiring both oxygen and energy. Although alcohol does not inhibit thiamin uptake by the mucosal cell, the vitamin is not released into the blood as a result of alcohol inhibition of the enzyme required for this step (sodium-potassium ATPase).[30]

Thiamin absorption is impaired in alcoholics with or without liver disease and returns to normal within eight weeks after use is discontinued.[68] The direct effect of alcohol on the absorption mechanism is confirmed by the observation that absorption is similarly depressed in normal subjects given alcohol before thiamin ingestion. As a result of ineffective absorption, thiamin deficiency is common among alcohol abusers. In one report nearly half of a group of chronic alcoholics (n=50) had below-normal red blood cell transketolase activity as compared to only 2% of healthy adults (n=1,152).[30]

Neurologic disorders marked by visual disturbances, abnormal gait (ataxia), mental confusion, and memory loss (e.g., Wernicke-Korsakoff syndrome) occur in thiamin deficiency regardless of associated alcoholism.[30,37] Degeneration of the peripheral nerves, with loss of normal reflexes and burning sensations, weakness, and pain in the lower extremities are classic signs of inade-

quate thiamin. Clinical beri-beri, with disturbed cardiac function, edema, and eventual cardiac failure, has been described in experimental as well as accidental thiamin deficiency. As pointed out by Iber and coworkers,[30] cardiac disease, loss of memory, and loss of vibratory sense in the lower extremities, suggestive of thiamin deficiency, frequently occur with advancing age. The diagnostic problem is complicated further by the fact that older people may have multiple vitamin deficiencies regardless of alcohol abuse.[36]

Although aged alcoholics or individuals with poor thiamin intake (over at least three months) often respond to thiamin therapy, both behavior changes and cardiac symptoms in older people can result from a variety of disease conditions. Long-term neurologic and psychologic follow-up of older people whose thiamin status was restored to normal is needed to provide information regarding both physiologic and behavior changes pertinent to thiamin problems in this age group.

VITAMIN AND MINERAL SUPPLEMENTS IN OLDER PEOPLE

Extent of Use

A large number of older people use vitamin and mineral supplements. Block and associates[10] analyzed previously uncoded data from the National Health and Nutrition Examination Survey I study to evaluate the use of these supplements. Persons age 65 years and older regularly took vitamin and mineral supplements twice as often as any other age group, with the exception of vitamin E, iron, and multiple vitamins. More recent studies have corroborated this, with estimates that approximately 33% to 69% of the older population regularly use vitamin and mineral supplements.[26,29,47] In addition, the data indicate that the elderly frequently take supplements in potentially toxic doses,[26,47] overestimate the benefits of the products, and do not select supplements that will correct existing dietary deficiencies.

Data from the 1987 National Health Interview Survey reported estimates of supplement use in a large representative sample of the U.S. population.[63] Included were 2,498 respondents from ages 65 to 74 and 1,742 respondents age 75 or older. In the 65 to 74 age group, multivitamin-mineral supplements were the most commonly consumed supplement (22%), followed in decreasing order of daily usage by calcium (12%), vitamin C (11%), vitamin E (7%), and vitamin A (2%). In those age 75 or older, the order changed somewhat: multivitamin-mineral supplements (22%), vitamin C (10%), calcium (9%), vitamin E (7%), and vitamin A (2%).

Elderly people taking vitamins and minerals tend to have misperceptions about vitamin and mineral supplements. More than half of 102 elderly subjects from rural congregate meal programs believed that taking supplements makes one feel better physically, 64% believed most elderly need dietary supplements, and 70% believed a "run-down" feeling indicates a need for vitamins and minerals.[46] Almost half of the subjects in the study were taking supplements inappropriately, interpreted as the use of a multivitamin-mineral supplement containing more than 150% of the U.S. Recommended Dietary Allowance (USRDA; the standard reference values of nutrients developed for and formerly used on food labels) or taking three or more individual supplements not prescribed by a physician.

Potentially toxic doses of vitamin A ($\geq$25,000 IU) were being taken by 3% of 11,888 residents of a retirement community in Southern California.[26] More than one-fourth of those who took vitamin E supplements and 23% of those who took vitamin C supplements were taking at least 10 times the RDA.

Twenty "overusers" of nutrient supplements (defined as taking at least one vitamin or mineral supplement exceeding 200% of the RDA without medical recommendation) took 44 types of products.[52] Supplement intakes greater than 25 times the RDA were reported for many overusers for vitamin E, vitamin B-12, thiamin, riboflavin, and vitamin C. One person took excess amounts of calcium (3 gm a day) and vitamin D (25,000 IU a day); another took a potentially toxic amount of iron (400 mg a day). Inappropriate reasons cited for taking supplements included preventing arthritis and infections by taking vitamin C, improving memory with niacin, and preventing constipation by taking vitamin E.

The older adult is a vulnerable target for the promised benefits of antioxidant supplements: the prevention of heart disease and cancer. The controversy generated by potential benefits versus harm of beta carotene and vitamins C and E supplementation has been considerable and is likely to continue. In a particularly succinct review, Herbert[29] explained that no supplement is a pure supplement. When present in the pharmacological (above-RDA) amounts found in some supplements, antioxidants tend to be redox agents, acting as antioxidants in some circumstances and as prooxidants in others. In high doses, antioxidants may actually produce harmful free radicals rather than protecting against free radicals. Pharmacological doses of antioxidant supplements can have harmful effects, including the promotion of cancer and heart, liver, and kidney disease.

Nutrient Toxicities

A panel of experts evaluating the potential danger of excessive ingestion of vitamins or minerals concluded that toxicities are unlikely to occur as a result of food intake except in those consuming the most unusual food pattern.[44] However, indiscriminate or inappropriate consumption of vitamin and mineral preparations predisposes the elderly to real hazards. Currently we do not know the maximum blood levels reached following ingestion of high potency supplements nor the period of time such levels are maintained. It is likely, however, that the kinetics of tissue disposal or excretion differ in older as compared to younger individuals based on the former group's reduced glomerular filtration rate and renal tubular secretion of metabolites. The fact that the aged adult is more susceptible to drug overdose and toxicity than a younger adult lends credence to such an argument.

ROLE OF THE NUTRITION PROFESSIONAL

Food and drug interactions are of increasing concern to nutrition professionals. A 1985 mandate by the Joint Commission on Accreditation of Healthcare Organizations recommends that a patient education plan for drug-nutrient interactions be implemented by dietetic services.[32] The responsibility of monitoring and providing information about potential food-drug interactions is shared by all health care professionals. However, the nutrition professional has the expertise to screen for medications with the potential for drug-nutrient interactions, to evaluate the elderly person's dietary pattern and nutritional status, and to counsel the patient accordingly.

A complete diet history is essential. In addition to the usual meal pattern, the nutrition professional needs to ask about any food idiosyncracies the person may have, any known allergies or food intolerances, and what food or nutrient supplements are currently being used. Armed with knowledge of the more common and more serious drug-nutrient interactions, the nutrition professional can ask more meaningful questions. All information should be communicated with other members of the health care team. If the older person is taking medications known to interact with nutrients or if nutritional status is likely to interfere with drug therapy, the pharmacist and physician should be consulted so that appropriate intervention can be planned.

The nutrition professional must also question the person about prescribed and OTC medications being taken currently, why they are used, what he or she knows about the drugs, and whether the patient is experiencing any drug-related problems. Ideally the person should be asked to bring in all drugs currently being taken, including OTC drugs, to compare with the record of medications known to have been prescribed. Always keep in mind that noncompliance with drug regimens and misuse of drugs may not be intentional. Lack of understanding of the importance of the drug and taking it as ordered, difficulties in scheduling times to take the drug compatible with the personal daily schedule, memory deficits, and physical limitations such as poor eyesight or inability to swallow often contribute to noncompliance.[2] It is not uncommon to see an older person omit dosages in an attempt to stretch the prescription or fail to have the prescription filled because of cost. Considerable skill is necessary to gain the trust and confidence of the person so that this very personal information will be divulged. Depending on the mental and physical status of the individual, it may be necessary to go to collateral sources, such as close family or friends, for information.

The older person needs to be educated about the possible side effects of drugs he or she is taking, including the effect diet may have on drug therapy. In counseling the older person, remember to keep instructions simple and to the point.[2] Provide relevant information in a logical sequence. Repeat information and ask the person to repeat what he or she has heard. Written instructions are helpful and should be in large print. Compliance aids such as medication reminders and calendars can add a feeling of security to an anxious patient.

The nutrition professional should be aware of his or her own limitations. New knowledge of drugs is constantly being presented. A patient is more likely to know the brand name than the generic name of a drug. The nutrition professional has the responsibility to identify any drug from its brand name and its generic name. This information is available from sources such as the *American Hospital Formulary, Physician's Desk Reference (PDR)*, and *U.S. Pharmacopeia Dispensing Information (USPDI)*. The clinical pharmacist is a tremendous resource for drug information. The nutrition professional must keep current on newly discovered uses, side effects, and interactions of drugs that are already on the market.

Summary

Using prescription and OTC drugs can be deleterious to nutritional status. The older adult population, with attendant multiple health problems and chronic conditions, is particularly vulnerable. They are the chief users of drugs in the United States. Alcohol use and abuse can produce harmful interactions with other drugs and compromise nutritional health. In addition, vitamin and mineral supplements can act as drugs and, if used in excess, are detrimental to nutritional and physical health. Supplements are often taken at higher-than-recommended levels, and, unfortunately, these supplements do not always supply the nutrients lacking in the diet.

❖❖❖
CASE STUDY

Mr. H, age 74, moved to another state to live with his daughter and sought a new physician. He told the doctor he had been taking a "water pill" for the past three years for his blood pressure. He brought in a bottle labeled "Hydrodiuril." In describing how he felt, he mentioned that he often felt fatigued and depressed, his heart seemed to race occasionally, and frequently he experienced muscle cramps. The doctor prescribed a potassium supplement. Because his lab results indicated elevations in total cholesterol and LDL cholesterol, the physician also prescribed Questran and instructed him to return in two months.

1. What are the generic names and actions of each of the drugs prescribed?
   a) Hydrodiuril
   b) Questran
2. Why was a potassium supplement prescribed?
3. What special instructions should Mr. H have been given regarding Questran?

Mr. H returned two months later. Recent lab reports indicated that he was experiencing some early signs of renal problems; his lipid profile had not improved. His blood pressure had increased from the first visit. In describing how he was feeling, Mr. H said he was feeling better, was less depressed, mentioned no more problems with leg cramps, and noted some annoyance with constipation. The physician changed his order from Hydrodiuril to Monopril and said that at his age, bowel irregularity was not unusual.

4. What is the drug classification of Monopril?
5. What is the likely reason for Mr. H's improvement in fatigue, depression, racing heart, and leg cramps?
6. What may be the cause of his constipation?

Within two weeks Mr. H was brought to the emergency room by his daughter. He had been experiencing muscle cramps, unusual fatigue, and general weakness for the past week. He was nervous and short of breath and now seemed very confused. The daughter brought along all the medications he was currently taking: Monopril, Questran, and a potassium supplement.

7. What do Mr. H's symptoms indicate?
8. What might be the likely cause?

Mr. H was admitted to the hospital. His admitting lab values were indicative of hyperkalemia. Monopril was continued; Questran and the potassium supplement were discontinued. An order for a consult with the dietitian was written.

9. What are some questions that the dietitian should ask?

Multiple drug intake can lead to drug-drug interactions and compromise nutritional status. The problem is exacerbated when the elderly person is consuming a marginal diet and/or when drugs are misused, whether intentionally or unintentionally. Drugs can interfere with nutrient intake, absorption, and metabolism, or they can enhance nutrient excretion. Conversely, food and dietary patterns can jeopardize drug activity and increase the hazards of drug therapy. Monitoring and providing counseling about potential food and drug interactions is a challenge for the nutrition professional.

REVIEW QUESTIONS

1. Why do older people take more prescription and over-the-counter drugs than do younger people? What factors contribute to multiple drug use in older people? What are the most common drugs used by the elderly living in the community and those living in long-term care facilities?
2. Why are older people more vulnerable to adverse drug reactions? What physiologic, sociologic, and psychologic factors influence drug use in the elderly?
3. Define pharmacokinetics and pharmacodynamics and discuss how each influences drug metabolism in the elderly. How do body fat, body water, plasma albumin concentration, and blood flow affect pharmacokinetics in the elderly?
4. What are the effects of drugs on nutritional status? How can nutritional status affect drug actions? What drugs can cause an increase in nutrient excretion? What effect does food have on drugs?
5. What are some of the most common drugs used to treat cardiovascular disease in the elderly and

what are the most common drug-nutrient interactions? Why are the number of psychotherapeutic drug prescriptions increasing? What nutritional effects do these types of drugs have in an elderly population?

SUGGESTED LEARNING ACTIVITIES

1. Prepare a list of common medications that affect nutritional status of the elderly by increasing appetite, decreasing appetite, impairing nutrient absorption, affecting nutrient metabolism, or affecting nutrient excretion. For each drug on the list provide an appropriate dietary recommendation.
2. Visit a drug store and record the sodium level of the following over-the-counter (OTC) medications: antacids, cough/cold remedies, and enema preparations. Prepare a one-page information sheet on sodium-containing OTC medications that can significantly contribute to sodium intake.
3. Interview two pharmacists and one health food store clerk about vitamin/mineral preparations targeted at older consumers. After this assignment, do you think these products are useful?
4. Go to the library and find three articles about nutrient-drug interactions with MAO inhibitor drugs. Prepare a comprehensive list of foods older people should avoid while taking these medications.

REFERENCES

1. Adams, W.L., and others: Alcohol-related hospitalizations in elderly people: Prevalence and geographic variation in the United States, J.A.M.A. 270(10):1222, 1993.
2. ASPEN Reference Group: Drugs. In: Lawrence, K.E., Roe, S.N., editors: Geriatric patient education resource manual, Rockville, MD, 1991, Aspen Publishers, Inc.
3. Avorn, J., and Gurwitz, J.W.: Drug use in the nursing home, Ann. Intern. Med. 123(3):195, 1995.
4. Barnea, Z., and Teichman, M.: Substance misuse and abuse among the elderly: implications for social work intervention, J. Gerontol. Soc. Work. 21(3/4):133, 1994.
5. Beers, M.H., and others: Characteristics and quality of prescribing by doctors practicing in nursing homes, J. Am. Geriatr. Soc. 41:802, 1993.
6. Beers, M.H., and others: Influence of hospitalization on drug therapy in the elderly, J. Am. Geriatr. Soc. 37:679, 1989.
7. Beers, M., and others: Psychoactive medication use in intermediate-care facility residents, J.A.M.A. 260:3016, 1988.
8. Begg, C.B., and Carbone, P.P.: Clinical trials and drug toxicity in the elderly: the experience of the Eastern Cooperative Oncology Group, Cancer 52:1986, 1983.
9. Bero, L.A., Lipton, H.L., and Bird, J.A.: Characterization of geriatric drug-related hospital readmissions. Med. Care 29(10):989, 1991.
10. Block, G., and others: Vitamin supplement use by demographic characteristics, Am. J. Epidemiol. 127(2):297, 1988.
11. Blumberg, J.B., and Suter, P.: Pharmacology, nutrition, and the elderly: interactions and implications. In: Chernoff, R., editor: Geriatric nutrition: the health professional's handbook, Gaithersburg, MD, 1991, Aspen Publishers, Inc.
12. Cadieux, R.J.: Drug interactions in the elderly, Postgrad. Med. 86(8):179, 1989.
13. Campion, E.W., deLabry, L.O., and Glynn, R.J.: The effect of age on serum albumin in healthy males: report from the Normative Aging Study, Geriatrics 43(1):M18, 1988.
14. Cooper, J.K.: Drug treatment of Alzheimer's disease, Arch. Intern. Med. 151:245, 1991.
15. Corey-Bloom, J., and Galasko, D.: Adjunctive therapy in patients with Alzheimer's disease, Drugs Aging 7(2):79, 1995.
16. Delafuente, J.C., and others: Drug use among functionally active, aged, ambulatory people, Drug Intell. Clin. Pharm. 26(2):179, 1992.
17. Drugs for psychiatric disorders, Med. Lett. 31:13, 1989.
18. Dufour, M., and Fuller, R.K.: Alcohol in the elderly, Annu. Rev. Med. 46:123–132, 1995.
19. Ebersole, P., and Hess, P.: Drug use and abuse. In: Toward healthy aging: human needs and nursing response, ed. 3, St. Louis, 1990, CV Mosby Co.
20. The Expert Panel: Summary of the Second Report of the National Cholesterol Education Program, J.A.M.A. 269(23):3015, 1993.
21. Food and Drug Administration: Guideline for the study of drugs likely to be used in the elderly, Rockville, MD, 1989, Food and Drug Administration Center for Drug Evaluation Research.
22. Food and Nutrition Board: Recommended dietary allowances, ed. 10, Washington, DC, 1989, National Academy of Sciences.
23. Gerbino, P.P., and Gans, J.A.: Antacids and laxatives for symptomatic relief in the elderly, J. Am. Geriatr. Soc. 30:S81, 1982.
24. Goldberg, P.B., and Roberts, J.: Pharmacologic basis for developing rational drug regimens for

elderly patients, Med. Clin. N. Amer. 67(2):315, 1983.

25. Gosney, M., and Tallis, R.: Prescription of contraindicated and interacting drugs in elderly patients admitted to hospital, Lancet 1:564, 1984.

26. Gray, G.E., and others: Vitamin supplement use in a southern California retirement community, J. Am. Diet. Assoc. 86(6):800, 1986.

27. Gurwitz, J.H., and Avorn, J.: The ambiguous relation between aging and adverse drug reactions, Ann. Intern. Med. 114(11):956, 1991.

28. Helling, D.K., and others: Medication use characteristics in the elderly: The Iowa 65+ rural health study, J. Am. Geriatr. Soc. 35(1):4, 1987.

29. Herbert, V.: The antioxidant supplement myth, Am. J. Clin. Nutr. 60:157, 1994.

30. Iber, F.L., and others: Thiamin in the elderly, relation to alcoholism and to neurological degenerative disease, Am. J. Clin. Nutr. 36(5):1067, 1982.

31. Iliffe, S., and others: Alcohol consumption by elderly people: a general practice survey, Age Ageing 20:120, 1991.

32. Joint Commission on Accreditation of Hospitals: Accreditation manual for hospitals, 1985, Chicago, 1984, The Commission.

33. Kee, J.L., and Hayes, E.R.: Pharmacology: a nursing process approach, Philadelphia, 1993, W.B. Saunders Co.

34. Lamy, P.P.: Nonprescription drugs and the elderly, Am. Fam. Phy. 39(6):175, 1989.

35. Lamy, P.P.: Nonprescription drugs and the elderly. In: Feldman, E.G., and Blockstein, W.L., editors: Handbook of nonprescription drugs, ed. 9, Washington, DC, 1990, American Pharmaceutical Association.

36. Leevy, C.M.: Thiamin deficiency and alcoholism, Ann. N.Y. Acad. Sci. 378:316, 1982.

37. LeSage, J.: Polypharmacy in geriatric patients, Nurs. Clin. N. Amer. 26(2):273, 1991.

38. Levine, M.A.: Rational and pharmacologically sound drug therapy for the elderly patient, Geisinger Bull. 37(2):34, 1988.

39. Lile, J.L., and Hoffman, R.: Medication-taking by the frail elderly in two ethnic groups, Nurs. Forum 26(4):19, 1991.

40. Lindley, C.M., and others: Inappropriate medication is a major cause of adverse drug reactions in elderly patients, Age Ageing 21:294, 1994.

41. Miller, M.J.: Drug use and misuse among the elderly. In: Young, R.F., and Olson, E.A., editors: Health, illness, and disability later in life: practical issues and interventions, Newbury Park, CA, 1991, Sage Publications.

42. Montamat, S.C., and Cusack, B.: Overcoming problems with polypharmacy and drug misuse in the elderly, Clin. Geriatr. Med. 8(1):142, 1992.

43. Montamat, S.C., Cusack, B.J., and Vestal, R.E.: Management of drug therapy in the elderly, New Engl. J. Med. 321:303, 1989.

44. National Nutrition Consortium: Vitamin-mineral safety, toxicity, and misuse, Chicago, 1978, American Dietetic Association.

45. Nichols, T.W.: Phytobezoar formation: a new complication of cimetidine therapy, Ann. Intern. Med. 95(1):70, 1981.

46. Oakland, M.J., and Thomsen, P.A.: Beliefs about and usage of vitamin/mineral supplements by elderly participants of rural congregate meal programs in central Iowa, J. Am. Diet. Assoc. 90(5):715, 1990.

47. Opdycke, R.A.C., and others: A systematic approach to educating elderly patients about their medications, Patient Educa. Couns. 19(1):43, 1992.

48. Parker, B.M., Cusack, B.J., and Vestal, R.E.: Pharmacokinetic optimisation of drug therapy in elderly patients, Drugs Aging 7(1):10, 1995.

49. Patrick, M., and others: Prescription for the high cost of drugs in nursing homes, Geriatr. Nurs. 12(2):88, 1991.

50. Pinto, J.T.: The pharmacokinetic and pharmacodynamic interactions of food and drugs, Topics Clin. Nutr. 6:14, 1991.

51. Piraino, A.J.: Managing medication in the elderly, Hosp. Prac. 30(6):59, 1995.

52. Ranno, B.S., Wardlaw, G.M., and Geiger, C.J.: What characterizes elderly women who overuse vitamin and mineral supplements? J. Am. Diet. Assoc. 88(3):347, 1988.

53. Roe, D.A.: Drug and nutrient interactions in elderly cardiac patients, Drug-Nutrient Interactions 5(4):205, 1988.

54. Roe, D.A.: Diet and drug interactions, New York, 1989, Van Nostrand Reinhold.

55. Roe, D.A.: Drug-nutrient interactions in the elderly. In: Munro, H.N., and Danford, D.E., editors: Nutrition, aging, and the elderly, New York, 1989, Plenum Press.

56. Roe, D.A.: Handbook on drug and nutrient interactions: a problem-oriented reference guide, ed. 4, Chicago, 1989, American Dietetic Association.

57. Samet, J., and others: Choice of cancer therapy varies with age of patient, J.A.M.A. 255(24):3385, 1986.

58. Semla, T.P., and others: Perceived purpose of prescription drugs: the Iowa 65+ rural health study, Drug. Intell. Clin. Pharm. 25(4):410, 1991.

59. Shannon, M.T., and Wilson, B.A.: Drugs and nursing implications, ed. 7, Norwalk, CT, 1992, Appleton-Century Crofts.

60. Stewart, R.B., and Cooper, J.W.: Polypharmacy in the aged, Drugs Aging 4(6):449, 1994.

61. Stewart, R.B., and others: Changing patterns of therapeutic agents in the elderly: a ten-year overview, Age Ageing 20:182, 1991.

62. Stuart, B., and Grana, J.: Are prescribed and over-the-counter medicines economic substitutes? Med. Care 33(5):487, 1995.

63. Subar, A.F., and Block, G.: Use of vitamin and mineral supplements: demographics and amounts of nutrients consumed. The 1987 Health Interview Survey, Am. J. Epidem. 132:1091, 1990.

64. Sulsky, S.I., and others: Descriptors of alcohol consumption among noninstitutionalized nonalcoholic elderly, J. Am. Coll. Nutr. 9(4):326, 1990.

65. Thomas, J.A.: Drug-nutrient interactions, Nutr. Rev. 53(10):271, 1995.

66. Thornburg, J.E.: Gerontological pharmacology. In: Wingard, L.B. Jr., and others, editors: Human pharmacology molecular-to-clinical, St. Louis, 1991, Mosby-Year Book.

67. Tobias, C.R., and others: Alcoholism in the elderly: how to spot and treat a problem the patient wants to hide, Postgrad. Med. 86:67, 1989.

68. Tomasulo, P.A., and others: Impairment of thiamin absorption in alcoholism, Am. J. Clin. Nutr. 21(11):1341, 1968.

69. Tregaskis, B.F., and Stevenson, I.H.: Pharmacokinetics in old age, Brit. Med. Bull. 46(1):2, 1990.

70. Whelan, G.: Alcohol-related health problems in the elderly, Med. J. Australia 162(6):325, 1995.

71. Widner, S., and Zeichner, A.: Alcohol abuse in the elderly: review of epidemiology research and treatment, Clin. Gerontologist 11(1):3, 1991.

72. Wilber, J.A.: The role of diet in the treatment of high blood pressure. J. Am. Diet. Assoc. 80:25, 1982.

73. Williams, L.: Mixing food and drugs, Dietetic Currents 22(3):15, 1995.

74. Williams, B.R., and Baer, C.L.: Essentials of clinical pharmacology in nursing, Springhouse, PA, 1990, Springhouse.

75. Williams, L., Davis, J.A., and Lowenthal, D.T.: The influence of food and the absorption and metabolism of drugs, Med. Clin. N. Amer. 77(4):815, 1993.

76. Williams, L., and Lowenthal, D.T.: Drug therapy in the elderly, S. Med. J. 85:127, 1992.

77. Woodhouse, K.W., and James, O.F.W.: Hepatic drug metabolism and ageing, Brit. Med. Bull. 46(1):22, 1990.

78. Young, R.C., and Blass, J.P.: Iatrogenic nutritional deficiencies, Annu. Rev. Nutr. 2:201, 1982.

11

Nutritional Assessment of Older Adults

Marie Fanelli Kuczmarski and Robert J. Kuczmarski

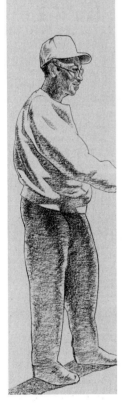

+++

Objectives

After studying the chapter, the student should be able to:

✔ *Understand the particular strengths and weaknesses of the various methods of nutritional assessment as applied to the evaluation of older people*

✔ *Recognize the problems inherent in using common nutrition assessment methods with the elderly*

✔ *Identify the biochemical methods used to evaluate protein, iron, and folate status of older people*

✔ *Understand the techniques of anthropometric assessment applicable to community settings and their value in evaluating nutritional adequacy in elderly people*

✔ *List the clinical signs of poor nutritional status often found in older people and the related nutritional or nonnutritional causes*

✔ *List the advantages and disadvantages of particular dietary assessment and screening methods with older clients*

INTRODUCTION

Nutritional status is defined as the health condition of a population or an individual as influenced by the ingestion and utilization of nutrients and nonnutrients.[2,21,41,79] Measures of nutritional status reflect the processes of dietary intake and digestion, absorption, transport, metabolism and storage, and the excretion of food components and their metabolic products. Health professionals recognize that many older adults in the United States are at risk of nutritional deficits, excesses, and imbalances in relation to metabolic and tissue needs, or, in other words, malnutrition.[21] Inadequate quantity and/or quality of food intake, poverty, social isolation, chronic diseases or conditions, physical disability, chronic prescription drug use, and advanced age (80+ years) are associated with increased risk of poor nutritional status.

Nutritional indicators used to assess an individual's status are quantitative and have been classified historically as anthropometric, biochemical, clinical, and dietary. The various applications of each of these four components are identified in table 11-1.[68] Examples of indicators within each component are listed in the box. Information concerning economic and sociodemographic status, cultural food practices and habits, and food beliefs also should be collected because these factors are known to affect nutritional status.

Nutritional status can range from optimal to malnutrition (fig. 11-1). **Marginal nutritional status** is a condition in which performance,

TABLE 11-1   *Nutritional Assessment Methods and Their Purpose*

Method	Purpose
Anthropometric	• Determine and monitor body weight to detect changes in weight
	• Determine and monitor body composition, especially body fat and water
	• Determine body fat distribution to assess risk for selected chronic conditions
Biochemical	• Determine and monitor nutritional risk for selected chronic conditions such as heart disease
	• Determine and monitor the level of recent dietary intakes of selected nutrients
	• Determine and monitor nutrient stores
	• Obtain functional measures of nutritional adequacy or deficiency
	• Confirm or refute nutritional diagnoses based on other assessment measures
	• Determine immune function
Clinical	• Determine presence of diagnostic signs or symptoms of nutritional deficiency or toxicity
	• Determine and monitor ability to perform ADLs
	• Evaluate and monitor dental health
	• Evaluate cognitive status
	• Determine whether signs or symptoms indicative of nutritional problems are reversed by nutritional intervention
Dietary	• Obtain actual food and beverage intakes to determine quality of diet
	• Monitor food consumption patterns of individuals or groups to identify changes and trends over time
	• Determine usage of supplements and their effect on nutrient intake
	• Evaluate feeding practices of institutionalized older adults

❖

COMPONENTS OF NUTRITIONAL ASSESSMENT FOR OLDER ADULTS

- *Anthropometric*
  Weight
  Stature/Knee Height/Total Arm
    Length/Arm Span
  Circumferences
  Skinfolds
  Bioelectrical Impedance
- *Biochemical*
  Cholesterol Levels
  Folate Status
  Iron Status
  Protein Status
- *Clinical*
  Signs and Symptoms
  Functional Status
  Cognitive Status
  Oral Health
  Use of Drugs
- *Dietary*
  Food and Beverage Intake
  Food Preferences
  Food Security/Insecurity
  Use of Supplements

health, or longevity may not be impaired even though nutrient stores are low. Individuals with marginal nutritional status are at risk for nutritional deficiency, particularly if subjected to physical, social, or emotional stressors that may further increase requirements or deplete body stores of nutrients or energy. **Overnutrition,** a form of malnutrition, results from an excess of available nutrients in relation to tissue needs. Obesity, an excess of body fat, is an example of energy overnutrition from fat, carbohydrate, protein, or alcohol sources. Another form of malnutrition is **undernutrition,** which results from a deficit of available nutrients with respect to tissue needs. An example of undernutrition that is prevalent among institutionalized elderly people is protein-energy malnutrition. **Nutritional imbalance** is a condition arising from insufficient or excessive intakes of one nutrient or nonnutrient (such as dietary fiber) relative to another; it may be associated with adverse health consequences, especially in older adults.

As shown in figure 11-1, a change in dietary intake initiates a sequence of events which may alter an individual's nutritional status. Biochemical indicators are the first parameters to reflect a change in dietary status, followed by anthropometric and clinical indicators.

Measures of nutritional status are used in applied settings (1) at the individual level in patient diagnosis, screening, intervention, and monitoring, and (2) at the population level for setting policy, in program evaluation, and in nutritional surveillance. Nutritional status indicators are used by a diverse group of professionals, including researchers, clinical practitioners, program managers, and policy makers. Consequently, those professionals should recognize that no single indicator for a given nutrient will meet the needs of all users. Selecting the best indicator depends on the purpose of the nutritional evaluation.

When a nutritional evaluation is initiated by an older adult's physician, it is with the consent of that individual. Informed consent must be obtained from an older adult when the evaluation is part of a research, intervention, or planning program which could be initiated by a university or college, government agency, or nonprofit community agency. Older adults should be informed as to who is conducting the evaluation, what the objective of the study is, how the data will be used, how confidentiality of information will be protected, and exactly what is expected of the participant.

NUTRITIONAL ASSESSMENT

Nutritional assessment is the integration and interpretation of anthropometric, biochemical, clinical, and dietary data to determine the nutritional and health status of individuals and population groups. A nutritional assessment can take one of three forms: surveys, surveillance, or screening. With **nutrition surveys,** data are collected within specified population groups either cross-sectionally or sequentially over specified

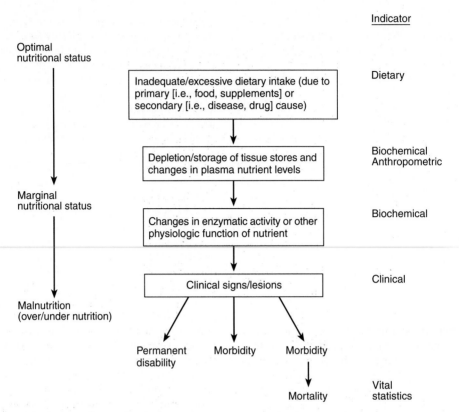

FIG. 11-1   Development of Malnutrition. When dietary intake is inadequate or excessive, the first changes are in the levels of nutrient stores in the tissues and plasma nutrient levels. Changes in enzyme activity and physiologic function follow. Clinical signs or lesions are the last to appear.

time periods. These data are used to establish baseline information and identify subgroups at risk for malnutrition for the purpose of ascertaining the nutritional status of the population examined. **Nutritional surveillance** is the continuous monitoring of nutritional status indicators for the purpose of detecting changes that indicate a need to initiate or evaluate intervention measures. Nutrition screening programs are more targeted and generally less comprehensive than surveys or surveillance systems. **Nutrition screening** is the process of determining characteristics or risk factors known to be associated with dietary or nutritional problems and then identifying individuals who

either have the condition or are potentially at high risk for the condition. Surveys and surveillance represent nutritional assessment approaches that are used at the community level for population groups, whereas screening applies to individuals in clinical settings and to more narrowly defined population subgroups.

Our knowledge of the complex relationships between nutrition and aging is still evolving. The assessment of older adults presents special challenges to health professionals because evidence which may be indicative of a nutritional problem in a young adult can also result from nonnutritional causes in the older adult. Interpretation of nutritional status data is sometimes difficult because selected reference values for older adults have not been established. Some of the physiologic changes that occur with age are indistinguishable from clinical signs of nutrient deficiencies. Finally, the frequent use of prescription drugs by older people can affect the interpretation of biochemical assays and may influence clinical signs and symptoms. This chapter provides an overview of the commonly used methods of nutritional assessment, information on resources for appropriate reference values, and descriptions of available screening tools for use with older adults.

ANTHROPOMETRIC ASSESSMENT

Anthropometry is the art and science of measuring the human body. It can be done in several ways (see chapter 5). Anthropometric measurements that are used frequently in clinical settings and nutrition surveys include weight, height, skinfolds, and circumferences. They are used to estimate or predict amounts of the various components of the body, such as fat or muscle mass, which can be more definitively evaluated in a research body composition laboratory. Anthropometric measurements are particularly useful in detecting moderate and severe degrees of malnutrition, notably imbalances of protein and energy. Detailed descriptions of the procedures for anthropometric methods have been published in the *Anthropometric Standardization Reference Manual*.[43] A video demonstrating the anthropometric measurements performed in the Third National Health and Nutrition Examination Survey (NHANES III) is also available.[78]

Body Weight

The most accurate body weight on ambulatory adults is obtained with a calibrated scale. However, as people age and enter the decades of the 80s and 90s, they often become bed-bound or chair-bound. For nonambulatory people, a calibrated wheelchair or bed beam-type scale should be used. In a clinical setting, the individual should be weighed wearing either a hospital gown or minimal underclothing. In community settings, people should be dressed in minimal

light indoor clothing. Heavy sweaters, jackets, handbags, pocket contents, and shoes should be removed before the person is weighed. The individual who records body weight should not only document the date of the measurement, but also the type of clothing worn and the hydration status of the older adult. Edema or severe dehydration can distort actual body weight measurements and lead to misinterpretation of relative weight for height values and weight changes.

Body Height

In comparison to body weight measurements, height or stature measurements can be more complicated. The stature of those older adults capable of standing upright can be measured with a stadiometer or against a calibrated nonstretchable tape attached to a vertical surface. Ideally, the person's heels, buttocks, shoulders, and head should be touching the stadiometer, and his or her eyes should be looking straight ahead so that the line of vision is perpendicular to the body in the Frankfort plane. Ideally, the person should also be barefoot: however, height can be measured in stocking feet. For some older adults with large amounts of adipose tissue, not all four body parts previously mentioned will come in contact with the stadiometer.

It is impossible to obtain an accurate height measurement with a stadiometer in older adults with kyphosis (dowager's hump) or scoliosis (curvature) of the spine or in nonambulatory older adults. Recumbent length, the distance from the crown of the head to the heel, can serve as a proxy measure of height, provided head and foot boards are available. Because the length of the long bones does not change with aging, when a standing height cannot be measured alternate methods, such as arm span,[40] total arm length (TAL),[49,51] or knee height,[12,16] can be used to predict stature. Arm span is double the distance from the person's sternal notch to the fingertips of one arm. Total arm length, the distance from the tip of the right acromial process of the scapula to the end of the styloid process of the ulna with the elbow bent at a 45 degree angle, is measured with a flexible steel tape. Knee height is the distance from the sole

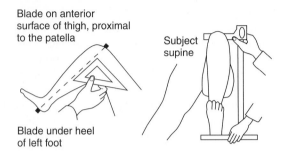

Blade on anterior
surface of thigh, proximal
to the patella

Subject
supine

Blade under heel
of left foot

FIG. 11-2   Measurement of Knee Height.

From PRINCIPLES OF NUTRITIONAL ASSESSMENT by Rosalind S. Gibson. Copyright © 1990 by Rosalind S. Gibson. Used by permission of Oxford University Press, Inc.

of the foot at the heel to the anterior surface of the thigh with the ankle and knee each flexed to a 90 degree angle. None of these alternative methods to estimate stature is flawless. Bowed legs, present in cases of progressive bone loss, can affect the accuracy of knee heights, while kyphosis can influence arm span measurements.

Knee height is highly recommended because it is an easier measure for health professionals and it has a lower interobserver error when compared to the arm measurements. Knee height can be measured with a broad blade caliper with the person either in a sitting or in a recumbent position. The shaft of the caliper should be parallel to the shaft of the tibia and pass over the anklebone just behind the head of the fibula. One of the blades of the caliper is positioned under the heel of the foot and the other over the anterior surface of the thigh above the condyles of the femur just proximal to the patella (fig. 11-2). Stature can be estimated from knee height using the following formulas:[12]

White Men's Stature = 59.01 +
    (2.08 × knee height [cm])
Black Men's Stature = 95.79 +
    (1.37 × knee height [cm])
White Women's Stature = 75.00 +
    (1.91 × knee height [cm]) –
    (0.17 × age [yrs])
Black Women's Stature = 58.72 +
    (1.96 × knee height [cm])

These equations were derived from data obtained from a nationally representative sample

of ambulatory adults (438 white men, 453 white women, 50 black men, 60 black women), 60 to 80 years old.[12] The equations for white adults were cross-validated using two independent samples of elderly white men and women. Thus, these equations will probably yield acceptable results with other groups of white older people. However, the sample of black older adults was limited, so use caution in interpreting results when applying these equations to elderly black populations.

Relative Weight for Height

Relative weight for height, the ratio of an individual's present weight to a reference weight based on the individual's height and gender, is a parameter used to assess anthropometric data. The most widely used weight references are the Metropolitan Life Insurance Company height and weight tables,[48] the table of average weight for height published by Master, Lasser, and Beckman,[46] and tables of weight for height derived from data collected in the NHANES.[22]

All of these references have limitations. The Metropolitan weight-for-height tables do not include values for people above age 59. The table by Master and associates is based on a sample of about 5,600 ambulatory, disease-free, noninstitutionalized white people in the United States and provides reference weights for adults 65 to 94 years of age. Although regarded by many as the best data currently available for the older adult population, these measurements were recorded 30 years ago with many observers and pieces of equipment that were not uniformly standardized. The NHANES I and II data were collected by trained technicians following standardized protocols from a representative national sample, but were restricted to people ages 74 and younger.

Table 11-2 is a reference table based on data from the NHANES I Epidemiologic Follow-up Survey that includes the 15th, 50th, and 85th percentiles of body weight for each inch of height for men and women ages 55 to 84 years.[17] This study population consisted of 562 black adults (272 men and 290 women) and 2,777 white adults (1,314 men and 1,463 women). These reference data provide three useful categories for distinguishing underweight, average weight, and overweight: below

TABLE 11-2 *Percentiles of Body Weight for Each Inch of Height, by Age and Sex: USA 1982–1984*

	Age														
	60–64 yr			65–69 yr			70–74 yr			75–79 yr			80–84 yr		
Percentile:	15th	50th	85th	15th	50th	85th	15th	50th	85th	15th	50th	85th	15th	50th	85th
Height (in.)															
Women															
58	103	130	166	103	128	164	101	126	160	100	122	154	98	118	148
59	107	133	169	106	132	167	105	129	163	104	126	158	102	121	151
60	111	137	172	110	135	170	109	133	166	107	130	161	105	125	154
61	115	140	176	114	139	173	113	137	169	111	133	164	109	129	157
62	118	144	179	118	142	176	117	140	173	115	137	167	113	132	161
63	122	147	182	121	146	180	120	144	176	119	140	170	117	136	164
64	126	151	185	125	149	183	124	147	179	122	144	174	120	139	167
65	130	154	188	129	153	186	128	151	182	126	147	177	124	143	170
66	133	158	192	133	157	189	132	154	185	130	151	180	128	146	173
67	137	161	195	136	160	192	135	158	188	134	154	183	132	150	176
68	141	165	198	140	164	196	139	161	192	137	158	186	135	153	180
69	145	168	201	144	167	199	143	165	195	141	161	190	139	157	183
70	148	172	204	148	171	202	147	168	198	145	165	193	143	160	186
Men															
60	128	142	161	123	140	158	120	138	154	118	135	149	116	131	143
61	131	146	166	126	144	163	123	142	159	121	139	154	119	135	147
62	134	150	170	129	148	168	126	146	164	124	143	158	122	139	152
63	137	154	175	132	152	172	129	150	168	127	147	163	125	142	157
64	140	158	180	136	156	177	132	154	173	130	151	168	128	146	161
65	143	162	184	139	160	182	135	158	178	133	155	173	131	150	166
66	146	166	189	142	164	186	138	162	183	136	159	177	134	154	171
67	149	170	194	145	168	191	141	166	187	139	163	182	137	158	176
68	152	174	198	148	172	196	144	170	192	142	166	187	140	162	180
69	155	178	203	151	176	201	147	174	197	145	170	191	143	166	185
70	158	182	208	154	180	205	150	178	201	148	174	196	146	170	190
71	161	186	213	157	184	210	153	182	206	151	178	201	150	174	194
72	164	190	217	160	188	215	156	186	211	154	182	206	153	178	199

Modified from Cornoni-Huntley, J.C., and others: An overview of body weight of older persons, including impact on mortality, J. Clin. Epidemiol. 44:743, 1991.

NOTE: based on weighted linear regression models using common slope with intercepts for each age group fitted by quadratic model; separate models for men and women.

the 15th percentile (underweight or lean); in the 15th to 84th percentile (average); above the 85th percentile (overweight or obese). Recognizing the need for more extensive weight and height data for older adults, the NHANES III measured approximately 5,300 people ages 60 years and older, and representative of the noninstitutionalized elderly population in the United States.[40] When available these data may provide the best reference values for older adults.

Changes in Body Weight

A person's usual weight and history of recent weight changes are important.[64] A study of elderly nursing home residents identified the indicators most often associated with unintentional weight loss of more than 10% of actual weight in six months. The six indicators present most often were, in descending order: reduced functional ability, intake of 50% or less of food served in the past three consecutive days, chewing problems, serum albumin below 35 g/l with normal hydration status, total cholesterol level below 160 mg/dl (4.1 mmol/l), and refusal of 50% or more of food replacement over the past seven days.[25]

Generally, the shorter the period for a given weight loss, the more likely nutritional health is compromised (see chapter 12). A significant weight change would be a loss of 1% to 2% of body weight in a week, 5% in a month, 7.5% in three months, or 10% in six months.[6,35] Weight losses greater than these percentages indicate severe malnutrition.[6] Before defining the severity of malnutrition, accuracy of the weight history and interpretation of the weight measurements with respect to the hydration status of the individual at the time of the measurements must be carefully considered.

Body Mass Index (BMI)

If weight and stature measurements are valid, body mass index (BMI) can be computed or determined from a nomogram (see fig. 11-3). The BMI has been shown to have a reasonable correlation with body fat in young adults. However, because of the progressive decrease in lean body mass and increase in body fat, along with a decrease in height, the BMI may result in miscalculated estimates of body fat in older adults. In white and black older adult populations, BMI has been shown to be inversely correlated with high density lipoprotein (HDL) cholesterol and positively correlated with hypertension.[73] Both high and low BMI have also been shown to be significantly related to the functional status of community dwelling older adults.[23]

The Nutrition Screening Initiative (NSI) is currently recommending intervention for older

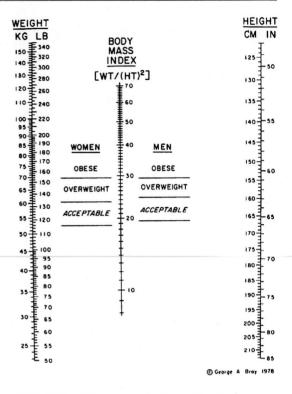

FIG. 11-3   Nomogram for Body Mass Index.

Copyright 1978 George A. Bray; courtesy Intern J Obesity.

adults with a BMI of less than 24 or greater than 27.[58] Individuals with a BMI of less than 24 may be at risk for poor nutritional status. Individuals with a BMI of more than 27 are obese and consequently are at risk for several conditions, including hypertension, diabetes, and osteoarthritis.

Guidelines issued by the U.S. government, which were based on analysis of mortality data, recommend that BMIs be in the range of 19 to 25 for the general adult population.[75,77] Contrary to previous guidelines, an increase in BMI with increasing age is no longer indicated.

Just as height measurement is adjusted for people with kyphosis, weight references also must be adjusted for people who have lost a body part as the result of surgery or trauma. For adjusting body weight according to the type of amputation, figures of segmental body weights are available.[56,60]

TABLE 11-3   *Mid-Upper Arm Circumference for Older Men and Women by Race*

	Percentile			Percentile		
	5th (cm)	50th (cm)	95th (cm)	5th (cm)	50th (cm)	95th (cm)
	Non-Hispanic white men			Non-Hispanic white women		
60–69 years	27.2	33.0	37.8	24.3	31.0	40.2
70–79 years	26.5	31.3	37.1	24.1	30.0	38.6
80+ years	23.5	29.5	35.1	21.5	28.3	35.5
	Non-Hispanic black men			Non-Hispanic black women		
60–69 years	25.9	32.9	39.9	25.4	33.6	42.9
70–79 years	25.7	31.6	38.5	25.0	32.2	42.8
80+ years	23.2*	30.0	36.7*	20.5*	29.1	36.1*
	Mexican American men			Mexican American women		
60–69 years	27.4	31.9	37.2	26.2	32.3	43.4
70–79 years	24.8*	30.5	35.2*	23.2*	29.8	40.7*
80+ years	23.2*	28.2	31.7*	21.2*	27.2	33.9*

*Represents a value which should be used with caution due to small sample size.
Source: Third National Health and Nutrition Examination Survey, 1988–1991.

Circumference Measurements

Circumference measurements are emerging as increasingly important data to collect on elderly people for several reasons. First, a shift in fat patterning from peripheral to central locations occurs with increasing age; in other words, fat shifts from the extremities to the trunk, notably in women, and from subcutaneous to deep adipose tissue in both men and women. The abdominal fat accumulation seems to be greater in men than in women, as shown by larger waist circumferences in men, and increases progressively with age. Fat patterning is an important determinant of HDL cholesterol, serum triglycerides, and the ratio of HDL to total cholesterol.[61,73]

The second reason to measure circumferences in older adults is the association between fat distribution and health outcomes.[38] Prospective studies have shown that the risk of disease increases steeply when the waist-to-hip ratio rises above 1.0 for men and 0.8 for women.[5]

Thirdly, circumference measurements require minimal expertise and very unsophisticated equipment—a calibrated, nonstretchable tape. The greatest problem is inconsistency among measurers on where the circumference tape is placed when taking the measurement.[15]

The mid-upper arm circumference is a measure of both the subcutaneous fat and muscle of the arm. Therefore, a change in this circumference reflects either a gain or loss in body muscle mass, a gain or loss in body fat, or both. Changes in mid-upper arm circumference measurements in adults can be used to monitor progress of nutritional interventions.

The circumference of the upper arm is measured at its midpoint, the distance halfway between the acromion and olecranon processes. The arm is bent at a 90-degree angle with the palm of the hand facing upward. Percentiles for mid-upper arm circumference measurements are available for people ages 60 years and older who were examined in the first phase of NHANES III (table 11-3). The 50th percentile represents the average value of a measurement, and the 5th and 95th percentiles are generally used as the lower and upper limits, respectively,

TABLE 11-4 *Triceps Skinfold for Older Men and Women by Race*

	Percentile			Percentile		
	5th (mm)	50th (mm)	95th (mm)	5th (mm)	50th (mm)	95th (mm)
	Non-Hispanic white men			Non-Hispanic white women		
60–69 years	7.5	13.1	26.0	12.5	24.3	37.9
70–79 years	6.4	12.4	24.4	11.1	21.8	35.4
80+ years	5.4	11.3	22.2	7.6	18.2	31.7
	Non-Hispanic black men			Non-Hispanic black women		
60–69 years	4.9	10.8	29.4	11.4	26.5	38.6
70–79 years	4.8	10.7	26.5	10.6*	24.1	38.4*
80+ years	5.4*	10.7	24.1*	7.1*	16.2	29.4*
	Mexican American men			Mexican American women		
60–69 years	6.6	11.4	22.1	14.2	24.6	35.6
70–79 years	5.5*	10.3	18.1*	10.9*	19.2	35.9*
80+ years	6.4*	10.3	17.4*	8.0*	14.4	26.8*

*Represents a value which should be used with caution due to small sample size.
Source: Third National Health and Nutrition Examination Survey, 1988–1991.

of acceptable values for a measurement. People with values at the extremes—less than the 5th or greater than the 95th percentiles—are more likely to have a nutritional disorder or disease than are people with values closer to the 50th percentile. Serial measurements can help to detect abnormal changes and to monitor the effectiveness of nutritional intervention.

Skinfold Assessments

Skinfold measurements have a number of inherent limitations when used in any age group. When coupled with the physical changes experienced by older people (including the apparent redistribution of fat, the decreased elasticity of the skin, marked alterations in skin thickness, and atrophy of subcutaneous adipocytes contributing to increased tissue compression), the caliper measurements may have a limited potential to reliably assess subcutaneous fat and accurately predict total body fat using regression equations. As mentioned in chapter 5, the body density equations typically used to predict total body fat may not apply to older people because of the noted changes in body composition.

The triceps skinfold thickness is measured on the back of the mid-upper arm over the triceps muscle. A calibrated skinfold caliper such as the Lange, Harpenden, or Holtain should be used for the measurement. The triceps skinfold represents a double fold of subcutaneous fat thickness. Table 11-4 presents the 5th, 50th and 95th percentile values obtained from the first phase of NHANES III. Individuals with a triceps skinfold measurement above the 95th percentile are generally considered obese, whereas those below the 5th percentile are considered underweight. In addition, the triceps skinfold measurement, along with the mid-upper arm circumference measurement, can be used to estimate body muscle mass. The formula for muscle area is:

[Mid-arm circumference –
(3.14 × Triceps skinfold)]^2 divided by 12.56[31]

Bioelectrical Impedance

Bioelectrical impedance analysis (BIA) has great appeal as an approach to measuring body composition because it is quick (less than two minutes), simple, relatively inexpensive, safe, and highly reproducible. There are no physical demands placed on the subjects, making it possibly an ideal method for measuring body composition in older adults.[13,14] With a single frequency BIA, an undetectable electrical current (50KHz, 800uA) is passed through the body by means of four electrodes placed on the hand and foot. The body's resistance to this current is measured and used to calculate total body water. Fat-free mass and percent of body fat may then be calculated.

The assessment of fat-free mass from BIA in older adults seems to be reliable, provided age-specific prediction formulas are used.[14,19] Regression equations for quantifying fat-free mass and fat mass of older adults have been published in the literature.[19,74] Use of equations based on measurements in younger populations can overestimate fat-free mass by approximately 6 kg[19] and at the same time underestimate fat mass and therefore are not applicable to elderly populations. Researchers have investigated an alternative impedance method for older adults based on the estimation of whole body composition from impedance measurements of body segments.[14] Further research is needed in developing and cross-validating prediction equations from impedance in older adults as compared to estimates obtained from multicompartmental models (see chapter 5).

A limitation of the BIA is the assumption that subjects are normally hydrated. Errors in estimation of fat mass can result from the variability in hydration levels. Serial BIA measures of body water in older adults would seem to be beneficial to assess risk for dehydration.

The risk for diabetes and osteoporosis increases with advancing age, thus increasing the risk for limb amputations and hip fractures. BIA may not be a valid measure of body composition in amputees or in people with metal pins in prosthetic hip replacements.

BIOCHEMICAL ASSESSMENT

Biochemical methods are more sensitive than anthropometric and clinical methods and reflect alterations in nutritional status before other methods can detect these changes (see fig. 11-1). When a nutrient deficiency occurs, tissue stores are gradually depleted. This depletion results in reductions in the levels of nutrients in reserve stores and body fluids, in the levels of metabolic products, and in the activity of nutrient-dependent enzymes.

Blood samples for biochemical analysis can be obtained by either fingerprick or venipuncture, depending upon the biochemical test selected. The number of assays available from a fingerprick sample are limited. In addition, this technique is subject to problems with hemodilution, hemoconcentration, and environmental contamination. A sufficient volume of blood can almost always be obtained with a venipuncture so analysis is not compromised. However, this procedure can be difficult in obese individuals whose veins in the upper arm are inaccessible or in elderly people in whom accessible veins may collapse. It is also necessary to recruit a qualified professional such as a phlebotomist to perform venipuncture.

Plasma and serum transport recently absorbed nutrients to the tissues and therefore provide an index of current dietary intake. Conversely, tissue stores reflect long-term nutrient status. The effect of recent dietary intake on plasma or serum nutrient levels can be reduced by collecting fasting blood samples.

Among older adults, protein-energy malnutrition, hyperlipidemia, and iron and folate deficiency anemias are common nutritional problems. The following section focuses on the biochemical indicators used to diagnose these problems. Selected criteria for biochemical measures are outlined in table 11-5.

Protein Status

The most reliable diagnostic indicators of protein-energy malnutrition in older adults include serum albumin, serum transferrin, hemoglobin, serum cholesterol, and total lymphocyte count.[50] Serum albumin and transferrin

TABLE 11-5 *Guidelines for Interpreting Biochemical Data*

Blood Biochemistries	Biochemical Values			Reference No.
Cholesterol status				
Total	≥240 mg/dl (High risk)			53
LDL	≥160 mg/dl (High risk)			53
HDL	<35 mg/dl (High risk)			53
Protein status	**Deficient**			
Serum albumin	<30 g/l			41
Serum transferrin	<200 mg/dl			41
Serum transthyretin	<11 mg/dl			37
Total lymphocyte count	<1,500 cells/mm³			34
Hemoglobin				41
Men	<12.6 g/dl			
Women	<11.9 g/dl			
Cholesterol	<160 mg/dl			69
Selected minerals				
Iron Status	**Depletion**	**Deficient erythropoiesis**	**Anemia**	29
Serum ferritin	<20 ug/dl	<60 ug/dl	<10 ug/dl	
Plasma iron	<115 ug/dl		<40 ug/dl	
Total iron binding capacity	>360 ug/dl	>390 ug/dl	>410 ug/dl	
Transferrin saturation	30%	<15%	<15%	
Erythrocyte protoporphyrin	30 ug/dl RBC	>100 ug/dl RBC	>200 gu/dl RBC	
MCV	<80 fl			
Serum Zinc	**Deficient**			41
A.M. + fasting sample	<70 ug/dl			24
Selected vitamins				
Folate Status	**Depletion**	**Deficient erythropoiesis**	**Anemia**	29
Serum folate	<3 ng/ml	<3 ng/ml	<3 ng/ml	
Erythrocyte folate	<160 ng/ml	<120 ng/ml	<100 ng/ml	
Vitamin B-12				29
Serum vitamin B-12	<150 pg/ml	<100 pg/ml	<100 pg/ml	
Vitamin A	**Low**	**Deficient**		24, 66
Plasma retinol	10–20 ug/dl	<10 ug/dl		
Vitamin C				24, 66
Serum ascorbic acid	0.20–0.29 mg/dl	<0.20 mg/dl		24, 66
Leukocyte ascorbic acid	8–15 mg/dl	<8 mg/dl		
Vitamin B-6				66
Serum vitamin B-6	<3.0 ng/ml			66
Red cell vitamin B-6	<12.0 ng/ml			

are good markers for evaluating visceral protein status. Visceral protein includes serum proteins, erythrocytes, granulocytes, lymphocytes, and solid tissue organs such as the liver, kidneys, pancreas, and heart. Total lymphocyte count is an indicator of immunocompetence. Hemoglobin can be used to detect anemia, which is commonly associated with malnutrition.

Serum albumin concentrations do not decrease with age to a significant degree (1%–6%) in healthy older people.[21] Serum albumin has a long half-life of 14 to 21 days. Thus, alterations of serum albumin take several weeks. Hypoalbuminemia or low serum albumin levels may be the consequence of a nutrition-related decrease in protein synthesis. However, various factors can influence serum albumin levels. Hypoalbuminemia may result from certain gastrointestinal and renal diseases, liver disease, hypothyroidism, congestive heart failure, infection, or zinc deficiency. In normally hydrated older adults, serum albumin levels should not be lower than 35 g/l.[21,37] Lipschitz and Mitchell suggest that a serum albumin value of less than 30 g/l can be used to differentiate malnourished from well-nourished older adults.[42]

Serum transferrin is located almost totally intravascularly and serves as an iron transport protein. In comparison to serum albumin, serum transferrin has a short half-life of 8 to 10 days and a smaller body pool. Therefore, it responds more rapidly to changes in protein status over short periods. Like serum albumin, serum transferrin concentrations are affected by other factors, such as pernicious anemia, iron overload, gastrointestinal, renal, and liver diseases, congestive heart failure, and inflammation. In concomitant protein-energy malnutrition and iron deficiency, a decrease in transferrin levels may be masked since transferrin synthesis is increased in response to increased iron absorption. Therefore, serum transferrin is not an appropriate index of protein status when both iron deficiency anemia and protein-energy malnutrition are present. Serum transferrin values of less than 200 mg/dl can be used to detect protein deficiency in older adults.[42]

Transthyretin (or prealbumin), a protein carrier for thyroxine, has a half-life shorter than either albumin or transferrin. Its half life is two to three days, and the pool size is small. Thus, this parameter undergoes rapid liver synthesis and is more responsive to physiologic changes. Transthyretin levels between 18 and 40 mg/dl are considered normal, whereas a level of 11 mg/dl or less indicates significant malnutrition.[37] Transthyretin level is affected by inflammation, surgery, nephrotic syndrome, and severe metabolic stress.

Total lymphocyte count (TLC) declines and lymphocyte response to antigens is impaired in malnutrition. TLC is determined using the following formula:

$$\text{TLC} = (\% \text{ lymphocytes} \times \text{white blood cell count}) \text{ in mm}^3$$

Unfortunately, the specificity (the ability of the index to identify and classify those people who are genuinely well-nourished) and sensitivity (the extent to which the index reflects nutritional status or predicts changes in nutriture) is low for TLC. This is because other factors, such as stress, sepsis, neoplasia, and the administration of steroids, affect the absolute lymphocyte count. The similarity between the effects of normal aging and the effects of protein-energy malnutrition also make the interpretation of routine immunological testing difficult. A TLC of less than 1,500 cells/mm^3 suggests protein depletion.[27,34]

There is much controversy about the cutoff values for hemoglobin that define anemia in older adults. A decline in hemoglobin may occur as a result of physiologic aging, although nutrient deficiencies and chronic disease may also be involved.[50,51] The lower normal limits for hemoglobin for people age 65 to 74 used in the NHANES II study were 11.9 g/dl for women and 12.6 g/dl for men.[41]

Evidence exists showing that low total serum cholesterol levels are predictive of excess mortality, independent of cancer incidence.[69] In addition, low total cholesterol levels in elderly people are associated with an increased risk of hemorrhagic stroke.[21] A total serum cholesterol value less than 160 mg/dl is also a marker for protein-energy malnutrition. This latter value is used in nutritional screening instruments such as the Level II Screen of the Nutrition Screening Initiative and SCALES to indicate the need for nutritional counseling or support intervention[52,58] (see table 11-8). These instruments will be discussed later in this chapter.

Hypercholesterolemia

High blood cholesterol, especially elevated low density lipoprotein (LDL) cholesterol and low HDL cholesterol, are risk factors for coronary artery disease. In older adult populations, lipoprotein cholesterol levels appear to be more predictive of coronary events than total serum cholesterol (see chapter 2). For example, a plasma total cholesterol level of 240 mg/dl or higher was reported to carry a small but nonsignificant increase in mortality risk from coronary heart disease (CHD), whereas HDL cholesterol levels below 35 mg/dl were significantly associated with a 2.5-fold increase in CHD mortality compared to HDL cholesterol levels of 60 mg/dl or higher.[18] The ratio of total cholesterol to HDL cholesterol was also strongly associated with CHD mortality in both older men and women. A one-unit increase in this ratio resulted in a 17% increase in relative risk.[18]

The National Cholesterol Education Program screening guidelines are considered appropriate for use with older adults. A total cholesterol level above 240 mg/dl and an LDL cholesterol level above 160 mg/dl are viewed as high risk.[53]

Iron Status

Iron deficiency is considered the most common nutrient deficiency in the world. Biochemical measurements of iron deficiency are provided in table 11-5. Iron deficiency among older people is generally associated with increased blood loss, excessive intake of aspirin or anti-inflammatory drugs for the relief of arthritic pain, or achlorhydria.

Three stages have been used to characterize the development of iron deficiency anemia.[29] The first stage, iron depletion, is characterized by a progressive reduction in the amount of storage iron, reflected by a decline in serum or plasma ferritin concentrations. The second stage, iron deficient erythropoiesis, is characterized by a complete depletion of iron stores.

Microcytic, hypochromic anemia is the third and final stage of iron deficiency. This stage is characterized by a reduction in the concentration of hemoglobin in the red blood cells, as well as decreases in the hematocrit and mean corpuscular volume (MCV). The biochemical cutoff values used to define each stage are provided in table 11-5.

Hemoglobin level is probably the most widely used screening test for iron deficiency anemia because it is inexpensive. However, this index has several limitations. Cigarette smoking is associated with higher concentrations of hemoglobin, while chronic infections, inflammation, hemorrhage, protein-energy malnutrition, vitamin B-12 or folate deficiency, and overhydration can result in low hemoglobin concentrations. In addition, regardless of age or income, African Americans may have hemoglobin values lower than those of white individuals. Hence, they may be misdiagnosed as having an iron deficit if the reference values are based on white population values.

Several factors can affect an index of iron status. Chronic diseases, such as infection, inflammation, and certain neoplastic diseases, lead to an anemia of chronic disease.[24] Its hallmark is normal or elevated iron stores in the presence of hypoferremia (see chapter 12). Elevated concentrations of serum ferritin can occur with liver disease, leukemia, or Hodgkin's disease, whereas serum ferritin may display normal or even slightly above-normal levels in vitamin B-12 or folate deficiency. Vitamin B-12 or folate deficiency can increase transferrin saturation and elevate MCV.

No single biochemical indicator has proven to be diagnostic of iron deficiency. To provide the best measure of iron status, several indices should be used simultaneously. In general, two or more abnormal values are considered indicative of impaired iron status. The selection of the most appropriate combination depends on the health of the individuals and the objectives of the assessment. Several combinations have been proposed. A panel of experts in nutrition proposed a four-variable model for assessing iron status, especially in older adults.[79] The four-variable model includes erythrocyte protoporphyrin, transferrin saturation, serum ferritin, and MCV. With this model either the ferritin or MCV value (or both), plus one additional value (either erythrocyte protoporphyrin or transferrin saturation) must be abnormal. This model may reduce the contribution of inflammatory conditions to prevalence estimates of iron deficiency.

Folate Status

Folate deficiency in older adults can be caused by low dietary intakes of folate, malabsorption syndromes, selected drugs, such as chronic aspirin use, and alcohol ingestion. Serum and erythrocyte folate concentrations are the most frequently used biochemical indicators of folate status. Serum levels reflect recent intake and acute folate status. Erythrocyte folate levels reflect body stores and are a more reliable index of folate status.

Similar to iron, there are three stages of folate deficiency: folate depletion, folate deficiency erythropoiesis, and folate deficiency anemia.[29] The cutoff values for serum and erythrocyte folate are provided in table 11-5. Low folate intake for more than a month may gradually reduce folate stores, resulting in folate depletion. Erythrocyte folate levels continue to decline as the stages of folate deficiency progress.

CLINICAL ASSESSMENT

The components of clinical assessment can include a medical history; physical examination to determine which physical signs and symptoms of nutritional disease are present; assessment of functional status, particularly skills related to purchasing, preparing, and eating foods; and an oral examination. When interviewing and examining older adults, health professionals should remember that (1) many elderly people may not report symptoms or changes in functional status because they accept their condition as a problem inherent in aging, and (2) some may be mentally confused and unable to clearly describe signs and symptoms. Clinical signs and symptoms are generally nonspecific and develop in the advanced stages of a nutritional deficiency.

Clinical Signs

A comprehensive listing of clinical signs indicative of nutritional disease can be found in table 11-6. An abbreviated checklist of clinical appearances suggesting nutritional problems includes the following: wasted appearance, edema, pale color, bruises, general weakness, apathy, tremors, skin lesions, rashes or scaly skin, and cracks or sores around the mouth. Remember that the symptoms and signs commonly found in the elderly population can have nonnutritional etiologic causes. For example, purpura (subcutaneous skin hemorrhages) is more commonly the result of aging of the skin and not the result of scurvy (a vitamin C deficiency) or vitamin K deficiency. Furthermore, night blindness may result from cataracts rather than vitamin A deficiency, and angular stomatitis can be caused by drooling of saliva rather than a riboflavin deficiency. In addition, clinical signs, observations made by a physician or other trained health professional, and **symptoms**—manifestations of a disease or condition experienced and reported by the patient—are not diagnostically specific and should be confirmed by other components of nutritional status assessment.

Functional Status

Changes in functional status represent an important symptom of nutritional status that need to be monitored. Two measures of independence/dependence commonly used to assess functional status are the Activities of Daily Living (ADLs) and the Instrumental Activities of Daily Living (IADLs). Dependence is defined as needing assistance for that activity most of the time, whereas independence implies that the activity can be performed without assistance. The inability to perform any ADLs and the nutrition-related IADLs signals the potential presence of poor nutritional status.[21]

Feeding is considered one of the six ADLs. Independent feeding is demonstrated by the ability to get food from the plate into the mouth, whereas dependence implies the need for assistance in the act of feeding because the person is not eating at all or requires parenteral feeding.[21]

TABLE 11-6   *Clinical Signs and Possible Nutrient Deficiency in Adults*

Clinical Signs	Consider Deficiency	Definition/Comment
Hair		
Easily pluckable, sparse	Protein, biotin Protein	
Straight, dull	Protein	
Coiled, corkscrewlike	Vitamin A, vitamin C	Caused by follicular and keratinization change
Skin		
Xerosis	Essential fatty acid	Dryness of skin/aging, loss of skin lubricants
Petechiae	Vitamin A, vitamin C	Pinhead-sized hemorrhages
Pigmentation	Niacin	Sign of pellagra distributed symmetrically in sun-exposed areas; also seen in hemochromatosis
Follicular keratosis	Vitamin A, possibly essential fatty acid	Keratin plugs in follicles, "goose flesh"
"Flaky-paint" dermatitis	Protein	
Subcutaneous fat loss, fine wrinkling	Protein-energy	Aging process
Poor tissue turgor	Water	Aging process
Edema	Protein, thiamin	Seen in protein-energy malnutrition with hypoalbuminemia and in wet beriberi resulting from thiamin deficiency
Purpura	Vitamin C, vitamin K	Also seen in vitamin E toxicity
Perifollicular hemorrhage	Vitamin C	
Pallor	Folacin, iron, vitamin B-12, copper, biotin	
Tendency toward excessive bruising (ecchymoses)	Vitamin C, vitamin K	Caused by increased fragility of capillary walls; aging process
Pressure sores	Protein-energy	
Seborrheic dermatitis	Essential fatty acid, pyridoxine, zinc, biotin	
Poor wound healing	Protein-energy, zinc, and possibly essential fatty acids	
Thickening of skin	Essential fatty acid	
Eyes		
Dully, dry (xerosis) conjunctiva	Vitamin A	Can lead to xerophthalmia in severe deficiency
Keratomalacia	Vitamin A	Softening of cornea
Bitot's spot	Vitamin A	Early evidence of deficiency
Corneal vascularization	Riboflavin	
Photophobia	Zinc	

Adapted from Heymsfield, S.B., and Williams, P.J.: Nutritional assessment by clinical and biochemical methods. In: Shils, M.E., and Young, V.R., editors: Modern nutrition in health and disease, ed. 7, Philadelphia, 1988, Lea & Febiger.

TABLE 11-6 *Clinical Signs and Possible Nutrient Deficiency in Adults—cont'd*

Clinical Signs	Consider Deficiency	Definition/Comment
Lips and oral structures		
Angular fissures, scars, or stomatitis	B-complex, iron, protein, riboflavin	Also seen with ill-fitting dentures
Cheilosis	B-6, niacin, riboflavin, protein	Also seen with ill-fitting dentures, exposure to sun or cold
Ageusia, dysgeusia	Zinc	Also associated with altered sense of smell
Swollen, spongy, bleeding gums	Ascorbic acid	If not edentulous
Tongue		
Magenta tongue	Riboflavin	
Fissuring, raw	Niacin	
Glossitis	Pyridoxine, folacin, iron, vitamin B-12	Also seen with food irritants, antibiotic administration, uremia
Fiery red tongue	Folacin, vitamin B-12	Seen if anemia is not pronounced
Pale	Iron, vitamin B-12	Seen in severe cases
Atrophic papillae	Riboflavin, niacin, iron	Also seen with ill-fitting dentures, food irritants, aging
Nails		
Spoon-shaped nails (koilonychia)	Chromium, iron	
Brittle, ridged, lined nails	Nonspecific	May be protein undernutrition
Heart		
Tachycardia, cardiomegaly, congestive heart failure	Thiamin	"Wet" beriberi associated with high output congestive heart failure
Decreased cardiac function	Phosphorus	
Cardiac arrhythmias	Magnesium, potassium	
Small heart, decreased output, bradycardia	Protein-energy	Prone to congestive heart failure during refeeding
Abdomen		
Hepatomegaly	Protein	Fatty liver/commonly seen in alcoholics
Wasting	Energy	Found in marasmus
Enlarged spleen	Iron	Found in 15% to 25% subjects with a significant degree of iron-deficiency anemia
Bones		
Bone pain	Calcium, vitamin D, phosphorus, vitamin C	Seen in osteomalacia

Continued.

TABLE 11-6   Clinical Signs and Possible Nutrient Deficiency in Adults—cont'd

Clinical Signs	Consider Deficiency	Definition/Comment
Muscles, extremities		
Wasting	Protein-energy	
Pain in calves, weak thighs	Thiamin	
Edema	Protein, thiamin	Also seen with sodium toxicity and hypertension
Muscular twitching	Pyridoxine	
Muscular pains	Biotin, selenium	
Muscular weakness	Sodium, potassium	
Muscle cramps	Sodium, chloride	
Neurologic		
Ophthalmoplegia, footdrop	Thiamin	Wernicke's encephalopathy
Disorientation	Thiamin, sodium, water	Korsakoff's psychosis; fabrication occurs in thiamin-deficient alcoholics
Decreased position, vibratory sense, ataxia, optic neuritis	Vitamin B-12	Subacute spinal cord degeneration
Weakness, paresthesia of legs (burning and tingling)	Thiamin, pyridoxine, pantothenic acid, vitamin B-12	Nutritional polyneuropathy, especially with alcoholism; "burning foot" syndrome with pantothenic acid deficiency
Hyporeflexia	Thiamin	Aging process
Mental disorders	Niacin, magnesium, vitamin B-12	In untreated B-12 deficiency, mental disorders may progress to severe psychosis
Convulsions	Pyridoxine, calcium, magnesium, phosphorus	
Depression, lethargy	Biotin, folacin, vitamin C	Aging process
Sleep disturbances	Pantothenic acid	Aging process
Peripheral neuropathy	Pyridoxine	
Other		
Diarrhea	Niacin, folacin, vitamin B-12	Also seen in vitamin C toxicity
Delayed wound healing and tissue repair	Vitamin C, zinc, protein-energy	
Anemia, pallor	Vitamin E, pyridoxine, vitamin B-12, iron, folacin, biotin, copper	
Anorexia	Vitamin B-12, chloride, sodium, thiamin, vitamin C	Also seen with vitamin A, zinc, or iron toxicity
Nausea	Biotin, pantothenic acid	
Fatigue, lassitude, apathy	Energy, biotin, pantothenic acid, magnesium, phosphorus, iron, potassium, sodium	

IADLs measure home management activities essential to independent living, including three nutrition-related activities: shopping, food preparation, and mode of transportation. Independence with respect to shopping means the individual takes care of all shopping needs and shops independently for small purchases. An individual who must be accompanied on any shopping trip or is completely unable to shop is dependent. An independent older adult can plan, prepare, and serve adequate meals without help or prepare adequate meals if the ingredients are supplied. Dependence implies that a person may be able to prepare meals or to heat and serve prepared meals but does not maintain an adequate diet or that a person must have his or her meals prepared and served. In terms of transportation, a dependent individual would travel on public transportation accompanied by another person, limit travel to automobile or taxi with assistance, or not travel at all. An independently living older person would travel on public transportation unaccompanied, drive his or her own car, or arrange his or her travel via taxi.[21]

Oral Status

Not only is the ability to select, secure, and prepare foods important, but adequate oral health is also essential for the ingestion and mastication of foods. Therefore, an assessment of the oral status of older adults is considered a critical feature of a nutritional status evaluation. The most common dental diseases and conditions in older people are dental caries, advanced gingivitis, inflammation of the periodontium because of dryness of the mouth, and oral lesions, including oral cancer.[4]

Oral screening can define the presence or absence of difficulties in chewing or swallowing food. The screening instrument can be used to determine reasons for chewing difficulties, such as poor fitting dentures, absence of teeth, a sore mouth, swollen gums, glossitis (red tongue without papillae), ulcers in the mouth, paralytic disease involving the face, or dry mouth. A more comprehensive assessment of both dentition and the oral mucosa requires a dentist, preferably one who specializes in geriatric dentistry.

Mental and Cognitive Status

In general, nearly 4% of older adults suffer from unrecognized dementia or chronic cognitive impairment.[4] Cognitive status refers to an individual's intellectual capability, including such areas as memory, language, reading, writing, and orientation to time, place, and person. Changed or diminished cognitive status can serve as an indicator of a nutritional problem.[26] The Folstein Mini Mental State Examination is considered by expert panels as the best screening procedure.[4] This validated instrument has been used to detect dementia, which is responsible for most of the loss of cognitive function.

Depression should also be regarded as an indicator of malnutrition because it can result in loss of appetite, inadequate food intake and subsequent weight loss, and even nutrient deficiency. It can be caused by metabolic disorders, drug toxicity, dehydration, protein-energy malnutrition, loss of spouse, sibling, or child, or change in lifestyle. Several useful screening instruments for depression are available.[3,8,63,65,82,83] Few data are available on the best methods for screening for depression in the elderly or the accuracy of screening.

DIETARY ASSESSMENT

The first stage of a nutrient deficiency is generally identified by a dietary evaluation (see fig. 11-1). The dietary evaluation should not only assess food consumption patterns but also assess food security or insecurity, food storage and cooking facilities, and use of therapeutic diets and supplements. **Food insecurity** is defined as the limited or uncertain availability of nutritionally adequate and safe foods or the limited or uncertain ability to acquire acceptable foods in socially acceptable ways.[2] In contrast, **food security** means people have access to enough food for an active, healthy life at all times.[2] Since homebound older adults are at greater risk for malnutrition, it has been recommended that food insecurity be assessed when surveying these older adults.[67] Examples of questions that can be asked to judge food security are found in the box.[7]

❖

SAMPLE FOOD SECURITY QUESTIONS

1. During the past month, did you skip any meals because there was not enough food or money to buy food?
2. How many days in the past month did you skip any meals because there was not enough food or money to buy food?
3. Which of the following reasons explain why you had this problem?
   a. You did not have transportation.
   b. You did not have working appliances for storing or preparing foods, such as a stove or refrigerator.
   c. You did not have access to a congregate meal site or home meal delivery program.

Before selecting a dietary assessment method, the following basic questions need to be answered:

- What is the objective of the dietary assessment?
- Is the dietary assessment being conducted on individuals or groups of people?
- What needs to be assessed: foods or intakes of energy and selected nutrients or both?
- How precise does the assessment need to be?

If the objective of the assessment is to determine whether a group of free-living older adults meets the Dietary Guidelines for Americans, a quantified food frequency questionnaire would be satisfactory. However, if the objective is to compare the energy and nutrient intakes of individuals who participate in a congregate meal program with nonparticipants, 24-hour dietary recalls would be the preferred method. Dietary records of multiple days would be appropriate when studying the relationship between nutrient intakes and food-related attitudes.

Obviously, the method chosen should be reliable, valid, and cost-effective. A **reliable** method is reproducible and generates typical intake patterns that are representative of the individual or group. **Validity** refers to accuracy. A valid method generates a "true" estimate of intake. Except in a metabolic laboratory setting where all food can be weighed and consumption levels closely monitored, the measurement of food intake tends to be imprecise.

Several issues related to the target audience also need to be considered when selecting a method. These issues include respondent burden, level of education and literacy of the individuals, and the degree of willingness and motivation of the individuals to cooperate. **Respondent burden** refers to the time spent for all aspects of the assessment, including the time required to be interviewed or to complete questionnaires and travel time to the site where the measurements are taken, if not in the home.

Information obtained during a dietary assessment may be incomplete or not reflect usual intakes. For example, people may underreport desserts and sweets or forget to mention alcoholic beverages. Regardless of the method used, some people may attempt to please the interviewer rather than report his or her actual intake. The quality of the dietary data obtained depends highly on the skill and patience of the interviewer and the understanding and cooperation of the individual being interviewed.

Assessing dietary intakes of older adults can be difficult because of impaired memory, reduced appetite, language barriers in selected ethnic groups, and low educational level. In some instances, reliable information must be obtained from a caregiver.[70] No firm evidence exists that long-term memory of diet is affected adversely in advancing age. Hankin[28] and Byers[9] reported that older adults, age 70 and older, performed as well as those less than 70 years old in recalling food intakes.[9,28] The ability to recall past dietary intakes may be more dependent on the person's awareness of what is being consumed than age. Some people eat almost mechanically, without thought to the types and amounts of food items consumed. This phenomenon has been suggested to occur more frequently in men than in women who plan, prepare, and serve meals. When interviewing older men at home, it is beneficial to have the spouse or other surrogate source who may prepare the meals present to assist in providing details about foods eaten at home.

Natow and Heslin have published guidelines for dietary assessment interviewing to help ensure a successful session.[56] A skilled interviewer will listen carefully, not interrupt the older adult unnecessarily, and allow sufficient time for the older adult to think and respond fully. The interviewer must not be judgmental or express either approval or disapproval at the older adult's responses. Another aspect to remember when interviewing older adults is to speak slowly and loudly if the elderly person has a hearing impairment. In addition, the interviewer should use simple and easy-to-understand language and take time to explain unfamiliar terms.

METHODS OF DIETARY ASSESSMENT

Prospective versus Retrospective Methods

With a prospective method, records of food intake are obtained at the time food is consumed. Retrospective methods rely on the ability of the person to recall food intake in the past and therefore rely on memory.[20] Remember, each method has strengths and weaknesses;[77] no single best method exists.

Prospective Method

Food diary or record. A **food diary** is a record of what is eaten at the time of consumption. The errors associated with memory lapse are less common with this method than with retrospective methods. This method requires more motivated and literate older adults who can hold a pen or pencil and write. The older adult needs to be instructed on how to record food intake and estimate portion sizes. Providing measuring aids to assist in estimating portions is recommended. Records must be checked by trained interviewers for completeness before nutrient analysis. With the food diary, food intakes may be altered during reporting periods. In fact, underreporting is common.

Although seven-day records are considered to provide the most representative summary of usual food intake, obtaining usable records beyond four days is often difficult because of respondent burden. Hence, the validity of the seven-day record to assess usual intakes of elderly people is questioned.[24] In a study conducted by Abernethy and Fanelli Kuczmarski,[1] a group of 36 women, ages 65 to 88 (mean age was 72.5), recorded four days of food intake successfully. This group was highly educated, with 36% completing more than 17 years of education and another 36% completing 14 to 16 years of education. These women stated that they did not feel this method was burdensome or time-consuming.[1]

Retrospective Methods

24-hour food recall. The 24-hour recall method is one in which an individual recalls all the foods and beverages consumed in the previous 24 hours. Thus, short-term memory is required. Using measuring aids and food models, the interviewer assists the subject in estimating portion sizes of foods consumed. Because the respondent burden is low and the time for administration is short, this method is widely accepted. Unlike the food diary, intakes are not consciously altered. Typically, individuals forget snack items, sweets, and alcohol. Therefore, trained interviewers need to be able to probe without leading the respondent.

The "flat slope syndrome" is associated with this method. Individuals whose actual food intake is low tend to overestimate the amount recalled, whereas individuals whose actual food intake is high tend to underestimate the amount recalled. In general, the 24-hour recall tends to underestimate mean intakes of older adults.[10,44] One study reported that recall of foods eaten was significantly improved when the elderly participants were notified that they would be asked to report intake from the previous day.[11]

It is widely recognized that a single 24-hour recall does not represent an individual's usual intake because of day-to-day or intraindividual variability. Serial 24-hour recalls are needed to provide an estimate of usual intakes of individuals. For groups of people, the 24-hour recall is considered reliable. The 24-hour recall is used by epidemiologists to study the relationship of diet and health in populations.

Food frequency questionnaires. Generally, food frequency questionnaires provide a qualitative description of how often foods are eaten in a specific period. They are easy to standardize and do not require highly trained interviewers for administration. In fact, many are self-administered by people who can read. Respondent burden is low, provided the number of food items is limited.

Food frequency questionnaires are extremely useful for describing food intake patterns for diet and meal planning, for studying the associations of types of foods and disease, and for developing nutrition education programs. However, they provide limited information about energy and selected nutrient intakes because portion sizes usually are not obtained. Despite this limitation, Smiciklas-Wright and her associates[71] noted the need for a valid and reliable food frequency questionnaire for assessing food intake of homebound older adults.

Obtaining information on total food consumption is difficult with food frequency questionnaires, because some foods are not included on the list. A controversial issue is the length of time that can be recalled. A rule of thumb is that food frequency questionnaires should not go beyond 30 days. Like the 24-hour recall method, the individual's ability to remember affects the accuracy of this method.

Semiquantified food frequency questionnaires (or simplified dietary history or list-based dietary history) include an estimate of the amounts of foods consumed, along with their frequency of use. Portion sizes are usually "standardized" amounts customarily eaten per serving by a given population group. Subjects select small, medium, or large size with respect to a stated "standard" portion. Energy and nutrient intakes can be estimated from semiquantified food frequency questionnaires. This method can be administered by professional nutritionists or other health workers or be self-administered.

Development of a semiquantified food frequency questionnaire for older adults has been described in detail by Hankin.[28] Photographs of small, medium, and large portion sizes of foods were used to estimate quantities. She has demonstrated that this method produces both valid and reliable results for this population group.

Kumanyika and associates[39] have validated a two-step picture sort approach to administering a semiquantitative food frequency questionnaire developed by the National Cancer Institute (NCI) to older adults. The NCI food frequency questionnaire contains 99 items that contributed 90% of the energy and more than 85% of several vitamin and mineral intakes reported by people interviewed in the NHANES II. The picture sort card contained a color picture of the food item on one side and on the reverse side, the medium size portion was displayed. Each older respondent was asked to sort the picture cards by frequency of consumption and then asked whether the usual portion consumed was smaller or larger than the medium size. This picture card approach appears to have advantages over the list-based form for older people with limited literacy or English-speaking skills or impaired vision.

Dietary History

The Burke-type dietary history method provides a more complete and detailed description of both qualitative and quantitative aspects of food intake than food diaries, 24-hour recalls, or food frequency questionnaires. Dietary intakes obtained by this method correlate well with other measures of nutritional status. Unfortunately, it is time consuming (one to two hours) and requires a highly trained nutritionist or dietitian and highly motivated participants. The required in-depth interview includes a typical day's eating pattern, occasional alternative foods, usual portion sizes, and any irregularities. A detailed list of foods is then reviewed as a cross-check to verify the eating pattern. The respondent also keeps a three-day measured food record. All of this information is used to derive usual daily food intake and estimates of usual nutrient intakes. This method is vulnerable to memory lapses and psychological tendencies to exaggerate or minimize self-described behaviors.[45]

Evaluation of Dietary Data

The food intake of individuals or groups can be evaluated against various standards of adequacy. The Dietary Guidelines for Americans[77] and the report entitled, "Diet and Health: Implications for Reducing Chronic Disease Risk"[54] included

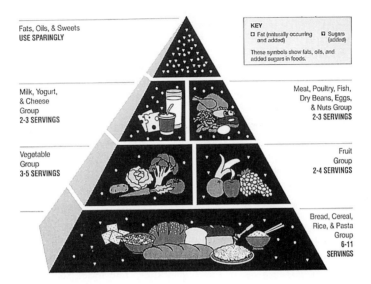

KEY
□ Fat (naturally occurring and added)   ▨ Sugars (added)
These symbols show fats, oils, and added sugars in foods.

Fats, Oils, & Sweets
USE SPARINGLY

Milk, Yogurt, & Cheese Group
2-3 SERVINGS

Meat, Poultry, Fish, Dry Beans, Eggs, & Nuts Group
2-3 SERVINGS

Vegetable Group
3-5 SERVINGS

Fruit Group
2-4 SERVINGS

Bread, Cereal, Rice, & Pasta Group
6-11 SERVINGS

FIG. 11-4   Food Guide Pyramid.

From Human Nutrition Information Service: USDA's food guide pyramid, Home and Garden Bull 249, Hyattsville, MD, 1992, U.S. Department of Agriculture.

recommendations to achieve an optimal and highly desirable dietary pattern for maintaining good health. This diet should provide:

- less than 30% of energy from total fat
- less than 10% of energy from saturated fat
- no more than 10% of energy from polyunsaturated fatty acids
- less than 300 mg of cholesterol a day
- more than 55% of energy from carbohydrates, especially complex sources
- less than 6 g of salt a day
- less than 1 ounce of alcohol a day.

Dietary habits can be evaluated against the Food Guide Pyramid.[33] As shown in figure 11-4 and the box, the Pyramid is an outline of the types and amounts or number of servings of foods to eat each day. The actual number of servings a person should consume depends on his or her energy needs. Consuming the lowest number of servings for each food group will provide approximately 1,600 kcal. This energy level will be appropriate for some older adults. Consuming the midpoint of the range of servings for each major food group will provide about 2,200 kcal, and the highest number of servings will provide approximately 2,800 kcal.[33]

Measurements of energy and nutrient intakes from dietary intake data, regardless of the dietary assessment method, can be difficult because of limitations of food composition tables and nutrient databases. For instance, sometimes the food items consumed, particularly if ethnic foods, may not be included in the databases used to analyze diets for energy and nutrient content. Other potential sources of error when estimating nutrient intakes can occur because of differences between the nutrient value contained in the database and in the food consumed because of where and how the food was grown, stored, processed, or prepared. The use of imputed nutrient values and inappropriate analytical methods and differences in the bioavailability of individual nutrients also introduce error in food composition data. Despite these weaknesses, measurement of energy and nutrient intake is probably the most widely used nutritional status indicator.

Energy and nutrient intakes can be compared to the Recommended Dietary Allowances (RDA).[55] Except for energy, the common assumption is that the recommended levels for essential nutrients provide a margin of safety.

❖

FOOD GUIDE PYRAMID: SERVING SIZES

Bread, cereal, rice, and pasta
1 slice of bread
1 ounce of ready-to-eat cereal
½ cup of cooked cereal, rice, or pasta
Vegetable
1 cup of raw, leafy vegetables
½ cup of other vegetables, cooked or
    chopped raw
¾ cup of vegetable juice
Fruit
1 medium apple, banana, orange
½ cup of chopped, cooked, or canned fruit
¾ cup of fruit juice
Milk, yogurt, and cheese
1 cup of milk or yogurt
1½ ounces of natural cheese
2 ounces of processed cheese
Meat, poultry, fish, dry beans, eggs, and nuts
2 to 3 ounces of cooked lean meat, poultry,
    or fish
½ cup of cooked dry beans, 1 egg, or 2
    tablespoons of peanut butter count as
    1 ounce of lean meat

From Human Nutrition Information Service: USDA's food guide pyramid, Home and Garden Bull 249 Hyattsville, MD, 1992, U.S. Department of Agriculture.

Some researchers compare nutrient intakes from dietary assessments to 100% of the RDA. If an older adult has nutrient intakes at or above 100% of the RDA, it is very likely that his or her nutrient needs are being met. Other researchers consider 67% of the RDA value to be adequate. However, an older adult consuming between 67% and 100% of the RDA is at risk for inadequate intakes. Consuming less than 67% of the RDA increases one's risk for nutritional problems, and in that situation additional indicators of nutritional status should be evaluated to verify a suspected nutritional problem.

The Healthy Eating Index developed by the U.S. Department of Agriculture is designed to provide a measure of the overall quality of an individual's diet.[36,76] The index measures the degree to which an individual's diet conforms to the Food Guide Pyramid serving recommendations for the five basic food groups, compliance with specific Dietary Guidelines, and the variety of foods in the diet. The serving recommendations from the Food Guide Pyramid were adjusted depending on the individual's energy requirements based on specific age and sex categories. Table 11-7 lists the components of the Healthy Eating Index and the criteria to achieve a perfect score of 10. The maximum score for the 10 components of the index is 100. If an individual's score is greater than 80, his or her diet is rated as good. A score between 51 and 80 indicates that the person's diet needs improvement, and a score less than 51 indicates a poor diet. The index score is directly associated with nutrient intake. For example, an index score between 71 and 80 is associated with the likelihood that at least 90% of the RDA for most nutrients will be met.

APPLICATIONS OF NUTRITIONAL ASSESSMENT

Nutritional assessment is important for older adults. Nearly 50% of the elderly population have undetected dental disease, and over 50% have some undetected disease or condition such as colon cancer, breast cancer, cardiovascular disease, impaired physical functioning, or nutritional problems.[4] Approximately 2% to 3% of older adults who have an undetected condition or disease can be diagnosed by routine laboratory tests. The most commonly undetected nutrition-related conditions for which assessment methods are available include: anemia, hyperlipidemia, diabetes, and electrolyte disturbances caused by diuretics and nonsteroidal anti-inflammatory agents.[4] The onset of diseases and subsequent complications can be lessened by early detection of risk factors or conditions and the initiation of nutritional intervention measures. As a result, older adults may maximize their independence in carrying out activities of daily living and lessen the number of illness-related days of restricted activity. Ultimately,

TABLE 11-7   Components of the Healthy Index and Criteria for Perfect Scores

Components	Perfect Score of 10	
	Men, 51+ Years	Women, 51+ Years
Food group	**Recommended servings**	
Grains	9.1	7.4
Vegetables	4.2	3.5
Fruits	3.2	2.5
Milk	2	2
Meat	2.5	2.2
	Men and Women, 51+ Years	
Dietary Guidelines		
Total fat	less than 30% energy from fat	
Saturated fat	less than 10% energy from saturated fat	
Cholesterol	300 mg or less	
Sodium	2,400 mg or less	
Variety	16 different foods over three-day period	

From: U.S. Department of Agriculture: The Healthy Eating Index, Washington, DC, 1995, U.S. Government Printing Office.

nutrition services can contribute substantial savings in health care costs.

The selection of nutritional indicators to assess nutritional status depends on several factors. These include: the objective of the assessment, the amount of time available for the assessment, and the level of personnel and money available to support the evaluation. Biochemical assessments generally involve invasive techniques and can be timely and expensive because of the cost related to the personnel required to draw blood samples and perform the assays. In comparison, anthropometric measurements can be easily obtained by trained personnel with relatively inexpensive tools. In addition, scales, calipers, height boards, and measuring tapes are transportable. If the objective is to obtain baseline data and then monitor the nutritional status of older adults in a day-care facility on a limited budget, the choice of indicators could be a 24-hour food recall, body weight and height measurements, and questionnaires dealing with eating practices, food preferences, presence of chronic diseases, and use of prescription drugs. Table 11-8 lists selected published nutritional assessment instruments, identifies the indicators used in each tool, and indicates appropriate settings for administering the instrument.

NUTRITION SCREENING INSTRUMENTS

Experts from various fields specializing in the care of elderly people have recommended various nutritional screening and assessment procedures.[4] The following section will discuss the instruments presented in table 11-8 which include the Nutritional Risk Index (NRI),[81] the Nutrition Screening Initiative's "Determine Your Nutritional Health" checklist and Level 1 and 2 Screen,[59] SCALES,[52] and the Mini Nutritional Assessment.[27]

TABLE 11-8 *Nutritional Assessment Screening Instruments for Older Adults: Indicators Measured and Target Populations*

| | Instruments | | | | | |
| | Nutrition Screening Initiative | | | | | |
	Checklist	Level 1 Screen	Level 2 Screen	NRI[1]	SCALES[2]	MNA[3]
Indicators measured						
Anthropometric						
Height		X	X			X
Weight		X	X			X
BMI		X	X			X
Weight change	X	X	X	X	X	X
Circumferences			X			X
Skinfolds			X			
Biochemical						
Albumin			X		X	
Cholesterol			X		X	
Clinical						
Clinical signs			X	X		
Functional status	X	X	X		X[4]	X
Oral status	X	X	X	X		
Mental status			X		X	X
Drug use			X	X		X
Dietary						
Food group intake	X	X	X			X
Nonalcoholic fluid intake						X
Alcoholic beverage intake	X	X	X			
Change in food intake	X		X	X		X
Eating alone	X		X			
Food insecurity	X	X	X		X	
Appetite		X	X	X		
Special diet		X	X	X		
Other						
Living environment		X	X			X
Smoking				X		
Self-assessed nutritional and health status				X		X
Target population						
Free-living[5]	X	X		X		X
Adult day-care center	X	X		X		X
Congregate meal site	X	X		X		X
Home-delivered meal program	X	X				
Long-term care facility				X	X	X
Medical office				X	X	X
Hospital				X	X	X

[1]Nutritional Risk Index (Ref. 81)
[2]SCALES = sadness, cholesterol, albumin, loss of weight, eating and shopping (Ref. 52)
[3]Mini Nutritional Assessment (Ref. 27)
[4]Only self-feeding skills
[5]Older adults residing in the community but not participating in congregate meal site programs or adult day-care centers

The NRI consists of 16 questions (see box) which focus on the mechanics of food intake, prescribed dietary restrictions, morbid conditions affecting food intake, discomfort associated with food intake, and significant changes in dietary habits. The NRI can be administered in a variety of settings by personnel with limited training, paraprofessionals, or allied health professionals. It is also suitable for use in telephone surveys.

Clinical validation studies have shown that the NRI is significantly correlated with established clinical and biochemical indicators of nutritional status, such as BMI, abdominal circumference, hemoglobin, and hydration status. Individuals scoring 7 or more on the NRI are considered to be at greater risk for poor nutritional status, poor health status in general, and greater use of health services than are individuals scoring less than 7.[81] The value of the NRI is its ability to assist professionals in identifying older adults in need of nutritional interventions or in-depth nutritional status assessment.

The checklist shown in figure 11-5 was developed as part of the Nutrition Screening Initiative (NSI), a multifaceted national effort to promote routine nutrition screening.[59] This initiative began in 1990 and is under the direction of the American Academy of Family Physicians, the American Dietetic Association, and the National Council on the Aging. The statements in the checklist, written at a fourth to sixth grade level, provide a vehicle for the older adult or caregiver to determine risk factors associated with the elderly person and a starting point for a general discussion about nutrition and health. Nutritional screenings based on the NSI model have been initiated by Departments of Aging in approximately 40 states.[57] Published reports indicate its usefulness in identifying older adults at greater risk for malnutrition, including those who take more than three drugs a day, eat alone, and have illnesses that result in changes in eating patterns.[30,47,57,62,72,84] The checklist has been translated to several languages, including Vietnamese, Chinese, Spanish, and Korean.[84]

Individuals receiving higher scores on the checklist are more likely to have (1) low nutrient

❖ **NUTRITIONAL RISK INDEX (NRI): QUESTIONS**

Do you wear dentures?
In the past month, have you taken any medicines prescribed by a doctor?
Have you ever had an operation in your abdomen?
In the past month, have you taken any medicines that were not prescribed by your doctor?
Do you have any troubles with your bowels that make you constipated or give you any diarrhea?
Are there any types of foods that you do not eat because they disagree with you?
Do you have trouble biting or chewing any type of food?
Do you now have an illness or condition that interferes with your eating?
Do you smoke cigarettes regularly now?
Are you on any type of a special diet?
Have you ever been told by a doctor that you were anemic (had iron-poor blood)?
Have you had any spells of pain or discomfort lasting three days or more in your abdomen or stomach in the past month?
Do you have an illness that has cut down on your appetite?
Have you had any trouble swallowing for at least three days in the last month?
Have you had any vomiting for at least three days in the last month?
Have you gained or lost any weight in the last 30 days? (NOTE: net gain/loss must exceed 10 pounds.)

Modified from Wolinsky, F.D., and others: Progress in the development of a nutritional risk index, J. Nutr. 120:1549, 1990.

intakes compared to the RDAs, (2) increased risk of adverse health conditions,[80] and (3) fair or poor perceived health status.[62] Like the NRI, the checklist is not intended to replace standard clinical or biochemical indicators; nor is it to replace accepted diagnostic approaches. Both

The Warning Signs of poor nutritional health are often overlooked. Use this checklist to find out if you or someone you know is at nutritional risk.

Read the statements below. Circle the number in the yes column for those that apply to you or someone you know. For each yes answer, score the number in the box. Total your nutritional score.

DETERMINE YOUR NUTRITIONAL HEALTH

	YES
I have an illness or condition that made me change the kind and/or amount of food I eat.	2
I eat fewer than 2 meals per day.	3
I eat few fruits or vegetables, or milk products.	2
I have 3 or more drinks of beer, liquor or wine almost every day.	2
I have tooth or mouth problems that make it hard for me to eat.	2
I don't always have enough money to buy the food I need.	4
I eat alone most of the time.	1
I take 3 or more different prescribed or over-the-counter drugs a day.	1
Without wanting to, I have lost or gained 10 pounds in the last 6 months.	2
I am not always physically able to shop, cook and/or feed myself.	2
TOTAL	

Total Your Nutritional Score. If it's —

0-2   **Good!** Recheck your nutritional score in 6 months.

3-5   **You are at moderate nutritional risk.** See what can be done to improve your eating habits and lifestyle. Your office on aging, senior nutrition program, senior citizens center or health department can help. Recheck your nutritional score in 3 months.

6 or more   **You are at high nutritional risk.** Bring this checklist the next time you see your doctor, dietitian or other qualified health or social service professional. Talk with them about any problems you may have. Ask for help to improve your nutritional health.

These materials developed and distributed by the Nutrition Screening Initiative, a project of:

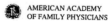
AMERICAN ACADEMY OF FAMILY PHYSICIANS

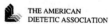
THE AMERICAN DIETETIC ASSOCIATION

NC OA   NATIONAL COUNCIL ON THE AGING, INC.

Remember that warning signs suggest risk, but do not represent diagnosis of any condition. Turn the page to learn more about the Warning Signs of poor nutritional health.

FIG. 11-5   Nutrition Screening Initiative Checklist.

Reprinted with permission by the Nutrition Screening Initiative, a project of the American Academy of Family Physicians, the American Dietetic Association and the National Council on the Aging, Inc., and funded in part by a grant from Ross Products Division, Abbott Laboratories.

are devices to be used to identify older individuals who are candidates for more detailed and extensive nutritional assessment measurements as well as health or social services intervention.

A score above 6 on the checklist indicates the need for more in-depth assessment, specifically the administration of either the Level 1 or Level 2 Screening Tool.[58] The Level 1 Screen is designed to be administered in community settings by professionals such as dietitians, trained caregivers, and health and social service professionals. This screen addresses body weight, BMI, changes in weight, eating habits, living environment, and functional status. The Level 1 Screen is designed to distinguish between two categories of older adults: those with documented, significant changes in body weight that require immediate referral to a health professional for more intensive nutritional assessment and those who do not have a quantifiable nutritional deficit severe enough to require a referral for specific medical care. The latter group may benefit from preventive interventions such as participating in congregate or home-delivered meal programs, shopping or transportation assistance, dietary counseling, socialization activities, and participation in food or economic assistance programs.

For individuals requiring more specific diagnostic information on nutritional status, the Level 2 Screening Tool should be administered. The Level 2 Screen is designed for use by physicians and other medical professionals to identify older adults with common nutrition-related problems such as protein-energy malnutrition, obesity, hyperlipidemia, and osteoporosis. It includes the indicators from the Level 1 Screen plus the following measurements:

- Anthropometric measures: mid-arm circumference, triceps skinfold, mid-arm muscle circumference;
- Biochemical tests: serum albumin, total serum cholesterol;
- Cognitive assessment: mental status exam;
- Emotional status assessment: Geriatric Depression Scale, Beck Depression Index;
- Chronic medication use: number and name of prescription and nonprescription drugs;
- Clinical signs of nutrient deficiency: skin changes, bone pain or fractures, oral tissue changes.[80]

Information obtained from the Level 2 Screen can be used in the development of nutritional support interventions for older adults in a variety of settings, such as nursing homes, adult day-care centers, doctors' offices, and hospitals.

Morley has developed a simple screening tool for dietitians and physicians called SCALES.[52] SCALES is an acronym for:

S—sadness (Yesavage Geriatric Depression scale),
C—cholesterol (less than 160 mg/dl),
A—albumin (less than 40 g/l),
L—loss of weight (2 pounds in 1 month or 5 pounds in 6 months),
E—eat (self-feeding problems), and
S—shopping (insufficient money to buy food and the inability to obtain and prepare it).

This instrument has demonstrated high specificity and sensitivity in detecting older individuals at nutritional risk, particularly protein-energy undernutrition.

The Mini Nutritional Assessment (MNA) was developed to accurately evaluate the nutritional status of older adults: normal or well-nourished, borderline or at nutritional risk, or undernourished[27] (see appendix C). The MNA consists of 18 questions focusing on anthropometric measurements, dietary questions (eight questions related to number of meals, food and fluid intake, and autonomy of feeding), global assessment (six questions related to lifestyle, medication, and mobility), and subjective assessment (self-perception of nutrition and health). (See table 11-8.) It was validated and cross-validated in elderly populations ranging from the very frail to the very healthy. This instrument takes less than 10 minutes to administer. Additional biochemical indicators, such as serum albumin, cholesterol, C reactive protein, and lymphocyte counts, may be included, lengthening the time to about 20 minutes for the blood drawing. With this tool, approximately 2% of older adults are misclassified with respect to their nutritional status. The MNA is available in 15 languages including Spanish, German, Japanese, Chinese, and English.

❖ ❖ ❖
CASE STUDY

Mrs. A is a 78-year-old woman living in an assisted-care facility. She is nonambulatory, but gets around reasonably well in a wheelchair. She prefers to prepare her own meals in her apartment and often refuses to eat in the facility's dining room. She has been diagnosed with severe osteoporosis, but has no other chronic health concerns. The nurse in the assisted-care facility has asked you to assess her nutritional status.

1. Describe the specific methods you would use to complete a thorough nutritional assessment of Mrs. A.

2. What standards would you use to evaluate the clinical, anthropometric, biochemical, and dietary data you collect?

3. What are some confounding factors that will make the interpretation of your findings difficult?

4. If your assessment leads to the identification of protein-energy malnutrition, what approach would you take in your attempt to improve Mrs. A's nutritional status?

Remember the special considerations when performing nutritional assessments of older adults. The normal process of aging, the presence of chronic conditions or diseases, and the frequent use of prescription drugs can affect the interpretation of nutritional assessment data. Nutritional assessment methods are available for older adults, although there is a lack of consensus on which and how many indicators are needed to accurately assess the nutritional status of older adults. Reference standards also require some refinement to meet the special considerations of some older adults.

Summary

Nutritional assessment is the integration and interpretation of anthropometric, biochemical, clinical, and dietary data to determine the nutritional and health status of individuals and populations. Nutritional status can range from optimal to severely malnourished. Many older adults in the United States are at risk of nutritional deficits, excesses, or imbalances as a result of aging changes, chronic disease, or poor or inappropriate dietary patterns.

Anthropometric measurements are used to estimate or predict amounts of the various components of the body such as muscle or fat. They are particularly useful in detecting moderate and severe degrees of protein-energy malnutri-

tion. Biochemical methods are the most sensitive indicators of nutritional status; however, they are not always specific for the nutrient involved. Biochemical parameters can be influenced by other factors such as chronic disease, hydration status, and inflammation. Nutritional inadequacies result in clinical signs which are useful in assessing nutritional status. It is important to recognize, however, that many of the clinical symptoms and signs seen in the elderly can have both nutritional and nonnutritional causes. In addition to physical signs, clinical assessment also includes evaluation of functional status, oral status, and mental and cognitive status of older adults.

Several methods are useful for the assessment of dietary intake in the elderly. Each method has strengths and weaknesses. Before selecting a dietary assessment method, it is necessary to identify the objective of the assessment and whether it will be conducted on a few individuals or on a large group. Once collected, dietary data must be evaluated against established standards of adequacy such as the Recommended Dietary Allowances or the Healthy Eating Index. Screening tools that take a relatively short time for completion are valuable in identifying older people at risk who are in need of nutritional counseling or services to prevent the development of overt malnutrition.

REVIEW QUESTIONS

1. Define nutrition assessment, nutrition surveillance, and nutrition screening. When is it appropriate to use each method? Why does nutrition assessment of older people pose problems for practitioners?
2. Distinguish between marginal nutritional status, malnutrition, and nutritional imbalance. What types of information are essential to establish the presence of these conditions?
3. What is anthropometry, and what anthropometric techniques are useful in assessing the elderly? How can aging influence body measurements? What is relative weight for height? Why are circumference measurements useful in nutrition assessment of older people?
4. What are the most reliable biochemical indicators of protein-energy malnutrition in the elderly? Why is the identification of iron deficiency important in the older person? What laboratory tests are most useful for identification of iron-deficiency anemia?
5. What are the differences between prospective and retrospective methods for collecting and assessing food intake information? What are the advantages and disadvantages of each type of method? What guidelines are useful for evaluating dietary intake information?
6. Identify several commonly used nutrition screening tools. Why is nutrition screening important? In what settings are particular nutrition screening tools most appropriate?

SUGGESTED LEARNING ACTIVITIES

1. Ask the director of a senior center if you may conduct a nutrition screening clinic. Half of the class should use the Nutritional Risk index and half of the class should use the "Determine Your Nutritional Health" checklist. Tabulate and compare your results. Prepare a class report that discusses the advantages and disadvantages of each method.
2. As part of your nutrition screening clinic, do a height and weight measurement for each participant. Record the difficulties encountered in obtaining these data in an older population. Determine the body mass index for each older person measured. Work with a registered dietitian to provide a follow-up activity for those with a body mass index outside of the range recommended by the Nutrition Screening Initiative or Nutritional Risk Index.
3. Go to the library and find all of the references that give normal values for biochemical measures of iron and folate status in older populations. Prepare a report that incudes a table to be used as a reference for biochemical assessment and discuss the limitations of current normal values for assessing iron and folate status of specific elderly individuals.
4. Obtain a 24-hour recall and a two-day written dietary record from an older relative or friend. Be sure to include one weekend day. Calculate the nutrient content using a computer program and list the number and size of portions from each food group. Evaluate the nutritional adequacy of the three-day record according to the Recommended Dietary Allowances, the Dietary Guidelines for Americans, the Food Guide Pyramid, and the Healthy Eating Index. Did all of these methods lead to the same conclusion? Develop a plan to assist your older client in making any dietary changes that would be appropriate.

REFERENCES

1. Abernethy, M.M., and Fanelli Kuczmarski, M.: Food intake and food related attitudes of older women: Implications for nutrition education, J. Nutr. Ed. 26:3, 1994.
2. Anderson, S.A.: Core indicators of nutritional state for difficult-to-sample populations, Besthesda, MD, 1990, Life Sciences Research Office, Federation of American Societies for Experimental Biology.
3. Beck, A.T., and Beck, R.W.: Screening depressed patients in family practice: A rapid technique, Postgrad. Med. Dec:81, 1972.
4. Beers, M.M., Fink, A., and Beck, J.C.: Screening recommendations for the elderly, Am. J. Public Health 81:1131, 1991.
5. Bjorntorp, P.: Obesity and the risk of cardiovascular disease, Ann. Clin. Res. 17:3, 1985.
6. Blackburn, G.L., and others: Nutrition in metabolic assessment of the hospitalized patient, J. Parenteral and Enteral Nutr. 1:11, 1977.
7. Briefel, R.R. and Woteki, C.E.: Development of food sufficiency questions for the Third National Health and Nutrition Examination Survey, J. Nutr. Ed. 24:24S, 1992.
8. Burman, M.A., and others: Development of a brief screening instrument for detecting depressive disorders, Med. Care 26:775, 1988.
9. Byers, T.E., and others: Dietary history from the distant past: a methodological study, Nutr. Cancer 5:69, 1983.

10. Campbell, V.A., and Dodds, M.L.: Collecting dietary information from groups of older people, J. Am. Diet. Assoc. 51:29, 1967.
11. Chianetta, M.M., and Head, M.K.: Effect of prior notification on accuracy of dietary recall by the elderly, J. Am. Diet. Assoc. 92:741, 1992.
12. Chumlea, W.C., and Guo, S.: Equations for predicting stature in white and black elderly individuals, J. Gerontol. 47:197, 1992.
13. Chumlea, W.C., and others: Bioelectrical and anthropometric assessments and reference data in the elderly, J. Nutr. 123:449, 1993.
14. Chumlea, W.C., Guo, S.S., and Vellas, B.: Anthropometry and body composition in the elderly, Facts and Research in Gerontology, Supplement 2:61, 1994.
15. Chumlea, W.C., and Kuczmarski, R.J.: Using a bony landmark to measure waist circumference, J. Am. Diet. Assoc. 95:12, 1995.
16. Chumlea, W.C., Roche, A.F., and Steinbaugh, M.L.: Estimating stature from knee height for persons 60 to 90 years of age, J. Am. Geriat. Soc. 33:116, 1985.
17. Cornoni-Huntley, J.C., and others: An overview of body weight of older persons, including impact on mortality, J. Clin. Epidemiol. 44:743, 1991.
18. Corti, M.C., and others: HDL cholesterol predicts coronary heart disease mortality in older persons, J.A.M.A. 274:539, 1995.
19. Deurenberg, P., and others: Assessment of body composition by bioelectrical impedance in a population aged >60 yrs, Am. J. Clin. Nutr. 51:3, 1990.
20. Dwyer, J.T.: Assessment of dietary intake. In: Shils, M.E., and Young, V.R., editors: Modern nutrition in health and disease, ed. 7, Philadelphia, 1988, Lea & Febiger.
21. Dwyer, J.T.: Screening older Americans' nutritional health: Current practice and future possibilities, Washington, DC, 1991, Nutrition Screening Initiative.
22. Frisancho, A.R.: New standards of weight and body composition by frame size and height for assessment of nutritional status of adults and elderly, Am. J. Clin. Nutr. 40:808, 1984.
23. Galanos, A.N., and others: Nutrition and function: Is there a relationship between body mass index and the functional capabilities of community-dwelling elderly? J. Am. Geriatr. Soc. 42:368, 1994.
24. Gibson, R.A.: Principles of nutritional assessment, New York, 1990, Oxford University Press.
25. Gilmore, S.A., and others: Clinical indicators associated with unintentional weight loss and pressure ulcers in elderly residents of nursing facilities, J. Am. Diet. Assoc. 95:984, 1995.
26. Goodwin, J.S., Goodwin, J.M., and Garry, P.J.: Association between nutritional status and cognitive functioning in a healthy elderly population, J. Am. Med. Assoc. 249:2917, 1983.
27. Guigoz, Y., Vellas, B., and Garry, P.J.: Mini Nutritional Assessment: A practical assessment tool for grading the nutritional state of elderly patients, Facts and Research in Gerontology, Supplement 2:15, 1994.
28. Hankin, J.H.: Development of a diet history questionnaire for studies of older persons, Am. J. Clin. Nutr. 50:1121, 1989.
29. Herbert, V.: The 1986 Herman Award lecture. Nutrition science as a continually unfolding story: the folate and vitamin B-12 paradigm, Am. J. Clin Nutr. 46:387, 1987.
30. Herndon, A.S.: Using the Nutrition Screening Initiative to survey the nutritional status of clients participating in a home-delivered meals program, J. Nutr. Elderly 14:15, 1995.
31. Heymsfield, S.B., and others: Anthropometric assessment of adult protein-energy malnutrition. In: Wright, R.A., Hemysfield, S., and McMan, C.B., editors: Nutritional assessment, Boston, 1984, Blackwell Scientific Publications, Inc.
32. Heymsfield, S.B., and Williams, P.J.: Nutritional assessment by clinical and biochemical methods. In: Shils, M.E., and Young, V.R., editors: Modern nutrition in health and disease, ed. 7, Philadelphia, 1988, Lea & Febiger.
33. Human Nutrition Information Service: USDA's food guide pyramid, Home and Garden Bulletin No. 249, Hyattsville, MD, 1992, U.S. Department of Agriculture.
34. Howard, J.H.: Nutritional parameters and assessment in the elderly, Top. Clin. Nutr. 11:77, 1996.
35. Jeor, S.T., and Scott, B.J.: "Weight" as a clinical indicator: adults, Top. Clin. Nutr. 7:44, 1991.
36. Kennedy, E.T., and others: The Healthy Eating Index: design and applications, J. Am. Diet. Assoc. 95:1103, 1995.
37. Kobriger, A.M.: Laboratory values in the elderly, Chilton, WI, 1995, Kobriger Presents.
38. Kuczmarski, R.J.: Need for body composition information in elderly subjects, Am. J. Clin. Nutr. 50:1150, 1989.
39. Kumanyika, S., and others: Picture-sort method for administering a food frequency questionnaire to older adults, J. Am. Diet. Assoc. 96:137, 1996.

40. Kwok, T., and Whitelaw, M.N.: The use of arm span in nutritional assessment of the elderly, J. Am. Geriatr. Soc. 39:492, 1991.

41. Life Sciences Research Office, Federation of American Societies for Experimental Biology: Nutrition monitoring in the United States: An update report on nutrition monitoring, DHHS Publication No. (PHS) 89-1255, Washington, DC, 1989, U.S. Government Printing Office.

42. Lipschitz, D.A., and Mitchell, C.O.: Nutritional assessment of the elderly: special considerations. In: Wright, R.A., Hemysfield, S., and McMan, C.B., editors: Nutritional Assessment, Boston, 1984, Blackwell Scientific Publications, Inc.

43. Lohman, T.G., Roche, A.F., and Martorell, R., editors: Anthropometric Standardization Reference Manual, Champaign, IL, 1988, Human Kinetics Books.

44. Madden, J.P., Goodman, S.J., and Guthrie, H.A.: Validity of the 24-hr. recall: analysis of data obtained from elderly subjects, J. Am. Diet. Assoc. 68:143, 1976.

45. Mahalko, J.R., and others: Comparison of dietary histories and seven-day food records in a nutritional assessment of older adults, Am. J. Clin. Nutr. 42:542, 1985.

46. Master, A.M., Lasser, R.P., and Beckman, G.: Tables of average weight and height of Americans aged 65 to 94 years, J. Am. Med. Assoc. 172:658, 1960.

47. Melnik, T.A., and others: Screening elderly in the community: the relationship between dietary adequacy and nutritional risk, J. Am. Diet. Assoc. 94:1425, 1994.

48. Metropolitan Life Insurance Company: 1983 Metropolitan height and weight tables, Statistical Bulletin 64:2, 1983.

49. Mitchell, C.O., and Lipschitz, D.A.: Arm length as an alternative to height in nutritional assessment of the elderly, J. Parenteral and Enteral Nutr. 6:226, 1982.

50. Mitchell, C.O., and Lipschitz, D.A.: Detection of protein-calorie malnutrition in the elderly, Am. J. Clin. Nutr. 35:398, 1982.

51. Mitchell, C.O., and Lipschitz, D.A.: The effect of age and sex on the routinely used measurements to assess the nutritional status of hospitalized patients, Am. J. Clin. Nutr. 36:340, 1982.

52. Morley, J.E.: Nutritional assessment is a key component of geriatric assessment, Facts and Research in Gerontology, Supplement 2:5, 1994.

53. National Institutes of Health: Expert panel on detection, evaluation, and treatment of high blood cholesterol in adults (Adult Treatment Panel II), NIH Publication No. 93-3096, Bethesda, MD, 1993, U.S. National Heart, Lung and Blood Institute.

54. National Research Council: Diet and health: implications for reducing chronic disease risk, Washington, DC, 1989, National Academy Press.

55. National Research Council: Recommended Dietary Allowances, ed. 10, Washington, DC, 1989, National Academy Press.

56. Natow, A.B., and Heslin, J.: Nutritional care of the older adult, New York, 1986, Macmillan Publishing Co.

57. NSI Technical Review Committee: Appropriate and effective use of the NSI checklist and screens, J. Am. Diet. Assoc. 95:647, 1995.

58. Nutrition interventions manual for professionals caring for older Americans, Washington, DC, 1992, the Nutrition Screening Initiative.

59. Nutrition screening manual for professionals caring for older Americans, Washington, DC, 1991, the Nutrition Screening Initiative.

60. Osterkamp, L.K.: Current perspective on assessment of human body proportions of relevance to amputees, Am. J. Diet. Assoc. 95:215, 1995.

61. Ostlund, R.E., and others: The ratio of waist-to-hip circumference, plasma insulin level, and glucose intolerance as independent predictors of the HDL_2 cholesterol level in older adults, New Engl. J. Med. 322:229, 1990.

62. Posner, B.M., and others: Nutrition and health risks in the elderly: the nutrition screening initiative, Am. J. Public Health 83:972, 1993.

63. Radloff, L.S.: The CES-D scale: a self-report depression scale for research in the general population, Appl. Psychiatr. Meas. 1:385, 1977.

64. Remig, V.M., Shumaker, N.S., and Jeor, S.T.: Weight as a clinical indicator, Top. Clin. Nutr. 8:16, 1993.

65. Robins, L.N., and others: National Institute of Mental Health Diagnostic Interview Schedule: its history, characteristics, and validity. Arch. Gen. Psychiatry 38:381, 1981.

66. Roe, D.A.: Geriatric Nutrition, ed. 3, Englewood Cliffs, NJ, 1992, Prentice Hall.

67. Roe, D.A.: In-home nutritional assessment of inner-city elderly, J. Nutr. 120:1538, 1990.

68. Roe, D.: Nutritional assessment of the elderly, World Rev. Nutr. Diet. 48:85, 1986.

69. Rudman, D., and Feller, A.G.: Protein-calorie undernutrition in the nursing home, J. Am. Geriatr. Soc. 37:173, 1989.

70. Samet, J.M.: Surrogate measures of dietary intake, Am. J. Clin. Nutr. 50:39, 1989.

71. Smiciklas-Wright, H., and others: Nutritional assessment of homebound rural elderly, J. Nutr. 120:1535, 1990.

72. Spangler, A.A., and Eigenbrod, J.S.: Field trial affirms value of DETERMINE-ing nutrition-related problems of free-living elderly, Am. J. Diet. Assoc. 95:489, 1995.

73. Stevens, J., Gautam, S.P., and Keil, J.E.: Body mass index and fat patterning as correlates of lipids and hypertension in an elderly, biracial population, J. Gerontol. 48:M249, 1993.

74. Svendsen, O.L., and others: Measurement of body fat in elderly subjects by dual-energy x-ray absorptiometry, bioelectrical impedance, and anthropometry, Am. J. Clin. Nutr. 53:1117, 1991.

75. U.S. Department of Agriculture: Report of the dietary guidelines advisory committee on the dietary guidelines for Americans, Washington, DC, 1995, U.S. Government Printing Office.

76. U.S. Department of Agriculture: The healthy eating index, Washington, DC, 1995, U.S. Government Printing Office.

77. U.S. Department of Agriculture and U.S. Department of Health and Human Services: Nutrition and your health: dietary guidelines for Americans, ed. 4, Home and Garden Bulletin No. 232, Washington, DC, 1995, U.S. Government Printing Office.

78. U.S. Department of Health and Human Services: Anthropometric procedures video. Produced by the National Center for Health Statistics, Centers for Disease Control and Prevention, 1996 (Stock No. 017-022-01335-5).

79. U.S. Department of Health and Human Services and U.S. Department of Agriculture: Nutrition monitoring in the United States: a progress report from the joint nutrition monitoring evaluation committee, DHHS Publication No. (PHS) 86-1255, Washington, DC, 1986, U.S. Government Printing Office.

80. White, J.V., and others: Nutrition screening initiative: development and implementation of the public awareness checklist and screening tools, J. Am. Diet. Assoc. 92:163, 1992.

81. Wolinsky, F.D., and others: Progress in the development of a nutritional risk index, J. Nutr. 120:1549, 1990.

82. Yesavage, J.A., and others: Development and validation of a geriatric depression screening scale: a preliminary report, J. Psychiat. Res. 17:37, 1983.

83. Zung, W.W.: A self-rating depression scale, Arch. Gen. Psychiatry. 12:63, 1965.

84. Zylstra, R.C.E., and others: Who's at risk in Washington state? Demographic characteristics affect nutritional risk behaviors in elderly meal participants, J. Am. Diet. Assoc. 95:358, 1995.

12 Nutritional Problems and Deficiencies in the Aging Adult

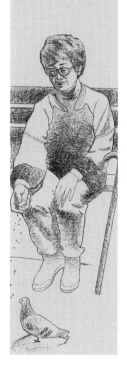

✦✦

Objectives

After studying the chapter, the student should be able to:

✔ *Identify the nutrition problems and deficiencies most commonly seen in older populations*

✔ *Recognize the prevalence and impact of nutritional anemias in aging adults*

✔ *Understand the mechanisms of adult bone loss leading to osteoporosis and list the treatments, including nutrition interventions*

✔ *Recognize the importance of undernutrition and weight loss in older people and strategies for prevention*

✔ *List common problems with gastrointestinal function in older people and understand the importance of dietary treatment*

INTRODUCTION

Both health and lifestyle influence nutrient intake and the development of nutrition problems in the older adult. Economic limitations and physical disability can limit both the amount and type of food consumed, hastening the development of protein-energy malnutrition. Chronic disease can exacerbate the deleterious effects of malnutrition or complicate the diagnosis of a nutrition-related disorder such as iron-deficiency anemia. Osteoporosis, a major cause of disability in older adults, is influenced by genetic factors and age-related changes in hormone secretion, but it also is strongly associated with lifelong calcium intake. In this chapter we will discuss nutrition-related problems in the older adult, their physiologic consequences, and strategies to prevent or ameliorate their occurrence.

NUTRITIONAL ANEMIAS

Causes of Anemia

Anemia results from a change in either the number or characteristics of the erythrocyte. A progressive anemia that leads to a decrease in the oxygen-carrying capacity of the blood and an oxygen deficit in the tissues can cause an increase in heart rate, shortness of breath, and weakness. Nutritional anemias are most commonly related to deficiencies of iron, folate, or vitamin B-12 and are reversed when the nutrient is restored. In older people anemias often are associated with protein-energy malnutrition, infection, inflammation, and chronic disease and may involve several nutrients. Erban[26] pointed out that hematologic abnormalities in older people should be recognized and assessed early, as they are frequently the earliest indicators of failing health or serious disease.

Types of Anemia

The two types of nutritional anemias usually found in older people result from (1) the inadequate production of erythrocytes stemming from an inadequate supply of iron (iron-deficient erythropoiesis) or (2) ineffective erythropoiesis caused by a lack of folate or vitamin B-12 required for the maturation of the red blood cell.[49] The majority of anemias identified in older people arise from an inadequate supply of iron for normal erythropoiesis. These anemias include iron-deficiency anemia and the anemia of chronic disease. Although both anemias are caused by a lack of sufficient iron for the normal production of red blood cells, in each case very different causes produce the change in iron supply. The most common type of anemia related to ineffective erythropoiesis is pernicious anemia.

Anemias Related to Inadequate Iron Supply

Iron-deficiency anemia. The nutritional anemia most easily identified and corrected in older people is iron-deficiency anemia, although vitamin deficiencies may complicate the problem. Iron-deficiency anemia is caused by (1) poor iron intake, (2) poor iron absorption, or (3) increased erythropoiesis resulting from chronic blood loss. Occult blood loss through the gastrointestinal tract is a frequent and critical cause of iron-deficiency anemia in older people. Excessive blood in the stool may go unnoticed and be discovered only on examination for anemia or other problems. Normal blood loss in the stool is less than 3 ml a day; losses above this level are pathologic. Blood losses of 50 to 75 ml impart a dark red or black color to the stool; however, significant losses below this amount are not usually obvious and require chemical analysis for detection.

Conditions associated with gastrointestinal bleeding include peptic ulcer disease, gastritis, diverticulitis, hiatus hernia, hemorrhoids, and cancer. Long-term use of aspirin, which irritates the gastric mucosa, can lead to significant blood loss.[49] Frequently individuals are free of symptoms and do not seek medical attention until the condition has progressed and the anemia is severe. One milliliter of blood from an individual with a hemoglobin level of 15 g/dl contains about 0.5 mg of iron; consequently, extended losses severely deplete iron stores.

Anemia of chronic disease. The anemia of chronic disease is usually associated with another disease or physiologic response to disease. Heart disease, renal disease, and inflammatory bowel disease can lead to this type of anemia. Inflammation resulting from rheumatoid arthritis, infection, an immune reaction, or cancer is related to anemia of chronic disease. Older adults with protein-energy malnutrition (PEM) develop an anemia characterized by low serum iron and transferrin saturation.[49]

Both iron-deficiency anemia and the anemia of chronic disease involve iron-deficient erythropoiesis, but their etiologies are vastly different. In iron-deficiency anemia, iron stores have been depleted as a result of blood loss or long-term deficient intake or absorption. In the anemia of chronic disease, the iron from degraded erythrocytes accumulates in the reticuloendothelial cells and is blocked from release; thus, inadequate iron is delivered to the bone marrow for incorporation into newly forming erythrocytes. In infection, body iron stores are blocked from release to make iron less available to the disease organism. These metabolic changes in infection and inflammation are part of the acute phase response mediated by interleukin 1. In the anemia of chronic disease, tissue iron stores are normal or may actually be elevated.[49]

Prevalence of Iron-Related Anemia

The prevalence of anemia varies according to age, sex, socioeconomic status, race, general health, and the hematologic standard used. Among healthy, economically advantaged older people in the Boston Nutritional Status Survey,[78] 9% of the men and 11% of the women had hemoglobin levels below 13.3 g/dl and 12.5 g/dl, respectively (these criteria for anemia were based on sex- and age-specific standards derived from the NHANES II study). Less than 3% of the anemic elderly had low serum ferritin and less than 5% had low serum iron. Among these independently living elderly, anemia was related to age. Only 8% of those below age 70 were anemic as compared to 18% of those in their 80s and 90s. Five percent of the anemic women and 10% of the anemic men had low serum vitamin B-12. In a survey of 80 older Canadians (ages 59 to 88) living in the community,[54] 21% of the women and 27% of the men had hemoglobin levels in the deficient range; however, a similar number also had deficient serum vitamin B-12 levels. Fewer than 4% had abnormally low ferritin, suggesting that a vitamin B-12 deficiency rather than a lack of iron was causing the anemia. In 193 health-conscious older people in Paris,[71] iron depletion was identified in 9% of the subjects. Among older men admitted to a veteran's hospital diagnostic clinic,[49] 58% had hemoglobin levels below 14 g/dl.

Institutionalized individuals with chronic disease are more likely to be anemic. A comparison of 50 independent-living and 50 institutionalized older people[14] revealed that only 4% of the men and 8% of the women living in the community had iron-deficiency anemia, whereas this was true of 40% of the institutionalized group.

Food intake and medications influenced the presence or absence of anemia among the elderly participants in the Boston Nutritional Status Survey.[78] Anemic elderly were more likely to be underweight based on body mass index measurements, and they had lower triceps skinfold thicknesses. Those with normal blood parameters had higher intakes of kilocalories and protein and better protein status. A striking finding was that the anemic elderly were taking more medications of the over-the-counter type, and Russell[78] questioned if medications such as aspirin might have contributed to the observed anemia. Overall food intake may play a major role in the development of anemia as individuals living alone, housebound elderly, and people over age 80 were more likely to be anemic; all of these circumstances are associated with lower food intake. Surprisingly, the number of diagnosed diseases was not higher among the anemic versus the nonanemic participants. Reduced food intake, weight loss, and self-medication may all be markers of a deteriorating health status associated with anemia.

Age and Hematologic Parameters

Currently, there is no evidence to suggest that different standards should be used to evaluate hematologic status in older people. An evaluation of healthy elderly people age 84 and over revealed that hematologic values are remarkably stable into advanced age.[92] All mean values were within the normal range. In the 20 participants who were studied over a five-year period, the variation in hemoglobin levels within individual subjects was only 0.55 g/dl.

The idea that age itself is a risk factor for anemia and that older people are likely to become anemic as they age leads to the false assumption that anemia is inevitable, which delays or precludes appropriate evaluation and treatment of the underlying cause. Normal ranges for the general population of adults appear to include about 80% of the general elderly population, which is likely to contain individuals with illness or conditions that lead to anemia.[26] Unfortunately, a recent survey[21] indicated that many clinicians expect an age-related decline in the parameters used to assess anemia. About half of the 232 physicians responding indicated that they would accept a difference of up to 2 g/dl from their usual standard for hemoglobin before initiating a stool test for occult blood in an elderly patient. Beard and coworkers[7] noted that some researchers support the development of

TABLE 12-1   Parameters Used to Identify Anemia and the Cause

Parameter	Advantages and Limitations with Older People
Hemoglobin	Does not support early intervention as levels drop relatively late in the development of anemia; low levels do not distinguish between iron deficiency or other anemias; levels are reduced by inflammation or infection and in folate or vitamin B-12 deficiency; level is increased in dehydration.
Mean corpuscular volume	Does not support early intervention because volume decreases only when iron deficiency has become severe; folate or vitamin B-12 deficiency causes an increase in volume; when both iron and vitamin B-12 deficiencies are present, there may be no change in volume.
Serum iron, transferrin, and transferrin saturation	Serum iron decreases fairly early in the development of iron-deficiency anemia; serum iron exhibits diurnal variation and decreases in infection and inflammation; transferrin levels are reduced by chronic disease, infection, inflammation, and protein-energy malnutrition.
Erythrocyte protoporphyrin level	Increases fairly early in the development of iron-deficiency anemia; levels increase in infection.
Serum ferritin	Decrease in level is an early indicator of declining iron status; extremely high levels indicate iron overload; levels are increased by chronic disease, liver disease, and inflammation.
Red blood cell count	Does not support early intervention as the total number of erythrocytes declines late in the development of iron-deficiency anemia; age-related changes in the bone marrow can reduce red blood cell production.
Acute phase response proteins (e.g., C-reactive protein)	Serum levels increase in infection and inflammation; may assist in differentiating iron-deficiency anemia and anemia of chronic disease.
Plasma transferrin receptors	Plasma transferrin receptors increase in iron-deficiency anemia but are not influenced by inflammatory diseases; may assist in differentiating iron-deficiency anemia and anemia of chronic disease.
Erythrocyte sedimentation rate	Red blood cells from elderly people with inflammatory disease have a higher sedimentation rate based on changes in blood proteins; may assist in differentiating iron-deficiency anemia and anemia of chronic disease.

age-specific criteria for anemia based on the fact that other developmental changes that occur in aging lead to differences in laboratory values between younger and older adults. In light of the known functional impairments associated with iron deficiency (see chapter 7), it would seem prudent to investigate all indicators of poor iron status.

Parameters for Evaluating Iron Status

Various parameters provide clues as to the cause and severity of an existing anemia. Individual methods and their general limitations for use with older people are described in table 12-1. Hemoglobin level is frequently used as an indicator of hematologic status because it requires only a small amount of blood and is a relatively inexpensive chemical test. Hemoglobin levels declined with age in the NHANES II study as did other indices of iron status.[7] When individuals with diseases likely to cause anemia were excluded, it appeared that the expected normal hemoglobin level was lower for men above age 70. Lipschitz,[48] who considers a hemoglobin level of 14 g/dl to represent the lower level of normal in men, noted that a large percentage of the men ages 65 to 74 in the NHANES II study would be classified as anemic if evaluated using this standard. In general the sex differences in hemoglobin and red blood cell counts observed in young adults tend to diminish in older adults. This is primarily the result of a decline in levels among older men, although a slight rise in levels has been observed in older women.[7]

Serum iron and transferrin levels are influenced more by body iron stores than by sex or age but are lower in elderly people with inflammatory diseases. In the NHANES II study,[67] fewer than 10% of older adults had a transferrin saturation below the normal range (less than 16%), although African American men were most likely to have a low saturation level.

Erythrocyte protoporphyrin levels have become recognized as indicators of faulty erythropoiesis. **Protoporphyrin** is a precursor of heme; if iron is unavailable for incorporation into hemoglobin, protoporphyrins will accumulate; thus, high levels indicate a developing anemia. Inflammation also elevates the erythrocyte protoporphyrin level, limiting the usefulness of this parameter in older people with chronic conditions. In the NHANES II study,[67] 10% of all men ages 65 to 74 had protoporphyrin levels that suggested a problem in hemoglobin synthesis.

Serum ferritin levels have been considered to provide a good estimate of iron stores (see chapter 7). In the general population[67] relatively few older adults (2% to 3%) have low serum ferritin levels (below 12 ng/ml). Conversely, about 5% appear to have iron overload as indicated by serum ferritin levels above 300 or 400 ng/ml, the upper limits of normal in women and men, respectively. Unfortunately, inflammation and several chronic diseases raise serum ferritin levels and can mask a true iron deficiency.[38] Holyoake and coworkers[38] evaluated serum ferritin and bone marrow iron stores in 472 consecutive referrals of elderly patients to a geriatric hospital. Of the 32 patients with serum ferritin between 12 and 45 ng/ml (consistent with normal iron status), 84% had no stainable iron in their bone marrow. Moreover, patients with ferritin levels up to 75 ng/ml had blood smears indicating iron deficiency.

At the other extreme, serum ferritin levels exceeding 1,000 ng/ml have been considered to be indicative of iron overload. A review of 95 patients with ferritin levels exceeding 1,000 ng/ml[43] revealed that for all but eight, the elevated ferritin was related to renal disease, liver disease, cancer, sickle cell disease, pneumonia, or recent blood transfusions. Those researchers[43] suggested that measures of transferrin saturation may provide a better basis for evaluation. If individuals have both a high ferritin and a high transferrin saturation, the possibility of iron overload needs to be seriously considered. Current analytic methods for ferritin are based on the measurement of its protein component, not its iron content. It appears that the chronic conditions noted above result in the synthesis of large amounts of ferritin with a lower concentration of iron than normal. A new analytic technique[37] that measures ferritin iron content and not merely the amount of ferritin, may assist in the diagnosis of iron status.

A further issue in the evaluation of iron status is the day-to-day variation within an individual. Ahluwalia and coworkers[3] evaluated the biologic variation in iron status parameters in relatively healthy women ages 70 to 79. Hemoglobin and serum ferritin levels appeared to have very little variation and a true estimate (within 20% of the true value) was obtained with one blood sample. In contrast, a true estimate of serum iron or transferrin saturation required blood samples on seven to eight days. Surprisingly, findings in a group of chronically ill, hospitalized elderly were similar to those in the healthy group.[7]

Diagnosis of Anemia

The correct and timely differential diagnosis of iron-deficiency anemia versus the anemia of chronic disease is critical to the health of the older adult. Iron deficiency not only is detrimental to general well-being, but also iron-deficiency anemia arising from chronic blood loss may be the first symptom of a serious medical problem.

The anemia of chronic disease and iron-deficiency anemia have somewhat different effects on erythrocytes and biochemical parameters of iron status (table 12-2).[7,48] Both conditions are characterized by low serum iron, low

TABLE 12-2 *Hematologic Parameters in Iron-Deficiency Anemia and the Anemia of Chronic Disease*

	Iron Deficiency Anemia	Anemia of Chronic Disease
Hemoglobin	<12 g/dl	<12 g/dl
Serum iron	<40 µg/dl	<60 µg/dl
Serum transferrin	>400 µg/dl	<250 µg/dl
Transferrin saturation (%)	<20%	<20%
Serum ferritin	<50 ng/ml	>100 ng/ml

Adapted from Lipschitz, D.A.: Impact of nutrition on the age-related declines in hematopoiesis. In Chernoff, R., editor: Geriatric nutrition. The health professional's handbook, Gaithersburg, MD, 1991, Aspen Publishers; and Beard, J.L., Ashraf, M.H., and Smiciklas-Wright, H.: Iron nutrition in the elderly. In: Watson, R.R.; editor: Handbook of nutrition in the aged, ed. 2, Boca Raton, 1994, CRC Press.

transferrin saturation, and high erythrocyte protoporphyrin levels, although Lipschitz[48] considers a low transferrin saturation to more likely indicate an iron deficiency. Iron stores are high in an anemia of chronic disease, and serum ferritin levels may exceed 100 ng/ml. In individuals with both inflammatory disorders and gastrointestinal iron loss, both types of anemia may be present; hence, ferritin levels between 50 ng/ml and 100 ng/ml often represent a combination of iron deficiency and an ongoing chronic disease.[49]

New research is focusing on other diagnostic indicators of inflammation that could assist in differentiating between iron-deficiency anemia and the anemia of chronic disease. Serum levels of proteins that are characteristic of the acute phase response to inflammation and infection may be one possible way of avoiding misdiagnosis of anemia.[18] In a study of 163 patients above age 60,[18] high levels of C-reactive protein were related to low serum iron and transferrin saturation levels and high serum ferritin levels. In a comparison of elderly women with rheumatoid arthritis (a chronic inflammatory disease) and other women similar in age,[4] a combination of serum ferritin, plasma transferrin receptors, and erythrocyte sedimentation rate successfully differentiated between iron-deficiency anemia and the anemia of chronic disease 81% of the time. Iron-deficiency anemia was verified by an increase in hemoglobin after supplementation with iron. Plasma transferrin receptor sites increase in iron-deficiency anemia but do not respond to inflammation. On the other hand, changes in blood proteins that occur in inflammation cause the red blood cells to clump together when tested for sedimentation rate. In this study[4] the women with anemia, whether iron-deficiency anemia or anemia of chronic disease, had lower incomes and were more functionally impaired based on measures of mental health, physical health, and the ability to perform activities of daily living.

Subclinical chronic disease may bring about changes in hematologic parameters in even the apparently healthy individual. One clinician[49] has emphasized that anemia is often multifactorial in frail older people who have multiple medical problems. An individual with rheumatoid arthritis is likely to be taking large amounts of aspirin that will cause blood loss; the same person, because of pain and stiffness, cannot prepare adequate meals. In such cases a bone marrow test indicating iron stores may be necessary for conclusive evidence of the cause of the anemia.

Age and Bone Marrow Function

Bone marrow, the site where red blood cells are manufactured and mature, is a tissue with a high cellular turnover and thus is particularly sensitive to nutritional deprivation. At the same time, age-related changes in the bone marrow can diminish hematopoietic capacity. Although the stem cells of the bone marrow retain their ability to divide throughout life, stem cells from older human donors have a reduced capacity to proliferate compared to cells from younger human donors.[48] This is particularly evident under conditions of stimulation; stem cells from older donors are less able to increase their production of hematopoietic cells.

Changes in bone marrow function become significant in times of physiologic or nutritional stress and contribute to anemia. Elderly people with unexplained anemia were found to have fewer bone marrow stem cells than healthy people of similar age, and healthy older people had fewer than younger people. Less efficient delivery of nutrients to proliferating cells may contribute to reduced erythrocyte production.[48] Bone marrow stem cells normally respond to high levels of erythropoietin by producing mature cells in shorter intervals of time. Older people in good health retain the ability to respond to increased erythropoietin whether released in response to blood loss or administered intravenously.[33] Decreased release of erythropoietin by the kidneys or the inability of the hematopoietic tissues to respond to erythropoietin may contribute to anemia in chronically ill older people.

Treating Iron-Deficiency Anemia

Treating iron-deficiency anemia requires careful evaluation, and the regimen should be supervised by a physician. Administering supplemental iron to individuals who actually are vitamin B-12 deficient has serious consequences, since the vitamin B-12 deficiency eventually will cause neural damage. Equally unwise is supplementation with iron and all vitamin cofactors necessary for red blood cell production and maturation. Excessive or inappropriate iron supplementation can cause gastrointestinal distress and excessive iron storage that can mask occult blood loss. When iron-deficiency anemia is diagnosed, 60 mg of iron daily as ferrous sulfate divided across the three meals should result in an increase in hemoglobin of 0.5 g/dl a week.[48] It may be necessary to begin with a lower level of iron to minimize common side effects, including nausea, vomiting, constipation, and diarrhea. Self-medication with iron can lead to hemochromatosis.

Pernicious Anemia

Basis of the problem. Pernicious anemia is a progressive, macrocytic anemia caused by a lack of intrinsic factor and subsequent vitamin B-12 deficiency. Pernicious anemia occurs in only 1% to 2% of the population, but the incidence increases with age.[11] The average age of onset is 60 years. Pernicious anemia is more common in women and rarely occurs in African American

adults.[49] The pathological aspects of this condition relate to both the anemia and the role of vitamin B-12 in maintaining neural tissue. Although the macrocytic anemia associated with a vitamin B-12 deficiency disappears when the vitamin is restored, the damage to the myelin covering of the spinal nerves cannot be reversed (see chapter 6).

The underlying cause of the pernicious anemia resulting from atrophic gastritis and the loss of intrinsic factor is not known. Pernicious anemia in people over age 75 has been associated with hypothyroidism and a family history of pernicious anemia. There is also evidence that an autoimmune reaction may cause pernicious anemia. Parietal cell antibodies that lead to atrophic gastritis have been identified in most patients with pernicious anemia, suggesting that the loss of both gastric acid and intrinsic factor secretion are related.

Criteria for diagnosis. A major problem in clinical practice is appropriate criteria for identifying pernicious anemia and vitamin B-12 deficiency. At one time it was believed that hematologic changes occurred early on in the deficiency and neurologic changes later, and never before the classic macrocytic anemia.[11] Current evidence indicates that neurologic damage associated with pernicious anemia or vitamin B-12 deficiency can occur in the absence of anemia and when serum vitamin B-12 levels still fall within the normal range. Carmel[11] emphasized that true vitamin B-12 deficiency is not only more common than is generally believed, but also it develops in a more subtle fashion. Among 80 consecutive patients diagnosed with pernicious anemia, 36% had serum vitamin B-12 levels above the deficient range; 19% had hemoglobin levels in the normal range; and 33% had normal-sized erythrocytes. Six patients had neurologic abnormalities, including numbness of the hands and feet, confusion, or bizarre behavior, despite the absence of anemia or macrocytic cells.

These findings about the early appearance of neurologic damage were confirmed in another group of patients with neuropsychiatric abnormalities related to vitamin B-12 deficiency.[45] Forty of the 141 patients studied had normal hemoglobin and red blood cell volume measurements, but exhibited sensory losses and psychiatric disturbances. Thirty-eight of the 40 patients were treated with vitamin B-12. All but 10 became free of symptoms, and all showed improvement. In some cases a correct diagnosis of the condition had been delayed for months or even years because vitamin B-12 deficiency was considered to be unlikely in the absence of anemia.

Martin and coworkers[52] stressed the urgency of identifying pernicious anemia and vitamin B-12 deficiency in elderly people. They studied 22 older men and women with low serum vitamin B-12 and a mean age of 78.5 years. For them the duration of their symptoms of deteriorating mental status was a major factor in their response to vitamin B-12 therapy. Those individuals who had exhibited changes in memory, judgment, and the ability to express ideas and thoughts for no longer than three months were able to return to normal function as evaluated on a cognitive rating scale. The patients whose symptoms had continued for less than 12 months showed some improvement, but those who had been deficient for more than 12 months continued to deteriorate in mental status. Martin and coworkers[52] concluded that a limited window of opportunity for intervention exists in older adults with mental dysfunction caused by vitamin B-12 deficiency. Vitamin B-12 deficiency is not related to the cognitive impairment associated with senile dementia of the Alzheimer type.

It is unclear why some older individuals develop neuropsychiatric abnormalities prior to hematologic abnormalities in vitamin B-12 deficiency. Iron deficiency in combination with vitamin B-12 deficiency may prevent the development of macrocytic cells.[49] Folate supplements administered inappropriately also alter the progression of symptoms in pernicious anemia.[45]

Although it is agreed that vitamin B-12 treatment should be initiated when low serum vitamin B-12 levels are observed, the usual standard of deficiency (74 pmol/l) is not effective in identifying older people with pernicious anemia.[45] Lindenbaum and coworkers[45] reported elevated serum levels of methylmalonic acid and homocysteine in untreated patients with pernicious anemia and inappropriately high levels of serum methylmalonic acid in a general population of older people in the Framingham study.[46] These metabolic intermediate compounds accumulate because subsequent metabolic reactions require vitamin B-12 as a cofactor. When the patients with pernicious anemia were supplemented with vitamin B-12, serum levels of both methylmalonic acid and homocysteine dropped markedly.[45] (See chapter 6 for further discussion of vitamin B-12 and methylmalonic acid levels.)

A critical need is a sensitive and cost-effective protocol for evaluating vitamin B-12 status. Vitamin B-12 deficiency has implications for both physiologic[46,57] and mental[45] well-being in older adults. Vitamin B-12 also is required for the normal function of osteoblasts, the cells that carry out bone formation. A two-year follow-up study of an older man with pernicious anemia and osteoporosis[57] indicated that administration of vitamin B-12 along with a drug that stimulates osteoblast activity could prevent further vertebral fractures.

Treating pernicious anemia. The usual treatment for pernicious anemia is intramuscular injection of 1,000 mg of vitamin B-12 every one to three months. Oral intakes of 500 to 1,000 mg a day carry little risk of toxicity and appear to be adequate to maintain normal function in patients with pernicious anemia.[36] Also, oral cobalamin is relatively inexpensive when compared to the cost associated with vitamin B-12 injections that must be administered in a clinic or by a home health nurse. Oral supplementation should be considered with appropriate monitoring and follow-up. Patients must also be advised of the need for continuing supplementation.

PROTEIN-ENERGY MALNUTRITION (PEM)
Causes of Protein-Energy Malnutrition

PEM in older people is caused by inadequate nutrient intake, increased nutritional requirements, or a combination of both. Infection and fever increase the need for protein and kilocalories to support the acute phase response. Trauma, such as a broken bone from a fall, or surgery induce a 40% increase in protein synthesis and breakdown.[60] Reduced food intake and lower nutrient reserves place the older individual at risk of subsequent protein-energy undernutrition when illness strikes or chronic disease develops. Morley[58] summarized available data indicating that 3% to 16% of older adults living in the community, 17% to 65% of older patients in acute care hospitals, and 26% to 59% of older residents of long-term care facilities are undernourished.

Lipschitz[48] has defined PEM as the metabolic response to stress associated with increased requirements for kilocalories and protein. Others refer to this syndrome as hypoalbuminemic malnutrition and use for diagnosis a serum albumin under 3 g/dl.[47] Older people are more susceptible to PEM than younger people and develop this disorder more rapidly and under conditions of less stress. Injuries, surgery, infection, and inflammatory conditions such as rheumatoid arthritis can result in PEM. In older people even a relatively minor illness of short duration, for example, a urinary tract or respiratory infection, can initiate the development of PEM. Such conditions frequently exist postoperatively. An inadequate intake of kilocalories and protein has the greatest effect on body systems with a high level of protein synthesis, including the hematopoietic system, the immune system, and liver metabolism of drugs and toxins.[47]

Metabolic Consequences and Disease Outcome in Protein-Energy Malnutrition

The initial reaction to metabolic stress plays a positive role in enabling the individual to make an optimal physiologic response to the infection or illness initiating the stress.[24] The breakdown of muscle protein as part of the acute phase response yields a supply of amino acids for the synthesis of new proteins essential for an appropriate immune response or for energy while nutrient intake is interrupted or reduced. Younger people with a greater muscle mass and protein reserve can have a reduced nutrient intake for up to 10 days with no apparent change in nutritional status or disease outcome.[48] After that, inadequate intakes of protein and energy lead to a significant lowering of serum albumin and impaired immunologic, hematologic, and hepatic function which adversely affect recovery. In contrast to younger people, older people experience the negative effects of reduced protein and energy intakes within two to three days, with increased morbidity and mortality.[48] A serum albumin below 3.5 g/dl was the best single predictor of mortality among 80 consecutive patients between the ages of 85 and 100 admitted to a major medical center.[2] This held true regardless of age or disease diagnosis. In those patients a low serum albumin was associated with infection and reduced immunologic capability.

PEM also carries increased risk of death for older adults living at home.[85] Involuntary weight loss that was not related to a terminal disease or an increased level of exercise was associated with increased mortality among older men discharged from a geriatric rehabilitation unit.[85] Moreover, when undernourished patients were readmitted, they were more likely to develop complications relating to infection (bronchitis or pneumonia) or skin integrity (decubitus ulcers or poor wound-healing).[84] In malnourished patients in extended care facilities, nutritional status may relate to energy and protein intake before rather than after admission. Poorly nourished patients could have had some degree of disability before entering the extended care facility, and they may have been limited in their ability to obtain food and prepare meals.

Hematologic Changes in Protein-Energy Malnutrition

One physiologic consequence of PEM is anemia and reduced hematopoietic function in the bone marrow.[49] Unfortunately, it is difficult to separate changes that result from normal aging complicated by chronic disease from changes that result from PEM, since they are remarkably similar. In fact Lipschitz[48] has suggested that protein deficiency may contribute to the changes in blood cell formation usually ascribed to aging. The anemia associated with

PEM parallels the anemia of chronic disease. In PEM hemoglobin ranges from 10 to 12 g/dl, and serum iron and transferrin levels are low. In contrast to iron-deficiency anemia, iron stores are normal or even elevated in the anemia associated with PEM.[15] Improved nutrient intake is directly related to positive metabolic changes in PEM. Increased intakes of protein and kilocalories bring about a rise in serum iron and transferrin within 48 hours, indicating a nutritional role in the hematopoietic impairment that occurs in PEM.[48]

Immunologic Changes in Protein-Energy Malnutrition

Immune function declines with advancing age and PEM may be additive, as PEM leads to more severe changes in immune function in older adults than in younger adults.[48] Older patients with PEM have fewer **neutrophils,** the white blood cells that act as phagocytes and engulf bacteria and foreign substances. Examination of the bone marrow reveals reductions in the number of stem cells and other cell precursors important in immune function. Poor protein and energy status leads to not only reduced numbers of white blood cells but also changes in their function.[77] Neutrophils, B cells, and T cells have decreased antigenic and bactericidal activities when nutrition is inadequate. Protein supplementation of the chronically ill older adult does increase bone marrow production of precursor cells necessary for normal immune function, although levels do not reach those of healthy elderly people.[48]

Protein-Energy Supplementation

Nutrition support providing adequate protein and kilocalories will prevent the development of PEM or ameliorate the problem when it has occurred. The best approach with older people at risk for PEM is to promote the consumption of a nutritionally dense, well-balanced diet. Increasing fat to 35% of total kilocalories will assist in raising energy intake in poorly nourished elderly people. Individuals should be encouraged to eat as much as they can, keeping in mind their dental status, functional status, and medical condition.[15] For frail elderly, those with long-standing PEM, or the critically ill, eating enough food to overcome existing nutritional deficiencies may not be possible, and dietary or liquid supplements or enteral feeding may be required. One care team[15] noted that only 10% of their older patients with PEM could eat a sufficient amount of food at meal time to correct their nutritional deficits. A goal for nutrient intake is 35 kcal/kg of body weight with 20% or more of total energy as protein.[47]

Between-meal or bedtime snacks of nutrient-dense foods, such as cheese and crackers, peanut butter and crackers, hard-cooked eggs, milkshakes or frappes, or a half sandwich, will supply protein and energy as well as vitamins and minerals. Commercial liquid supplements can add nutrients when food intake is low. In a study of older British women admitted to the hospital following a hip fracture,[23] a liquid supplement given at bedtime reduced both the length of the hospital stay and the incidence of complications. Six months after these women were discharged from the hospital, complication rates were still significantly lower in the group that received the supplement (40% had complications) than in the group that did not (74% had complications).

Increasing energy and protein intakes in hospitalized older people may be difficult if their usual food intake provides only about 1,000 kcal per day, and they are unable to consume additional food or liquids. Carbohydrate and protein powders that do not change the flavor, color, or texture of foods can be added to soup, cereal, juice, milk, or other soft foods to increase nutrient density.

Unfortunately, the biochemical and physiologic markers of PEM do not always respond to protein-energy supplementation. Among malnourished, homebound older people, commercial liquid supplements effectively raised serum albumin levels and led to increases in body weight.[48] Yet despite these indicators of improved nutritional status, immune function remained abnormal and hemoglobin levels did not increase. Lipschitz[48] concluded that poor nutritional status can aggravate existing abnormalities in immune function in older people. Although nutrient repletion of those who are severely malnourished leads to some improvement in immune response, it does not restore function to normal. Changes in immune and hematopoietic function observed in healthy or mildly malnourished elderly people are not related to—nor are they responsive to—protein or energy supplementation.[77]

Pressure Ulcers

Pressure ulcers are a common problem among immobile and debilitated older people.[47] Current data[63] indicate that the prevalence of pressure ulcers among patients newly admitted to nursing homes ranges from 17% to 21%. In older people cared for at home under the supervision of health care professionals, 9% to 19% have pressure ulcers. Pressure ulcers are especially frequent in patients over the age of 70. Although various factors are involved in their development, nutrition plays an important role in both their occurrence and healing.[63]

A primary cause of **pressure ulcers,** sometimes referred to as decubitus ulcers, is the pressure created by the weight of the body on the tissues covering a bony prominence. People who are bed-bound or chair-bound and unable to reposition themselves are at risk for pressure ulcers. The severity of pressure ulcers ranges from Stages I and II, in which the skin is red and cracked, to Stages III and IV in which the skin is broken and a deep crater-like ulcer has formed. Various indicators of compromised nutritional status are associated with the development of pressure ulcers. Bergstrom and Braden[8] reviewed the case histories of 200 newly admitted patients to a skilled nursing facility. Within three months 39% had developed pressure ulcers of Stage II or worse, and dietary intake was lower in those individuals. Patients developing pressure ulcers consumed only 80% of the RDA for protein and 53% of the RDA for energy. The patients who did not develop pressure ulcers were meeting the RDA for protein but not for energy (intake was about 70% of the RDA). Pressure ulcers also are more frequent in older people with serum albumin below 3.5 g/dl,[32] although lower albumin levels may be caused by protein and fluid loss relating to the ulcer rather than prior nutritional status.

Several recommendations have set a level of nutritional support required to heal pressure ulcers. The Agency of Health Care Policy and Research[16] suggests an energy level of 30 to 35 kcal/kg and a protein level of 1 to 1.25 g/kg. Other clinicians[10] have recommended protein intakes equaling 24% of total kilocalories. This level of protein intervention resulted in the healing of even stage IV ulcers among 28 malnourished elderly (their mean age was 72 years). A similar group fed a diet with 14% protein had no ulcer healing. The greatest change in ulcer size and healing occurred in the patients with the highest energy and protein intakes. Pressure ulcers are associated with a fourfold increase in mortality, and patients with ulcers are hospitalized for longer periods of time.[63] In light of these facts, nutrition intervention should be implemented to preserve skin integrity or promote healing if ulcers are already present.

MANAGEMENT OF BODY WEIGHT

Obesity is a recognized health problem in most of the industrialized societies but underweight in adults has received less attention. At younger ages obesity increases mortality; however, the relationship between obesity and increased risk of death at older ages is less clearcut. Conversely, underweight, which tends to improve one's health outlook as a young adult, becomes a serious threat to health in an older adult. Situations involving extreme obesity or the loss of protein and fat indicative of PEM leave no doubt as to the need for intervention, although implementation may prove difficult and the outcome uncertain. An unresolved question is the extent to which obesity or unintentional weight loss can be ameliorated in the older individual.

Obesity and Health

At all ages morbid obesity with extreme adipose tissue accumulation is detrimental to health, but at older ages it carries particular risk of functional disability and a lower quality of life. On the other hand, the relative health risk of mild to moderate overweight in older adults is less clear.[59] Durnin[24] proposed that a moderate degree of fatness is of nutritional benefit to the older individual when food intake is interrupted and metabolic needs elevated as a result of illness or surgery. Fat also protects vital organs from injury and this protective role may be especially important in the older adult at risk of falling.[59]

In older people it is difficult to establish an ideal body mass index (BMI) that minimizes risk of mortality or morbidity.[82] The Nutrition Screening Initiative[62] recommended a BMI between 22 and 27 in the elderly (see chapter 11). A recent evaluation of elderly men between the ages of 70 and 80[82] found no differences in mortality between a BMI of 20 and 33. There was no increase in mortality among the women at even higher levels of obesity. Over age 75 there appears to be an actual loss of body weight and body fat which may relate to normal aging. Based on these observations, one clinician[82] suggested that a slight obesity may not justify intervention, particularly in those age 75 or over. Morley and Glick[59] define morbid obesity as a body weight that is above 130% to 140% of average weight. This level of obesity carries an increased risk of death even into very old age. Moderate overweight, 110% to 130% of average weight, seems to carry minimal additional risk of mortality in most older people. Morley and Glick[59] consider weight reduction to be essential for people over age 64 whose body weight is greater than 130% of average weight. Diabetic elderly whose weight exceeds 110% of average weight should be advised to lose weight.[59] The location of one's fat may be more important to good health than the amount. Increased fat around the waist (increased waist-to-hip ratio) is associated with a greater risk of hypertension, stroke, and diabetes.

Weight Gain

The general pattern of weight gain, as well as the absolute body weight attained, influences health at older ages. A study published more than 25 years ago[1] suggested that individuals who were underweight as children but gained weight rapidly as adults were more likely to develop serious cardiovascular disease by age 50 than those who were somewhat overweight from childhood. Evaluation of the body weight history of participants in the Baltimore Longitudinal Study of Aging (BLSA)[50] suggested that variations in body weight were associated with a deterioration in glucose tolerance and a greater concentration of body fat on the trunk. The rate of weight change per year ranged from -4.3 kg to +2.6 kg, although the average change was -0.02 kg a year. Substantial weight gain over adulthood may influence functional capacity and the ability to remain independent. People who were overweight in their 30s were more likely to have osteoarthritis of the knee when reaching their 70s.[27]

Another aspect of disease risk is the pattern of weight loss followed by weight gain that occurs in many individuals. Stable weight over time is associated with best health.[51] All patterns of weight change, whether they be weight gains, weight losses, or a combination of the two, are associated with increased mortality risk. In the Framingham Heart Study,[51] individuals who had a high degree of fluctuation in their BMI had a higher mortality risk regardless of their level of obesity or overall trend in body weight. In fact the Framingham workers[51] concluded that the relative risk associated with continued fluctuations in body weight was as great as that associated with static obesity.

Intervention for Weight Reduction

Possible benefits of weight reduction. A rising BMI is associated with increased morbidity related to noninsulin-dependent diabetes mellitus, coronary heart disease, and hypertension. Restricted-activity and bed-rest days also increase at higher levels of overweight. A weight loss goal considered to be realistic, achievable, and consistent with a reduction in disease risk for most overweight people is 10% of body weight; however, a recent expert panel[56] acknowledged that a lack of background information precludes the establishment of body weight reduction goals for elderly people.

The possible advantages of weight loss should be measured against the possible physical and emotional stress imposed by a weight loss program. Severely limiting energy intake when protein, vitamin, and mineral status is already precarious may further compromise general well-being. Also, Stunkard[83] reported that even modest energy restriction resulted in a loss of 1 g of lean body tissue for every 3 g of fat in healthy young adults. This effect of weight reduction has not been evaluated in older adults. Very-low-calorie diets, leading to severe negative nitrogen balance, or weight loss drugs are not appropriate for the older individual.[59]

In older people with chronic disease, an improvement in metabolic or physiologic status is a more appropriate goal than actual pounds lost. The loss of even 2.3 to 4.5 kg (5 to 10 lbs.) will help to lower blood pressure, improve serum lipoprotein patterns, and decrease insulin resistance with improvement in glucose tolerance.[56] Weight loss in this range also protects heart muscle mass.[56] A change in waist-to-hip ratio is also of importance to health goals. A reasonable approach is a well-balanced diet, increased exercise level, and lifestyle changes as appropriate.

Energy intake and food selection. Little information exists to guide weight reduction programs in older people. Morley and Glick[59] recommend an energy intake of at least 1,000 kcal daily, and even this level is likely to reduce the resting metabolic rate. It is difficult to consume adequate levels of micronutrients on this caloric intake, and a supplement providing the RDA for vitamins and the trace elements is recommended. For individuals who are bed-bound or chair-bound and have a low lean body mass, an intake as low as 1,000 kcal may not result in weight loss, although it may prevent weight gain.

A well-balanced diet that is lower in fat and higher in carbohydrate can help to reduce energy intake. A recent intervention trial with women ages 45 to 69 indicated that decreasing dietary fat from 39% to 22% of total energy resulted in a loss of about 2.4 kg over three months.[34] This is particularly noteworthy because the women were not counseled to reduce their total dietary intake, merely their intake of fat. Their decrease in fat intake was substantial and lowered daily energy intake from 1,738 kcal to 1,300 kcal. This was achieved in part by substituting lower fat dairy products and salad dressings for higher fat products, and pretzels and similar low-fat grain products for potato chips and high-fat grain products. Overall, intakes of fruit and grain products increased. Decreasing fat intake to 22% of total energy has not been recommended for older adults; however, some decrease in dietary fat will, over time, contribute to weight loss or help prevent weight gain.

Exercise program. Because a major factor contributing to weight gain in older adults is a low level of physical activity, creating an energy deficit with consistent exercise should be a first step in a weight management program. Walking for 30 minutes has been estimated to use about 180 kcal in a 170-lb. man and about 140 kcal in a 130-lb. woman. A walk of two to three miles several times a week is a reasonable goal for older people in good health.[59] Even a short daily walk at a slow pace will assist in weight control. Strength training also adds to energy expenditure and is beneficial in preserving muscle mass. For older people who are unable to walk, upper body exercises will add to energy expenditure.[59] Implementing an exercise program with sedentary older adults requires professional supervision with a gradual increase in activity over time.

Lifestyle. Active participation in a variety of activities helps prevent unwanted weight gain. Spending an afternoon walking around the mall expends more energy than sitting in a favorite chair. Among employed adult men, those who watched television more than three hours a day were twice as likely to be obese as those who watched television only one to two hours a day.[87] This held true regardless of age, level of physical fitness, and hours of exercise weekly. Efforts to develop spare time pursuits involving some physical activity should begin early in adult life.

Involuntary Weight Loss

Rapid, involuntary weight loss in an older adult is a sign of a deteriorating physical condition or a serious disease.[24,28] Under these circumstances, both lean body mass and body fat will be lost. An older individual with a substantial amount of body fat will lose a relatively small amount of lean tissue and a relatively large amount of fat when there is an energy deficit.

Conversely, those with little body fat will break down lean tissue to meet energy needs resulting in muscular, cardiac, and visceral wasting.

Involuntary weight loss has many causes. Physiologic and metabolic changes can reduce the absorption or assimilation of nutrients. Chronic infections and severe cardiovascular and pulmonary disease increase metabolic demands and can induce weight loss. Dementia or disability that interferes with self-feeding or makes swallowing difficult can decrease food intake. Hyperthyroidism, causing an elevation in metabolic rate (see chapter 5), results in weight loss. Cytokinins, released in the presence of tumors or infections, are elevated in cancer, uncontrolled diabetes, and pulmonary disease and contribute to the anorexia and cachexia associated with these problems.[28] A disturbed body image characteristic of anorexia nervosa has been identified in older people with low food intake.[59]

Because of the vulnerability of older people to weight loss, body weight should be evaluated regularly, particularly in those with poor food intake or chronic disease. Fischer and Johnson[28] suggest the use of additional anthropometric measurements, since edema, tumor growth, or preexisting obesity can mask weight loss (see chapter 11). Body weight should be measured once a month and the current weight compared to the previous weight. If an individual appears to be losing weight, weekly measurements may be required to identify the problem and define intervention strategies. Older adults living in the community and their caregivers should be alerted to the diagnostic significance of involuntary weight loss.

Involuntary weight loss is not uncommon among older people. A four-year follow-up study[89] of 247 men above age 64 indicated that mortality rates were more than doubled in the men reporting involuntary weight loss versus those who did not lose weight (mortality rates were 28% and 11%, respectively) (fig. 12-1). The most frequent causes of death were cancer, cardiac disease, and infection. This study also points to the importance of voluntary weight loss in older people. The mortality rate of those losing weight by dieting was similar to those with involuntary weight loss (36% versus 28%).

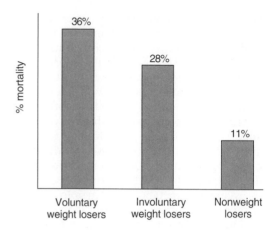

FIG. 12-1 Weight Loss and Mortality in Older Male Outpatients. Older men who lost body weight whether by dieting (voluntary weight loss) or other causes (involuntary weight loss) had a higher risk of death over the next two years than those who did not lose weight.

Data from Wallace, J.I., and others: Involuntary weight loss in older outpatients: incidence and clinical significance, J. Am. Geriatr. Soc. 43:329, 1995.

Wallace and coworkers[89] noted that voluntary weight loss is usually difficult to achieve and health professionals need to monitor those older adults who have exceptional success with dieting. A loss of 4% or more of body weight, regardless of cause, was associated with a higher mortality in these men. In older men and women above the age of 83,[68] those with a BMI below 22 were less likely to be able to remain living at home and more likely to be hospitalized.

Institutionalized older adults are at particular risk of weight loss.[28] In a two-year follow-up of 335 institutionalized older people,[25] 30% had a weight loss of at least 4.5 kg from their admission weight. Several patients had extreme weight loss, with one losing 12 kg the first year and 18 kg the second year. The survival rate was lower among those losing at least 4.5 kg. Monitoring body weight is especially important in patients with cognitive disorders or physical disabilities causing feeding problems. Fogt and coworkers[29] have defined significant weight loss as 1% to 2% of body weight in one week, 5% of body weight in one month, or 10% to 20% of body weight over time. Wallace and others[89] suggest that loss of 5% of body weight over a period of 6 to 12 months indicates the need for further evaluation. The Nutrition Screening Initiative[62] considers the loss of 10 pounds over six months to be nutritionally significant and a basis for referral to a health professional.

OSTEOPENIA IN THE AGING ADULT
Definitions

About age 30 to 40, both men and women start to lose bone and begin to develop osteopenia or bone with a below-normal level of bone mineral. Bone loss accelerates dramatically in women after menopause, and older women are at increased risk for bone fractures. Men lose bone more gradually but become vulnerable to bone fracture in very old age. As noted in chapter 10, the World Health Organization has established several categories of bone mineral density useful for diagnosis and intervention.[69]

- Normal bone mineral density is a bone mineral content that is not more than 1 standard deviation below the mean value of young adults.
- Low bone mass, or osteopenia, is a bone mineral content between 1 and 2.5 standard deviations below the mean value of young adults. Individuals in this category would benefit from preventive health measures to avoid further loss and, to the extent possible, restore bone mass.
- Osteoporosis is a bone mineral content that is more than 2.5 standard deviations below the mean value of young adults; fractures either have occurred or are likely to occur.

Although these standards are helpful, defining osteoporosis is still difficult because of individual differences. Some people with bone mineral consistent with the diagnosis of osteoporosis do not suffer fractures whereas others with low bone mass do. The National Institutes of Health consensus conferences on osteopenia[69] have defined **osteoporosis** as a disease characterized by low bone mass and changes in bone architecture that lead to increased fragility and risk of fracture. Although all people lose some bone as a consequence of aging, not all develop osteoporosis. Osteoporosis involves a decrease in both bone mineral and bone matrix. In addition to bone fractures that occur despite minimal or no trauma, osteoporosis results in bone pain, spinal deformity, and loss of height.

Public Health Aspects

Osteoporosis has enormous implications for both personal well-being and the health care system. By age 65 one in three women will have vertebral fractures; by age 90 one in three women and one in six men will have had a hip fracture.[72] A hip fracture often results in loss of independence; half of these patients are unable to return to their former residence and thus become dependent on nursing home care. The direct and indirect costs associated with osteoporosis are estimated to exceed $6 billion a year.[72] As the number of people above age 85 continues to grow, so will these costs.

Bone as a Tissue

Bone is composed of a protein and collagen matrix and mineral in the form of hydroxyapatite with a formula of $Ca_{10}(PO_4)_6OH_2$.[90] The hydroxyl group can be replaced by a fluoride ion to form fluoroapatite which is more resistant to resorption than hydroxyapatite. The matrix portion accounts for about one-third of bone weight, and the mineral deposits account for about two-thirds of bone weight.[90]

The mature skeleton has two types of bone: cortical bone and trabecular bone. Cortical bone is dense and compact and has a slow turnover. It consists of circular layers arranged around a blood vessel. Cortical bone appears as a solid mineralized area on a normal x-ray. It is found in the skull, the jaw, and the shafts of the long bones. About 80% of the skeleton is cortical bone.[41,90] Trabecular bone, sometimes referred to as spongy or cancellous bone, has a greater surface area than cortical bone and is more metabolically active. It is made up of numerous interwoven horizontal and vertical bars, called trabeculae, which form partitions filled with marrow and fat. Trabecular bone has a lacelike structure on magnification. It is found in the vertebrae, in the flat bones of the ribs and pelvis, and in the ends of the long bones such as the femur. Trabecular bone forms about 20% of the skeleton.[41,90]

Once thought to be relatively inert, bone is now recognized to be a dynamic tissue that undergoes constant remodeling throughout life. While old bone is being broken down at one location, new bone is being formed at another. **Osteoclasts** are the cells that are instrumental in bone resorption; these cells secrete acids that dissolve bone mineral and recruit phagocytes to remove remaining proteins. **Osteoblasts,** the active cells that form new bone, synthesize the protein matrix and accumulate the calcium and phosphorus deposited in the matrix.[81]

In young adults bone resorption and formation are tightly coupled. An advancing series of osteoclasts forms a cavity, which the osteoblasts fill in with new bone. Under normal circumstances bone formation equals bone resorption, and bone mass is maintained. The first change to occur in bone remodeling is incomplete replacement of the bone that was resorbed, resulting in the age-related bone loss that begins about ages 30 to 40.[75] The accelerated bone loss that occurs in women immediately after menopause is associated with increased bone turnover. Both bone resorption and accretion escalate, but osteoclasts increase to a greater extent and create cavities in the bone that cannot be filled.[41] Loss of bone and the changing geometric pattern of the bone contribute to a loss in bone strength.

Bone Development and Loss

Factors influencing bone mass. Many factors contribute to bone formation and bone loss. Some of these are under an individual's control, whereas others are genetic or physiologic in nature. The characteristics listed in the box are associated with lower bone mass.[81,90]

The most obvious predisposing factor for bone loss is being female. Over adult life, women lose about 35% of their cortical bone and 50% of their trabecular bone; men lose only about two-thirds as much.[75] African Americans have greater bone density than white people of similar age and sex and have been considered to be less susceptible to bone loss and osteoporosis. Increased mechanical stress on the bone is

---

CHARACTERISTICS ASSOCIATED WITH A LOWER BONE MASS

Genetic
Female
White or Asian race
Family history of bone disease
Extremely short or tall stature
Physiologic or Endocrine
Hyperparathyroidism
Hyperthyroidism
Diabetes mellitus
Premature menopause
Leanness
Environmental
Low calcium intake
Low exposure to sunlight
Low physical activity
Use of alcohol
Smoking

---

believed to contribute to the higher bone density of obese women as compared to lean women, although a second hypothesis relates to the hormone supplied by adipose tissue.[90] In postmenopausal women, the estrogen supplied by adipose tissue may contribute to the preservation of bone mass, putting the obese older woman at an advantage over the more lean. Hyperparathyroidism and use of glucocorticoids accelerate urinary calcium loss and decrease bone mass. In contrast, thiazide drugs reduce the excretion of calcium, and users have a reduced incidence of hip fractures.[72] The impact of estrogen deficiency on bone mass has implications for bone health in young women with ovarian dysfunction because of very low energy intake or extreme levels of physical exercise.

Bone development in early life. Bone density in old age is the sum total of the bone acquired during the years of growth minus the bone lost after maturity. Because a low bone mass is a major determinant of bone fracture, a high bone mass at maturity is believed to offer the best protection against age-related bone fractures. An evaluation of rural counties in China[39] in which farming was the predominant lifestyle suggests that a generous intake of calcium during the period of bone growth and throughout adulthood offers long-term benefits. In one county women drank milk tea with their meals and consumed cheese and other dairy products. In another county they drank milk tea with meals but did not eat other dairy foods. In a third county no milk or dairy foods were available. Calcium intakes among the three groups of women were 724 mg, 369 mg, and 230 mg, respectively. Differences in bone mass were already apparent at age 30. As described in figure 12-2, those with a greater bone mass at younger ages had a greater amount of bone remaining in later life despite bone loss.

In the NHANES III study,[88] the median calcium intakes of teenage women ranged from 685 mg to 745 mg; the RDA for this age group is 1,200 mg. These adolescent girls now developing their skeletal mass will be at high risk for low bone mass in later life if calcium intakes remain at these levels.

Patterns of bone loss. Age of onset and patterns of bone loss differ between cortical and trabecular bone, and these differences contribute to the sequence of fractures associated with each bone type. Cortical bone loss begins about age 40 in men and women and proceeds slowly at a rate of about 0.3% to 0.5% a year. The rate of loss increases to 2% to 3% per year immediately after menopause and then gradually returns to lower levels.[75] It has been estimated[69] that women lose as much as 15% of their bone in the six to seven years after menopause.

The pattern of trabecular bone loss is less well defined. It generally is agreed that trabecular losses begin at least 10 years earlier than cortical losses in both sexes, probably about age 30 to 35.[72] Losses of trabecular bone appear to be continuous at a rate of 1% a year with no acceleration after menopause, although excessive losses in younger women following oophorectomy have been reported. Losses may be less rapid in natural menopause, when estrogen withdrawal is more gradual. If trabecular bone loss does accelerate after menopause, the duration of the increased loss is shorter than for cortical bone. The earlier onset of trabecular bone loss is paralleled by the earlier onset of vertebral fractures, fractures of the forearm, and tooth loss.[90]

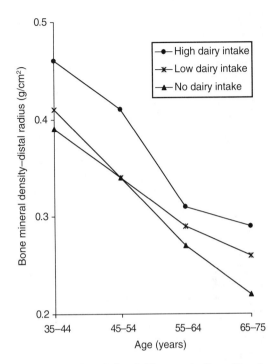

FIG. 12-2 Age-Related Changes in Bone Density in Chinese Women Consuming Different Levels of Dairy Products. The women with higher intakes of dairy products and calcium throughout their lifetime had a greater bone density at older ages despite age-related bone loss.

Data from Hu, J.F., and others: Dietary calcium and bone density among middle-aged and elderly women in China, Am. J. Clin. Nutr. 58:219, 1993.

How Osteoporosis Develops

Two distinct types of osteoporosis exist, and they differ in age of onset, relation to menopause, clinical symptoms, and hormonal patterns (table 12-3).[72,75] Postmenopausal osteoporosis (type I) is found in women 10 to 15 years after menopause; it also occurs in men, albeit less frequently. The first clinical symptoms are fractures of the vertebrae, which cause spinal deformity, back pain, and a decrease in stature. The escalation in trabecular bone loss that sometimes occurs in postmenopausal osteoporosis is believed to result from the hormonal changes that accompany estrogen withdrawal.

TABLE 12-3   Comparison of Postmenopausal and Senile Osteoporosis

	Postmenopausal Osteoporosis	Senile Osteoporosis
Age of onset (yrs)	50 to 65	Over 70
Type of bone lost	Trabecular	Trabecular and cortical
Rate of bone loss	Rapid	Slow
Calcium absorption	Below normal	Below normal
Major cause	Menopause (estrogen withdrawal)	Aging (impaired bone remodeling and 1,25(OH)$_2$D production)

Adapted from Riggs, B.L., and Melton, L.J.: Involutional osteoporosis, New Engl. J. Med. 314:1676, 1986.

Accelerated bone mobilization and high serum calcium levels suppress parathyroid hormone (PTH) and elevate calcitonin. This in turn depresses renal 1-α-hydroxylase activity, the production of 1,25(OH)$_2$D, and calcium absorption. Although all women become deficient in estrogen after menopause, not all develop osteoporosis. Women who develop osteoporosis lose bone at three times the rate of women who do not.[90] Other factors interacting with or exacerbating the estrogen deficiency are unknown. (See chapter 7 for a review of hormonal regulation of calcium metabolism.)

Senile osteoporosis (type II) differs from postmenopausal osteoporosis in several ways.[75] First, it occurs later in life, at age 70 or after, and it is more common among men than type I osteoporosis. Two major characteristics that contribute to the development of senile osteoporosis are (1) a decrease in active osteoblasts, which widens the gap between bone resorption and formation and (2) a decreased production of 1,25(OH)$_2$D, which impairs calcium absorption and enhances bone calcium mobilization. Continued bone resorption leads to fractures of the hip and pelvis. Vertebral fractures form a wedge shape, resulting in kyphosis, or "dowager's hump."

All factors contributing to bone mass are cumulative; thus, increased bone mass at maturity, increased bone loss related to smoking or use of alcohol, or the accelerated bone loss occurring after menopause all influence total bone density in advanced age. As bone loss continues throughout life, an increasing proportion of individuals have bone mass levels that fall below the threshold associated with bone fracture. People with fractures have lower bone mass than age-matched controls, regardless of where the fracture occurs or where bone density is evaluated. For reasons that are not clear, osteoporotic fractures occur less frequently in developing countries than in industrialized countries.[61] It is interesting to speculate as to the role of vitamin D in this observation, as many women in developing countries are involved in agriculture and spend many hours in the sun.

Treating Osteoporosis

Many therapies are being examined with the goal of reversing bone loss. Although particular regimens hold promise, many are both costly and experimental. Therapeutic agents act by either decreasing bone resorption or stimulating bone formation.

Decreasing Bone Resorption

Hormone replacement therapy. About a third to a half of all bone lost in women results from menopause and estrogen withdrawal.[76] Bone loss after menopause can be effectively reduced with hormone replacement therapy. Estrogen slows the activation of new osteoclasts, although it does not inhibit the activity of existing osteoclasts; nevertheless, the loss of both cortical and trabecular bone is reduced.[75] When initiated at menopause, estrogen replacement prevents the early phase of bone loss when bone mass is lost most rapidly. The ages at which estrogen replacement is effective and the number of years of hormone replacement required to yield a long-term effect on bone are still being debated.

A major consideration of women and their physicians making the decision to initiate or discontinue hormone replacement therapy is the risk of breast or endometrial cancer. Estrogen replacement has been reported to increase the risk of endometrial cancer by 0.1% per year.[90] In a 10-year prospective study of postmenopausal nurses, Colditz and colleagues[19] found about a 30% increase in the risk of breast cancer and an increased risk of endometrial cancer among current users of estrogen, and risk increased with age. Past use, even if long term, did not increase risk two years[19] after therapy was discontinued. Decisions regarding hormone replacement therapy need to be made on an individual basis.

Biphosphonates. Biphosphonate compounds such as alendronate are strong inhibitors of osteoclast activity and bone resorption. Clinical trials of up to two years[19] indicate that this drug can increase both bone mass and bone strength in postmenopausal women with low bone density. Biphosphonates appear to suppress bone remodeling, with a decline in bone resorption followed by a decline in bone formation. This sequence is similar to what is seen with hormone replacement therapy, and overall low bone turnover does not increase fracture risk.

Stimulating Bone Formation

Fluoride. Fluoride stimulates osteoblastic activity and at low levels increases trabecular bone mass. At high levels, however, fluoride is very toxic, causing gastric distress and bone pain. Early clinical trials with sodium fluoride were disappointing as the new bone was poorly formed and highly vulnerable to fracture. The development of a new form of sodium fluoride that is less bioavailable and is released slowly has overcome these negative effects. In a four-year clinical trial,[65] osteoporotic patients had a 20% increase in bone mass in the spine and a 9% increase in the hip. Among those receiving the slow-release sodium fluoride, 85% remained free of new fractures as compared to 57% of those given a placebo.

Calcitonin. Calcitonin reduces the life span and the number of osteoclasts and lowers bone resorption. Calcitonin derived from fish is 50 to 100 times more biologically active than calcitonin derived from mammals.[74] Treatment with salmon calcitonin for 10 days a month over a two-year period[74] led to increases in both cortical and trabecular bone, and total body bone mineral in osteoporotic women. It appears that calcitonin not only prevents bone resorption but also may stimulate bone formation, which offers an advantage over hormone replacement therapy and the biphosphonates.

Calcitriol. Synthetic $1,25(OH)_2D$ (calcitriol) increases calcium absorption and over time increases bone density in osteoporotic patients.[30] Vitamin D also exerts an effect on the osteoblasts and stimulates bone remodeling and the accretion of bone mass. Unfortunately, when calcitriol supplementation is discontinued, bone remodeling continues with accelerated resorption. Patients with high calcium intakes can develop vitamin D toxicity with hypercalcemia and hypercalciuria. For this reason patients receiving calcitriol are told to limit their calcium intake to 500 mg a day.[30]

Currently, many therapeutic agents are being developed to preserve or restore bone mass in older men and women. Although clinical trials demonstrate positive results, each drug has limitations as to the type of bone that is targeted or the length of time that treatment is effective. Except for calcitriol which has been used successfully for five to six years,[30] other drugs seem to lose their ability to influence bone after two to three years of use.

Prevention of Osteoporosis

Major attention must be directed toward osteoporosis prevention in both younger and older adults. Primary factors to be considered in lifelong promotion of bone health include calcium intake, vitamin D status, exercise, and avoidance of smoking and alcohol.

Calcium intake. The effect of added calcium on the bone health of postmenopausal women in the absence of estrogen remains controversial. Clinical trials using daily supplements of 400 mg to 1,500 mg of calcium have produced mixed

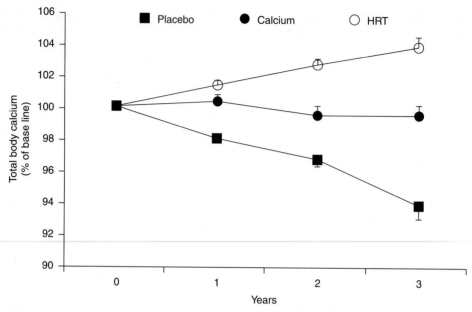

FIG. 12-3   Changes in Total Body Calcium in Postmenopausal Women. Postmenopausal women taking daily supplements of 1,700 mg of calcium and 400 IU of vitamin D lost less body calcium over a three-year period than those receiving a placebo; the women taking the calcium and vitamin D supplements and receiving hormone replacement therapy (HRT) gained body calcium over the study period.

From Aloia, J.F., and others: Calcium supplementation with and without hormone replacement therapy to prevent postmenopausal bone loss, Ann. Intern. Med. 120(2):97, 1994. (Used with permission.)

results.[22] Dawson-Hughes,[22] in a comprehensive review, pointed to some of the reasons for these differences. The period after menopause is a major factor in a woman's response to supplemental calcium. Within the first five years after menopause, bone is less responsive to added calcium and, although bone loss may be reduced, it will not be arrested. Another issue in comparing studies is the length of time the supplement was consumed. It may take as long as two years for increased levels of calcium to modify the bone remodeling cycle, and ethical considerations become increasingly urgent as nonsupplemented subjects continue to lose bone. Finally, added calcium influences various regions of the skeleton (e.g., spine, hip, and forearm) differently.

Two recent clinical trials have addressed calcium supplementation in early menopause and late menopause. Aloia and coworkers[5] evaluated

bone mineral loss in 118 healthy white women within six years of menopause (early menopause). They were given 1,700 mg of calcium and 400 IU of vitamin D daily or a placebo. Half of the supplemented group also received hormone replacement therapy. Calcium supplementation alone retarded the loss of total body calcium (see fig. 12-3) and specifically retarded bone loss from the hip, although there was no effect on loss from the spine. Daily calcium loss fell from 46 mg a day to 12 mg. Hormone replacement therapy plus calcium was more effective in preventing bone loss, leading Aloia and coworkers[5] to conclude that women with marked osteoporosis or at high risk of osteoporosis would benefit from hormone replacement therapy plus calcium. However, all women will reduce their loss of cortical bone with appropriate intakes of calcium.

TABLE 12-4   *Choosing a Calcium Supplement*

Factor	Examples
Price: Choose a form and brand that provides the most elemental calcium for the lowest cost per tablet.	Cost for a one-month supply of 1,000 mg per day ranges from $1.20 to $49. Generic calcium carbonate preparations are less expensive than brand name preparations; calcium gluconate preparations cost more than calcium carbonate and calcium citrate.
Dosage: Doses above 500 mg can lead to gastrointestinal discomfort by enhancing acid secretion or can lead to constipation.	Calcium preparations vary from 200 mg to 600 mg per dose.
Bioavailability: Calcium preparations must be soluble at the pH of the stomach; using a simple home test, tablet should dissolve in 6 oz. of white vinegar at room temperature within 30 minutes.	Calcium carbonate is soluble at an acid pH but insoluble at a neutral pH, making it less appropriate for achlorhydric patients; calcium citrate is more soluble, especially in effervescent forms and a good choice for achlorhydric patients; calcium gluconate is reasonably well absorbed and used for intravenous preparations.
Safety: Bone meal and dolomite contain toxic contaminants such as lead, arsenic, or mercury; multiple doses of products containing vitamin D may lead to potentially toxic intakes.	Particular brand name products may be more consistent in content and less likely to contain unwanted contaminants; some products contain magnesium or potassium and renal patients on restricted intakes need to check ingredients.

Adapted from Levenson, D.I., and Bockman, R.S.: A review of calcium preparations, Nutr. Rev. 52(7):221, 1994.

Reid and coworkers[70] studied the effect of daily intakes of 1,750 mg of calcium (750 mg from diet and 1,000 mg from a supplement) on the bone health of women who had completed menopause 9 to 10 years prior (late menopause). At most bone sites, the placebo group lost bone at the rate of 1% a year, whereas the calcium-supplemented group lost about one-third to one-half of that amount. This reduction in loss, if cumulative, could maintain bone mass above the threshold level associated with fracture. Calcium supplements appear to reduce calcium losses and the risk of developing osteoporosis. Considerations when helping older people choose a calcium supplement are described in table 12-4.

Vitamin D. Vitamin D is another nutrient receiving attention as a contributor to bone health. Intakes above the RDA have been shown to assist in reducing the loss of cortical bone.

Supplementation of very elderly women (their mean age was 84) with 1,200 mg of calcium and 800 IU of vitamin D resulted in a 43% drop in the rate of hip fractures over 18 months.[13] These 3,300 healthy women residing in nursing homes or apartment houses were able at the outset to walk on their own. A 2.7% increase in bone mass at the hip occurred in the supplemented women, whereas a 4.6% decrease in bone mass was observed in the placebo group. Hypercalcemia or renal calcium deposits did not occur in those receiving the increased level of vitamin D. These results suggest that intervention can be successful in older people of all ages.

Exercise. Health professionals have known for some time that bed rest or immobilization precipitates the loss of mineral from the bones. Weightlessness, as experienced by modern astronauts, results in significant bone loss. The general explanation given for bone loss under these circumstances has been the absence of gravitational pull and weight-bearing exercise acting on bone tissue.[41] Thus, walking, jogging, and running have been encouraged to maintain bone health. However, current thought suggests that weight loads generated by the pull of muscles, as occurs in weight training, may stimulate bone formation to an even greater extent than weight loads that are more evenly distributed. For example, the weight load exerted on the lower vertebrae while jogging is about two times body weight; the force exerted during weight lifting (usually considered to be a nonweight-bearing activity) can be five to six times body weight.[81]

Regular walking influences whole body bone density and bone mass in the legs and trunk. Women who walk more than 7.5 miles a week have a higher bone mass than women who walk less than one mile a week.[42] Walking appears to have less effect on bone mass in the spine. It is important to advise clients that exercise programs must be continued for gains in bone mineral mass to be sustained. In older women who had achieved a 5% gain in bone mass through intensive training,[20] bone mass returned to baseline levels within 13 months of discontinuing training.

Avoidance of alcohol and cigarettes. Both alcohol and smoking have a toxic effect on bone. Ethanol directly inhibits osteoblastic activity and appears to exacerbate the deleterious effect of a low-calcium intake.[90] The mechanism by which smoking adversely affects bone mass is unclear.

Counseling the Osteoporotic Patient

Diet planning for an osteoporotic patient will depend on the level of bone loss and associated chronic disease. General dietary guidelines include:[6]

- a high-calcium intake emphasizing food and/or supplements with high bioavailability (see table 12-4),[44]
- an adequate level of vitamin D from food, sun exposure, and/or supplements,
- a prudent intake of protein, sodium, and fiber to minimize calcium losses, and
- avoidance of alcohol, caffeine, and interfering vitamin or mineral supplements.

Bales and Gold[6] call attention to the psychosocial well-being of the osteoporotic patient. This condition responds relatively slowly to dietary, medical, and exercise interventions. Patients can become depressed, since their prognosis is uncertain. An appropriate dietary pattern that includes calcium-rich foods may be a difficult adjustment if these items were not a regular part of the diet. Continuing dietary care of osteoporotic patients within the context of their ongoing medical care is critical for successful management of their disease.

Future Research

Two groups requiring increased attention to their bone health are men[61] and African Americans.[66] Nordin[61] pointed out that men who used to die of cardiovascular disease at younger ages are now surviving to develop osteoporosis. A decline in secretion of the male sex steroid hormones and growth hormone and the subsequent effect on bone contributes to the decrease in bone mass in older men. Because men start out with larger amounts of bone than women, bone fractures are less common; however, Seeman[80] predicts that by the year 2025 almost half of all hip fractures will occur in men.

A recent report[66] indicated that elderly African Americans may be at greater risk for bone loss and fracture than previously thought. Community-living African Americans ages 68 to 93 were found to have low serum vitamin D and high serum PTH levels, which suggest poor calcium balance. No clinical studies have evaluated bone metabolism in aging African Americans, and this work is long overdue.

Osteomalacia

How osteomalacia develops. Osteomalacia, the adult form of rickets, is found in older adults. Osteomalacia and osteoporosis are both characterized by an inadequate amount of bone mineral; however, their etiologies differ.[31] People with osteomalacia have a normal amount of protein matrix, but it is not mineralized because of vitamin D deficiency and inadequate calcium absorption. In contrast, osteoporotic bone has lost both mineral and matrix as a result of hormonal, nutritional, and lifestyle factors. In osteoporosis, bone loss usually begins in the vertebrae or hip; in osteomalacia, bone loss is most apparent in the peripheral skeleton. Both disorders can exist in the same individual, but techniques now being used to evaluate bone mineral mass cannot distinguish the presence of protein matrix. A bone biopsy and histologic examination of tissues are required to confirm a diagnosis of osteomalacia.

In the young person with vitamin D deficiency, calcium levels are insufficient to mineralize newly formed bone matrix. In the older person, the situation is compounded by the fact that a fall in serum calcium and phosphorus not only fails to mineralize the matrix formed in bone remodeling but also stimulates the secretion of PTH, which leads to the resorption of existing bone.[31] The extensive bone loss observed in osteomalacia likely relates to the elevated secretion of PTH.

Clinical symptoms of osteomalacia include generalized bone pain, which in time becomes localized, and bones that become extremely sensitive to pressure. Changes in the vertebrae cause a loss in height, and the bones of the pelvis and sternum may become deformed. Muscle weakness is apparent in advanced osteomalacia as a result of low serum calcium and affects the pelvic and shoulder areas. Individuals may have trouble climbing stairs or raising their arms to comb their hair. Unfortunately, the pain is often assumed to be caused by arthritis, and muscle weakness tends to be expected in older people. Careful diagnostic evaluation of bone pain is critical to differentiate between osteoporosis and osteomalacia.

Causes of osteomalacia. Osteomalacia is less prevalent in the United States than in some other countries, and this has been attributed to the vitamin D-fortification of milk. Nevertheless, institutionalized or homebound older people who do not go outdoors and do not consume vitamin D-fortified dairy products are at risk of vitamin D deficiency and osteomalacia. Liver or renal disease that interferes with the conversion of vitamin D to its active form can lead to osteomalacia.[31] Malabsorption of fat can contribute to vitamin D deficiency.

Excessive use of antacids that contain aluminum hydroxide and bind dietary phosphate has been associated with this condition. In one clinical report[40] an earlier diagnosis based on radiological findings had considered the bone problem to be osteoporosis and so the use of aluminum hydroxide-containing antacids had continued with a further deterioration of bone health. Withdrawal of the antacids and a high calcium intake with adequate vitamin D will halt the bone loss. Continued use of phenytoin for control of seizures can lead to osteomalacia, as this drug interferes with the hydroxylation of vitamin D in the liver.[31]

Despite the fact that osteomalacia could contribute to bone loss and hip fracture, it does not appear to be generally associated with osteoporosis. Nevertheless, vitamin D deficiency leading to elevated serum PTH can exacerbate the bone loss associated with osteoporosis.

NUTRITION PROBLEMS ASSOCIATED WITH GASTROINTESTINAL FUNCTION

Functional changes in the gastrointestinal tract have both a direct and indirect effect on nutritional well-being in the older adult. Xerostomia or dysphagia can make eating difficult and effectively reduce food intake. Problems in bowel function and real or perceived constipation often lead to use of laxatives that increase losses of fluid and important electrolytes. The health professional working with older adults must be alert to these conditions and offer appropriate dietary guidance (see chapter 4 to review these conditions).

Food Intake and Changes in the Oral Cavity

Xerostomia. Xerostomia, or dry mouth, a common problem among older people, can arise from several causes, including a change in function of the central nervous system, certain prescription drugs such as antidepressants, antihypertensive agents, and bronchodilators, and radiation and chemotherapy cancer treatments.[53] Infections and ulcers in the oral cavity and increased tooth decay are consequences of dry mouth. Difficulty in lubricating, masticating, tasting, and swallowing food are critical effects of this condition.

Rhodus and Brown[73] compared the nutrient intakes of independently living and institutionalized adults with xerostomia and control subjects of similar age. Mean age was 68 to 69 years in all three groups. The institutionalized individuals with xerostomia had lower intakes of all nutrients than their counterparts living in the community. Energy intake was only 1,190 kcal in the institutionalized patients with dry mouth, as compared to 1,739 kcal in their counterparts living in the community. Older people with normal salivary secretion were consuming 2,164 kcal each day. None of the control subjects had less than the recommended levels of energy, protein, vitamins A and C, thiamin, and riboflavin, and only 5% were low in calcium and iron. In contrast 25% to 90% of those with xerostomia fell below the RDA for these nutrients. Diets were most inadequate for vitamin B-6, calcium, potassium, and zinc. BMI was significantly lower, and the number of individuals with inadequate serum albumin was higher among those with xerostomia. General health was similar across all groups. Xerostomia is an important risk factor for less than adequate nutrient intake.

Developing a care plan for patients with xerostomia involves both preventive and palliative measures.[53] If the condition is drug-related, a different drug with less severe side effects might be substituted. When the xerostomia is irreversible, attention to appropriate food choices, adequate hydration, and saliva stimulants is important. Foods that are spicy, acidic, or salty that could further irritate the tissues of the oral cavity should be avoided. To facilitate chewing and swallowing, moisten or dilute foods with milk, gravy, or sauces. Encourage a generous intake of water and other fluids low in sugar and noncaffeinated. Small, frequent sips of water help to moisten the mouth. Sugarless hard candy or chewing gum stimulates the secretion of saliva and reduces discomfort and irritation. Artificial saliva preparations with glycerine coat and lubricate the mucosa, and fluoride gels reduce the risk of dental caries. Coating the lips and dentures with petroleum jelly can be helpful in making the patient more comfortable. Mouth washes containing alcohol and alcoholic beverages should be avoided.

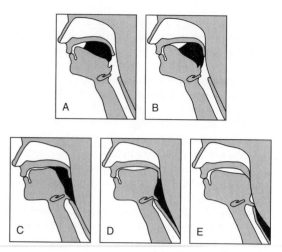

FIG. 12-4 Sequence of Events in Swallowing. **A,** Food is moved to rear of mouth. **B,** Soft palate rises and obstructs nasal passage. **C,** Epiglottis closes to obstruct trachea. **D,** Bolus passes through upper esophageal sphincter. **E,** Bolus moves down esophagus.

Adapted from Rushmer, R.F., and Hendron, J.A.: The act of deglutition: A cinefluorographic study, J. Applied Physiology 3:622, 1951. (With permission of the American Physiological Society.)

Dysphagia. Dysphagia is caused by changes in the central nervous system and deterioration of neuromuscular control. A cerebrovascular accident or stroke, Parkinson's disease, or organic brain syndrome can disrupt neural control of the muscles involved in swallowing and tongue movement. Diabetic neuropathy can lead to swallowing disorders. Dysphagia is characterized by difficulty passing food from the oral cavity to the stomach. As described in figure 12-4, swallowing is a complex process involving three phases:[86]

- In the oral phase, food is masticated, mixed with salivary secretions, and prepared for swallowing; the liquid or food bolus is then moved to the rear of the mouth.
- In the pharyngeal phase, the food is forced into the throat; for a moment breathing stops, the soft palate rises to prevent food from entering the nasal passages, the epiglottis closes to prevent food from entering the trachea, and the upper esophageal sphincter relaxes.

- In the esophageal phase, the food bolus or liquid enters the esophagus and moves down the passage; the lower esophageal sphincter relaxes and the food enters the stomach; the soft palate and epiglottis return to their normal positions, and breathing resumes.

Dysphagia has implications for both nutritional and physical health. This condition can limit the type and quantity of foods and liquids consumed, contributing to malnutrition or dehydration. Liquids, particularly thin liquids such as water, coffee, or tea, may be even more difficult to handle than solid foods. An immediate danger is choking and aspiration of food into the lung with development of pneumonia.[86] Thus, care in feeding and the selection of appropriately prepared foods are paramount. Evaluation and a treatment plan require a team approach that includes the physician, nurse, speech and language pathologist, and nutritionist.

Matthews[55] developed the following guidelines for working with dysphagic adults:

Positioning: The individual should be sitting at a 90-degree angle both when eating and for about 30 minutes before and after eating to take advantage of gravity flow and to properly align the esophagus for swallowing.

Food of appropriate consistency: Thick liquids, pureed meats in sauce or gravy, and foods that easily form a bolus in the mouth are preferred; sticky foods, foods with stringy fibers such as celery, foods with small seeds or pits, and foods with two consistencies (e.g., soups containing small pieces of meat or vegetables) increase the risk of choking and aspiration.

Environment: A relaxed, unhurried atmosphere is important, so the individual can take small amounts of food at a time and eat at a pace he or she finds comfortable. (Further suggestions and additional readings can be found in a journal article by Tripp and Cordero.)[86]

Health professionals working with older people must be alert to the need for ongoing evaluation of swallowing ability in both community-living and institutionalized older adults. In a survey of 136 community residents over age 87,[9] 16% reported bouts of coughing and choking when eating and drinking, or having

to swallow more than once to remove the same bite of food from the mouth. Institutionalized older adults may be inappropriately assigned to a diet based on suspected swallowing problems, or their ability to swallow may improve following an acute illness. An evaluation of 212 nursing home residents by a speech and language pathologist indicated that 91% were given diets modified to a greater extent than necessary.[35] The majority of these elderly people were receiving tube feedings or pureed diets. Following reevaluation and a gradual adjustment to the new diet level, many of those on tube feedings were advanced to pureed diets, and those formerly on pureed diets were successfully eating mechanical soft diets (regular foods with ground meat). The ability of these elderly people to have an improved quality of life underscores the need for ongoing evaluation of patients with feeding problems.

Dyspepsia. Abdominal discomfort following food ingestion can have many causes. Drugs such as digitalis, levodopa, or aspirin may be at fault. Overconsumption of food or alcohol can produce gastrointestinal distress. The reflux of gastric acid into the esophagus can be a source of discomfort and may indicate a hiatal hernia. Discomfort from burning sensations caused by irritation of the gastric mucosa or distention often leads to constant swallowing in an effort to relieve the distress. However, swallowing air can exacerbate the problem and lead to more discomfort. Psychologic stress and tension can cause gastric distress.[12]

Although chronic indigestion may signal the presence of ulcers or other organic disorder, some individuals experience chronic dyspepsia with no identifiable cause. Although we have no cure, symptoms can be reduced by avoiding alcohol, aspirin, other known stomach irritants, and large, heavy meals. Severe gastric distress can be treated with H_2-blockers, drugs that reduce the secretion of gastric acid and pepsin.[12] Chronic dyspepsia, nausea, or vomiting should be evaluated carefully for possible organic disease. Indigestion and gastrointestinal dysfunction are not normal consequences of advancing age.

Problems in Bowel Function

Disruption of normal bowel function, whether diarrhea or constipation, causes distress in older people. Both conditions have important implications for nutritional well-being. Diarrhea results in loss of nutrients and can be a symptom of a serious condition. Chronic constipation often causes anorexia, and fecal impaction is associated with nausea and, in some instances, spurious diarrhea.

Diarrhea. Diarrhea in an older person needs immediate evaluation. Osmotic diarrhea can stem from using magnesium hydroxide-containing antacids or eating lactose-containing foods if the person is deficient in lactase. Malabsorption syndromes involving fat or gluten-sensitive enteropathy are accompanied by diarrhea. Diarrhea related to fecal impaction requires immediate medical intervention. Infectious diarrhea is more common in older people than younger people, and because of decreased gastric acidity and intestinal motility, pathogens can remain in the gastrointestinal tract for a long time. Diarrhea is also a characteristic symptom of gastrointestinal cancer. An important aspect of treatment is the replacement of fluids followed by the restoration of bland foods to the diet, such as cooked cereals, bread, crackers, baked potato, or eggs. Fried or spicy foods, candy, and caffeinated or alcoholic beverages should be avoided. A normal diet should be tolerable within two or three days.

Management of constipation. Many older people have constipation over a period of years or even decades and regard it as a serious health problem. In fact among the frail homebound elderly studied by Wolfsen and coworkers,[91] many considered constipation to be a major health problem and, of this group, half rated it as one of their three top concerns. An issue of importance is the treatment strategies used to manage constipation. The overwhelming majority of this homebound elderly group choose to use laxatives, although 17 of the 62 also tried to make a dietary change. Of the 23 subjects who made dietary changes either in combination with laxatives or alone, only five added a high fiber food. A few people took molasses every day, and 10 people added a fruit. However, the fruit usually added was prunes, which are low in fiber but contain phenolphthalein. Phenolphthalein is the pharmacologic ingredient in irritant laxatives that can lead to neural changes in the wall of the colon and loss of colonic muscle motility.

Although laxative use has long been associated with fluid and electrolyte losses, a recent report suggests a relationship between laxative use and protein status. In a longitudinal study of 2,529 older people in Iowa, age 71 or older,[64] those using laxatives regularly were three times as likely to have a serum albumin below 3.5 g/dl. This remained true after adjusting for age, disability, prescription drug use, BMI, presence of anemia, or institutionalization. In that hypoalbuminemia is a predictor of disease and mortality in older individuals, this relationship deserves further study.

Constipation can often be alleviated and usually prevented by (1) increasing dietary fiber, (2) increasing fluid intake to 2,000 ml a day, and (3) getting more exercise which stimulates colonic motility. These measures are less likely to be effective if long-term laxative use has resulted in loss of colonic motility or muscle coordination.

Dietary fiber and bowel habits. Dietary treatment of constipation usually involves increasing fiber intake, either with fiber-rich foods or fiber supplements. Eating 10 to 20 g of wheat bran daily (4 to 8 g of dietary fiber) was shown to alleviate constipation in up to 60% of an older institutionalized population.[12] However, increasing dietary fiber to this extent initially will result in flatulence, abdominal distress, and in some cases, even more irregular bowel habits than when using laxatives. It is best to increase fiber intake gradually to allow adaptation to the higher fiber level. All increases in dietary fiber should be accompanied by a generous intake of fluids. Bran supplements or preparations containing psyllium can obstruct the esophagus and are not appropriate for older people with dysphagia or esophageal problems. Stool bulking agents are not appropriate for severely debilitated older patients. Using bran supplements in institutional settings has been reported to be successful in reducing the need for laxatives, adding to the general comfort of

❖ ❖ ❖

CASE STUDY

Miss S is a 77-year-old Caucasian woman who was admitted to the hospital with a hip fracture. Her admission assessment revealed the following information:

Dietary: currently consumes approximately 90% of the RDA for calcium, energy, and protein.

Biochemical: serum PTH and vitamin D concentrations below normal limits.

History: before retiring she worked in a factory, often working 12-hour shifts from sunup to sundown; she smoked 15 to 20 cigarettes a day since she was a teenager; she had moderate alcohol intake (one to two drinks a day) during her adult years.

1. Based on the above information, what is her most likely diagnosis?
2. What additional information would confirm the diagnosis?
3. How could the lifestyle factors revealed in her history have impacted the development of her bone disease?
4. What would be the most likely medical treatment prescribed for Miss S?
5. Develop a dietary protocol for Miss S that includes recommendations for all nutrients related to bone health.

---

many older patients and resulting in significant cost savings.[12] Before initiating dietary treatment of irregular bowel habits, it is imperative that organic causes of constipation (e.g., bowel obstruction or fecal impaction) be eliminated as possible factors.

Encouraging an individual to eat foods high in fiber is a desirable alternative to fiber supplements for older people who can eat reasonable amounts of food. Fruits, vegetables, whole-grain breads and cereals, and legumes not only contribute dietary fiber but also important vitamins and minerals. Unfortunately, daily fiber intake is often less than optimal in both institutionalized older people and those living in their own homes. In the NHANES III study[88] over half of the women over age 60 ate less than 13 g of fiber a day. The current recommendation of the National Cancer Institute suggests a fiber intake of 20 g to 30 g a day to be achieved by eating a variety of foods.[88] Findings from the NHANES I study[79] indicated that people who reported problems with constipation ate fewer servings of dried peas and beans, fruits, and vegetables. Twenty-one percent of those who never ate legumes were constipated, compared to 9% of those who ate legumes about once a day.

Older individuals with chewing or swallowing problems may not eat high-fiber foods regularly. Matthews[55] pointed out that green peas, baked beans, and lentils can be cooked to a soft con-

sistency or made into soup so they can be eaten fairly easily by those who are edentulous or have some degree of dysphagia. Whole-grain muffins, cookies, and hot breads may be attractive to older people who are less receptive to whole-grain breads or cereals. Wheat bran becomes more palatable when incorporated into baked products, soups, casseroles, or meat loaf.

Summary

Age-related degenerative changes exacerbated by chronic disease make the older individual increasingly vulnerable to nutrient-related chronic disorders, regardless of health status. Nutritional anemia in the aged person can have many different causes. Although iron-deficiency anemia is most often the result of occult blood loss, chronic infection, disease, protein-energy malnutrition, or changes in the bone marrow can impair erythropoiesis. Pernicious anemia, uncommon in younger people, is associated with macrocytic anemia, neural damage, and behavior changes in older people. A strategy for identifying vitamin B-12 deficiency in the absence of anemia is urgently needed. Hematologic parameters falling below normal ranges in older adults demand aggressive evaluation and intervention. PEM in older people is caused by inadequate nutrient intake, increased nutritional requirements, or both. Consequences of PEM include loss of muscle mass, decreased immune function, involuntary weight loss, and anemia. Protein-energy supplementation will reverse some, but not necessarily all of the manifestations of PEM. Avoidance of inappropriate weight gain and the appropriate loss of even small amounts of excessive body weight can reduce morbidity and mortality in older people.

Osteoporosis, characterized by a loss of bone matrix and mineral with a loss of bone strength, is a major cause of bone fracture and associated disability, particularly in older women. Bone mass at maturity, intakes of calcium and vitamin D, genetic disposition, level of physical activity, presence of metabolic disorders that enhance PTH secretion and urinary calcium loss, and estrogen status all influence bone health at older ages. Functional disorders of the gastrointestinal tract, including xerostomia, dysphagia, and dyspepsia, cause discomfort and may lead to a reduction in food intake. Problems in bowel function and constipation often lead to use of laxatives that increase fluid and electrolyte loss. Encouraging older individuals to eat foods high in dietary fiber is an important dietary recommendation that can alleviate bowel problems.

REVIEW QUESTIONS

1. Describe the different etiologies, criteria for diagnosis, and treatments of iron-deficiency anemia and anemia of chronic disease. Are there any potential harms associated with treating anemia of chronic disease with iron supplements?
2. What causes pernicious anemia? Why is it more prevalent in older people? What hematologic changes are associated with pernicious anemia? What treatment should be prescribed for a person with pernicious anemia?
3. What are the positive and negative outcomes associated with weight loss in older people? What is the appropriate approach for weight loss in an older person? How would you decide if weight loss should be recommended for an older individual?
4. Why are chronic disorders hard to diagnose and treat in older people? Why is osteoporosis so "costly"? What factors influence bone density? Do cortical bone and trabecular bone differ in patterns of loss? What is the difference between osteoporosis and osteomalacia?
5. What are the causes of xerostomia? What effect does xerostomia have on nutritional status? What

dietary recommendations are appropriate for a person with dysphagia? Why does dysphagia increase the risk for aspiration of food into the lungs? Describe the treatment of constipation in the elderly.

SUGGESTED LEARNING ACTIVITIES

1. Design a standard-of-care protocol to be used for older adults with protein-energy malnutrition living in an assisted-care facility. Include criteria for diagnosis and monitoring, potential complications, treatment including dietary recommendations, and plan for follow-up.
2. Your 86-year-old uncle has recently been diagnosed with osteoporosis. He tells you that men do not get osteoporosis, that it is a "woman's disease." How would you respond to him? Plan a three-day diet program for your uncle, including calcium-rich foods even though he is lactose intolerant.
3. Beginning with the identification in an older person of a below-normal hemoglobin level, develop an algorithm of further dietary, clinical, and biochemical measurements and standards that you would use to determine the type of anemia—iron-deficiency anemia, anemia of chronic disease, or pernicious anemia—that was the cause of the low hemoglobin.
4. Prepare a one-page nutrition education tool on the benefits of a high-fiber diet, including examples of high-fiber foods and easy ways to incorporate them into the meal plan of older people.

REFERENCES

1. Abraham, S., Collins, G., and Nordsieck, M.: Relationship of childhood weight status to morbidity in adults, Public Health Rep. 86:273, 1971.
2. Agarwal, N., and others: Predictive ability of various nutritional variables for mortality in elderly people, Am. J. Clin. Nutr. 48:1173, 1988.
3. Ahluwalia, N., and others: Day-to-day variation in iron status indexes in elderly women, Am. J. Clin. Nutr. 57:414, 1993.
4. Ahluwalia, N., and others: Iron deficiency and anemia of chronic disease in elderly women: a discriminant-analysis approach for differentiation, Am. J. Clin. Nutr. 61:590, 1995.
5. Aloia, J.F., and others: Calcium supplementation with and without hormone replacement therapy to prevent postmenopausal bone loss, Ann. Intern. Med. 120:97, 1994.

6. Bales, C.N., and Gold, D.T.: Nutrition education for osteoporosis patients: an innovative approach to care of the chronically ill elderly, J. Nutr. Educ. 23:120, 1991.
7. Beard, J.L., Ashraf, M.H., and Smiciklas-Wright, H.: Iron nutrition in the elderly. In: Watson, R.R., editor: Handbook of nutrition in the aged, ed. 2, Boca Raton, 1994, CRC Press.
8. Bergstrom, N., and Braden, B.: A prospective study of pressure sore risk among institutionalized elderly, J. Am. Geriatr. Soc. 40:747, 1992.
9. Bloem, B.R., and others: Prevalence of subjective dysphagia in community residents aged over 87, Br. Med. J. 300:722, 1989.
10. Breslow, R.A., and others: The importance of dietary protein in healing pressure ulcers, J. Am. Geriatr. Soc. 41:357, 1993.
11. Carmel, R.: Pernicious anemia; the expected findings of very low serum cobalamin levels, anemia, and macrocytosis are often lacking, Arch. Intern. Med. 148:1712, 1988.
12. Cashman, M.D.: The aging gut. In: Chernoff, R., editor: Geriatric nutrition. The health professional's handbook, Gaithersburg, MD, 1991, Aspen Publications.
13. Chapuy, M.C., and others: Vitamin D_3 and calcium to prevent hip fractures in elderly women, New Engl. J. Med. 327:1637, 1992.
14. Chen, L.H., and Cook-Newell, M.E.: Anemia and iron status in the free-living and institutionalized elderly in Kentucky, Inter. J. Vit. Nutr. Res. 59:207, 1989.
15. Chernoff, R.: Nutritional support in the elderly. In Chernoff, R., editor: Geriatric nutrition. The health professional's handbook, Gaithersburg, MD, 1991, Aspen Publishers.
16. Chernoff, R.: Policy: nutrition standards for treatment of pressure ulcers, Nutr. Rev. 54(1[II]):S43, 1996.
17. Chestnut, C.H.: Alendronate treatment of the postmenopausal osteoporotic woman: effect of multiple dosages on bone mass and bone remodeling, Amer. J. Med. 99:144, 1995.
18. Chiari, M.M., and others: Influence of acute inflammation on iron and nutritional status indexes in older inpatients, J. Am. Geriatr. Soc. 43:767, 1995.
19. Colditz, G.A., and others: Prospective study of estrogen replacement therapy and risk of breast cancer in postmenopausal women, J.A.M.A. 264:2648, 1990.
20. Dalsky, G.P., and others: Weight-bearing exercise training and lumbar bone mineral content in postmenopausal women, Ann. Intern. Med. 108:824, 1988.
21. Daly, M.P., and Sobal, J.: Anemia in the elderly; a survey of physicians' approaches to diagnosis and workup, J. Fam. Pract. 28:524, 1989.
22. Dawson-Hughes, B.: Calcium supplementation and bone loss: a review of controlled clinical trials, Am. J. Clin. Nutr. 54:274S, 1991.
23. Delmi, M., and others: Dietary supplementation in elderly patients with fractured neck of the femur, Lancet 335:1013, 1990.
24. Durnin, J.V.G.A.: Anthropometric methods of assessing nutritional status. In Horwitz, A., and others, editors: Nutrition in the elderly, New York, 1989, Oxford University Press.
25. Dwyer, J.T., and others: Changes in relative weight among institutionalized elderly adults, J. Gerontol. 42:246, 1987.
26. Erban, J.K.: Hematologic problems of the elderly. In Reichel, W., editor: Care of the elderly. Clinical aspects of aging, ed. 4, Baltimore, 1995, Williams and Wilkins.
27. Felson, D.T.: Weight and osteoarthritis, Am. J. Clin. Nutr. 63(suppl):430S, 1996.
28. Fischer, L., and Johnson, M.A.: Low body weight and weight loss in the aged, J. Am Diet. Assoc. 90:1697, 1990.
29. Fogt, E.J., Bell, S.J., and Blackburn, G.L.: Nutrition assessment of the elderly. In: Morley, J.E., Glick, Z., and Rubenstein, L.Z., editors: Geriatric nutrition. A comprehensive review, ed. 2, New York, 1995, Raven Press.
30. Gallagher, J.C.: Prevention of bone loss in postmenopausal and senile osteoporosis with vitamin D analogues, Osteoporosis Int. Suppl. 1:S172, 1993.
31. Gambert, S.R., and Schultz, B.M.: Osteomalacia. In: Watson, R.R., editor: Handbook of nutrition in the aged, ed. 2, Boca Raton, FL, 1994, CRC Press.
32. Gilmore, S.A.: Clinical indicators associated with unintentional weight loss and pressure ulcers in elderly residents of nursing facilities, J. Am. Diet. Assoc. 95:984, 1995.
33. Goodnough, L.T., Price, T.H., and Parvin, C.A.: The endogenous erythropoietin response and the erythropoietic response to blood loss anemia: the effects of age and gender, J. Lab. Clin. Med. 125:57, 1995.
34. Gorbach, S.L., and others: Changes in food patterns during a low-fat dietary intervention in women, J. Am. Diet. Assoc. 90:802, 1990.
35. Groher, M.E., and McKaig, T.N.: Dysphagia and dietary levels in skilled nursing facilities, J. Am. Geriatr. Soc. 43:528, 1995.

36. Hathcock, J.N., and Troendle, G.J.: Oral cobalamin for treatment of pernicious anemia, J.A.M.A. 265:96, 1991.

37. Herbert, V., Shaw, S., and Jayatilleke, E.: High serum ferritin protein does not distinguish iron overload from inflammation, but a new assay, high serum ferritin-iron, does, Am. J. Clin. Nutr. 61:119, 1995.

38. Holyoake, T.L., and others: Use of plasma ferritin concentration to diagnose iron deficiency in elderly patients, J. Clin. Pathol. 46:857, 1993.

39. Hu, J.F., and others: Dietary calcium and bone density among middle-aged and elderly women in China, Am. J. Clin. Nutr. 58:219, 1993.

40. Insogna, K.L., and others: Osteomalacia and weakness from excessive antacid ingestion, J.A.M.A. 244:2544, 1980.

41. Kiebzak, G.M.: Age-related bone changes, Exp. Gerontol. 26:171, 1991.

42. Krall, E.A., and Dawson-Hughes, B.: Walking is related to bone density and rates of bone loss, Amer. J. Med. 96:20, 1994.

43. Lee, M.H., and Means, R.T.: Extremely elevated serum ferritin levels in a university hospital: associated diseases and clinical significance, Am. J. Med. 98:566, 1995.

44. Levenson, D.I., and Bockman, R.S.: A review of calcium preparations, Nutr. Rev. 52(7):221, 1994.

45. Lindenbaum, J., and others: Neuropsychiatric disorders caused by cobalamin deficiency in the absence of anemia or macrocytosis, New Engl. J. Med. 318:1720, 1988.

46. Lindenbaum, J., and others: Prevalence of cobalamin deficiency in the Framingham elderly population, J. Am. Clin. Nutr. 60:2, 1994.

47. Lipschitz, D.A.: Approaches to the nutritional support of the older patient, Clin. Geriatr. Med. 11(4):715, 1995.

48. Lipschitz, D.A.: Impact of nutrition on the age-related decline in hematopoiesis. In: Chernoff, R., editor: Geriatric nutrition. The health professional's handbook, Gaithersburg, MD, 1991, Aspen Publishers.

49. Lipschitz, D.A.: Nutrition-related anemias in the elderly. In Morley, J.E., Glick, Z., and Rubenstein, L.Z., editors: Geriatric nutrition. A comprehensive review, ed. 2, New York, 1995, Raven Press.

50. Lissner, L., and others: Body weight variability in men: metabolic rate, health, and longevity, Int. J. Obesity 14:373, 1989.

51. Lissner, L., and others: Variability of body weight and health outcomes in the Framingham population, New Engl. J. Med. 324:1839, 1991.

52. Martin, D.C., and others: Time dependency of cognitive recovery with cobalamin replacement: report of a pilot study, J. Am. Geriatr. Soc. 40:168, 1992.

53. Martin, W.E.: The oral cavity and nutrition. In: Morley, J.E., Glick, Z., and Rubenstein, L.Z., editors: Geriatric nutrition. A comprehensive review, ed. 2, New York, 1995, Raven Press.

54. Martinez, O.B.: Indices of vitamin, iron, and hematological status of a selected sample of elderly Canadians, Nutr. Res. 8:1345, 1988.

55. Matthews, L.E.: Techniques for feeding the person with dysphagia, J. Nutr. Elderly 8:59, 1988.

56. Meisler, J.G., and St. Jeor, S.: Summary and recommendations from the American Health Foundations expert panel on healthy weight, Am. J. Clin. Nutr. 62(suppl):474S, 1996.

57. Melton, M.E., and Kochman, M.L.: Reversal of severe osteoporosis with vitamin B-12 and etidronate therapy in a patient with pernicious anemia, Metabolism 43(4):468, 1994.

58. Morley, J.E.: Nutrition. In: Abrams, W.B., Beers, M.H., and Berkow, R., editors: Merck manual of geriatrics, ed. 2, Whitehouse Station, NJ, 1995, Merck Research Laboratories.

59. Morley, J.E., and Glick, Z.: Obesity. In: Morley, J.E., Glick, Z., and Rubenstein, L.Z., editors: Geriatric nutrition. A comprehensive review, ed. 2, New York, 1995, Raven Press.

60. Nelson, K.M., and others: Protein and energy balance following femoral neck fracture in geriatric patients, Metabolism 44(1):59, 1995.

61. Nordin, B.E.C., and others: Treatment of osteoporosis in the elderly, Clin. Geriatr. Med. 10(4):625, 1994.

62. Nutrition Screening Initiative: Nutrition interventions manual for professionals caring for older Americans, Washington, DC, 1992, Nutrition Screening Initiative.

63. Osterweil, D., Wendt, P.F., and Ferrell, B.A.: Pressure ulcers and nutrition. In: Morley, J.E., Glick, Z., and Rubenstein, L.Z., editors: Geriatric nutrition. A comprehensive review, ed. 2, New York, 1995, Raven Press.

64. Pahor, M., and others: Use of laxatives medication in older persons and associations with low serum albumin, J. Am. Geriatr. Soc. 42:50, 1994.

65. Pak, C.Y.C., and others: Treatment of postmenopausal osteoporosis with slow-release sodium fluoride, Ann. Intern. Med. 123:401, 1995.

66. Perry, H.M., and others: A preliminary report of vitamin D and calcium metabolism in older African Americans, J. Am. Geriatr. Soc. 41:6121, 1993.

67. Pilch, S.M., and Senti, F.R., eds.: Assessment of the iron nutritional status of the U.S. population based on data collected in the Second National Health and Nutrition Examination Survey, 1976–1980, Bethesda, MD, 1984, Life Sciences Research Office, Federation of American Societies for Experimental Biology.

68. Rajala, S.A., and others: Body weight and the three-year prognosis in very old people, Inter. J. Obesity 14:997, 1990.

69. Recker, R.R., and others: Patient care of osteoporosis, Clin. Geriatr. Med. 11(4):625, 1995.

70. Reid, I.A., and others: Effect of calcium supplementation on bone loss in postmenopausal women, New Engl. J. Med. 328:460, 1993.

71. Research Group on Aging (GERBAP): Extensive laboratory assessment of nutritional status in fit, health-conscious, elderly people living in the Paris area, J. Amer. Coll. Nutr. 13(6):646, 1994.

72. Resnick, N.M., and Greenspan, S.L.: Senile osteoporosis reconsidered, J.A.M.A. 261:1025, 1989.

73. Rhodus, N.L., and Brown, J.: The association of xerostomia and inadequate intake in older adults, J. Am. Diet. Assoc. 90:1688, 1990.

74. Rico, H., and others: Total and regional bone mineral content and fracture rate in postmenopausal osteoporosis treated with salmon calcitonin: a prospective study, Calcif. Tissue Int. 56:181, 1995.

75. Riggs, B.L., and Melton, L.J.: Involutional osteoporosis, New Engl. J. Med. 314:1676, 1986.

76. Riggs, B.L., and Melton, L.J.: The prevention and treatment of osteoporosis, New Engl. J. Med. 327(9):620, 1992.

77. Roebotham, B.V., and Chandra, R.K.: Relationship between nutritional status and immune function of elderly people, Age Ageing 23:49, 1994.

78. Russell, R.M.: Anemia. In: Hartz, S.C., Russell, R.M., and Rosenberg, L.H., editors: Nutrition in the elderly. The Boston nutritional status survey, London, 1992, Smith-Gordon and Company.

79. Sandler, R.S., and others: Demographic and dietary determinants of constipation in the U.S. population, Am. J. Public Health 80:185, 1990.

80. Seeman, E.: The dilemma of osteoporosis in men, Am. J. Med. 98(suppl 2A):2A-76S, 1995.

81. Snow-Harter, C., and Marcus, R.: Exercise, bone mineral density, and osteoporosis, Exercise Sport Sci. Rev. 19:351, 1991.

82. Steen, B.: Obesity in the aged. In: Watson, R.R., editor: Handbook of nutrition in the aged, ed. 2, Boca Raton, FL, 1994, CRC Press.

83. Stunkard, A.J.: Conservative treatments for obesity, Am. J. Clin. Nutr. 45:1142, 1987.

84. Sullivan, D.H., and Walls, R.C.: Impact of nutritional status on morbidity in a population of geriatric rehabilitation patients, J. Am. Geriatr. Soc. 42:471, 1994.

85. Sullivan, D.H., Walls, R.C., and Lipschitz, D.A.: Protein-energy undernutrition and the risk of mortality within 1 y of hospital discharge in a select population of geriatric rehabilitation patients, Am. J. Clin. Nutr. 53:599, 1991.

86. Tripp, F., and Cordero, O.: Dysphagia and nutrition in the acute care geriatric patient, Top. Clin. Nutr. 6:60, 1991.

87. Tucker, L.A., and Friedman, G.M.: Television viewing and obesity in adult males, Am. J. Public Health 79:516, 1989.

88. U.S. Department of Health and Human Services: Dietary intake of vitamins, minerals, and fiber of persons ages 2 months and over in the United States: Third National Health and Nutrition Examination Survey, Phase I, 1988–91, Advance Data from Vital and Health Statistics, Number 258, Nov. 14, 1994, Hyattsville, MD, National Center for Health Statistics.

89. Wallace, J.I., and others: Involuntary weight loss in older outpatients: incidence and clinical significance, J. Am. Geriatr. Soc. 43:329, 1995.

90. Wardlaw, G.M.: Putting osteoporosis in perspective, J. Am. Diet. Assoc. 93:1000, 1993.

91. Wolfsen, C.R., Barker, J.C., and Mitteness, L.S.: Constipation in the daily lives of frail elderly people, Arch. Fam. Med. 2:853, 1993.

92. Zauber, N.P., and Zauber, A.G.: Hematologic data of healthy very old people, J.A.M.A. 257:2181, 1987.

Nutrition, Physiologic Function, and Chronic Disease

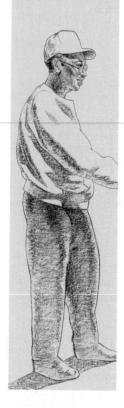

++

Objectives

After studying this chapter, the student should be able to:

✔ *Understand the relationship between the function of organ systems and aging, chronic disease, and physiologic stress*

✔ *Recognize the types of disruptions in brain physiology that cause reversible and irreversible dementia*

✔ *List the factors that contribute to age-related changes in glucose metabolism, and appreciate the importance of dietary therapy in diabetes mellitus*

✔ *Understand the effects of aging, nutrition, and activity on cardiovascular function and the development of hypertension in the elderly*

✔ *Identify factors associated with age, disease, and nutrition that affect renal, pulmonary, and immune function*

INTRODUCTION

Physiologic change continues throughout life. During the period of growth, increases in body size are readily apparent and are indicators of internal changes in physiologic function. Beyond maturity, changes in physical dimensions occur more slowly, but internal changes in body composition and organ function continue to take place. In previous chapters we discussed age-related changes in body composition, including muscle mass, bone mineral mass, and fat.

Organ systems demonstrate different patterns of change over the course of adulthood. Several patterns of change are described below:

• Remains stable with little or no change. Resting heart rate and fasting blood glucose exhibit very little change into advanced age.

• Declines steadily in healthy people. Basal metabolism and vital capacity decrease at a slow but steady rate through middle age and beyond; secretion of growth hormone demonstrates a slow but steady decline per decade of age.

- Declines precipitously and can be accelerated by disease. Maximal breathing capacity declines rapidly and loss in function is exacerbated by emphysema or pulmonary disease; bone mass is lost at an accelerated rate in women after menopause.

In older people it is not always possible to recognize the difference between biologic changes related to aging and those related to disease. Disease may accentuate an aging effect; for example, an excessive accumulation of abdominal fat can exacerbate an age-related change in glucose tolerance. On the other hand, maximum oxygen consumption may actually increase in an elderly person who has been sedentary and initiates an exercise program.

Chronic disease often influences the symptoms associated with a particular disorder in older people, making recognition more difficult.[45] In chapter 12 we noted that chronic inflammation causing an increase in ferritin synthesis can obscure an iron deficiency. A disease also can present different symptoms in elderly people. As described in chapter 5, hyperthyroidism in an older individual often results in lethargy, cardiac failure, or confusion. At one time we believed that aging changes were inevitable. We now recognize that successful aging is possible, and based on the concept of primary prevention, healthy lifestyle patterns can be designed to prevent disease before it starts. When chronic diseases do become apparent, intervention strategies related to diet, exercise, or appropriate medications will slow or prevent their progress. In this chapter we discuss aging changes in major organ systems and nutrition strategies for prevention and intervention.

AGING IN ORGAN SYSTEMS
Changes in Physiologic Function

A major characteristic of physiologic aging is a decrease in the ability to respond to changes in either the internal or external environment. The rate of recovery or return to homeostasis is slowed in the older individual. This alteration in response could stem from a decrease in the sensitivity of control receptors or from actual changes in tissue and organ function. Figure 13-1 describes the age-related decline in major organ

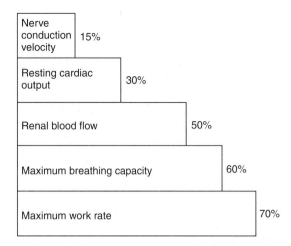

FIG. 13-1   Average Loss in Physiologic Functions Between Ages 30 and 80. Major organ systems, including the heart, lungs, and kidneys, undergo a loss in function as a result of normal aging (e.g., by age 80 kidney function is only 50% of its level at age 30). These changes were observed in men in the Baltimore Longitudinal Study of Aging.

Data from U.S. Department of Health and Human Services: Normal human aging: the Baltimore Longitudinal Study of Aging, NIH Publication No. 84-2450, Washington, DC, 1984, U.S. Government Printing Office.

systems observed in men ages 30 to 80.[75] The loss in function by age 80 is shown as a percentage of the level of function at age 30. These data came from the Baltimore Longitudinal Study of Aging (BLSA) being conducted by the National Institute on Aging. Although these values represent cross-sectional comparisons of function in different age groups, the long-range goal of the BLSA is to record the changes occurring within individuals over their adult lives.

Physiologic responses differ in their level of change according to the degree of coordination that is required among organ systems. Nerve conduction velocity, a function involving one organ system, decreases by about 15%. Resting cardiac output, which requires both neural and muscular coordination, declines by 30%. When the desired response involves many organ systems, as, for example, maximum work rate, the age-related decline is substantial (70%).[75]

In general, changes in physiologic function are most evident when simple behaviors are compared to more complex behaviors. An older person may walk with comparative ease on a level surface, but climbing stairs, which demands more complicated muscular motions and a greater oxygen expenditure, may require heavy effort and lead to tachycardia and labored breathing. Food preparation that requires both visual and motor coordination, such as peeling vegetables, may become difficult. Loss of neuromuscular control is believed to contribute significantly to the loss of muscle coordination.

Despite changes in physiologic capacity, most older people function quite well on a day-to-day basis under normal conditions. For most organ systems the level of maximum functional performance is 7 to 11 times the average physiologic demand;[75] thus, some degree of loss can occur with no noticeable effects. However, when extreme demands are placed on the system or when functional losses are excessive, problems become evident. As discussed in a later section, physiologic considerations such as reduced kidney function enter into dietary recommendations for older people.

Variability Among Individuals

Normal aging results in functional changes in the same direction in most people, but the rate of change is unique to each individual. In fact, the variability among individuals of the same age may actually exceed the variability among people of different ages.[75] Both genetic constitution and lifelong experiences that influence physical well-being exert an effect. Since no two people experience the same combination or intensity of influences, by age 60 all individuals are remarkably different. On this basis older people differ more from one another than do younger people. Such differences underscore the need to assess each older person as an individual.

AGING AND NEUROENDOCRINE FUNCTION
Mental Function

The assumption that changes in the nervous system and loss of mental function are normal consequences of aging is false.[42] Yet ascertaining the degree of loss of mental function in a particular individual can be of practical importance. When to relinquish one's driver's license often is an excruciating decision for the older person or for the family of an older driver when reaction time has deteriorated below a safe level. The results of a test of cognitive skills developed to measure response time, memory, and reasoning suggest that mental capacity begins to decline about age 45, but greater changes occur after age 65.[71] However, not all people experience the same degree of change. Those beyond the usual retirement age of 65 with test scores similar to younger people were most likely to be working, whereas those scoring lower than younger people were in many instances retired. This finding suggests that lifestyle rather than age influences mental function. Do people stop working because they realize they are no longer able to function at the same level, or do people lose mental acuity because they no longer have the mental stimulation associated with work responsibilities? Continuing research in both behavioral and biological aspects of neural function may provide an answer to this question.

Brain and Neural Tissue

Structural aspects. Cells in the central nervous system, unlike cells in some other organ systems, cannot reproduce. Cells in the liver or lung, if damaged or injured, can regenerate to some extent. Brain cells, if injured, usually die and disappear.[42] At one time health professionals believed that normal aging was characterized by brain atrophy and a significant loss of neurons. Brain weight declines by about 10% between ages 30 and 90, but massive losses of neurons occur only in those with brain diseases such as senile dementia of the Alzheimer type (SDAT).[38] In normal older people, neither brain size nor cell number is related to mental function. Brain cells are not lost equally across all areas of the brain; in some areas losses are minimal and in other areas quite significant. These losses likely influence the observed changes in some functions and not others.

The aging brain also retains the ability to form additional dendrites in the remaining neurons.[42]

This increase in **dendrites,** the tree-like branches that transmit impulses to and from the nerve cell body, makes possible new connections and may compensate for the loss in number of nerve cells. This growth in dendrites allows the formation of new pathways for neural transmission and may explain the ability of some older people to maintain a high level of cognitive function despite the loss of nerve cells.

Biochemical aspects. Biochemical as well as structural changes take place in the brains of older people even in the absence of neurologic diseases. Conduction of neural impulses requires the release of a chemical transmitter such as dopamine, serotonin, or acetylcholine by the neuron. Sufficient numbers of transmitter molecules must be present in the synapse (the space between the nerve cells) to activate the adjoining cell. Normal aging is associated with a lower level of neurotransmitters in brain tissue. This lower level of neurotransmitters could result from a decrease in synthesis. Two common neurotransmitters, dopamine and norepinephrine, are derived from tyrosine; serotonin is derived from tryptophan. The enzymes required for these biochemical conversions, tyrosine hydroxylase and aromatic amino acid decarboxylase, are present in lower amounts in the neurons of older people.[62] Conversely, other enzymes, including monoamine oxidase, that are detrimental to brain function are present in higher amounts. Increases in monoamine oxidase are associated with the loss of motor function in Parkinson's disease.[42]

The production of neurotransmitters can fall by 20% to 30% with no significant change in brain function, demonstrating the functional reserve capacity of the normal brain. However, when neurotransmitter synthesis drops below 50% of the normal level, some degree of dementia ensues.[42]

Disorders of the Nervous System

Of all the age-related changes that can present difficulties for older individuals and their families, none causes greater anxiety than the loss of mental function. In most healthy older people, occasional forgetfulness may be the only obvious change in mental function. In about 10% of older people, forgetfulness progresses to mild or moderate confusion. About 15% of older people have severe dementia, or so-called senile dementia, with loss of cognitive function and disturbances in behavior and mood.[72]

Age is the single most important risk factor for dementia.[72] SDAT is the most common cause of dementia in older people and accounts for more than half of all cases.[72] Loss of brain cells resulting from a cerebral hemorrhage or interruption of the blood supply to a particular region of the brain accounts for 20% to 30% of all cases.[72] Delirium or severe dementia can arise from acute electrolyte disturbances involving changes in serum sodium or potassium levels, thyroid dysfunction, drug toxicity, or illnesses that decrease the oxygen supply to the brain, which occurs in pneumonia or cardiac failure. Dementia occurring for the latter reasons usually is reversible following amelioration of the metabolic disturbance or infection. Changes in cognitive function stemming from SDAT or other excessive loss of brain cells are irreversible.

Senile dementia of the Alzheimer type (SDAT). Four million Americans have SDAT and the associated costs of long-term care exceed $90 billion a year.[6] SDAT is characterized by (1) a loss of cells from the cerebral cortex and other areas of the brain that control higher level function, and (2) the appearance in brain tissue of senile plaques (nerve cells surrounding a protein core) and neurofibrillary tangles of helical filaments. Although senile plaques and neurofibrillary tangles occur in normal aging, they are fewer in number. In SDAT the levels of all neurotransmitters are markedly lower.

SDAT is more common among women, although this may be because women live longer than men. Nevertheless, female gender might be a risk factor, since family history is involved in about half of SDAT patients.[72] The roles of viruses or environmental contaminants, particularly aluminum, have been studied, but no specific involvement has been identified.

In the early stages people with SDAT experience recent memory loss, personality changes, and increasing difficulty with daily activities, including finding their way around or preparing meals. In the latter stages these patients cannot perform any activity of daily living and become totally dependent on family caregivers or are admitted to a long-term care facility. Patients with SDAT appear to have elevated energy requirements, and weight loss is a problem.[60] Feeding can be difficult as patients become indifferent to their environment or develop compulsive eating and attempt to eat inedible objects. (Tips for feeding the SDAT patient were discussed in chapter 8.)

Parkinson's disease. About 1 million Americans have Parkinson's disease.[78] Although this disorder is uncommon among people under age 50, the incidence increases with age and peaks about age 75. Parkinson's disease is caused by a loss of neurons from the base of the brain whose function is production of the neurotransmitter dopamine. Dopamine is important in the control of muscle movement. When dopamine is no longer produced in sufficient quantities, the characteristic symptoms of Parkinson's disease—muscular rigidity, tremors, difficulty with balance, and a shuffling gait—become evident.

The usual treatment has been administration of the drug levodopa, which is converted to dopamine in the central nervous system.[78] As more neurons are lost, the patient is forced to take ever-increasing amounts of the drug to keep symptoms in check. Levodopa can bring about undesirable side effects, including mental confusion and gastrointestinal distress. Unfortunately, administered levodopa becomes less effective over time. Current research is directed toward drugs that will slow the rate of neuronal loss and thereby reduce the levels of levodopa required for control. Elderly adults with Parkinson's disease have low body weight and low body fat despite the recommended level of kilocalories.[15] Alterations in muscle metabolism and involuntary muscle movements no doubt contribute to their apparently elevated energy requirements.

Endocrine System

Many components of the endocrine system undergo changes with age, but these changes do not proceed in a uniform direction (table 13-1).[66] Some secretory endocrine organs become less active as a result of disease or reduced hormone utilization or excretion. For

TABLE 13-1 *Age-Related Changes in Serum Hormone Levels*

Increased Levels	Decreased Levels	No Change
Norepinephrine	Triiodothyronine	Epinephrine
Antidiuretic hormone	Estradiol (in women)	Cortisol
Insulin	Testosterone (in men)	Thyroxin
Parathyroid hormone	Growth hormone	
	Aldosterone	

Modified from Solomon, D.H.: Introduction. Organ systems: metabolic and endocrine disorders. In: Abrams, W.B., Beers, M.H., and Berkow, R., editors: Merck manual of geriatrics, ed. 2, Whitehouse Station, NJ, 1995, Merck Research Laboratories.

example, a reduction in lean body mass and need for thyroid hormone is considered to be the basis for the age-related decline in the secretion of triiodothyronine and its metabolic conversion to thyroid hormone. Age-associated increases in norepinephrine are thought to reflect a compensatory response of the hypothalamic-neurohypophyseal axis to the decreased number of hormone receptors in target tissues. Serum hormone levels are the end result of all structural and metabolic changes in endocrine-related tissues.

Nutritional status can influence endocrine activity.[51] Changes in the synthesis of plasma proteins that serve as transport molecules for hormones influence not only blood hormone concentrations but also the rates of conversion to active forms. Conversely, endocrine function has an important influence on nutritional status. Mild decreases in the secretion of growth hormone and changes in serum testosterone may contribute to the decline in nitrogen retention observed in some older people.[51] The role of insulin in protein utilization and storage could be especially critical in aged individuals with borderline intakes or excessive losses of protein. Altered endocrine function could influence the ability to adapt to changes in nutrient intake. Current research on endocrine function in aging focuses on the hypothalamic-neurohypophyseal axis, which regulates hormone secretion, and possible changes in sensitivity to messages received by the hypothalamus or target tissues.

Clinical Significance of Changes in Hormone Levels

Hormonal changes that have far-reaching effects on the health and well-being of elderly people include those involving the sex steroid hormones, parathyroid hormone, and insulin. Changes in estrogen secretion after menopause in women and decreasing levels of testosterone in older men disrupt bone metabolism and bone health. Inappropriately high serum levels of parathyroid hormone contribute to bone loss and development of osteoporosis, although adequate vitamin D or exposure to sunlight may in some instances reduce PTH levels. Because nutrition also plays an important role in bone health at all ages, osteopenia was discussed in chapter 12. Changes in the endocrine pancreas and reduced effectiveness of available insulin leads to the development of diabetes mellitus.

INSULIN SECRETION, CARBOHYDRATE METABOLISM, AND GLUCOSE TOLERANCE

The ability to metabolize carbohydrate deteriorates with age. It is estimated that 18% of the population between the ages of 65 and 75 have diabetes mellitus, either diagnosed or not diagnosed, and another 23% have impaired glucose tolerance.[26] Diabetics over the age of 65 are three times more likely to be hospitalized than nondiabetics and are more likely to be institutionalized.[26] In a young adult abnormal glucose tolerance is associated with the development of overt diabetes. In an older adult, differentiating age-related changes from the pathologic sequence of disease is more difficult, as is deciding on the appropriate treatment. Only about 10% of all diabetics are insulin-dependent, and most of these are younger adults.[14] The prevalence of noninsulin-dependent diabetes mellitus (NIDDM) increases with age, and over half of all patients with diabetes are over age 65.[26]

Age and Changes in Glucose Tolerance

Elevated plasma glucose following a meal occurs with increasing frequency across the adult years. Medical researchers[14] estimate that two-hour postprandial plasma glucose increases 5 mg/dl each decade after age 50. In contrast, fasting plasma glucose changes very little over adulthood, increasing only 1 to 2 mg/dl each decade beyond middle age. In the elderly adult, diabetes can be somewhat asymptomatic, with fatigue, loss of energy, or weight loss as the only signs. At times peripheral neuropathy, with tingling or numbness in the hands or feet, or blurred vision are the first signs of NIDDM in older adults.[14] The diagnosis of diabetes often occurs at the time of a routine medical examination or when the patient is being treated for another medical problem.

Diagnosis of Diabetes

The normal fasting plasma glucose is below 115 mg/dl. A positive diagnosis of diabetes follows (1) a random plasma glucose equal to or greater than 200 mg/dl accompanied by the classic symptoms of diabetes, including polydipsia and polyuria; (2) a fasting plasma glucose equal to or greater than 140 mg/dl; or, (3) a plasma glucose greater than or equal to 200 mg/dl two hours after eating 75 g of glucose (an oral glucose tolerance test).[14] Normal plasma glucose two hours after consuming 75 g of glucose is less than 140 mg/dl. Individuals with two-hour plasma glucose levels between 140 and 199 mg/dl have impaired glucose tolerance. Davidson[14] notes that the oral glucose tolerance test is rarely needed, nor is it recommended for elderly adults. Older people with impaired glucose tolerance are more likely to develop vascular disease, leading to a stroke or coronary attack, than those with normal glucose levels. In this group it is estimated that about half will continue to have impaired glucose tolerance, about 30% will return to normal, and about 20% will develop diabetes.

As the number of older people increases, primary care physicians are being called upon to make decisions about the care of those demonstrating impaired glucose tolerance. In younger individuals elevated plasma glucose leads to microvascular complications and disturbances in visual function, and glucose control retards these changes.[52] In older adults with somewhat elevated plasma glucose, drug or dietary intervention that often requires a major change in lifestyle may also confer benefit. Kahn and coworkers[43] suggest that plasma glucose levels in older people be evaluated using age-corrected standards by which an individual is compared to others of similar age. This assumes, however, that changes in glucose tolerance represent normal aging. If impaired glucose tolerance is considered pathologic and predictive of diabetes mellitus, then any adjustment for age is inappropriate. In fact, changes in body weight and composition and exercise patterns contribute significantly to age-related changes in glucose tolerance and carbohydrate metabolism.[34]

Hyperglycemia does increase cardiovascular risk independent of age, blood pressure, serum cholesterol, body mass index (BMI), or smoking. In a 14-year follow-up of 2,471 older adults, Barrett-Connor and coworkers[2] found that either a history of diabetes or a fasting plasma glucose of 140 mg/dl or higher resulted in a twofold increase in fatal ischemic heart disease in men and a threefold increase in women. This finding suggested that diabetes mellitus or hyperglycemia set aside the natural resistance of women to fatal heart disease. Fasting plasma glucose levels above 140 mg/dl mandate evaluation and therapy.[52]

Basis for Change in Glucose Tolerance

Normal glucose regulation. Plasma glucose levels are regulated by the hormones insulin and glucagon which are secreted by the beta and alpha islets of the pancreas, respectively. Usually glucose is the primary energy source for the brain and red blood cells; consequently, it is important that adequate plasma levels be maintained between meals and overnight. Liver cells are very sensitive to the amounts of insulin and glucagon drained into the portal vein.[43] When plasma glucose levels fall, the secretion of glucagon will lead to a breakdown of liver glycogen and gluconeogenesis to restore plasma levels. After ingestion of food and the subsequent rise in plasma glucose, insulin is released, which

suppresses hepatic glucose production and promotes glucose uptake by muscle and adipose cells. Glucose uptake and storage by the liver is not dependent on insulin. Glucose tolerance is altered by (1) reduced uptake of glucose in peripheral tissues, (2) inappropriate hepatic release of glucose, and (3) inappropriate release of glucagon or reduced release of insulin.

Insulin sensitivity of peripheral tissues. Decreased sensitivity of muscle and adipose cells to insulin has long been regarded as a major cause of impaired glucose tolerance in older people, although the mechanism leading to this change is unclear. The rate at which glucose enters these cells is slowed despite normal or in some cases elevated plasma insulin levels.[43] Reduced glucose movement into the cell could be related to a change in the number or effectiveness of cell receptor sites for binding insulin. However, Kahn and coworkers[43] found similar numbers of receptors on cells from older and younger people, and age did not change the affinity of receptors for insulin. The rate of glucose oxidation inside the cell may be a factor in glucose transport.[37]

Insulin sensitivity in the liver. Reduced hepatic insulin sensitivity may play a role in the impaired glucose tolerance or the development of diabetes in older people. In healthy elderly people, hepatic release of glucose is rapidly suppressed by even small increases in insulin secretion, but changes in hepatic response to insulin do occur in NIDDM.[4]

Pancreatic function. Changes in glucose tolerance could relate to hormone secretion and control. Although some workers[4] have reported normal or increased serum insulin concentrations in older age, others have observed reduced levels. There does appear to be a reduction in the first phase of insulin secretion (the rapid release of insulin occurring immediately after ingestion of glucose), along with an inability to sustain normal insulin secretion.[4] A defect in first-phase insulin secretion is associated with the inappropriate plasma glucose levels observed in those with NIDDM. These alterations in beta-cell function may contribute to the decline in glucose uptake by the peripheral cells, but their overall significance is uncertain.[43]

Factors Contributing to Altered Carbohydrate Metabolism

Changes in dietary pattern and lifestyle have been associated with changes in carbohydrate metabolism. Low carbohydrate intake, high body fat, particularly abdominal fat, and limited exercise have all been implicated in age-related changes in glucose disposal.

Carbohydrate intake. At one time low carbohydrate intake by older people was linked to their impaired glucose tolerance. However, a study of 175 older people living in Rotterdam[22] suggests that the type of carbohydrate eaten is more important than the amount. Feskens and colleagues[22] did a four-year follow-up of community-living elderly people between the ages of 64 and 87 who had normal glucose tolerance when the study began. After four years, 59 of the 175 older subjects had developed impaired glucose tolerance. Although total carbohydrate intake was similar in both groups (215 g and 217 g), those who maintained normal glucose tolerance consumed more of their carbohydrate as legumes; those whose glucose tolerance deteriorated consumed more of their carbohydrate as pastries, and high use of pastries more than tripled the risk of impaired glucose tolerance. In those elderly people neither age nor intake of saturated fatty acids was related to the detrimental effect of pastry on glucose metabolism.

Body mass index (BMI). Obesity and enlarged adipose cells have been related to the insulin resistance of muscle and adipose cells and impaired glucose tolerance in people of all ages. A BMI of 27 versus 24 was associated with a twofold increase in risk of impaired glucose tolerance in the older Rotterdam residents described earlier.[22] In those with a higher BMI, both fasting and two-hour postprandial plasma glucose levels were elevated.

A loss of body fat can improve glucose homeostasis. Reaven and others[59] reported that an average weight loss of 9 kg reduced the degree of hyperglycemia among 12 obese patients age 71 years. Improvement occurred despite the fact that none reached their ideal body weight. Conversely, a weight gain of even 10 pounds between ages 40 and 60 can double the risk of impaired glucose metabolism.[34]

Enlarged fat cells are less sensitive to insulin than smaller fat cells. Yet it is important to recognize that impaired glucose tolerance in older people is, at least in part, independent of fat cell size and obesity. In the elderly glucose entry into adipose cells is enhanced at high plasma glucose concentrations, as is the case in normal young adults; rate of glucose entry is not influenced by plasma glucose concentration in obese young adults.[10]

The location of body fat influences glucose tolerance. Among 60 healthy people who ranged in age from 23 to 83 years,[7] intra-abdominal or visceral fat, measured by magnetic resonance imaging, accounted for 51% of the insulin resistance observed in a glucose tolerance test. This relationship held true regardless of age, sex, or BMI. In people with a central obesity, skeletal muscle cells seem to be more resistant to insulin and glucose transport, although the basis for this resistance is not understood. The release of free fatty acids from the abdominal fat into the portal vein may slow the degradation of released insulin and thereby contribute to the elevated insulin levels observed in those with excessive abdominal fat.

Exercise. Exercise improves insulin effectiveness through changes in the skeletal muscle. In 46 men ages 45 to 75 years,[35] fitness level, measured by exercise time to exhaustion, contributed 47% of the variance in plasma insulin levels after consuming glucose. Insulin levels fell in older men ages 70 to 79 who participated in an intensive endurance exercise program for six months, although their glucose levels changed only slightly. In contrast, resistance training completed by older men of similar age did not affect plasma insulin.[33] Because elevated plasma insulin levels increase the risk of diabetes, a significant drop in insulin secretion resulting from improved insulin action in skeletal muscle contributes significantly to health. In a follow-up study of 2,000 healthy people over age 50,[34] those using exercise as their means of avoiding weight gain reduced their risk of diabetes by half.

Endurance training may be an effective intervention for impaired glucose tolerance. When 18 older subjects with impaired glucose tolerance completed a 12-week endurance training program at the Human Nutrition Research

Center on Aging in Boston,[36] oral glucose tolerance returned to normal in 8 of the 18, and plasma glucose levels dropped in all, despite no change in body fat (fig. 13-2). Serum insulin levels remained unchanged, indicating that available insulin became more effective.

Age. Regardless of other factors, age per se still appears to exert a significant effect on glucose tolerance. Among 743 healthy men and recently added women in the BLSA,[65] fasting and two-hour postprandial plasma glucose levels increased with age, although to a greater extent in men. The percentage of body fat and waist-to-hip ratio also increased with age and were positively related to plasma glucose levels; physical fitness, measured by maximum oxygen consumption, was related to plasma glucose only in men. These associations did explain the changes in glucose tolerance observed between the young (ages 17 to 39) and middle-aged (ages 40 to 59) men and women; however, they did not account for the further decline in glucose tolerance observed in the oldest age group (ages 60 to 92). Carbohydrate intake did not appear to influence these results, because intakes actually increased by 8 g a day per decade. Visceral fat, not obvious using the waist-to-hip measurement, could have contributed to the changes in the oldest age group. As noted by Cefalu and coworkers[7] in their evaluation, the waist-to-hip measurement is less accurate in evaluating intra-abdominal fat than x-ray methods.

Continuing research is looking at the role of particular nutrients in glucose metabolism. Magnesium, a nutrient low in the diets of many older people, is a necessary cofactor for important enzymes that control glucose oxidation, and it also exerts an effect on the beta cells of the pancreas. Both insulin response and uptake of glucose by skeletal muscle and adipose cells improved in older people (mean age was 78) supplemented with magnesium.[56] This improvement in the ability to handle glucose, however, may represent a pharmacologic rather than a physiologic effect because the older subjects were supplemented with 4.5 g of magnesium a day for four weeks. (The RDA for magnesium is 350 mg for men and 280 mg for women.) Higher plasma vitamin E levels were related to

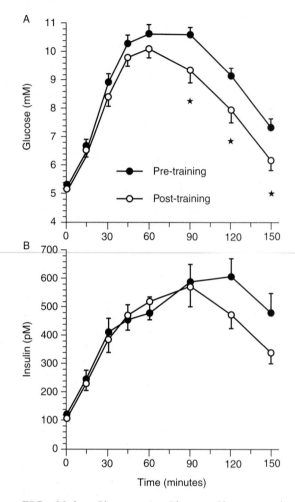

FIG. 13-2 Changes in Plasma Glucose and Insulin Levels in Older People Following an Exercise Program. Older people with impaired glucose tolerance who completed a 12-week exercise program had significantly lower plasma glucose levels at 90 minutes and beyond on a glucose tolerance test demonstrating improved utilization of glucose. Body composition and plasma insulin levels did not change significantly.

Hughes, V.A., and others: Exercise increases muscle GLUT-4 levels and insulin action in subjects with impaired glucose tolerance, Am. J. Physiol. (Endocrinol. Metab. 27):E855, 1993. (Used with permission of the American Physiological Society.)

improved glucose utilization in both elderly patients with NIDDM and healthy older people.[57] Vitamin E as part of its antioxidant function may stabilize membranes and so facilitate glucose transport.

Diabetes Mellitus in Older People

NIDDM in older patients is accompanied by hyperglycemia but is usually not complicated by ketoacidosis. Ketones are present in the urine if the disease is poorly controlled, but they do not accumulate in the serum. Insulin-dependent diabetes mellitus, with accompanying ketoacidosis, is less common in older individuals but does occur in those who no longer produce any significant amount of insulin. Morley and Perry[52] emphasized that appropriate glucose control contributes measurably to the older patient's quality of life. Microvascular changes develop rapidly in older patients and lead to many problems: ocular complications with loss of color vision or total sight; neural complications with increased pain, loss of cognitive function, or depression; renal complications; increased susceptibility to infection; and impaired circulation in the lower extremities with the risk of gangrene and resulting amputations. Progressive neuropathy sometimes results in loss of mobility or fecal incontinence and unwanted institutionalization.

Management of the Older Diabetic Patient

Management of the older individual with NIDDM usually involves dietary modification, exercise, weight reduction if indicated, and a hypoglycemic drug if necessary. Morley and Perry[52] recommend that treatment be implemented when fasting plasma glucose exceeds 140 mg/dl on two separate occasions or when plasma glucose exceeds 200 mg/dl at least two hours after the most recent meal.

Dietary management. The American Diabetes Association has released new recommendations for medical nutritional therapy for people with diabetes.[55] Emphasis is placed on individualizing the diet as far as possible to meet social, ethnic, and lifestyle preferences and to achieve disease management goals. These goals include 1) maintaining as near optimum blood glucose levels as possible, 2) achieving optimum serum lipid levels, and 3) controlling blood pressure. It appears that people with diabetes have protein requirements similar to the general population, and protein intakes of 10% to 20% of total kilocalories are recommended. The division of the remaining kilocalories between carbohydrate and fat is based on the particular patient. For all patients saturated fat should provide less than 10% of total kilocalories and polyunsaturated fat should provide no more than 10% of total kilocalories. If protein provides 10% to 20% of total energy, this leaves 60% to 70% of total energy to be divided between monounsaturated fat and carbohydrate.

For those individuals with normal body weight and reasonable lipoprotein levels, the Dietary Guidelines for Americans that suggest less than 30% of energy from fat and 55% to 60% of total energy from carbohydrate are appropriate. For NIDDM patients with high serum triglycerides, providing 20% of kilocalories from monounsaturated fats, thus lowering kilocalories from carbohydrate, may assist in glycemic control and modification of serum lipoproteins.[31] Grundy[31] recommends a high-carbohydrate, low-fat dietary pattern for obese individuals newly diagnosed with NIDDM who are attempting to lose weight or who may have been unsuccessful at weight loss but are maintaining good glucose control. For older nonobese individuals with a long history of NIDDM, high carbohydrate intake may aggravate elevated blood glucose and serum triglycerides. A reduced level of dietary carbohydrate and an increased level of fat as monounsaturated fat may support treatment goals. For people with diabetes as well as for the general population, a liberal intake of fiber (20 g to 30 g daily) from a variety of foods and a sodium intake limited to 2,400 mg to 3,000 mg a day is appropriate.[55]

A major change in the new recommendations of the American Diabetes Association is the focus on the amount rather than the type of carbohydrate.[55] Formerly, patients were urged to avoid simple sugars such as sucrose, which were believed to play a role in elevating blood glucose. In fact, many complex carbohydrate-containing foods, such as potatoes and bread, have a similar effect on blood glucose levels. Allowing a wider variety of foods and foods that have been a part of the diet for many years contributes to patient satisfaction and the likelihood that the diet will be followed. Coulston[13] pointed out that elderly diabetics who moved from a calorie-controlled diabetic diet to a regular diet had a slight change in fasting serum glucose (from 121 mg/dl to 131 mg/dl), but their glycosylated hemoglobin level was virtually unchanged (7.8% versus 8.1%). Glycosylated hemoglobin is a measure of the average serum glucose level over the previous weeks and rises significantly in uncontrolled diabetes.

A recent study from the Human Nutrition Research Center on Aging in Boston evaluated dietary treatment of older people with impaired glucose tolerance.[37] Hughes and coworkers[37] reported that a high-carbohydrate diet, unless accompanied by a high level of exercise, may promote deterioration of glucose tolerance in older people. Their older subjects with impaired glucose tolerance were given a diet providing 60% of kilocalories as carbohydrate, and one group also participated in an aerobic exercise program. Insulin-stimulated glucose utilization did not improve in either group, although glucose oxidation increased in both groups. The exercise group increased their muscle glycogen stores, which contributed to glucose utilization; however, their serum lactate levels also increased. Lactate can serve as a precursor for liver gluconeogenesis and add to the further deterioration of glucose tolerance. Hughes and colleagues[37] recommended prudent use of a high-carbohydrate diet with older people at risk for developing NIDDM.

Exercise and weight loss. When possible, even modest weight loss of 10 to 20 pounds (4.5 to 9 kg) should be encouraged.[52] However, older people placed on diets that are very low in kilocalories and require many dietary changes are at increased risk of malnutrition.[52] An exercise program involving 20 to 30 minutes of brisk walking each day improves glucose metabolism and cardiovascular fitness. Older diabetics undertaking a walking program need to be advised about proper footwear and care of their feet.

Oral hypoglycemic agents. The sulfonylureas such as tolazamide and glyburide are prescribed in NIDDM.[14] Because these drugs stimulate the release of insulin from the beta cells, they are not useful if all beta-cell function is lost. In contrast to insulin, oral hypoglycemic agents have no direct effect on plasma glucose levels. Individuals whose plasma glucose cannot be controlled with diet, exercise, and oral hypoglycemic agents, or who have nonfunctional beta cells, must be treated with insulin. (The management of insulin-dependent diabetes mellitus is beyond the scope of this book; interested readers should consult a therapeutic nutrition text.)

AGING AND CARDIOVASCULAR FUNCTION

Cardiovascular structure and function in older people are the result of age-related changes complicated by lifestyle factors and chronic disease. Occult forms of disease such as coronary artery disease can exaggerate the functional changes in the heart thought to be due to aging, leading to erroneous conclusions about the age effect.[45] Moss[53] describes a long distance runner who at the age of 77 ran the mile in less than seven minutes. The evaluation of age-related versus disease-related changes is complicated further by difficulties in diagnosis. Although at least 50% of all people age 60 and older have severe coronary artery disease, only half exhibit clinical symptoms.[45] Coronary artery disease, along with possible age-related changes in the coronary arteries, contributes to the considerable loss in cardiovascular performance observed among some elderly people.

Structural Changes in the Cardiovascular System

The aging heart can atrophy, develop moderate or marked hypertrophy, or remain unchanged. Cardiac atrophy occurs only with severe wasting disease and does not represent normal aging; neither does marked cardiac hypertrophy, which usually is the result of severe hypertension.[45] Mean heart weight, when related to body surface area or body size, does not change with age in healthy men. In women heart weight increases slightly between the ages of 40 and 70. This increase in women may be related to the small rise in blood pressure sometimes associated with menopause. Modest increases in the thickness of the left ventricular wall occur in individuals with normal blood pressure who are free of disease. This change in thickness is believed to result from an increase in cardiac cell size, not from an increase in fatty or fibrous tissue. Fat deposition in the human heart is related to total body fat and not to age.[46]

Age-related changes take place in the major arteries independent of atherosclerotic disease.[45] The aorta increases in diameter and length, and the arterial walls stiffen and lose their elasticity. Increases in elastin and collagen and the deposition of calcium contribute to these changes. Whether changes take place in the smooth muscle of the major arteries is not known.

Changes in Cardiovascular Function

For most healthy older people, cardiac function at low or moderate levels of activity is sufficient to meet physiological needs. Resting heart rate does not change with age. Cardiac output at resting levels does not fall in physically active older people who do not have heart disease. Although cardiac output need not change with advancing age, it does in many elderly individuals as a result of coronary artery disease or hypertension. A reduction in lean body mass and a subsequent lower tissue demand for oxygen could also bring about a lower cardiac output.[46]

Age-related changes in cardiovascular function become most obvious under conditions of strenuous exercise, when the workload of the heart increases fourfold to fivefold above resting levels.[45] In younger people, added adrenergic stimulation increases the strength of the contraction of the cardiac muscle, but decreases the duration of the contraction, thus increasing the heart rate. Plasma epinephrine and norepinephrine levels are higher in older adults than in younger adults under conditions of vigorous exercise, suggesting an increase in adrenergic activity; however, the aging cardiovascular system is less responsive to adrenergic stimulation

and less able to react to excessive physiologic demands. Although older individuals cannot increase their heart rate to the extent that younger individuals can, older people can increase their stroke volume, or the amount of blood delivered with each beat of the heart, thereby increasing cardiac output.

The ability to perform physical work or vigorous exercise depends on a constant and sufficient supply of oxygen to working muscles and tissues. This places demands on both the respiratory and cardiovascular systems, since sufficient oxygen must be taken into the body and delivered to the cells and tissues. Maximum body oxygen consumption, along with maximum work capacity, declines with age, although to a variable extent. The maximum oxygen consumption of older people who exercise regularly actually exceeds that of younger people who are sedentary.[45] This suggests that physical conditioning retards the age-related decline in cardiovascular performance or, conversely, that a lack of physical activity rather than the aging process brings about cardiovascular decline.

The decrease in maximum oxygen consumption observed in healthy older people also may be caused by changes in the peripheral tissues rather than by changes in the heart. Loss of lean body mass reduces the maximum amount of work performed and, in proportion, the level of oxygen required. In fact, when maximum oxygen consumption is evaluated on the basis of creatinine excretion, an indicator of total body muscle, the differences between older and younger groups are greatly diminished.[46] Regular physical exercise is important in maintaining cardiovascular function and promoting successful aging.

Older people with advanced coronary artery disease tolerate poorly stress stemming from either physiologic or emotional causes. These individuals may function well under ordinary conditions but develop tachycardia with emotional stress, fever, or exercise. This points to the importance of medical evaluation of older people before they start an exercise program. Also, those who have been sedentary must take a gradual approach to increasing the length and intensity of exercise.

If cardiac function is impaired, the reduced cardiac output compromises the function of other organ systems. In those with cardiovascular disease, cerebral blood flow and renal blood flow are lower. A diminished supply of blood and oxygen to the brain has been implicated in the loss of mental function in some older people.[45] Removal of waste products is less efficient when the glomerular filtration rate falls. A decline in cardiovascular performance has far-reaching consequences for the functional capability of the aging individual. Therefore efforts throughout adulthood to retard development of coronary artery disease and maintain a high level of fitness should be a priority.

Aging and Cardiovascular Disease

Because of the progressive nature of cardiovascular disease, the incidence is highest among the elderly, and cardiovascular disease is the leading cause of death in this age group. Atherosclerosis is the underlying cause of coronary heart disease in older people and contributes to both morbidity and functional disability. Although diet is recognized as playing a role in determining blood lipid levels and may contribute to the development of diabetes and hypertension associated with atherosclerotic vascular disease, the effects of diet in the prevention and treatment of atherosclerosis in older people have received little attention.

Cholesterol and Lipid Metabolism in Older People

Serum cholesterol levels. Serum total cholesterol, examined in the NHANES II and NHANES III studies, has been decreasing in all age groups, including those age 65 and older.[41] In general, high density lipoprotein (HDL) cholesterol and very-low-density lipoprotein (VLDL) cholesterol levels have not changed. This indicates that the fall in serum total cholesterol is the result of a drop in the low density lipoprotein (LDL) cholesterol. Changes in serum total cholesterol and specific lipoprotein fractions and their significance in people age 65 and older are areas of active discussion. The proportion of older people with desirable serum total cholesterol increased after age 74 in the

❖

STANDARDS FOR EVALUATING SERUM LIPOPROTEIN LEVELS

Total Cholesterol

Desirable:	<200 mg/dl (5.2 mmol/l)
Borderline-high:	200–239 mg/dl (5.2–6.2 mmol/l)
High Risk:	≥240 mg/dl (6.2 mmol/l)

LDL Cholesterol

Desirable:	<130 mg/dl (3.4 mmol/l)
Borderline-high:	130–159 mg/dl (3.4–4.1 mmol/l)
High Risk:	≥160 mg/dl (4.1 mmol/l)

HDL Cholesterol

Desirable:	≥35 mg/dl (0.9 mmol/l)
High Risk:	<35 mg/dl (0.9 mmol/l)

Adapted from U.S. Department of Health and Human Services: Second report of the expert panel on detection, evaluation, and treatment of high blood cholesterol in adults, NIH Publication No. 93-3095, Washington, DC, 1993, U.S. Government Printing Office.

NHANES III study[21] (see box for evaluation standards for lipoprotein levels). In men ages 50 to 59, 60 to 74, and 75 years and over, 29%, 32%, and 48%, respectively, had desirable serum total cholesterol levels. Older women are less likely to have serum total cholesterol levels in the desirable range as only 26% of the women ages 50 to 59, 20% of the women ages 60 to 74, and 28% of the women age 75 and over had desirable levels.

These trends in serum cholesterol in older age groups were also apparent in the Boston Nutritional Status Survey (fig. 13-3).[47] The increased life expectancy of women, despite their higher serum total cholesterol, is likely influenced by their levels of particular lipoprotein fractions. In the Boston survey, the older women had the highest HDL cholesterol. The Boston investigators[47] also measured apolipoprotein A-1 (the major protein in HDL) and apolipoprotein B

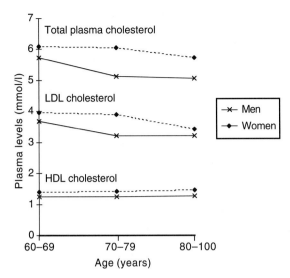

FIG. 13-3 Plasma Total Cholesterol, LDL Cholesterol and HDL Cholesterol in Elderly People (Boston Nutritional Status Survey). In community-living older people mean total plasma cholesterol and LDL cholesterol levels continue to decline with advancing age; HDL cholesterol levels exhibit less change.

Data from Lamon-Fava, S., and others: Effects of dietary intakes on plasma lipids, lipoproteins, and apolipoproteins in free-living elderly men and women, Am. J. Clin. Nutr. 59:32, 1994.

(the major protein in LDL). Apolipoprotein A-1 was higher in the women, and apolipoprotein B was higher in the younger men (ages 60 to 69). It has been suggested that apolipoproteins A-1 and B are better predictors of cardiovascular risk than are HDL and LDL cholesterol levels, although this is still a matter of debate. The importance of HDL-cholesterol levels to the longevity of elderly people is reinforced by the fact that only 3% of the Boston participants, age 80 and over, had high-risk levels of HDL-cholesterol (less than 35 mg/dl). In these older people, optimum vitamin A intakes and plasma levels and lower BMI were associated with favorable plasma lipid profiles. Vitamin A does increase apolipoprotein A-1 synthesis in animal models and may have a similar effect in humans.

Longitudinal changes in serum cholesterol levels. An evaluation of plasma lipid levels over a nine-year period in 157 healthy, older people in the New Mexico study[28] revealed decreases in total cholesterol, HDL cholesterol, and LDL cholesterol in both men and women. The mean age of the participants when the study began was 70 years. Garry and coworkers[28] noted that decreases in dietary fat were significantly related to the fall in plasma lipids. The proportion of kilocalories from fat decreased from 37% to 31% in the women and from 37% to 34% in the men between 1980 and 1989. Mean energy intakes were below recommended levels and equaled only 25 kcal/kg in the women and 28 kcal/kg in the men. Calculated energy requirements for these subjects were 30 kcal/kg for the women and 31 kcal/kg for the men. Despite the relatively good health enjoyed by this older group, a large abdominal circumference contributing to a higher waist-to-hip ratio was associated with lower HDL cholesterol.[11]

Serum lipoprotein levels and coronary risk. The relationship between serum lipoprotein status, aging, and coronary risk is unclear. Srinath and coworkers[67] pointed out that the decline in serum LDL and VLDL cholesterol in people over age 85 may reflect an actual decrease in these lipoproteins or the removal through death of individuals with higher levels. One factor for consideration when evaluating the influence of serum cholesterol on mortality risk is relative risk versus attributable risk.[32] The relative risk for coronary heart disease mortality between the groups with the highest total cholesterol levels and the groups with the lowest total cholesterol levels decreases with age, suggesting that older people have less to gain by lowering their serum total cholesterol. At the same time, attributable risk, the difference in absolute rates of heart disease between groups with higher or lower serum total cholesterol, actually increases with age, indicating that older people could benefit from lipid-lowering strategies.

Dietary Intervention in Older People with Elevated Serum Lipids

The American Heart Association Step 1 diet limits total fat to less than 30% of energy intake, reduces saturated fatty acids to less than 10% of energy intake, and limits dietary cholesterol to

TABLE 13-2   *Effect of a Low-Fat Diet and Weight Loss on Plasma Cholesterol in Older Men*

	Baseline	3 Months	9 Months
Low-Fat Diet Group*			
Total Cholesterol (mmol/L)	5.39	4.56	4.82
LDL Cholesterol (mmol/L)	3.57	3.03	3.19
HDL Cholesterol (mmol/L)	1.04	0.83	0.88
Low-Fat Diet + Weight Loss Group*			
Total Cholesterol (mmol/L)	5.41	4.56	4.33
LDL Cholesterol (mmol/L)	3.42	2.98	2.72
HDL Cholesterol (mmol/L)	1.11	0.93	1.06

*Both groups followed the American Heart Association Step 1 Diet for 3 months at an energy intake to maintain body weight; at that time energy intake was reduced in the weight loss group.

Modified from Dengel, J.L., Katzel, L.I., and Goldberg, A.P.: Effect of an American Heart Association diet, with or without weight loss, on lipids in obese middle-aged and older men, Am. J. Clin. Nutr. 62:715, 1995.

300 mg a day. This diet has been used with older people. Older men with a mean age of 61 to 62 years followed this diet for three months with energy intakes calculated to maintain body weight.[17] The usual diets of these men contained 35% fat and 380 mg of cholesterol a day. After the first three months the men had a 16% decrease in total cholesterol, a 14% decrease in LDL cholesterol, and a 17% decrease in HDL cholesterol (table 13-2). At that time the group was divided with half continuing on the energy intake calculated to maintain body weight and half placed on an energy intake calculated to bring about weight loss. Over the next nine months, serum lipids remained the same in the men who maintained their weight; however, in the men who lost weight, HDL cholesterol returned to about the original level and LDL cholesterol declined an additional 7%. Weight loss in these men was about 20 lb.

The American Heart Association Step 1 diet was also effective in lowering total and LDL cholesterol in postmenopausal women (their mean age was 61)[18] who were not receiving hormone replacement therapy (fig. 13-4). Total cholesterol dropped by 14 mg/dl, but LDL cholesterol dropped by 11 mg/dl. Although the average decrease in LDL cholesterol was only

6%, Denke[18] pointed out that for several women this change was sufficient to avoid drug therapy and allowed them to be maintained on diet alone. A major finding in this study was the significant variability of response to the intervention diet. Only 10% of the variability could be explained by adherence to the diet. Obese women appeared to be less sensitive to dietary modification, and the women who lost weight had a greater decrease in LDL cholesterol. It would have been helpful if the diet had been continued for longer than two months. Based on Denke's experience, variability in response to dietary intervention is greater in women than men. Nevertheless, it appears that at least half of postmenopausal women can achieve good to excellent reductions in elevated serum LDL cholesterol through dietary means.

Basis for Intervention Decisions

Both age and risk factors should be considered when planning an intervention strategy for an older adult.[1] In the healthy young-old, aggressive dietary intervention and drug therapy as needed is warranted and may delay the onset of heart disease and accompanying disability. According to Stone,[69] the question of intervention in the 75-year-old patient is less clear-cut.

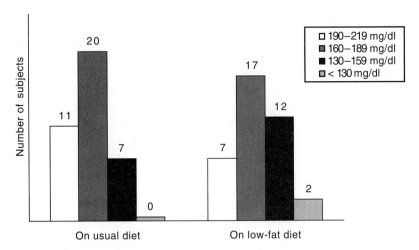

FIG. 13-4 Changes in LDL Cholesterol in Older Women Adopting a Low-Fat Diet. Older women with moderately elevated serum LDL cholesterol were able to decrease their levels by reducing their fat intake from 41% to 27% of total kilocalories.

Data from Denke, M.A.: Individual responsiveness to a cholesterol-lowering diet in postmenopausal women with moderate hypercholesterolemia, Arch. Intern. Med. 154:1977, 1994.

Although lowering serum cholesterol may, in fact, reduce cardiovascular risk in this patient, there have been no clinical trials to provide conclusive evidence that this will happen. Secondly, large numbers of community-living elderly people over age 70 have total cholesterol levels above 200 mg/dl. Kannel[44] recommends that individuals with low HDL cholesterol be targeted for intervention, especially if additional risk factors include systolic hypertension, smoking, or impaired glucose tolerance. Factors discouraging intervention in the elderly adult include life-threatening illnesses, dementia or degenerative neurologic disorders, or undernutrition. It would also appear inappropriate to attempt radical dietary changes in an elderly person for whom the burden of change or the loss of favorite foods might outweigh any possible benefit.

Arguments against interventions in hypercholesterolemic elderly people often refer to the fact that serum cholesterol levels below 140 mg/dl are associated with increased mortality from noncardiovascular causes. Goichot and coworkers[30] conducted an evaluation of 380 older people in the community with a mean age of 76 to determine the prevalence and related nutritional factors associated with hypocholesterolemia. Only 12 had serum total cholesterol below 140 mg/dl, and nutrient intake was not appreciably different in those individuals, although they tended to eat more carbohydrate and less fat. This group also had low serum thyroxin levels, low cognitive scores, and low BMI. Goichot and colleagues[30] concluded that very low serum cholesterol is associated with poor health status and occurs despite an apparently adequate nutrient intake. A standard of 140 mg/dl may be too low to identify individuals with deteriorating health status.

Hypertension in Older People

Elevated blood pressure puts an increased strain on the heart and cardiovascular system. In western societies both systolic and diastolic blood pressures tend to rise until age 60. Beyond that age systolic blood pressure sometimes continues to rise whereas diastolic blood pressure remains the same or may actually decline.[27] Hypertension is defined as a systolic blood pressure of 140 mm Hg or higher or a diastolic blood pressure of 90 mm Hg or higher. Isolated systolic hypertension is a systolic pressure of 140 mm Hg or higher and a normal diastolic pressure under 90 mm Hg.[27] More than 50% of older Americans ages 65 to 74 have elevated blood pressures.[54] Older African Americans are more likely to have hypertension than older whites or Mexican American elderly. In the NHANES III study 72% of the African American elderly had elevated systolic and/or diastolic blood pressure as compared to 53% of white elderly and 55% of Mexican American elderly. There were no major differences in prevalence of hypertension between men and women. Isolated systolic hypertension was identified in 65% of the people age 60 and over and increased with age. Only 26% of the older adults with hypertension had their blood pressure controlled to normal levels.

Blood pressure is more closely related to stroke or myocardial infarction in people age 65 and older than in people ages 35 to 64.[54] In the Framingham Heart Study, risk of cardiovascular disease was strongly related to systolic blood pressure, and risk increased at levels even below 140 mm Hg. Incidence of cardiovascular disease increased with a diastolic blood pressure of 75 mm Hg or higher in men and 95 mm Hg or higher in women. Elevated blood pressure also increases risk of renal failure, cardiac failure, and peripheral vascular disease. Because an older person is more likely to experience a stroke or heart attack than a younger person, blood pressure reduction at every level of blood pressure has a greater benefit in elderly people than in younger people. A blood pressure intervention study involving nearly 4,700 people age 60 and older[54] resulted in a 36% reduction in strokes and a 27% reduction in myocardial infarction. This is a reduction of 55 cardiovascular incidents per 1,000 people.

The widespread prevalence of hypertension among older people has led to the belief that a rise in arterial blood pressure is a part of normal aging and carries little risk. Evidence to suggest that this rise is at least in part environmental or cultural rather than biologic comes from the observation that in primitive societies, neither systolic nor diastolic blood pressure rises with age.[27] Hypertension has several causes in older people. Atherosclerotic disease increases the rigidity and decreases the distensibility of the large arteries. Reduced distensibility of the aorta to the volume of blood delivered from the left ventricle is a major factor in the development of isolated systolic hypertension. Enhanced activity of the renin-angiotensin system, increasing the release of aldosterone, also increases vascular resistance. Reduced activity of the prostaglandin system, which normally decreases vascular resistance and lowers blood pressure, contributes to the development of hypertension. Alterations in the sympathetic nervous system and baroreceptors increase vasoconstriction and blood pressure. Hyperthyroidism, thiamin deficiency with clinical or subclinical beriberi, and fever raise systolic blood pressure. Renal disease causes a rise in arterial pressure and will aggravate existing hypertension.[27]

Hypertension is a significant medical and nutritional problem among older people. Unabated hypertension leads to hypertrophy of the left ventricle of the heart and, eventually, cardiac failure and impaired renal function. Hypertension in an elderly adult is sometimes a newly developed condition, arising for the first time at an older age.

Factors Contributing to Hypertension

Obesity. Body mass influences blood pressure into advanced age. Among 255 Dutch elderly ages 65 to 79,[50] BMI was positively associated with both systolic and diastolic blood pressures; at the same time, creatinine excretion, an indicator of muscle mass, was inversely related to systolic blood pressure. In those older people a normal body weight seemed to offer some protection against hypertension despite a high sodium intake. Both the relative degree of adiposity and its location influence blood pressure. A higher waist-to-hip ratio was associated with hypertension among 42,000 women ages 55 to 69.[25] Women with greater abdominal adiposity had a higher risk of hypertension even after accounting for body weight. Hyperinsulinemia raises blood pressure by increasing reabsorption of sodium by the kidneys and raising activity of the sympathetic nervous system, which increases vasoconstriction.[68] Elevated secretion of insulin may be one link in the pathogenesis of hypertension in obesity and NIDDM, as it is common to all three conditions.

Weight reduction lowers blood pressure. The loss of even 5 kg can bring about a 5 mm Hg decline in systolic blood pressure, and if coupled with even mild sodium restriction, this decrease in systolic pressure can reach 11 mm Hg.[68] A decline of this degree may reduce dependence on drug therapy and the associated effects on nutritional health.

Alcohol. Use of more than 2 ounces of alcohol a day elevates blood pressure in adults of all ages.[12] Reducing alcohol use brings about reductions in both systolic and diastolic blood pressures in hypertensive individuals, and blood pressures return to their former levels when alcohol consumption is resumed. Alcohol abuse may contribute to the prevalence of hypertension in some older groups.

Exercise. Intervention studies suggest that aerobic exercise reduces blood pressure in hypertensive adults of middle age. However, in a recent clinical trial, Blumenthal and coworkers[3] found no difference in systolic or diastolic blood pressure between mildly hypertensive subjects participating in supervised exercise three times a week and nonexercising control subjects. Those authors suggest that the positive effects of exercise reported by others may have resulted from associated weight loss; body weight did not change in the exercise group that did not have a decrease in blood pressure. It would be interesting to speculate whether a decrease in insulin levels or insulin resistance resulting from the exercise program contributed to the changes in blood pressure observed by other investigators. Insulin levels were not measured in this study. Despite the uncertainty of the mechanism by which exercise may influence blood pressure, the overall benefits of exercise in promoting health justify its use.

Dietary intake. Daily intakes of several minerals, including sodium, potassium, calcium, and magnesium, have been related to blood pressure. An excessive intake of sodium leads to elevated blood pressure in sensitive individuals.[12] It also appears that African Americans and older people are more sodium sensitive than white adults and younger people; they often respond to moderate sodium restriction of 2 g sodium per day (5 g sodium chloride).[76] Sodium restriction to this level sometimes makes it possible to control blood pressure using fewer medications. Given the lower ability of aged kidneys to conserve sodium, clinicians[73] advise against reducing sodium intake below 2 g a day.

Potassium intake is inversely related to blood pressure. Löwik and coworkers[50] proposed that increased dietary potassium helped prevent hypertension among elderly Dutch men in their study by increasing urinary sodium. Higher intakes of potassium may lower the release of renin and the subsequent angiotensin conversion and secretion of aldosterone. A recent clinical trial[70] examined the effect of raising potassium intake from food sources on blood pressure in hypertensive adults. Potassium intake increased from 1,500 mg to 2,400 mg in the experimental group. After one year, blood pressure and body weight had not changed in either group; however, 38% of those who increased their potassium intake no longer required drugs to control their hypertension as compared to only 9% of the control subjects. Physical symptoms related to elevated blood pressure or side effects of hypertension medications declined by almost half. It is curious that intervention trials in which potassium was administered in supplement form have not reported an effect of potassium on blood pressure.[61] Whether another substance also found in fruits and vegetables influences blood pressure is an area for further study. How potassium acts to control blood pressure is still unclear, but the fact that increasing intake of potassium-rich foods can reduce dependence on hypertension medication further supports the recommendation to eat more fruits and vegetables for long-term health.

Dietary calcium levels are still of interest in relation to blood pressure, although the connection is controversial. An evaluation of the NHANES I study data suggested that hypertensive individuals consumed less calcium than normotensive individuals, but later attempts to influence blood pressure using calcium supplements yielded equivocal results.[61] A four-year follow-up of 60,000 health professionals indicated a significant difference in incidence of hypertension between the women consuming at least 800 mg of calcium a day and those consuming 400 mg or less.[61] It has been proposed that a calcium intake of 800 mg blunts the effect of sodium on blood pressure. Maintaining an appropriate calcium intake makes sense in the interest of general and bone health.

Low intakes of magnesium are associated with higher blood pressure levels. Among older women with mild to moderate hypertension who were not receiving hypertension medication, supplementation with 485 mg of magnesium for six months was associated with a 3.4 mm Hg decrease in diastolic blood pressure.[77] In another case the substitution of sodium chloride with a mineral salt low in sodium and high in potassium and magnesium led to a decrease in both systolic and diastolic blood pressure in older people with untreated mild to moderate hypertension.[29] A major finding in this study was the fact that discontinuation of the special salt led to a rise in blood pressure to original levels; unfortunately, it is not possible to separate the actions of the three nutrients involved. A factor to be considered in future studies should be the magnesium status of the subjects prior to supplementation. Magnesium supplements may lower blood pressure only in those individuals with a preexisting deficiency.[61]

Treatment of Hypertension

Only in recent years has elevated blood pressure in older people been treated aggressively. Borderline isolated systolic hypertension (a systolic blood pressure between 140 and 159 mm Hg and a diastolic pressure below 90 mm Hg) often goes untreated. In the Framingham Heart Study 80% of the participants above age 60 with borderline isolated systolic hypertension had a rise in systolic blood pressure to at least 160 mm Hg and a rise in diastolic blood pressure to at least 90 mm Hg.[64] Only 45% of the normotensive subjects had a rise in blood pressure. The rise in blood pressure in those with borderline isolated systolic hypertension increased their risk of cardiovascular disease and cardiovascular death. For older people with systolic blood pressure between 140 and 159 mm Hg, lifestyle interventions as compared to drug intervention

may be sufficient to lower blood pressure to normal. Tjoa and Kaplan[73] emphasize a cautious approach in developing a care plan for the older individual, keeping in mind the physiologic characteristics of this group and the difficulties related to any lifestyle adjustments recommended. Guidelines developed by the Joint National Committee on Detection, Evaluation, and Treatment of High Blood Pressure[76] for lifestyle modifications for reduction of blood pressure include:

- initiate modest weight reduction (a goal of even 5 kg is appropriate)
- limit sodium intake to 2–3 g (5–6 g sodium chloride)
- limit alcohol consumption to 1 ounce a day or less (24 ounces of beer, 8 ounces of wine, or 2 ounces of whiskey)
- initiate a regular walking program or other aerobic exercise
- consume five servings of fruits and vegetables daily
- maintain recommended daily intakes of calcium and magnesium.

Drug therapy for treating hypertension in older people usually involves diuretics, but all classes of antihypertensive medications are well tolerated (see chapter 10).

AGING AND RENAL FUNCTION
Overview of Renal Function

Renal function is of great importance to the nutritional and physical health of the older individual. The kidneys have general responsibility for removing waste and regulating the volume and composition of the extracellular fluids. Changes in renal function limit a person's capacity to handle both normal situations or situations of stress brought on by illness or disease. We pointed out in chapter 7 that aging kidneys are less able to conserve water during periods of fluid deprivation or excrete excess water when necessary. Older kidneys are less able to concentrate urine, which means a greater volume of urine is necessary to remove high levels of hydrogen ions (acid) or nitrogenous waste. Similarly, intakes of sodium and potassium become important as levels in excess are less easily excreted and existing supplies less easily conserved. Changes in the endocrine functions of the kidney, which include the hydroxylation of 25-OH-D to 1,25(OH)$_2$D, and the secretion of renin in response to reduced blood volume have important implications for bone health and fluid regulation.

Renal Function in Older People

Kidney function can deteriorate with age because of both a loss of nephrons and a change in blood flow. The pathophysiology of these changes, however, is open to question. The long-held notion that aging led to an inevitable loss of nephrons and deterioration in renal function is not supported by findings from the BLSA.[75] In the 254 men who were followed for 24 years,[75] one-third demonstrated no change in renal function based on measurement of the glomerular filtration rate (GFR), even up to age 80. In fact, a small group showed an increase in GFR over time. Despite these findings among the generally healthy BLSA men, it is known that degenerative changes in renal structure and function do occur in some individuals beginning about age 40. Kidney weight decreases by as much as 30% by age 80, with primary losses occurring in the capillary bed where filtration occurs. These structural changes contribute to an age-related decline in GFR of about 1 ml per minute per year after age 30.[63] In the BLSA the GFR fell from 140 ml per minute in men ages 25 to 34 to 97 ml per minute in those ages 75 to 84.[75]

Hyperperfusion and Hyperfiltration

The wide variation in kidney function among older people has given rise to the idea that detrimental changes are caused, at least in part, by disease or pathologic events rather than normal aging. When the number of functioning nephrons decreases as a result of disease or infection or when the filtration load of the kidneys increases, the kidneys respond with an adaptive hyperperfusion and hyperfiltration.[48] The filtration load of the kidneys increases in hypertension, in uncontrolled diabetes when blood glucose levels are elevated, or with high protein intakes leading to increased levels of urea and other nitrogenous waste. Under such conditions

the renal cells undergo hypertrophy and increase in size. The GFR rises by vasodilation of the arterioles that deliver blood to the nephrons. These responses occur in situations of stress and are discontinued when the need to increase both blood flow and filtration is alleviated. For example, the GFR rises after a meal high in protein and then returns to normal. However, when this adaptive increase in the GFR is long in duration as a result of continued high protein intakes, systemic hypertension, or infection, the capillary membranes are damaged, and the development of fibrous tissue and deposition of mineral salts ensues.[48] The inability of many older people to increase their GFR suggests that they are already in a state of hyperperfusion and hyperfiltration and no longer have a renal reserve. On the other hand, an evaluation of healthy younger and older women indicated that in older people with normal blood pressure and no evidence of kidney disease, renal reserve is preserved until at least age 80.[24]

Avoiding excessive protein intake when kidney function is compromised might restore some degree of renal reserve or slow the progression of renal deterioration. Currently, there is no strong evidence to suggest that high protein intakes increase the risk of renal disease; however, results from the NHANES I Epidemiologic Follow-Up Study[19] suggest that increased dietary protein may accelerate the progression of existing renal disease, leading to end-stage renal disease. Of 2,572 white older people evaluated in 1971 to 1975, 175 were considered to have renal disease based on a physician's report or the presence of albumin in the urine. A 14-year follow-up revealed that a 15 g increase in daily protein was associated with a 25% increase in mortality among the men with early indicators of renal disease. Protein intake was not related to mortality risk in the men free of renal disease or in the women regardless of renal status. A history of diabetes was associated with more deaths in those with renal disease. This relationship between diabetes and renal disease emphasizes the importance of glycemic control in older people with NIDDM. Maintaining normal blood pressure also offers some protection to the aging kidney.[48]

Any loss in kidney function has implications for both the conservation of nutrients and the excretion of potentially harmful waste products. Important molecules actively reabsorbed in the kidney tubule include glucose, amino acids, ascorbic acid, and plasma proteins. An excessive protein intake that produces high levels of nitrogenous waste and hydrogen ions may burden a less efficient kidney. It has been suggested that protein intake not exceed two times the Recommended Dietary Allowance in people of all ages.[12] Megadoses of water soluble vitamins, taken on the assumption that what is not needed can be readily excreted, may accumulate and result in high blood levels while awaiting excretion. Drug dosages also need to be adjusted in light of altered excretion rates.

Renal Failure

Chronic renal failure is not uncommon in older adults because renal disease often is associated with other chronic diseases. Cancer, advanced atherosclerosis, congestive heart failure, use of drugs toxic to the kidney, diabetes, and uncontrolled hypertension lead to chronic renal failure. Elderly people managed on maintenance dialysis frequently are malnourished. Amino acids and water soluble vitamins are lost in the dialysate, and in peritoneal dialysis, protein and albumin are lost as well. Elderly dialysis patients require 1 to 1.2 g/kg of protein with a high biologic value and an energy intake of 35 kcal/kg to prevent negative nitrogen balance.[5]

Many individual factors contribute to malnutrition in elderly patients on dialysis. Anorexia, changes in taste, numerous medications that interfere with the absorption of nutrients, and other illnesses increase the risk of poor nutritional status. Inner city elderly confined to their homes other than for visits to the dialysis facility were found to have general weakness and fatigue that precluded other outside activities.[39] Mean hematocrit in that group was 0.28, despite regular administration of erythropoietin. The lower level of normal for hematocrit in men is 0.42 and in women is 0.37. As the number of elderly people on maintenance dialysis continues to rise, nutritionists and health care professionals will need to intensify their efforts to maintain optimum nutritional health in this group.

AGING AND PULMONARY FUNCTION

Structural and Functional Changes

Aging changes affect not only the physiologic function of the lungs but also the ability of the lungs to defend themselves.[74] Whether the mechanisms that lead to these changes are caused by environmental influences or loss of respiratory reserve resulting from the aging process itself is still unclear. Maintenance of pulmonary function is directly related to survival. Impaired pulmonary function as measured using a spirometer (this measures the amount of air that can be moved in and out of the lungs) is associated with an increased risk of death from heart disease, chronic obstructive pulmonary disease, and lung cancer. In the BLSA, individuals with the greatest loss of pulmonary function had a mortality rate from coronary artery disease that was four to six times higher than those with well-preserved pulmonary function.[74]

The functions of the lungs are the ventilation of the alveoli and the exchange of oxygen and carbon dioxide across the alveolar membrane. Inflammatory injuries to the lungs resulting from smoking or oxidation reactions with other environmental toxins or smoke lead to obstruction of airways and interfere with tissue repair.

Structural changes in the lungs cause a decrease in elasticity and loss of alveolar surface area. Alveolar membranes weaken and stretch, and air sacs become larger with the collapse of small airways. This results in a decrease of as much as 30% in the surface area for gas exchange. Gas exchange is also less efficient because of the thickening and reduced permeability of the alveolar membranes and the reduced flow of blood through the alveolar capillaries. Consequently, oxygen partial pressure in arterial blood decreases. Because the chest wall stiffens and is less easily expanded, the work of breathing is increased. Total lung capacity does not change, although the proportion of alveolar space that is ventilated with each breath decreases and residual volume increases. Even when corrected for sex, height, and weight, the volume of air moved in and out of the lung with each breath decreases with age.[74]

Healthy older people who are relatively free of lung disease can still be vulnerable to complications with diseases such as pneumonia that reduce oxygen levels. Age-associated alterations in the central nervous system decrease the sensitivity of the chemoreceptors that recognize changes in blood and tissue levels of oxygen and carbon dioxide. In younger people hypoxia and hypercapnia bring about increases in breathing and heart rates, which increase the supply of oxygen and reduces the elevated levels of carbon dioxide. In older people response rates are about half those in younger people and are independent of changes in the lung itself. Older adults in whom lung function is compromised are especially limited in their ability to respond to a decreased oxygen supply because of their diminished capacity to ventilate the lungs as well as their reduced neural drive to breathe.[74]

Pulmonary Disease

Chronic obstructive pulmonary disease (COPD) is the fourth leading cause of death among people age 65 and older, and its incidence is rising. Both genetic predisposition and environmental exposure contribute to COPD, but cigarette smoking is involved in over 80% of all cases.[74] COPD represents a group of diseases including chronic bronchitis, emphysema, and asthma; all result in obstruction of the airways with shortness of breath, difficulty in breathing, and loss of respiratory reserve.

Nutrient intervention in older people with COPD is both critical and highly specific.[16] The inflammatory response and associated catabolism of muscle mass appears to affect the diaphragm and respiratory muscles, especially the muscles involved in forceful expulsion actions such as coughing. PEM and a decline in antibody production allows bacterial growth and increased lung infection. Malnutrition also leads to decreased production of surfactant, the lipoprotein that promotes elasticity in the lung and reduces the surface tension of lung fluids, thereby increasing the area for gas exchange. Although undernutrition is a concern, hypercaloric intake is equally undesirable and may result in metabolic or respiratory difficulties. Excessive intake of carbohydrate increases lipogenesis and carbon dioxide production which

causes additional respiratory muscle fatigue or carbon dioxide accumulation. High-protein meals stimulate an increased rate of breathing. Lipids as an energy source reduce carbon dioxide production for older patients with compromised pulmonary function, but the lipemia following a high-fat meal interferes with gas exchange in the lungs. Thus, balance among these nutrients must be individually defined and the older person's condition constantly monitored.

An evaluation of 90 older people with COPD[23] indicated that patients with deteriorating pulmonary function as indicated by increasing blood levels of carbon dioxide had a lower body weight. Weight loss seemed to occur in some patients despite what appeared to be an appropriate energy intake. Fiaccadori and coworkers[23] suggested that the increased work of the lungs may have elevated energy needs. Older people with breathing difficulties may also have low food intake as a direct result of their disease or the appetite-reducing effect of prescribed drugs such as theophylline. As increasing numbers of older COPD patients are being cared for at home, there is an urgent need for health professionals with related expertise within home health agencies.

AGING AND IMMUNE FUNCTION

Infectious diseases are more frequent and often more severe in older people. Many chronic disorders common in the elderly, including diabetes, cancer, and COPD, increase susceptibility to infections. Risk of infection increases with age as the response of the immune system progressively declines. The cause of these changes in immune response is an area of much debate. Although normal aging could play a role, nutritional status also may be involved. Altered immune function observed in PEM is similar to that observed in aging individuals.

Changes in Immune Function

The components of the immune system include (1) nonspecific immunity, the action of the leukocytes or white blood cells as part of the inflammation response to injury and infection;

(2) humoral immunity, the action of the lymphocytes and B-cells in stimulating the production of antibodies or immunoglobulins in response to the presence of antigens or foreign proteins; and (3) cell-mediated immunity, the action of T-cells that assist in the antigen-antibody response and attack virus, bacteria, and foreign bodies. The inflammation response (nonspecific immunity) changes to a limited extent in advanced age. When changes in nonspecific immunity are observed, they are usually related to chronic disease. In uncontrolled diabetes, hyperglycemia interferes with the action of the white blood cells. Vascular disease reduces the blood flow to various areas of the body, reducing resistance to infection and compromising wound healing.[20]

Humoral immunity declines with age because of changes in T-cell function, not because of changes in B-cells. The total amount of immunoglobulins in the serum remains the same although the distribution among the various types changes somewhat. Older people have a lower antibody response to the microorganisms causing influenza and pneumonia, which is borne out by the higher rates of death from pneumonia and infectious disease among the oldest-old. Conversely, a higher level of autoantibodies are produced by older individuals, which, according to one clinician, reflects a breakdown in regulation of the immune system.[20] The progressive decline in cell-mediated immunity and T-cell function has been associated with many degenerative diseases common to older people, including cancer, arthritis, and vascular disease.

Several researchers[8,9,40] have commented on the importance of nutrition in the maintenance of immune function. Immune cells are very sensitive to oxidation because they have a large amount of polyunsaturated fatty acids in their membranes, and, as might be expected, they have a high concentration of antioxidants. Marginal deficiencies of vitamins C and E, selenium, zinc, or glutathione could have an adverse effect on immune function.[8]

Although it is known that nutrient deficiency impairs immune function, excessive nutrient intake does not always enhance it. Daily zinc intakes of 4 to 10 times the RDA have been

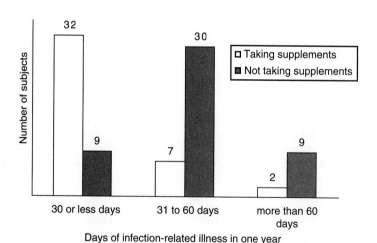

FIG. 13-5   Infection-Related Illness and Micronutrient Supplementation. Apparently healthy elderly people living in the community and taking vitamin and trace mineral supplements had fewer sick days from infection-related illnesses than those taking a placebo.

Data from Chandra, R.K.: Effect of vitamin and trace-mineral supplementation on immune responses and infection in elderly subjects, Lancet 340:1124, 1992.

❖ ❖ ❖

CASE STUDY

Mr. H, who is 80 years old, was recently diagnosed with hyperglycemia at his annual physical examination. His fasting glucose was 158 mg per dl. He has no other symptoms of diabetes. He has a history of cardiovascular disease and became concerned about his fat intake. For 15 years he has been consuming a self-prescribed diet that includes only 15% fat. He is about 20% above his ideal weight of 63 kg, and his serum triglycerides are seriously elevated. His LDL cholesterol is 136 mg/dl, and his HDL cholesterol is 62 mg/dl.

1. What types of intervention will likely be effective in treating his hyperglycemia? In what situation would oral hypoglycemic agents be helpful?
2. What modification of his current low-fat diet would you suggest to achieve and maintain normal blood glucose levels? How would you proportion fat, carbohydrate, and protein? What micronutrients might be important to glycemic control?
3. Based on his current lipoprotein levels, how would you assess his cardiovascular risk? What levels of particular fatty acids would be appropriate?
4. What would be your recommendations regarding exercise and weight control to assist in maintaining normal blood glucose levels?
5. Develop a three-day menu incorporating your dietary recommendations. Using a computer program, calculate total protein, fat, carbohydrate, and saturated, polyunsaturated, and monounsaturated fat, and pertinent micronutrients noted in question #2.

shown to suppress immune function.[8] Nevertheless, a double blind study of 96 healthy elderly people living at home[9] indicated that a vitamin and mineral supplement within the dietary range increased resistance to infection (fig. 13-5). The supplement contained approximately the RDA for vitamins A, C, and D, the B complex vitamins, and iron, copper, zinc, and selenium, and about four times the usual intakes of vitamin E and beta carotene. Over a period of one year the elderly people taking the supplement had an increased number of T-cells and level of antibody response to influenza vaccine. Responses were greater in the older people whose blood nutrient levels were deficient when the study began, but all subjects demonstrated increases in nutrient levels following supplementation. In terms of general health, the supplemented group reported only 23 days of infection-related illness over the course of the year as compared to 48 days in the elderly people receiving the placebo. The need for antibiotic drugs was also reduced by almost half in the supplemented group.

Changes in immune function accompany PEM in all age groups.[49] A change in delayed-type hypersensitivity has been used as a predictor of outcome in hospitalized older patients.[40] The implications of PEM for resistance to infection was evident in a review of 69 elderly patients classified as well-nourished or undernourished when admitted to a geriatric unit.[58] BMI and arm muscle area were used to establish level of nutrition. Over the course of the hospital stay (the median length of stay was 16 days), 73% of the undernourished group developed pneumonia or other serious infection as compared to 39% of the well-nourished group. Nutrition intervention may prevent, at least in part, what have been assumed to be age-related changes in immune function.

Summary

Significant age-related changes in physiologic function can decrease the ability of organ systems to respond to environmental stress. The rate at which functional changes occur varies greatly among individuals and is influenced by both genetic inheritance and lifestyle. Intervention strategies related to nutrition, exercise, or appropriate medications are useful in ameliorating these changes, which are often complicated by chronic disease.

Although loss of mental function is not a normal consequence of aging, the results of testing suggest a decline in mental capacity in some older people. Severe brain disease, such as senile dementia of the Alzheimer type (SDAT), leads to a serious loss of mental function. SDAT accounts for more than half of all cases of dementia in older people and is characterized by a loss of cerebral cortex cells. Some other causes of confusion or dementia in older people that can be reversed with appropriate treatment are acute electrolyte disturbances, thyroid dysfunction, or drug toxicity.

The prevalence of diabetes mellitus or impaired glucose tolerance increases with age. Since impaired glucose tolerance is less likely to progress to overt diabetes in older people than in younger people, there is a question as to whether a deterioration in the ability to metabolize glucose is a part of normal aging and related to changes in body weight and composition and exercise patterns. Cardiovascular function is altered by age, lifestyle factors, and chronic disease. Much of the decrease in cardiovascular performance seen in later life can be avoided by continued endurance exercise. Cardiovascular disease, the leading cause of death among the elderly, is linked to the effect of diet on blood lipids. A decrease in dietary fat can lead to a beneficial fall in plasma lipids in some older people, especially if combined with weight loss; however, aggressive intervention to lower serum lipids in individuals over the age of 75 remains controversial. Elevated blood pressure is closely related to stroke or myocardial infarction in the elderly and even slightly elevated blood pressure should not go untreated. Factors that contribute to hypertension are obesity, alcohol abuse, a lack of exercise, excessive sodium intake in sensitive individuals, and possibly suboptimum intakes of calcium, potassium, and magnesium.

Degenerative changes in renal structure and function often begin to occur after age 40. Because the aged kidney is less able to concentrate urine, a generous intake of fluid becomes important. Chronic renal failure in the elderly is often associated with other chronic diseases such as diabetes, and renal dialysis and associated malnutrition often result. Age-related changes in pulmonary physiology bring about a reduced surface area for gas exchange and aggravate existing heart and lung disease. The response of the immune system in the elderly progressively declines and may be related to chronic disease as well as nutritional status. Despite age-related changes in physiologic function, most older people manage fairly well under normal conditions. Promoting optimum nutrient intake, appropriate exercise, and avoidance of excessive use of alcohol and smoking can slow functional losses and contribute to a higher quality of life.

REVIEW QUESTIONS

1. Describe the three types of changes in physiologic function that occur as people age. How might chronic disease complicate the biologic changes related to aging?

2. Describe some structural and biochemical changes in the brain that often accompany aging. What are the physical changes in the brain associated with SDAT? What are causes of reversible as compared to irreversible changes in mental function?

3. Is the change in glucose tolerance seen with advancing age a normal age change, or is it a pathologic age change? Defend your answer. How do weight gain, weight loss, and body mass index influence glucose tolerance? What are the differences between impaired glucose tolerance and noninsulin-dependent diabetes mellitus? What are the goals and recommendations for medical nutritional therapy outlined by the American Diabetes Association?

4. What dietary, lifestyle, and physiologic factors contribute to changes in cardiovascular function in advanced age? What intervention strategies are appropriate for older people and how successful are they? What are factors to be considered when deciding whether or not to implement aggressive intervention?

5. Why is hypertension a significant risk factor for heart disease, even into advanced age? What physiologic changes contribute to altered blood pressure with aging? What dietary and lifestyle factors contribute to the development of hypertension? What role do the minerals sodium, potassium, calcium, and magnesium play in the management of hypertension?

6. Distinguish between hyperfiltration and hyperperfusion. What factors or situations lead to these

changes in function? What dietary recommendations would you have for an older person who has compromised kidney function?

SUGGESTED LEARNING ACTIVITIES

1. Examine NHANES II and NHANES III publications that present biochemical and clinical data across age categories for factors related to coronary heart disease. Summarize the parameters measured. Compare the findings among younger and older adults. What are the implications for dietary and lifestyle interventions?

2. Obtain printed information on postmenopausal hormone replacement therapy from a gynecology clinic. Summarize the pros and cons of the different replacement strategies as related to cardiovascular disease and bone health.

3. Starting with a food source, follow the conversion of tyrosine into dopamine and norepinephrine, and tryptophan into serotonin. Note the enzymes required which may be affected by aging. List the vitamin or mineral cofactors required for each biochemical step. Based on the NHANES III data presented in Chapter 10, are older people at nutritional risk?

4. Define the plasma lipoprotein fractions, including the apolipoproteins, and list the levels associated with the risk of cardiovascular disease. Describe the etiology of atherosclerosis as it relates to the types of lipoproteins in the blood. Develop a one-page handout for older people that explains how blood lipids can contribute to atherosclerosis and provides dietary advice for promoting appropriate lipoprotein levels. Be sure to use words and terms that can be easily understood.

5. Visit an outpatient kidney dialysis unit in your community and interview the dietitian. You might ask her what proportion of her patients are above the age of 60 and what types of diets have been prescribed. If possible, talk with some of the older patients about any problems or difficulties they are having in following their diet.

REFERENCES

1. Albrink, M.J.: Advisability (or lack of it) of lipid-lowering diets for the elderly. In: Prinsley, D.M., and Sandstead, H.H., editors: Nutrition and aging, New York, 1990, Alan R. Liss.

2. Barrett-Connor, E., and others: Why is diabetes mellitus a stronger risk factor for fatal ischemic heart disease in women than in men; the Rancho Bernardo study, J.A.M.A. 265:627, 1991.

3. Blumenthal, J.A., Siegel, W.C., and Appelbaum, M.: Failure of exercise to reduce blood pressure in patients with mild hypertension; results of a randomized controlled trial, J.A.M.A. 266:2098, 1991.

4. Broughton, D.L., and Taylor, R.: Review: deterioration of glucose tolerance with age: the role of insulin resistance, Age Ageing 20:221, 1991.

5. Brown, W.W., and Wolfson, M.: Diet as culprit or therapy: stone disease, chronic renal failure, and nephrotic syndrome, Med. Clin. N. Am. 77(4):783, 1993.

6. Butler, R.N.: Cognitive failure: delirium and dementia. In: Abrams, W.B., Beers, M.H, and Berkow, R., editors: Merck manual of geriatrics, ed. 2, Whitehouse Station, NJ, 1995, Merck Research Laboratories.

7. Cefalu, W.T., and others: Contribution of visceral fat mass to the insulin resistance of aging, Metabolism 44(7):954, 1995.

8. Chandra, R.K.: Antioxidant nutrients and immune response. In: Rosenberg, I.H., editor: Nutritional assessment of elderly populations, Measure and function, New York, 1994, Raven Press.

9. Chandra, R.K.: Effect of vitamin and trace-element supplementation on immune responses and infection in elderly subjects, Lancet 340:1124, 1992.

10. Chen, M., and others: Pathogenesis of age-related glucose intolerance in man: insulin resistance and decreased β-cell function, J. Clin. Endocrinol. Metab. 60:13, 1985.

11. Chumlea, W.C., and others: Fat distribution and blood lipids in a sample of healthy elderly people, Int. J. Obesity 16:125, 1992.

12. Committee on Diet and Health, Food and Nutrition Board: Diet and health. Implications for reducing chronic disease risk, Washington, DC, 1989, National Academy Press.

13. Coulston, A.M.: Nutrition management in nursing homes. In: Morley, J.E., Glick, Z., and Rubenstein, L.Z., editors: Geriatric nutrition. A comprehensive review, ed. 2, New York, 1995, Raven Press.

14. Davidson, M.B.: Diabetes mellitus and other disorders of carbohydrate metabolism. In: Abrams, W.B., Beers, M.H, and Berkow, R., editors: Merck manual of geriatrics, ed. 2, Whitehouse Station, NJ, 1995, Merck Research Laboratories.

15. Davies, K.N., King, D., and Davies, H.: A study of the nutritional status of elderly patients with Parkinson's disease, Age Ageing 23:142, 1994.

16. DeMeo, M.T., and others: Nutrition in acute pulmonary disease, Nutr. Rev. 50(11):320, 1992.

17. Dengel, J.L., Katzel, L.I., and Goldberg, A.P.: Effect of an American Heart Association diet, with or without weight loss, on lipids in obese middle-aged and older men, Amer. J. Clin. Nutr. 62(4):715, 1995.

18. Denke, M.A.: Individual responsiveness to a cholesterol-lowering diet in postmenopausal women with moderate hypercholesterolemia, Arch. Intern. Med. 154:1977, 1994.

19. Dwyer, J.T., and others: Diet, indicators of kidney disease, and later mortality among older persons in the NHANES I epidemiologic follow-up study, Amer. J. Public Health 84(8):1299, 1994.

20. Eickhoff, T.C.: Vaccines and immunization. In: Abrams, W.B., Beers, M.H, and Berkow, R., editors: Merck manual of geriatrics, ed. 2, Whitehouse Station, NJ, 1995, Merck Research Laboratories.

21. Federation of American Societies for Experimental Biology, Life Sciences Research Office: Third report on nutrition monitoring in the United States, Washington, DC, 1995, U.S. Government Printing Office.

22. Feskens, E.J.M., Bowles, C.H., and Krombout, D.: Carbohydrate intake and body mass index in relation to the risk of glucose intolerance in an elderly population, Am. J. Clin. Nutr. 54:136, 1991.

23. Fiaccadori, E., and others: Hypercapnic-hypoxemic chronic obstructive pulmonary disease (COPD): influence of severity of COPD on nutritional status, Am. J. Clin. Nutr. 48:680, 1988.

24. Filser, D., and others: Renal functional reserve in healthy elderly subjects, J. Am. Soc. Nephrol. 3:1374, 1993.

25. Folsom, A.R., and others: Incidence of hypertension and stroke in relation to body fat distribution and other risk factors in older women, Stroke 21:701, 1990.

26. Fonseca, V., and Wall. J.: Diet and diabetes in the elderly, Clin. Geriatr. Med. 11(4):613, 1995.

27. Frohlich, E.D.: Hypertension. In: Abrams, W.B., Beers, M.H, and Berkow, R., editors: Merck manual of geriatrics, ed. 2, Whitehouse Station, NJ, 1995, Merck Research Laboratories.

28. Garry, P.J., and others: Longitudinal study of dietary intakes and plasma lipids in healthy elderly men and women, Am. J. Clin. Nutr. 55:682, 1992.

29. Geleijnse, J.M., and others: Reduction in blood pressure with a low sodium, high potassium, high magnesium salt in older subjects with mild to moderate hypertension, B.M.J. 309:436, 1994.

30. Goichot, B., and others: Low cholesterol concentrations in free-living elderly subjects: relations with dietary intake and nutritional status, Am. J. Clin. Nutr. 62:547, 1995.

31. Grundy, S.M.: Dietary therapy in diabetes mellitus: is there a single best diet, Diabetes Care 14:796, 1991.

32. Grundy, S.M.: Management of high blood cholesterol in the elderly: based on the Second Adult Treatment Panel Report of the National Cholesterol Education Program. In: Rosenberg, I.H., editor: Nutritional assessment of elderly populations. Measure and function, New York, 1994, Raven Press.

33. Hersey, W.C., and others: Endurance exercise training improves body composition and plasma insulin responses in 70- to 79-year-old men and women, Metabolism 43(7):847, 1994.

34. Holbrook, T.L., Barrett-Connor, E., and Wingard, D.L.: The association of lifetime weight and weight control patterns with diabetes among men and women in an adult community, Inter. J. Obesity 13:723, 1989.

35. Houmand, J.A., and others: Effects of fitness level and the regional distribution of fat on carbohydrate metabolism and plasma lipids in middle- to older-age men, Metabolism 40:714, 1991.

36. Hughes, V.A., and others: Exercise increases muscle GLUT-4 levels and insulin action in subjects with impaired glucose tolerance, Am. J. Physiol. 264(Endocrinol. Metab. 27):E3855, 1993.

37. Hughes, V.A., and others: Long-term effects of a high-carbohydrate diet and exercise on insulin action in older subjects with impaired glucose tolerance, Am. J. Clin. Nutr. 62:426, 1995.

38. Hyman, B.T., and others: Alzheimer's disease, Annu. Rev. Public Health 10:115, 1989.

39. Ifudo, O., and others: Dismal rehabilitation in geriatric inner-city hemodialysis patients, J.A.M.A. 271:29, 1994.

40. James, S.J., Castle, S.C., and Makinodan, T.: Decline in immune function with age: interaction with specific nutrient deficiencies. In: Morley, J.E., Glick, Z., and Rubenstein, L.Z., editors: Geriatric nutrition. A comprehensive review, ed. 2, New York, 1995, Raven Press.

41. Johnson, C.L., and others: Declining serum total cholesterol levels among U.S. adults, J.A.M.A. 269:3002, 1993.

42. Joynt, R.J.: Normal aging and patterns of neurologic disease. In: Abrams, W.B., Beers, M.H., and Berkow, R., editors: Merck manual of geriatrics, ed. 2, Whitehouse Station, NJ, 1995, Merck Research Laboratories.

43. Kahn, S.E., and others: The glucose intolerance of aging: implications for intervention, Hospital Practice 30:29, April 1991.

44. Kannel, W.B.: Justification for management of blood lipids in the elderly. In: Rosenberg, I.H., editor: Nutritional assessment of elderly populations. Measure and function, New York, 1994, Raven Press.

45. Lakatta, E.G.: Normal changes of aging. In: Abrams, W.B., Beers, M.H., and Berkow, R., editors: Merck manual of geriatrics, ed. 2, Whitehouse Station, NJ, 1995, Merck Research Laboratories.

46. Lakatta, E.G.: The aging heart: aging, lifestyle, and disease, Ann. Intern. Med. 113:456, 1990.

47. Lamon-Fava, S., and others: Effects of dietary intakes on plasma lipids, lipoproteins, and apolipoproteins in free-living elderly men and women, Am. J. Clin. Nutr. 59:32, 1994.

48. Lindeman, R.D.: The aging renal system. In Chernoff, R., editor: Geriatric nutrition. The health professional's handbook, Gaithersburg, MD, 1991, Aspen Publishers.

49. Lipschitz, D.A.: Screening for nutritional status in the elderly, Prim. Care 21(1):55, 1994.

50. Löwik, M.R., and others: Nutrition and blood pressure among elderly men and women (Dutch Nutrition Surveillance System), J. Am. Coll. Nutr. 10:149, 1991.

51. Morley, J.E., and Glick, Z.: Endocrine aspects of nutrition and aging. In Chernoff, R., editor: Geriatric nutrition, The health professional's handbook, Gaithersburg, MD, 1991, Aspen Publishers.

52. Morley, J.E., and Perry, H.M.: The management of diabetes mellitus in older individuals, Drugs 41:548, 1991.

53. Moss, A.J.: Diagnosis and management of heart disease. In: Reichel, W., editor: Care of the elderly. Clinical aspects of aging, ed. 4, Baltimore, 1995, Williams and Wilkins.

54. National High Blood Pressure Education Program Working Group: National high blood pressure education program working group report on hypertension in the elderly, Hypertension, 23:275, 1994.

55. New recommendations and principles for diabetes management, Nutr. Rev. 52(7)238, 1994.

56. Paolisso, G., and others: Daily magnesium supplements improve glucose handling in elderly subjects, Am. J. Clin. Nutr. 55:1161, 1992.

57. Paolisso, G., and others: Pharmacological doses of vitamin E and insulin action in elderly subjects, Am. J. Clin. Nutr. 59:1291, 1994.

58. Potter, J., and others: The nutritional status and clinical course of acute admissions to a geriatric unit, Age Ageing 24:131, 1995.

59. Reaven, G.M., and others: Beneficial effect of moderate weight loss in older patients with non-insulin-dependent diabetes mellitus poorly controlled with insulin, J. Am. Geriatric. Soc. 33:93, 1985.

60. Renvall, M.J., and others: Body composition of patients with Alzheimer's disease, J. Am. Diet. Assoc. 93:47, 1993.

61. Reusser, M.E., and McCarren, D.A.: Micronutrient effects on blood pressure regulation, Nutr. Rev. 52(11):367, 1994.

62. Rossor, M.N.: The central nervous system, neurochemistry of the aging brain and dementia. In: Brocklehurst, J.C., editor: Textbook of geriatric medicine and gerontology, London, 1985, Churchill Livingstone.

63. Rowe, J.W.: Renal changes and disorders. In: Abrams, W.B., Beers, M.H., and Berkow, R., editors: Merck manual of geriatrics, ed. 2, Whitehouse Station, NJ, 1995, Merck Research Laboratories.

64. Sagie, A., Larson, M.G., and Levy, D.: The natural history of borderline isolated systolic hypertension, New Engl. J. Med. 329:1912, 1993.

65. Shimokata, H., and others: Age as an independent determinant of glucose tolerance, Diabetes 40:44, 1991.

66. Solomon, D.H.: Age-related endocrine and metabolic changes. In: Abrams, W.B., Beers, M.H., and Berkow, R., editors: Merck manual of geriatrics, ed. 2, Whitehouse Station, NJ, 1995, Merck Research Laboratories.

67. Srinath, V., and others: Diet in the prevention and treatment of atherosclerosis, Clin. Geriatr. Med. 11(4):591, 1995.

68. Stein, P.P., and Black, H.R.: The role of diet in the genesis and treatment of hypertension, Med. Clin. N. Am. 77(4):831, 1993.

69. Stone, N.J.: The 75-year-old patient with hypercholesterolemia: to treat or not to treat? Nutr. Rev. 52(8):S31, 1994.

70. Supplemental dietary potassium reduced the need for antihypertensive drug therapy, Nutr. Rev. 50:144, 1992.

71. Thomas, P.: Aging and the brain, stopping the brain drain, Harvard Health Letter 16(12):6, 1991.

72. Timiras, P.S.: Alzheimer disease compared with normal aging of the brain, Ann. Intern. Med. 113:461, 1990.

73. Tjoa, H.I., and Kaplan, N.M.: Treatment of hypertension in the elderly, J.A.M.A. 264:1015, 1990.

74. Tockman, M.S.: The effects of age on the lung. In: Abrams, W.B., Beers, M.H., and Berkow, R., editors: Merck manual of geriatrics, ed. 2, Whitehouse Station, NJ, 1995, Merck Research Laboratories.

75. U.S. Department of Health and Human Services: The Baltimore longitudinal study of aging, NIH Publication No. 84-2450, Washington, DC, 1984, U.S. Government Printing Office.

76. U.S. Department of Health and Human Services: The fifth report of the joint national committee on detection, evaluation, and treatment of high blood pressure, NIH Publication No. 93-1088, Washington, DC, 1993, U.S. Government Printing Office.

77. Witteman, J.C.M., and others: Reduction of blood pressure with oral magnesium supplementation in women with mild to moderate hypertension, Am. J. Clin. Nutr. 60:129, 1994.

78. Yahr, M.D., and Pang, S.W.H.: Movement disorders. In: Abrams, W.B., Beers, M.H., and Berkow, R., editors: Merck manual of geriatrics, ed. 2, Whitehouse Station, NJ, 1995, Merck Research Laboratories.

14

Nutrition and the Continuum of Care for Older Adults

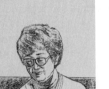

✦✦

Objectives

After studying this chapter, the student should be able to:

✔ *Recognize the impact of projected increases in the elderly population on future needs for health care and other support services for older people*

✔ *Understand the concept of long-term care and the importance of food and nutrition services in both community-based long-term care and nursing facilities*

✔ *Identify the federal legislation that sets the standards for food and nutrition services in community-based nutrition programs and nursing facilities*

✔ *Recognize the impact of community-based nutrition services on the food intake, nutritional status, and quality of life of the older participants*

✔ *Identify food management issues important to the implementation of food and nutrition services in community-based long-term care programs and nursing facilities*

✔ *List approaches and methods that are important when developing nutrition education programs for older people*

INTRODUCTION

Our health care system is receiving increasing attention from both politicians and the general public. In recent years health care costs have increased more rapidly than wages or the costs of other goods and services.[24] Another issue related to the growing health care crisis is the projected increase in the elderly population, particularly the group age 85 and older. By the year 2010, about one in four Americans will have reached their 65th birthday.[24] These trends raise concerns about the health care needs of older people and the resources that will be necessary to meet these needs. Currently, the elderly account for about 30% of all health care costs and are three times more likely than young adults to be hospitalized.[3] One aspect of health care that heretofore has been given limited attention is health promotion and disease prevention. The public health initiative Healthy People 2000[57] has as a priority the maintenance of health and functional independence in all people. Nutritional well-being is the cornerstone of physical and mental well-being at all levels of health, and nutrition intervention should be a fundamental component of care within all health programs. In this chapter we will look at the role of food and nutrition services in long-term care and how we can help older people both in the community and in nursing facilities meet their health and nutritional needs.

AGING AND THE CONTINUUM OF CARE
Concept of Long-Term Care

Older people differ greatly in their general health, degree of chronic disease, functional ability, mental capacity, and mental outlook. Thus, a full range of health, medical, nutrition, social, and personal services—a **continuum of care**—must be in place to support independent living or personal well-being at the highest possible level for older people with different needs.[3] The continuum of care must include different types of facilities, services, providers, and levels of care that can maintain the older individual over a period of years as needed. The continuum of health care should provide access to all services needed for acute medical conditions, chronic conditions, and disease prevention. All older people require preventive health care, including a regular physical examination, nutritional assessment, and nutrition education, along with a sufficient amount of appropriate food.[55]

As people grow older and experience physical and functional changes, various services and facilities can support nutritional and physical well-being. When an older person can no longer drive or handle bundles of groceries, grocery delivery, assistance with shopping, or congregate or home-delivered meals may solve the problem. If an individual cannot prepare meals, homemaker services offered through a home health agency or a move to a retirement community where meals are provided in a central dining room can be a solution. When help is needed with Activities of Daily Living (ADLs), such as eating, dressing, or bathing, services can be provided at home by a home health worker or family members, or the older person might move to an assisted living facility. Older people who are confined to bed or have multiple and serious health problems and disability and require ongoing skilled medical care will likely need to live in a nursing home. Providing medical, social, and personal care services to older people on a continuing basis is often referred to as **long-term care**.[3] In the past, long-term care was usually provided in an institutional setting such as a nursing home. Today, we are exploring new options for community-based long-term care that involve both traditional services, such as home-delivered meals, and new services, such as adult day care.

Ideally, health care and other support services should be coordinated, allowing an individual to obtain new services or discontinue services as his or her medical or functional condition improves or worsens. Unfortunately, in most communities health care services and support services are provided by different agencies. An evolving system for overseeing the assignment of comprehensive services for older people is case management.

Case management provides ongoing assessment, planning, and monitoring by a health professional or social service professional who arranges for services and handles referral to other providers or facilities as needed.[3] This ensures the provision of continuous services and facilitates the movement of the older client from one type of care to another as his or her needs change.

An unresolved issue within the continuum of care is payment for the services required. At one time home health and support services for community-based long-term care were not covered by Medicare and had to be paid for out-of-pocket. Medicare funds could be used only for hospital care, home care during convalescence, or long-term care in a nursing facility.[29] For many older people the cost of home care services was beyond their income, making institutionalization their only alternative. Current changes in the laws governing the use of Medicare funds have provided waivers for states to use these funds to provide community-based services that prevent or delay institutionalization.[3] Such services might be provided by nurses, personal care aides, or nutrition programs. Unfortunately, needed services are not available in all geographic locations; rural areas are most likely to be underserved. In the following sections we will discuss the types of services and facilities that make up the continuum of care.

COMMUNITY-BASED LONG-TERM CARE
Types of Community Services

Many different types of in-home and community-based services have been developed for older people. These services include medical, social, and support services and involve many different service providers (see box).[29] Medical and social services are usually provided by nurses, physical therapists, mental health therapists, nutritionists, social workers and other professional staff members. Support services may be carried out by a home health aide, home nursing assistant, or volunteer. Support services can be formal or informal. Formal services are delivered by home health care agencies, medical

❖

IN-HOME SERVICES IN COMMUNITY-BASED LONG-TERM CARE

Health Services

Nursing—Assessing medical condition; monitoring medications; instructing older resident or caregiver on self-care, care of catheter or other medical device; supervising other providers, such as companies bringing oxygen equipment.

Nutrition—Assessing nutritional status; monitoring food intake; supervising medical nutrition therapy such as parenteral feeding; instructing older resident or caregiver on appropriate diet.

Occupational or speech-language therapy—Assessing need for help with self-feeding or kitchen devices to facilitate food preparation; helping with swallowing problems.

Physical therapy—Assessing need for rehabilitative exercise; instructing older resident or caregiver on exercise plan.

Support Services

Personal care—Assisting with bathing, dressing, or other ADLs.

Home management—Grocery shopping, meal planning and preparation, housekeeping, home-delivered meals.

Social Services

Case management—Arranging and coordinating in-home services; ordering equipment; setting up transportation; handling financial arrangements; helping with housing or alternative placement as needed.

Mental health—Assessing cognitive status; providing counseling.

equipment companies, hospitals, or government agencies, and generally payment is required. Informal services are provided by family members, neighbors, or friends. Formal services, such as medical or support services, required for several weeks or months following discharge from a hospital, are often paid by Medicare, Medicaid, or private health insurance. These services must be supervised or coordinated by a home health agency that meets state and federal guidelines for participation in the Medicare program.[29] Long-term in-home services to older people who would otherwise require institutionalization are paid for by the recipient, by family members, or by Medicare in those states that have obtained a waiver to fund such in-home services.

One model of community-based long-term care is the New York program called Nursing Home Without Walls.[29] This program provides home health aides who deliver personal care to homebound elderly and assist with meal preparation or housekeeping chores as needed. Case managers plan and implement services and handle financial arrangements. An integral part of the program is patient monitoring by a home health nurse. More in-home services are now being provided by government agencies such as area agencies on aging. Area agencies on aging are funded under the Older Americans Act, the major piece of federal legislation providing services for older people. These services are administered by the Administration on Aging in the Department of Health and Human Services through a complex connection of agencies that forms the National Aging Services Network.[3] The particular services provided vary from state to state but may include home health services, personal care, homemaker assistance, adult day care, transportation, and home-delivered meals. Charges for services are usually based on a sliding fee scale. The Elderly Nutrition Program is the largest single program providing community-based long-term care to older Americans, and it will be discussed later in this chapter.

Role of Family Care

Despite the expansion of formal community-based services, the family continues to provide most of the care needed by older people. An estimated 70% of the care of impaired elderly people is provided by relatives, neighbors, and friends.[44] Informal care is often preferred because it is more personal, continuously available, and perhaps most importantly, less costly. Family care may continue for an extended period of months or even years until an acute

illness or other crisis makes home care impossible. An older individual with impaired mobility may be cared for adequately by a spouse or adult child who handles meal preparation and household chores. Debilitating illness that confines the older person to bed can result in short-term or permanent institutionalization if formal in-home services by a home health nurse or supervised home health aide are not available or are not sufficient to meet the person's needs. Unfortunately, formal services are not available in all communities or, if available, may not be financially accessible to a family attempting to care for an older parent. Providing meals or personal care on weekends might be handled by working family members if home-delivered meals or homemaker or personal care services are available Monday through Friday.

Increasing life expectancy will lessen the ability of a spouse or children to care for older family members and will expand the role of government agencies. Based on current trends, women will outlive their husbands, and as family size decreases, fewer children will be available to provide care for their aging parents (see chapter 1).[52] Moreover, the children of the oldest-old are likely to be retired and living on a fixed income and may have health problems themselves that preclude the care of elderly parents. Adults in middle age will be financially and emotionally challenged, caring for their children, parents, and grandparents.

Need for Community Services

The use of formal home- and community-based services is influenced by age, living arrangements, and functional status defined by limitations in ADLs and Instrumental Activities of Daily Living (IADLs).[58] Thirty-two percent of people between ages 65 and 74 who have difficulty walking or have at least one ADL or IADL limitation use at least one formal service; this increases to 43% in those age 85 or older.[58] Among older adults with at least three ADL limitations, 47% use formal services. The help received from family members should not be underestimated, since only 24% of those with two ADL limitations who live with others use formal services, compared to 56% of those who live alone. A newly developed community-based service to assist older people and their families is the adult day care center.[61] An adult day care center provides supervision, personal care, and appropriate activities in a structured environment. Older people spend the day at the center and return to their home in the evening. Services and activities are designed to maintain physical and mental function and, to the extent possible, restore function and communication skills in an impaired older adult. The adult day care center offers an ideal setting for nutrition screening and intervention with an older client and family members.

For both state and federal government agencies, the cost of in-home and community-based care is a growing issue. In past years the government-funded insurance programs, Medicare and Medicaid, favored institutional care rather than community-based care. However, the increasing costs of institutionalization as well as the rising number of elderly requiring care have focused increased attention on in-home services. At the same time, government planners remain concerned about the development of new programs financed by tax dollars that might replace the in-home services now provided at no cost by family members.[44] Short and Leon[50] reported that in-home meal and housekeeping services are used by 1.4 million people over age 65. Services used to a lesser extent included telephone checks and transportation. Increasing emphasis on in-home care not only has created a growing demand for services, but also has increased the complexity of services required. This includes nutrition services. In one location 44% of those requesting home-delivered meals were in need of special diets.[38] An Ohio study[38] emphasized the importance of coordinating medical and nutrition services for homebound elderly people with chronic obstructive pulmonary disease who were receiving oxygen therapy and for chronically ill patients receiving parenteral feeding.

Housing Options Across the Continuum of Care

Many housing and resident options exist for older people with different needs. Although many older people want to remain at home, other accommodations may become necessary with changes in physical, mental, or functional abilities. Assessment by health, nutrition, and social service professionals is needed to assist with decisions that will best meet the requirements of each individual.

Home modification. An older person with functional disabilities can have structural renovations made on his or her current house to provide a safe and barrier-free environment.[18] Occupational therapists and physical therapists can recommend changes suited to the individual's capabilities. Relocating one's bedroom and bathroom to the first floor may solve a major problem for an older person living in a two-story house who can no longer manage the stairs. Installing rails in the bathroom for safety or widening doors for wheelchair accessibility may support continued independent living. A surface cook-top reduces the hazards associated with reaching over an open flame or hot raised burner unit. A microwave oven or toaster oven for heating foods will eliminate the need for handling heavy utensils or transferring hot foods from a cooking utensil to a serving dish. A beeper-type device worn by the older person provides a means of summoning help if needed. Unfortunately, structural adaptations can be costly and out of reach for many older people with limited financial resources.

Apartments in congregate housing. Living independently does not have to mean living alone.[18] Apartment complexes for elderly people with low to moderate incomes are managed by churches, social service or community agencies, and government agencies. In most cases recreation and help with accessing personal or transportation services are available. In some congregate housing units, meals are provided in a common dining room and housekeeping is taken care of. Congregate housing allows older people to retain their own apartment but still have easy access to some support services.

Assisted-living housing. Assisted-living housing offers more personal care and supervision than congregate housing. Residents can receive help with bathing, dressing, toileting, or other ADLs as needed. Meals are provided in a common dining room and emergency assistance is available on a 24-hour basis. It is sometimes difficult to distinguish between board-and-care facilities and assisted-living facilities.[18] Both provide help with personal care and 24-hour supervision. Board-and-care facilities are sometimes referred to as rest homes, homes for the aged, or adult group homes. Board-and-care homes often include many older people living on public assistance.

Continuing-care retirement community. A housing option for older people that is growing in popularity is the continuing-care retirement community which provides all options of care ranging from meal services only, to assisted-living facilities offering personal care, to skilled nursing care.[59] Older people usually join the community while they are still in good health and live independently, although options for meal services in a community dining room are usually available. As the need for personal care or nursing care arises, the resident moves from one level of care to another. Such communities place a strong emphasis on promoting health and nutrition services directed toward disease prevention.

Nursing homes. Currently, about 16,000 nursing homes in the United States care for 1.9 million people.[28] This represents about 53 nursing beds for every 1,000 people above age 65. The probability of nursing home placement increases with age. Only 17% of those age 65 to 74 are in a nursing home as compared to 60% of those over age 85. It has been projected that almost half of all people above age 64 will be admitted to a nursing home sometime in their aging years. Nursing homes provide 24-hour nursing care under the supervision of a physician. Koren[28] emphasized that nursing facilities should not be looked on as hospitals for chronically ill older people. Instead, they should be considered places where older people live and receive health care and many other services. Most residents in nursing facilities are confined to a bed or wheelchair and require skilled nursing services and supervised medications. Recent legislation, the Omnibus Budget Reconciliation Act of 1987 (OBRA),[40] addressed the fact that the typical nursing home resident has a complex set of problems and requires assessment by an interdisciplinary team. Basic team members include the physician, nurse, and social worker, but a nutritionist, pharmacist, physical therapist, or occupational therapist are other important members.

THE ELDERLY NUTRITION PROGRAM
Pertinent Legislation

The amended version of the Older Americans Act of 1965 is the major funding source for nutrition and social service programs for people age 60 and over. When establishing the Elderly Nutrition Program (ENP) in 1972, Congress pointed to the fact that many elderly people do not eat adequately because 1) they cannot afford to do so; 2) they lack the skills to select and prepare nourishing, well-balanced meals; 3) they have limited mobility, which may impair their capacity to shop and cook for themselves; and 4) many feel rejected and lonely, which can obliterate the incentive to prepare and eat a meal alone. Although these factors remain important, the continued aging of the older population and the increasing prevalence of functional disability have added to the complexity of the services needed.[55]

When first established in 1972, the ENP was designed to provide nourishing meals in a social setting. In 1978 amendments provided for the integration of nutrition and social services, including transportation services, and established a home-delivered meals component with separate funding.[20] Earlier guidelines restricted the number of meals that could be home-delivered and emphasized meals served in a congregate setting. The ENP receives its primary funding under Title III of the Older Americans Act and is sometimes referred to as the Title III Nutrition Program. Funding for nutrition and support services for Native Americans, Alaskan Natives, and Native Hawaiians are provided under Title VI of the Older Americans Act.[42]

The growing number of frail and homebound elderly has brought about an ever-increasing demand for meals delivered to the home. Home-delivered meals have increased at the rate of 12% per year, and nearly half of all meals

TABLE 14-1   *Title III Meal Pattern*

Food Type	Recommended Portion Size
Meat or meat alternate	3 ounces of cooked edible portion
Vegetables and fruits	Two ½ cup servings
Enriched or whole grain bread or alternate	One serving (one slice of bread or equivalent)
Butter or margarine	1 teaspoon
Dessert	½ cup
Milk	½ pint (one cup)

From the U.S. Department of Health, Education and Welfare: Guide to effective project operations: The Nutrition Program for the Elderly, Corvallis, OR, 1973, Oregon State University.

funded by the ENP are home-delivered.[55] The total budget for the nutrition program, including federal, state, and local funds and participant contributions, is about $1 billion a year.[55] The most recent annual statistics for Title III indicate that 127 million meals were served to 2.3 million elderly people at congregate sites, and more than 113 million meals were delivered to 877,000 homebound elderly.[42] Under Title VI about 1.3 million meals were served to 41,000 Native American, Native Hawaiian, and Native Alaskan congregate meal participants, and 1.5 million meals were home-delivered to 47,500 members of these groups.[42] Every day more than 16,000 meal sites operate in all 50 states.[55]

General Organization

Under the framework of the Older Americans Act, each state is required to establish area agencies on aging which are responsible for planning, organizing, and implementing nutrition and social services in a given geographic area. A nutrition project serving a designated area administers a variable number of congregate meal sites and home-delivered meal programs, depending on the size of the area and its population density. Funds are appropriated by the federal government according to the number of people age 60 or over residing in the state. At least 15% of total operating funds must be contributed from state or local sources.[42] Many programs have expanded their funding base through local fund-raising efforts and grants secured from charitable foundations. Meal

recipients are also encouraged to make a donation toward the cost of the meal received; however, no one can be required to pay for the meal.

Under federal guidelines a hot or cold meal must be served or delivered five days a week, usually at noon. In rural and sparsely populated areas, meals may be served only one to four days a week. Generally, neither congregate meal sites nor home-delivered meal programs operate on weekends.

Nutrient Content of ENP Meals

Nutrient requirements. Guidelines developed for the ENP require that each meal provide one third of the recommended dietary allowance (RDA) for this age group.[2] The Title III Meal Pattern (table 14-1) indicates both the types and the amounts of food to be included in each meal; it was developed to assist in menu planning. Based on the RDAs for men and women over age 50, a meal providing approximately one-third of the daily energy requirement should contain about 600 kcal to 800 kcal.[46] When two meals are served or delivered on the same day, the combined nutrients in both meals should equal at least two-thirds or 67% of the RDA.[2]

Since the ENP was established in 1972, our nutrition perspective has widened to include an emphasis on dietary patterns that will prevent disease as well as ensure nutritional adequacy. The Dietary Guidelines for Americans recommend limiting fat to no more than 30% of total kilocalories; however, a recent review[46] mentions several reasons why a somewhat higher fat content in ENP meals could be justified. First, most programs provide only one meal each day, and for many participants, especially the home-bound, this may be their only major meal; thus, providing a higher level of food energy by increasing total fat may be appropriate. For older individuals with chronic diseases for whom unintended weight loss is a serious threat, a meal containing 35% fat can be of benefit. Also, gravies and sauces are often necessary to maintain temperature and moisture in meals that are held and transported for an extended time period. Nevertheless, a meal containing only 30% fat will benefit the healthy young-old who attend congregate meals. The vast differences in health status between some older adults who attend congregate meals and many chronically ill adults who receive home-delivered meals accentuate the complexity associated with menu planning and food management in the ENP.

Emphasis on nutrient density. Because the ENP meal is the major source of nutrients for many participants, maximizing the protein and micronutrient content is critical. Fruits and vegetables, which may be consumed only infrequently at other meals, are important sources of the carotenoids, vitamins B-6 and C, folate, potassium, magnesium, and fiber. Dark green and deep yellow vegetables, citrus items, and potatoes are particularly good nutrient sources.

Bread and cereal products prepared from enriched grains are acceptable; however, whole-grain items improve intake of fiber, vitamins, and trace minerals such as zinc and chromium. Whole-grain foods may be especially important for physically impaired older people who consume mostly preprepared foods at other meals. Whole-grain breads and pasta can be introduced gradually to improve acceptance.

Because rising food costs limit the size and frequency of servings of meat, fish, liver, or poultry, other sources of high-quality protein, vitamin B-6, iron, and zinc need to be considered. Legumes, lentils, peanut butter, or tofu (if well accepted) are possible alternatives. If cheese or other milk-based foods are the primary protein source, iron and zinc must be provided elsewhere in the meal. Whole-grain items and a dessert containing eggs, peanut butter, or iron-rich fruits could add micronutrients. Vegetable protein

products made from soybeans are low in fat and relatively inexpensive; as meat extenders, they contribute high quality protein.[46] It is wise, however, to monitor the sodium content of these products.

Older people generally consume less than the recommended level of calcium (see chapter 7), suggesting that menu items made from milk be emphasized. The fluid milk provided with the meal is more likely to be consumed if low-fat milk and buttermilk are available. Milk and dairy products also can be used in cooking. Nonfat dry milk or grated lower fat cheeses can fortify soups, sauces, or mashed potatoes, increasing the calcium, protein, and riboflavin content. (Cheese is sometimes available to ENP meal sites as a government commodity.)

Dessert should be a significant source of nutrients as well as a pleasant climax to the meal. A citrus fruit or banana or a baked fruit dessert made with whole grains contributes important vitamins and minerals. Pudding, custard, or ice cream provides calcium and high-quality protein for those who do not drink milk. In a home-delivered meal program,[56] meals containing milk-based desserts fortified with nonfat dry milk had twice the calcium content of meals with desserts consisting of canned fruit or baked products prepared from a mix. Moist, flavorful baked products prepared with whole grains, oatmeal, raisins, applesauce, pumpkin, sweet potato, or banana contain iron, B-complex vitamins, and trace minerals.

A Title III program in California[63] successfully lowered the sugar and fat and increased the dietary fiber in its meals. The program emphasized fresh and juice-packed fruits rather than syrup-packed fruits, replaced 2% fat milk with 1% fat milk, and increased use of legumes. New items such as tofu and low-fat cottage cheese were added to lasagna, meat loaf, and meat sauce to reduce the amount of meat needed; this allowed the purchase of higher quality cuts of meat that were lower in fat. Oats were mixed into meat loaf to add more fiber. These menu changes were well received by the program participants, although for some individuals the increased use of legumes resulted in some intestinal distress. Wilson and Barry[63] mentioned that brown rice had a higher acceptance level than they had anticipated. These changes, however, required extensive staff training in new cooking techniques and the standardization of recipes. Despite the cooperation of food vendors in seeking out healthy and economical food choices, these menu changes resulted in a 4% increase in food costs.

Special diets. At one time it was proposed that all Title III nutrition programs offer special diets; however, related food costs, limitations of the caterer or meal provider, and/or the lack of an appropriate nutrition professional to supervise and implement the service make this a difficult goal to attain.[46] Modified meals lower in fat, sodium, or kilocalories involve fairly simple changes and are currently offered by 49% of congregate programs and 63% of home-delivered programs.[42] The use of home-delivered meals by chronically ill elderly people with specific medical problems increases the need for home delivery of therapeutic diets. For example, increasing numbers of older people with end stage renal disease are being maintained on renal dialysis and require medical nutrition therapy (see chapter 13). Such meals might be purchased from a hospital food service department, but the cost of these meals, if available, far exceeds the cost of the other meals bought or produced by the nutrition program. For participants with diabetes mellitus or others who must limit their energy intake, the ENP meal is likely to be acceptable if portion size is controlled, skim or low-fat milk is available, and fruit is offered as a dessert. Little or no salt should be added in meal preparation; those wishing to add salt may do so at the table. Preprepared entrees and soup or gravy mixes high in sodium should be avoided. Margarine or butter should be added to vegetables in only limited amounts.

Serving procedures influence the adaptability of meals to various diets. At congregate meal sites it may be possible to ask participants if they wish to have added gravy or sauce when the item is served. Salad dressing can be placed in a small plastic cup when meals are home-delivered.

Food Service Management in the ENP

Nutrition programs may choose to prepare their own meals or purchase meals from a caterer. This decision will depend on (1) the availability of food preparation facilities, (2) the proximity of meal sites to one another, and (3) the availability of potential contractors. When there are several meal sites in a particular locality, meals can be prepared in a central kitchen operated by the nutrition project or a contractor and distributed to nearby sites. In rural areas where meal sites are at some distance from one another, each meal site may prepare its own meals, or meals may be purchased from a local vendor. In any given area the savings accrued through volume buying or large-scale food production must be evaluated in terms of the cost of transporting the prepared food to the serving locations and the equipment required to maintain the food at appropriate temperatures. Nearly half (43%) of all congregate meal sites prepare their own meals, and about a third purchase meals from contractors. Most of the programs serving Native Americans prepare their home-delivered meals at congregate sites.[42] Although it might be expected that meals prepared on site would be preferred by congregate participants, meals containing the same foods delivered from a central kitchen were generally rated as good.[22]

A major consideration in selecting a food service option is total meal cost, which includes the costs of food, labor, and administration. Food and labor are the principal costs and together make up 75% to 80% of the total meal cost. A recent national survey of Title III and Title VI meal programs authorized by the Administration on Aging reported that the average meal cost was $5.17 for congregate meals and $5.31 for home-delivered meals.[42] Costs were slightly lower, 38 cents lower for congregate meals and 81 cents lower for home-delivered meals, in programs serving at least 1,000 meals a week. In a Florida study[35] of five programs serving from 100 to 2,500 meals daily, cost per meal decreased as number of meals produced increased. Larger programs can buy food more efficiently and receive better prices based on the larger quantity of food they buy. Larger programs also can use personnel more effectively. Rural programs, programs in the South and Midwest, and projects using a central food kitchen have lower meal costs.[42] On the other hand, the cost of meal delivery, especially home delivery, is often higher in rural areas.

Volunteer help in setting up tables and serving food at congregate meal sites or packaging and delivering home meals makes a significant financial contribution to many programs.[35] Despite the fact that food preparation at most congregate sites is not supervised by a food service professional, meal costs for the Title III program ($5.17 for a congregate meal) are surprisingly similar to the costs of lunch meals produced commercially. The National Restaurant Association reports that the average person cost of lunch ranges from $4.86 to $5.20 in cafeterias and "family-type" restaurants.[42]

Transporting Prepared Food

When food is prepared at a central location and transported to congregate meal sites or when packaged meals are delivered to individual homes, loss of nutrients, microbial growth, and deterioration in appearance, texture, and flavor are potential problems. The longer the time between when the food is fully cooked and when it is eaten, the greater is the loss in quality and the greater is the chance of inappropriate changes in temperature.

Holding time. The total length of time that food is held at serving temperature after final heating includes the time at the preparation site before or after packaging, the transportation time to the serving location, and the time the food is held at the meal site or in the home before it is eaten.[34] McCool and Posner[34] recommend that food be held less than two hours after final heating. Total holding time is influenced by the size of the geographic area served by the nutrition project and the length of the delivery route for home-delivered meals. Heavy traffic, poor roads in rural areas, and adverse weather conditions significantly increase holding time. Transportation time can be reduced by increasing the number of delivery vehicles, thereby shortening delivery routes. If existing constraints result in holding times beyond the two-hour limit, hot prepared meals should be discontinued and frozen or shelf-stable items used in their place. Losses in food quality as a result of extended holding time may have influenced one report indicating that congregate meal participants preferred meals cooked on-site.[22]

Losses of ascorbic acid and the B-complex vitamins accelerate when food is held at serving temperature for long periods. A British evaluation[56] of six home-delivered meal programs serving 4,200 meals daily reported that cooked vegetables were held about 24 minutes before being placed in insulated delivery containers and an additional 23 minutes transpired before the first meal was delivered. The time between delivery of the first and last meal was about 90 minutes. In this situation total holding time for the meals delivered last was 137 minutes, or 17 minutes beyond the recommended time of 120 minutes. Losses of vitamin C averaged 31% to 54% during the holding period before delivery, and up to 19% during delivery. Because of the substantial losses of ascorbic acid from hot vegetables, a citrus juice or fruit in which ascorbic acid is more stable may be a better menu choice. Vitamin B-6 and folate also are lost rapidly when vegetables are held at serving temperatures for long periods.[62] Losses of vitamin B-6 may reach 26% and losses of folate may reach 57% after two hours of holding time. In contrast, retinol, thiamin, riboflavin, and niacin are relatively stable. Nutrient losses through holding time should be considered when developing menus for meal programs.

Packaging of food. Packaging materials for transporting hot and cold foods must maintain food at safe and acceptable temperatures, prevent contamination, be reasonable in cost, and be easily handled by both staff and older recipients. Desirable characteristics of meal delivery packaging are listed in the box.

Food served at congregate meal sites usually is transported in bulk containers and portioned on-site or served cafeteria style. Bulk containers with an electrical power source that can be preheated and thermally controlled are available but expensive. Home-delivered meals are individually packaged, keeping hot and cold items separate. The need for appropriate packaging is particularly pertinent in relation to temperature control; hot and cold items are delivered under weather conditions ranging from 100° F in summer to −30° F in winter. To prevent microbial growth, cold items must be maintained at a temperature below 45° F and hot items must be maintained at a temperature above 140° F.[35]

❖
IDEAL MEAL
DELIVERY PACKAGING

Food containers
Impervious to moisture
Firm (will not bend easily)
Easily stacked
Deep enough so that liquids do not spill
Resistant to heat transfer
Safe for reheating food in conventional or
    microwave oven
Easily sealed
Environmentally safe for disposal
No sharp edges
No transfer of odor, flavor, or residue to food
Easily opened by older recipient or volunteer
Carrying case
Easily cleaned with water and detergent
Stain and grease resistant
Impervious to moisture
Lightweight and easy to handle
Easily stacked
High degree of insulation
Tight-fitting latches or doors
Appropriate size and shape for delivery vehicle
Side bars or rails to prevent bulk food
    containers from tilting

An English study[56] suggests that even electrically preheated carrying cases may not maintain hot foods at the appropriate temperature when holding time extends beyond two hours. When a long delivery route caused holding time to exceed two hours, the temperature of the last hot meal delivered was 106° F, well below the critical temperature of 140° F. However, the hot food may not have been heated to the recommended temperature of 165° F before being placed in the container. A manual developed for nutrition program managers[46] emphasizes the importance of preheating or precooling carrying containers before they are filled with bulk food or portioned meals.

Innovations in food technology are producing new types and methods of food packaging and preservation, including more aseptic packaged goods, irradiated foods, and controlled- and modified-atmosphere packages. Such food items have increased holding properties for consideration in home-delivered meals. Ultrapasteurized fluid milk that can be stored safely without refrigeration is available in both bulk and one-cup containers. The introduction of these foods will continue to have an impact on both congregate and home delivery meal programs. Frozen meals also reduce the potential of foodborne illness resulting from inappropriate handling of hot or chilled food.

Congregate Meal Programs

Establishing meal sites. Congregate meal sites have been set up in community or recreation centers, municipal buildings, public housing, senior citizens centers, and churches. Important criteria in selecting a location for a congregate meal site are accessibility and familiarity to older people in the community. Programs located in senior centers with ongoing activities are more likely to be well attended. An appropriate location has a major concentration of elderly people within walking distance or accessible public transportation. Title III social service funds are used to provide transportation to congregate sites; however, the need is greater than can be accommodated with existing funds.

Importance of social component. The opportunity for socialization is one of the reasons given for participation in ENP congregate meals; in fact, when participants in a recent national survey were asked what they liked most about the program, more than 70% mentioned meeting with the other participants.[42] The ENP may be particularly important to older people living alone, since more than twice as many participants (60%) live alone as compared to the number of older people in the general population who live alone (25%).[42] More than half of congregate meal site attenders reported that activities at the meal site are either their only source of social activity or a major source. Social support and referral to other needed services can be critical for homeless or other disadvantaged older people.

Home-Delivered Meals

Early history. The concept of home-delivered meals began early in this century. In 1905 the invalid kitchens of London began sending hot meals to housebound patients. The first meal delivery program in the United States began in Philadelphia in 1954.[36] That program operated through a settlement house serving an area of about five square miles and delivered meals to 50 homebound clients each day. In less than 45 years we have gone from 50 clients[36] a day to about 877,000 clients[42] receiving home-delivered meals, and the number of older people requesting meals continues to grow.

Program development. Meal delivery programs were first organized by community nonprofit organizations and health and social service agencies such as hospitals, churches, nursing homes, and visiting nurses associations. In community-sponsored programs, meals sometimes are delivered by volunteers who pay their own transportation costs, whereas in the ENP most of those delivering meals are paid for their time and mileage.

Meal delivery programs operate Monday through Friday. A hot meal is delivered at noon, and sometimes a cold meal is included to be eaten later. Some programs deliver additional frozen or cold meals before the weekend or a holiday. About half of all programs offer the option of weekend meals, but only 22% offer supper meals.[6] Delivery of cold or frozen meals requires that the recipient have a working refrigerator or freezer and a means of reheating a frozen meal. No program provides meals on all days or for all meals of the day.

Meal delivery procedures. For homebound elderly people the social interaction with the individual delivering the meal is very important. This may be the only person they see that day, and the visit, although brief, reinforces the fact that someone cares about them. The reputation of a program rests on the reliability and personal qualities of those delivering the meals, and their selection and training are critical. Because they will be entering the homes of older people who are vulnerable both physically and emotionally, careful screening is important. Those who deliver meals must be trained to handle any

irregular situation. If a recipient does not answer the door, the volunteer or staff member should know the person or agency to call, since this could indicate an emergency. The need for referral is particularly important if the meal recipient lives alone. Delivery staff should be alert to any physical or mental change in the older recipient and relay this information to the appropriate individual.

Profile of ENP Participants

Eligibility requirements. Under the Older Americans Act, all people age 60 and older and their spouses, even if under age 60, are eligible to participate in the ENP. To receive home-delivered meals, the older individual must be confined to his or her home because of disability or other extenuating circumstance. A two-person household may need home-delivered meals if one person is caring for an invalid spouse or other family member and has little time to prepare meals. However, the authors of the Older Americans Act emphasized that special attention be directed to older people who, because of low income, social isolation, or physical disability, were more likely to have nutrition problems.

Success in reaching the target population. A national evaluation conducted between 1993 and 1995[41,42] determined the overall impact of the ENP on the nutrition and well-being of older people, and, in particular, its success in reaching target groups. The results indicate that ENP participants include a large proportion of individuals at high nutritional risk based on age, income, social isolation, or race or ethnic group. In the U.S. population age 60 and older, the average age is about 72 whereas the average age of congregate meal participants is 76, and the average age of home-delivered meal participants is 78.[42] The oldest Title III participant interviewed in the national evaluation was 101 years of age, and the oldest participant in the Title VI program was 103. Congregate and home-delivered meals also reach low-income older people. Although 15% of all people over age 59 have incomes at or below the poverty level, nearly one-third of older people attending congregate meals and one-half of those receiving home-delivered meals are at or below the poverty level. Racial and ethnic minorities who tend to be at nutritional risk make up 25% to 27% of all Title III participants but only 14% of the general population age 60 and older.

Older people in rural areas can be at a disadvantage with fewer available nutrition and social services. Support programs do not exist in all rural areas, and travel distances may interfere with participation. It is interesting to note that 28% of congregate participants reside in rural areas, suggesting that programs in rural communities have been successful in establishing transportation services or are attracting older people who have cars. In contrast, only 16% of home-delivered participants live in rural areas.[42] Moreover, in rural areas home-delivered meal services tend to cluster in county seats with a greater population density of older people than in remote rural areas with fewer old people, despite the fact that the more isolated areas have higher proportions of older people with incomes below the poverty level.[13] This points to the need for the introduction of new technologies that will enable the delivery of shelf stable food items by the postal service or commercial delivery services.

Health status and functional ability of participants. Both Title III and Title VI programs are reaching elderly people with chronic health problems and functional disability. Both congregate and home-delivered participants have two to three chronic health conditions, and many of these conditions, which include heart disease, anemia, and diabetes, require or benefit from dietary intervention.[42] Home-delivered participants are more likely to have difficulty with everyday tasks such as meal preparation than congregate participants. Both groups are at nutritional risk as a result of eating few fruits, vegetables, or milk products, taking three or more prescription or over-the-counter drugs a day, and eating alone most of the time[41] (these are criteria used by the Nutrition Screening Initiative described in chapter 11). Older people served by the ENP are for the most part more functionally impaired than is typical of the over-60 population, and this is especially true for the home-delivered participants. The greater degree of impairment among those receiving home-delivered meals would also be suggested by their

older age (78 years for the home meal participants versus 72 years for the older population in general).

Nutritional Impact of the ENP

Meal nutrient content. ENP meals are expected to provide one-third of the RDA, but the average meal contains up to 112% of the RDA for certain nutrients.[41] Because nutrient calculations are based on the RDA for men, the level of nutrients in the meal will in some cases meet an even greater proportion of the recommended intake for women. The meal components present at the lowest level as compared to the RDA are energy, vitamin B-6, magnesium, and zinc (relative amounts were 33% to 38% of the RDA). Protein, vitamin E, thiamin, niacin, folate, calcium, and iron fell within 40% to 60% of the RDA.[41] Vitamins A, C, D, and B-12 and potassium levels met 70% or more of the RDA. The ENP meals are relatively nutrient dense, providing a greater proportion of the recommended level of many micronutrients as compared to the proportion of kilocalories. Both congregate and home-delivered meals provided 35% to 36% of total energy as fat; however, in light of the low energy intake of many older people, reducing total fat with a likely reduction in total kilocalories may not be wise for this population.[42]

Despite the fact that ENP meals usually contain well above one-third of the RDA for most nutrients, meals in a particular locality can fall below this level. In home-delivered meals obtained from a caterer over a five-day period, nutrients falling below one-third of the RDA were energy (32%), calcium (23%), thiamin (29%), and riboflavin (30%).[4] The meals did contain more than half the recommended level of protein, vitamin A, and niacin. The marginal levels of several important nutrients were related to the meal supplier's failure to follow the Title III Meal Pattern. Evaluation of 30 meals collected over a six-year period (Table 14-2) indicated that only the requirements for one serving of a bread or grain item and one serving of butter or margarine were met in all meals. The requirement for one cup of milk was not met in any of the meals evaluated, and this likely contributed to the below-recommended levels of

TABLE 14-2   *Number of Catered Home-Delivered Meals Meeting Title III Guidelines***

Food Item	Number of Meals (%)
Meat (3 ounces) or alternate	9 (30%)
Fruits and vegetables (two ½-cup servings)	20 (67%)
Bread or alternate (one slice)	30 (100%)
Whole-grain bread or alternate (optional)	10 (33%)
Butter or margarine (1 teaspoon)	30 (100%)
Dessert (½ cup)	20 (67%)
Milk (1 cup)	0 (0)

*Based on evaluation of 30 meals over six years.
Modified from Asp, E.H., and Darling, M.E.: Home-delivered meals: food quality, nutrient content, and characteristics of recipients, J. Am. Diet. Assoc. 88:55, 1988.

calcium and riboflavin. Program managers responsible for quality assurance must regularly evaluate the meals actually supplied by contractors and enforce contract menu specifications.

Nutrient intakes of Title III participants. Title III participants receive a substantial proportion of their daily nutrient intake from the congregate or home-delivered meal. Overall, congregate participants obtained 45% of their total dietary intake from the Title III meal.[41] The nutrients contributed at the highest level (47% to 50% of total daily intake) were protein, vitamins A, D, E, and B-12, and zinc. About 44% of total kilocalories were consumed at the congregate meal site. The nutrients contributed at the lowest level were thiamin, folate, and iron, as only 40% of the daily intake was contained in the congregate meal.

Home-delivered participants consume less food than congregate participants but receive a greater proportion of their daily nutrient total (47%) from the Title III meal (congregate participants receive 45% of their total intake from the Title III meal).[41] For home-delivered participants, protein, vitamin A, and vitamin B-12 were contributed in the highest amount (47% to 49% of total daily intake) and thiamin, folate, and iron were contributed in the lowest amount (36% to 37% of total daily intake) in the noon meal. The home-delivered meal contributed 39% of total energy. It might be expected that the ENP meal would contribute a higher proportion of the total daily intake of home-delivered participants who are dependent on relatives, friends, or neighbors to bring food or groceries for other meals. The fact that congregate participants also receive a significant proportion of their total nutrient intake from the ENP meal suggests that older people who can leave their homes still depend on the ENP for a major portion of their nutrient total. In fact, 45% of congregate participants reported that the ENP is their major source of food.[42]

Title III participants consume better diets on the days that include a congregate or home-delivered meal and consume better diets than nonparticipants similar in age and socioeconomic background.[41] Congregate participants have better diets overall than home-delivered participants. Nutrients falling below 100% of the RDA in both participant and nonparticipant groups were vitamin E, vitamin B-6, calcium, magnesium, and zinc. Total kilocalories also were below the RDA in all groups; nevertheless, for each of these parameters participants reached a higher level than nonparticipants and congregate participants were at lower risk than home-delivered participants (fig. 14-1). Although participants reported only about 92% of the RDA for calcium, nonparticipants reported only 73% to 75% of the RDA.[41] The importance of serving fluid milk in the Title III meal is indicated by the fact that meal participants reached the RDA for vitamin D whereas nonparticipants reached only 84% of the RDA. The below-recommended levels of dietary vitamin D reported by nonparticipants is especially critical in light of reports that the RDA for vitamin D is already too low to support bone health (see chapter 6). Low dietary intake of vitamin D puts homebound individuals at particular risk because they are less likely to go outdoors and spend time in the sun. For all vitamins and minerals except vitamin E, thiamin, niacin, and iron, participants had significantly higher intakes than nonparticipants.

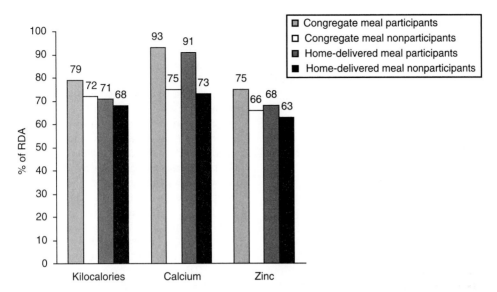

FIG. 14-1   Meal participants have a higher energy intake and reach a higher percentage of their RDA for most nutrients than nonparticipants similar in age and socioeconomic status; home-bound elderly people have lower nutrient intakes than elderly people who can leave their home.

Data from Ponza, M., Ohls, J.C., and Millen, B.E.: Serving elders at risk. The Older Americans Act Nutrition Programs: National Evaluation of the Elderly Nutrition Program 1993–1995, Vol. I, Title III Evaluation Findings, Princeton, NJ, June, 1996, Mathematica Policy Research.

The comparison group of nonparticipants used in this evaluation consisted of individuals from Medicare lists, and statistical methods were used to control for existing differences in age, income, race, and years of education. The researchers decided not to use for comparison individuals on Title III waiting lists because those older people might differ in age and health from individuals who are now being served.[41] One could speculate, however, that older people who have requested meals but are still waiting have nutrient intakes that are even lower than the comparison group actually used.

Issues relating to dietary adequacy. The results from the national evaluation indicate that the ENP makes a significant contribution toward helping older people reach an appropriate level of nutrient intake. Nevertheless, there continue to be unanswered questions regarding the level of nutritional support provided to participants and the relative needs of congregate versus home-delivered participants. Homebound older people are especially vulnerable to poor nutritional status as they are completely dependent on food provided to them by others. Their dietary adequacy is influenced not only by the nutrient content of the meal(s) delivered by programs such as the ENP, but also by the food resources available on nondelivery days and for meals not included on delivery days. Although family members or neighbors presumably provide assistance, some homebound older adults may not have family or friends to depend on. Nearly half of home-delivered recipients save part of their noon meal for later. Program meal leftovers are sometimes used as a part of another meal; however, 16% of home-delivered participants save part of their delivered meal for use as an entire other meal on that day or on a weekend day.[42] Home health nurses who visited older clients receiving home-delivered meals reported finding food stockpiled in the refrigerator or even stored at room temperature.[4] For an older individual dependent on food delivery, building a food reserve may represent a need for food security. These patterns of saving food for a later time emphasize the importance of available refrigeration for those receiving home-delivered meals and the need for nutrition education about meal storage. If refrigeration is not available, perishable items not consumed immediately should be discarded.

Evaluation of dietary records on both delivery and nondelivery days obtained from 95 rural and urban home-meal participants in California[51] indicated that many were at nutritional risk. Although no significant pattern of differences existed between urban and rural participants, rural men and women had somewhat lower energy intakes. The ranges of energy and micronutrient intake in this group were wide, with energy intake falling as low as 647 kcal, vitamin C as low as 12 mg, folate as low as 20 µg, and potassium as low as 735 mg. Seventy percent of meal recipients fell below two-thirds of the RDA for three nutrients, and 25% fell below this level for up to 12 nutrients. The rural men were significantly underweight compared to the urban men (body mass index was 21 versus 24), but the rural and urban women had a similar body mass index, 25 versus 26. The rural elderly were more dependent on family members for assistance with shopping and cooking, whereas the urban elderly were more likely to have help from neighbors or paid workers.

Despite the fact that the population of homebound and functionally impaired elderly continues to rise, funding for the ENP has remained generally level, and some programs have not been able to meet the demand for meals. Increasing requests for both congregate and home-delivered meals have resulted in waiting lists, pointing to a growing unmet need. Congregate meal programs are less likely to have waiting lists than home-delivered meal programs (9% of congregate versus 41% of home-delivered programs report waiting lists).[42] Also, waiting lists for congregate meals are shorter; congregate meal programs report average waiting lists of 52 individuals, but home-delivered meal programs report waiting lists of 85. The mean length of time on a waiting list is two to three months. In some cases the waiting list is equal to about one-third of the number of meals being served.

A recent evaluation of congregate participants and comparable nonparticipants in California

proposed that congregate participants are less in need of a Title III meal.[37] Neyman and coworkers[37] collected three-day food records from 70 congregate participants and 65 nonmeal participants who were active in other programs at local senior centers. Body mass index ranged from 24.9 to 27.7 in both sex and participant groups, and groups were similar in health status. There were no differences in intake of energy or nutrients between participants and nonparticipants. Moreover, nutrient intake did not differ on weekdays that did or did not include a congregate meal. Mean values of hemoglobin, red cell folate, and serum albumin, vitamin A, vitamin E, iron, zinc, and folate all fell within the normal range. Based on the parameter of three or more nutrients falling below 67% of the RDA, 28% of participants and 23% of nonparticipants were classed as having poor diets. The nonparticipants commented that they preferred to eat at home and did not need the Title III meal; they believed that they would be taking a meal away from someone who did need it. Among participants the most common reason given for participation was "to socialize with others," and the meal itself was secondary.

The California congregate meal participants appeared to be at lower risk than congregate participants interviewed in the national study, but there are some differences between the groups. Both the meal participants and nonparticipants in the California study[37] were younger than the national sample[42] of congregate participants (73 years of age for the California group versus 76 years for the national sample). Also, the majority of participants and nonparticipants in the California study were white and well educated; 80% had at least a high school education and over half completed college. Although many did not indicate their income, only 6% of nonparticipants and about 26% of participants had incomes below $10,000 a year.

In contrast to this relatively healthy group of California elderly, food insecurity is a problem among large numbers of Title III participants, including congregate meal participants.[42] In the national evaluation, 10% of congregate participants and 16% of home-delivered participants reported an occasion within the last month of having no food, having no money to buy food, or having to choose between buying food or buying medications. These percentages represent about 240,000 congregate participants and 130,000 home-delivered participants nationwide.[42]

The relative need for meals by congregate and home-delivered participants will continue to be a source of tension within the ENP. Congregate meals serve an important role in community-based long-term care in supporting appropriate nutrient intake and preventing in frail elderly people the downhill spiral that leads to increasing functional disability. At the same time, home-delivered meals play a role in maintaining the functionally impaired older adult at the optimum level and postponing or preventing nursing home placement.[42] Both roles and programs are important within an integrated network of long-term care services.

Future Directions for the ENP

Number of meals provided. The usual five-day-a-week pattern of meal service offered by both congregate and home-delivered meal programs does not meet the nutritional needs of older people with no other food resources. Balsam and Rogers[6] reported that 50% of home-delivered meal programs provided weekend meals as compared to only 17% of congregate programs. Changing trends in health care will continue to add to the demands placed upon the ENP as older people are discharged more quickly from acute care hospitals to continue their convalescence at home. An increasing number of surgical procedures, such as removal of cataracts, are being performed on an outpatient basis, and older people who live alone are dependent on neighbors or service agencies to provide care until they can resume the normal schedule of self-care. As a result of changes in welfare policies and trends toward deinstitutionalization, the number of socially impaired elderly[6]—the homeless, those who live in single-room occupancy, those who are physically abused or neglected, alcoholics, or those recently deinstitutionalized—continues to grow. Outreach efforts are needed to seek out those individuals and develop geographically accessible programs.

Nutritional and quality standards. The current nutrition standards for meal planning are based on the RDAs for people age 51 and older and the Dietary Guidelines for Americans.[2,46] As the ENP participants continue to age, medical and health problems will accentuate the need for medical nutrition therapy, nutrition intervention, and the services of a nutrition professional at the local level. To maximize nutrient content, meal planners must recognize not only the nutritional contributions of particular foods but also the overall nutrient requirements of older individuals as related to both physiologic and pathologic factors. The nutrition professional also can address cost containment, continuing food safety, and overall meal quality. Poor taste, a disagreeable texture, or unpopular cooking methods were given as reasons for discarding food portions by Canadian home-delivered recipients over age 75.[15] Salads were the most unpopular item. Problems in chewing fresh vegetables could have been a factor in this response. Such issues require the attention of a professional with nutrition training.

Food and meal services. The anticipated growth in the homebound elderly population will necessitate the development of more cost-effective and safe ways of providing meals to the shut-in. Some programs have experimented with frozen meals prepared ahead and delivered weekly. In one report[5] the reduction in cost associated with weekly delivery of five or more frozen meals was estimated to range from 16% to as much as 50%. As programs move to occasional delivery of frozen meals, it will be important to seek ways to provide daily social contact, either in person or by telephone, for the homebound adult who no longer receives daily meal delivery. It will be important to monitor food freezing practices at ENP sites that produce their own meals. Meal programs with freezers that were not intended for freezing large quantities of food at one time need guidelines as to the number of frozen meals that can be safely produced.[54]

Meal programs that lack facilities to freeze meals might purchase commercially produced meals for home delivery.[53] A survey of Kansas elderly[21] indicated that people age 76 and older were more accepting of frozen meals than younger people. When asked to rate commercial frozen meals available from the supermarket, baked and fried chicken, chicken and noodles, turkey and dressing, beef patties, roast beef, liver, ham, macaroni and cheese, and spaghetti meals scored 4.0 or higher (1 = I would eat this meal only if there were no other choices; 5 = I would eat this meal every chance I had). Few of these older subjects had microwave ovens; most heated frozen meals in a toaster oven or conventional oven. Gregoire and coworkers[21] pointed out that because microwave ovens operate on a timer and turn off automatically, they might be more safe for operation by an elderly person.

For homebound older people who can cook, groceries can supplement either frozen or hot meals. In one study[26] with rural elderly, groceries were delivered weekly to supplement two home-delivered hot meals. Recipes and preparation suggestions were included with the groceries. Fresh vegetables and fruits, dairy products, and high-protein foods were emphasized. The weekly delivery of perishable food items allowed these homebound elderly to manage with only one major food delivery a month by a relative or neighbor to replenish staple items. Canned, dehydrated, irradiated, and freeze-dried foods that can be stored at room temperature for a year or more could replace meal delivery or provide a food reserve for weekends or emergencies.

MEAL SERVICES IN LONG-TERM CARE FACILITIES
Nutritional Adequacy and Food Service Management

Federal regulations governing food service in nursing facilities eligible for Medicare and Medicaid reimbursement address both the nutritional quality of the food to be provided and the scheduling of meals:[10]

- Meals and snacks must provide 100% of the RDA.
- Meals and snacks must adhere to the physician's nutrition therapy orders.
- At least three meals must be served.
- Bedtime nourishment must be offered unless the physician orders otherwise.

- There may be no more than 14 hours between the evening meal and breakfast.
- Individual food preferences must be followed as closely as possible; if a patient refuses a food, an alternative food from the same food group must be offered.

To facilitate implementation of these nutritional recommendations, states have developed menu patterns expected to provide the level of kilocalories and nutrients required. As Coulston[10] pointed out, however, fiscal restraints influence the quality of the food provided. Although the financial reimbursement to long-term care facilities by state and federal governments is increased periodically as the costs of patient care increase, an individual facility decides how all funds are allocated, and food budgets may not be increased. In fact, if other costs exceed the reimbursement level, the food budget may actually be decreased, resulting in food of lesser quality and nutrient content.

An important consideration when planning meals in a long-term care facility is nutrient density. A benchmark study of 14 nursing homes in Wisconsin[49] reported that the RDAs for calcium, iron, thiamin, riboflavin, and niacin were not met unless patients consumed more than 2,000 kcal a day. At the median energy intake of 1,620 kcal in the men and 1,361 kcal in the women, only protein and vitamins A, C, and B-12 met the RDAs. At an energy intake of 2,000 kcal, menus still contained less than the recommended level of magnesium, zinc, vitamin B-6, and folate. More than half of the 108 women studied consumed less than 55% of the RDA for those four nutrients. A goal for menu planning should be meeting the RDAs for protein and all micronutrients without exceeding the RDA for energy. This will likely require reducing the number of cake and pastry desserts and increasing the number of portions or portion sizes of meat, fish, and poultry; dried peas, beans, and nuts; green leafy vegetables; bananas; and whole-grain cereals. Such changes, however, will also increase food costs.

Energy intakes of institutionalized elderly individuals have been reported to be lower than those of community-living older people; however, these findings are not consistent.[47,60] In a comparison of Dutch women,[60] the institutionalized group had a mean energy intake of 1,552 kcal, whereas those living in the community were eating 1,839 kcal. The women living in the nursing facility were four years older with a mean age of 81; the community group had a mean age of 77. Problems with self-feeding influence the amount of food eaten, but this effect may differ among individuals. Older patients who must be fed are considered at high risk for low energy intake and weight loss, but a surprising finding by Sanders and coworkers[48] was that dependent eaters had a higher energy intake (1,497 kcal) than independent eaters (1,252 kcal) of the same age. Perhaps the effort required for eating was difficult for the independent eaters despite the fact that they were considered capable of self-feeding. Anorexia, unfamiliar foods, or poor health could have contributed to the poor food intake among the independent eaters.

The overall quality of care provided by the nursing facility may enter into the patterns of food intake and energy balance observed in nursing home residents. Abbasi and Rudman[1] described two nursing homes with similar case loads and types of residents. In one, only 8% of the residents were underweight and only 10% had become eating-dependent over the previous six months. In contrast, 32% of the residents in the other nursing home were underweight and 29% had become eating-dependent. The researchers pointed out that the nursing home with better nourished residents had a 30% higher staff-to-resident ratio and overall spent 25% more money per resident. This increased expenditure could include more food or higher quality food. As noted earlier, changes in institutional budgeting can result in less money spent for food. Another critical finding was that undernutrition was strongly related to the subsequent loss of ability to feed oneself.

In nursing facilities providing quality care, energy and nutrient intakes of residents may be similar to or even higher than intakes of elderly living in the community. In the Boston Nutritional Status Survey,[47] the median energy intake of older men living in their own homes was 1,852 kcal and for older men in nursing facilities

it was 1,906 kcal. Among the women this difference was even greater as the women in the community ate 1,468 kcal a day and the women in the nursing facilities ate 1,718 kcal. Sahyoun[47] attributed some of this difference to the methods used to collect dietary information. The individuals living at home kept three-day dietary records and may have underreported their food intake. Among the institutionalized subjects, dietary data were gathered by the researchers who observed food intake. Nevertheless, the lower food intake reported by the elderly women in the community could reflect problems with grocery shopping, meal preparation, or food money. Over half of the women in the community and about three times as many women as men were over age 80.

Recent amendments to OBRA[17,40] have set new guidelines for nutrition management and intervention in Medicare- and Medicaid-approved nursing facilities. These regulations go beyond assuring an appropriate and adequate food supply to mandating the nutrition support required to achieve the highest possible level of function or rehabilitation in nursing home residents. These regulations focus on:[17,40]

- The rights of residents. Residents have the right to refuse treatment. This includes the right to choose what they eat, when they eat, where they eat, and if they are willing to follow a therapeutic diet.
- The need to maintain and enhance the quality of life of residents. They must be treated with dignity, and all efforts must be made to achieve the highest practical level of physical, functional, and psychosocial well-being. The resident must receive a nourishing, palatable, and well-balanced diet that meets his or her dietary requirements. A major influence on the quality of life is the ability to self-feed, and maintaining or restoring self-feeding must be a major priority of the health care team. Patient care must include the aggressive treatment of pressure sores, medical nutrition therapy as needed to maintain appropriate body weight and nutritional status to the extent possible, and sufficient fluids to prevent dehydration.

- A nutrition assessment of the resident must be completed regularly following a standardized protocol. An initial assessment must be conducted within 14 days of admission and every three months thereafter. The health care team completing the assessment should include the primary nurse, the physician, a social worker, the dietitian, and other professionals such as a speech pathologist or dentist as needed. A plan of care should be developed that sets measurable goals for progress or for preventing deterioration with a timetable for implementing treatment and the responsibilities of each team member.

This emphasis on promoting resident well-being, preventing weight loss or implementing weight gain, and maintaining or restoring self-feeding has resulted in new initiatives in dietary intervention.

Resident Satisfaction with Meals

A major food issue in long-term care facilities was emphasized by Gallagher[16] who observed that "above all, we want the residents to eat." This requires that food tastes good, looks attractive, and is served in a pleasant environment. Tablecloths or tray liners in soft colors not only increase the appeal of the food served but also help those with impaired vision to distinguish plates and cups from the table surface. A glass of milk can be difficult to see placed on a white tablecloth.

Physiologic changes in older people's ability to swallow sometimes require texture-modified diets that may be easier to swallow. Major problems with texture-modified diets and pureed foods can be appearance, which can limit acceptability by the older person, and low nutrient density. Special attention to recipe development can turn pureed dishes into attractive and popular menu items. Experimenting with a pastry bag and thickening agents will improve the quality and appeal of such dishes as pureed tuna on pumpernickel or angel food cake with pureed strawberry sauce.[16] Efforts to make pureed food attractive can enhance food intake. It is important, however, to control the addition of nonnutritive thickeners or water when preparing a pureed food. If portion size is based on volume following the addition of a significant amount of water, nutrient intake will be severely reduced even though the entire portion is consumed.[25] If a blender is used to puree foods from the regular menu without the addition of water, the nutrient density per portion will not decrease. Johnson and coworkers[25] pointed to the importance of quality control measures and staff supervision in the preparation of pureed foods for older people at nutritional risk. It is also important to implement a care plan that incorporates therapy by a speech pathologist which may alleviate the need for pureed food.

Current recommendations suggesting the limited benefits of special diets for older nursing home residents may also encourage greater food intake. Coulston[10] raised questions as to the demonstrated clinical usefulness of sodium-restricted diets or fat-modified diets in nursing home residents above 75 years of age. Any therapeutic benefits need to be weighed against the impact on nutrient intake of a diet that discourages food intake. In a review of 217 patients in four nursing homes in Wisconsin,[8] almost half had a serum albumin less than 3.5 g/dl, and one-third were losing weight at a rate greater than one pound a month. In those with low serum albumin 75% were on a restricted diet, 18% were energy restricted, and 35% were sodium restricted. Among those losing weight, 59% had some dietary restriction and 20% were limited in kilocalories. The mean BMI in these patients was 23.5, and 58% fell below recommended weight for height. Although therapeutic diets may play an important role in the outpatient or acute care setting, such diets do not appear to be justified in the malnourished patient. Coulston[10] recommends that a special diet be prescribed only when not using one will risk the patient's health. (Use of diabetic diets in nursing home residents was discussed in chapter 13.)

Long-term care facilities are also directing their attention to the dining environment. Elmstahl and coworkers[14] told about redecorating the dining room of a nursing facility to closely resemble a dining area of the 1940s. For the residents the 1940s were a time when they were very active in social events. Following the change in decor, food intake improved. It is interesting to note that these older people did not gain weight despite an increase in energy intake. This was attributed to the increase in physical activity that resulted from their improved psychological outlook.

Bonnel[7] established a model called Managing the Work of Eating for use in improving the dining environment in nursing facilities. For frail elderly people eating is work and requires more effort and attention than is true for younger people. There are four components in this model:

Negotiating the Environment: The physical arrangement of the dining room must be planned for safety, allowing space between tables to accommodate wheelchairs, walkers, and canes. Minimizing background noise from staff and using placemats to reduce sound promotes residents' conversation.

Coping with Frailty: Staff should be available to provide assistance with tasks requiring dexterity of the hands and fingers, such as opening cartons of milk or jelly and helping to cut meat for residents who are weak. Providing a way for timid residents to ask for help such as a table "flag" would promote eating of all food served.

Dealing with Colleagues: Seating individuals at small tables encourages conversation, and staff should introduce new residents to the others at the table. Placing residents at tables according to their level of function will ensure that individuals who are eager to talk with others are not surrounded by residents who are confused or withdrawn.

Responding to the System: A resident food council should be established to communicate to staff the concerns of residents who may not feel at ease raising a complaint or offering a suggestion. The council could also tell residents about ideas for change suggested by the nursing or dietetic staff.

NUTRITION EDUCATION FOR OLDER ADULTS

Eating an appropriate amount of nourishing food every day is an important aspect of self-care. Optimum nutrient intake combined with regular physical activity as part of a healthy lifestyle is a powerful influence on physical and mental well-being and the prevention or delay of chronic disease. Thus, nutrition education should be an important component of ongoing health promotion services for older people and their caregivers.

Food and Nutrition Knowledge of Older People

One influence on dietary intake is nutrition knowledge and the ability to select a nutritionally adequate diet from the food choices available. People develop a food pattern and acquire food knowledge through a lifetime of experience. For those adults with few years of formal schooling, nutrition knowledge generally is acquired through informal sources such as newspapers or magazines and friends or acquaintances. Nutrition education should build on the nutrition knowledge clients already have and provide appropriate information useful in daily food selection.

According to the results of formal nutrition knowledge tests, many older adults have only a limited knowledge of the foods required for good health. In a study of 165 people above age 64 living in Oregon,[43] participants were asked to name the four groups of foods required for a balanced diet. Almost none failed to mention protein foods or the need for fruits and vegetables, but more than one-fourth did not name the grain or dairy groups. This may reflect less attention on the part of nutrition educators in past years to these food groups. Also, it might be more useful to ask older people about the specific food items they think should be included in a meal or in the daily food pattern rather than about food groups.

Older people are generally very concerned about maintaining their health and independence, and this makes them especially vulnerable to claims of renewed vitality or relief from chronic complaints by using nutritional supplements. The money needed to buy costly vitamin or mineral supplements might better be used to buy wholesome food. Among 102 Iowa elderly[39] 49% used vitamin and mineral supplements regularly, and about one-fourth were following recommendations from health magazines. Of the 20 individuals who were taking supplements on their physician's advice, eight were taking an inappropriate amount (more than 150% of the RDA) along with additional individual supplements not prescribed by the physician. Elderly women are more likely to believe in nutritional supplements, whereas elderly men are more likely to trust the nutritional value of ordinary foods.

Nutrition educators must be sensitive to older individuals who are most likely to overuse nutritional supplements. Older Iowa women classified as users, nonusers, or overusers of supplements (they consumed 200% or more of the RDA)[45] did not differ on the basis of age, education, income, or perceived dietary adequacy. Overusers of supplements were more likely to live alone and have medically diagnosed health problems. Overuse of particular supplements among these women included vitamin B-6 (more than 10 times the RDA); thiamin, riboflavin, and vitamin C (more than 40 times the RDA); iron (400 mg per day); vitamin D (25,000 IU per day); and calcium (3 g per day). Such levels consumed on a continuous basis will result in serious toxicity or prevent the absorption of other important nutrients.

Sources of Nutrition Information

The appropriateness of nutrition-related decisions made by older people are influenced by their source of nutrition information. In general, older people rely on less formal sources of nutrition information, including magazines, newspapers, cookbooks, and television programs. Older women are more likely to use food labels for nutrition information than older men. A telephone survey of older people in Wyoming[33] indicated that 81% received their nutrition information from newspapers, 66% to 70% from books, magazines, and television, and 52% from physicians or nurses. Only 25% ever talked to a dietitian or nutritionist, and only 18% took advantage of materials or programs offered by extension home economists. Rural elderly may have less access to the services of a dietitian or lack transportation to extension programs.

Implementing Nutrition Education: The Learning Process in Older People

Older adults do express an interest in nutrition education.[19,23] Learning in the older adult is influenced by psychological, physiological, and environmental factors.[27] Older people bring to a learning situation a set of attitudes developed over a lifetime, and these attitudes and ideas must be respected. In the past teaching environments with authoritarian standards were considered most effective, and childhood school experiences may not have been pleasant. Thus, the first step in encouraging older people to participate is to emphasize the informality of the session.

Learning reflects an effort on the part of an individual to meet his or her perceived needs. Although children in a school setting may be resigned to learning facts that they may not consider important to their personal situation, the older learner wants to make immediate use of the information presented. The older woman on a limited food budget will have little interest in the nutritional value of fresh broccoli that she cannot afford to buy. The older African American man who is lactose intolerant will not benefit from ideas for using fluid milk unless he can purchase lactase preparations for treating the milk first. The ability of the listener to act on the suggestions being presented should be an important criterion when selecting material for nutrition education.

Physiologic limitations can influence learning in the older adult. Visual problems make it more difficult to see objects without blurring or distinguish between colors. Whenever possible use real food items as visual aids and arrange for good lighting. Use large print on posters or handouts. Many older people have some degree of hearing loss. When speaking to a group or counseling an individual, select a location free of distracting noises. Use words that are easily recognized.

Older adults bring to a learning situation perceptions of themselves, their abilities, and their limitations. Nutrition education can be a positive experience in a relaxed, noncompetitive atmosphere in which information is presented at the pace appropriate for the learner rather than the educator. A supportive environment directed toward individual needs is most likely to attract the older adult.

Innovative Approaches to Nutrition Education

Nutrition education programs for older adults are widespread; however, few have been evaluated as to outcome or positive changes in the food patterns of the participants. In many instances evaluation has focused on an increase in nutrition knowledge that may or may not result in a change in food behavior. One factor that may influence whether or not nutrition information is applied in making food choices is the topic presented. Topics for nutrition education suggested by rural elderly were vitamins, weight control, special diets (e.g., low fat or diabetic), cholesterol issues, and the nutritional value of foods.[30] Among older Boston residents,[19] food safety in the home and the effect of food processing on food nutrient content were the topics of greatest importance. Salt intake, sugar intake, and weight control were also issues of concern in the Boston group. Older people need reassurance as to the safety and nutritional adequacy of the food supply.

Identifying topics for nutrition education. Several formats[9,23,32] have been suggested for getting ideas for nutrition topics prior to beginning a nutrition education program for older adults. Iszler and coworkers[23] found focus groups to be successful with older men and women. Those older people emphasized the need for specific information about foods, pointing out that advice to "choose low fat foods" provides little help with day-to-day choices unless particular foods are identified. Another successful approach involved having older people keep a food diary and then helping them to identify changes that would improve their nutritional pattern.[32] Kumanyika and coworkers[31] developed a method using food pictures of designated portion sizes to help older people identify their previous food intake. This picture-sort method would be especially appropriate for older adults with low literacy or for those with arthritis or conditions such as Parkinson's disease that make writing difficult. A

group of 48 elderly diabetics[9] found it helpful to identify barriers that presented difficulties in following an appropriate diet. For example, those diabetics found it difficult to choose foods at parties when most of the foods available are high in sugar. A first step in working with individuals and groups is assessing their information needs.

Nutrition education classes. Congregate meal sites offer tremendous potential for the dissemination of food and nutrition information. Currently, 87% of Title III programs and 70% of Title VI programs offer nutrition education programs.[42] Of 116 frail adults living in a rural community, 40% were interested in a nutrition education program.[23] About half preferred a class setting in which all participants were about their same age and gender, although one-third thought it would be nice to have different ages and points of view represented. Older people prefer a series of shorter classes instead of one or two classes lasting one or two hours. Meeting more often and talking with others provide motivation to continue positive behavior changes. Focus group participants also pointed out that too much information at one time can be confusing and continuing classes allow the opportunity to have information repeated with time for questions. Older people prefer a verbal and visual format for nutrition education that includes talks, demonstrations, videos, or movies rather than lectures.[30]

Written materials and mailings. Older people consider written materials to be important and helpful sources of nutrition information. Among a group of frail elderly with a median age of 75 to 79, written materials rather than classes were considered to be the most interesting and helpful sources of nutrition information.[30] Home-based learning is receiving growing attention as a means of providing food and nutrition information to homebound older adults or those who may lack transportation. Written materials describing nutritious, shelf stable food items might be helpful for Title III or Title VI home-delivered meal participants who have someone shop for them occasionally to purchase food for weekends when meals are not delivered. For older people who can leave their homes, a combination of methods might be most appropriate. A class at which a home learning packet was distributed would allow older adults to receive an overview of the material, and a second class some time later would provide an opportunity to ask questions.

A series of three nutrition education packets with information about dietary fat, dietary fiber, and making healthy food choices at the supermarket was mailed at two-week intervals to 335 older people in rural communities.[11] A follow-up survey indicated no significant change in nutrition knowledge or in food choices at home. Crockett and coworkers[11] noted that these individuals were eating a relatively healthy diet prior to the nutrition intervention and thus dietary changes may have seemed to be less important to them. Also, the study period of six weeks may have been too short to allow dietary changes to occur.

As the older population continues to rise in educational level, written materials and home learning will likely become a highly utilized method for nutrition education. Of concern, however, is the fact that African American elderly are less likely to have a high school education; we must continue to focus on nutrition education methods that are applicable to low literacy groups. As the older population becomes more diverse, it is urgent that we provide nutrition education materials in Spanish that focus on ethnic foods to meet the needs of the Hispanic elderly. Videos that could be borrowed and returned by mail carry potential for use in home learning.

Dietary Advice for Older People

For most older people, dietary advice should emphasize the same foods considered to be appropriate for younger people. The Food Guide Pyramid and Healthy Eating Index that encourage use of meat, poultry, fish, and legumes, dairy products, fruits and vegetables, and grains are suitable guides for all age groups. Nutrition education for older people should strike a balance between the need for recommended levels of all nutrients and attention to the Dietary Guidelines for Americans that encourage limiting intake of fat and saturated fat. Daily menus low in fat, which over time include fewer portions of meat or eggs, are less likely to meet recommended levels of iron, vitamin B-6, and zinc.[12] Greater use of legumes can add to the supply of these nutrients. A reasonable approach to the use of meat, especially lean meat, as an important component of the diet may help to ensure adequate intakes of important nutrients. Maintaining recommended levels of all vitamins and minerals may be more important to ongoing health and well-being in elderly people than strict adherence to current guidelines for low dietary fat. A future goal should be the development of dietary guidelines for older people that promote optimum intake of all nutrients to ensure continuing good health, vitality, and quality of life.

Summary

The projected increase in the number of older people raises many questions about who will care for elderly people with functional disabilities who can no longer care for themselves. At one time government agencies believed that placing older people in institutional settings such as nursing homes was the most economical and appropriate way to provide day-to-day care for physically impaired or chronically ill elderly people. As the potential number of older people who need care and the projected costs of institutional care continue to escalate, health planners have begun to explore ways of providing community-based long-term care that will allow older people to remain at home and delay or prevent institutionalization. In-home services provided by nurses, physical therapists, occupational therapists, home health aides, personal care aides, and home-delivered meals programs can assist the older individual in remaining independent. Medical services, home management services such as grocery shopping or meal preparation, or personal care services such as help with bathing or dressing can be paid by Medicare if a state has received a waiver to support home care services. Various types of housing, including congregate housing or assisted-living housing, offer alternatives for the older person who cannot remain at home but does not require skilled nursing care.

❖ ❖ ❖
CASE STUDY

Mrs. J is 85 years old, uses a walker to move about, and even with her glasses has a problem distinguishing numbers or reading small print. She is a widow and lives alone. She receives home-delivered meals which provide a hot meal at noon Monday through Friday and two extra cold meals on Friday that include a sandwich, salad, fruit, milk, and dessert. Mrs. J has hypertension and is on a diuretic; she has been told to cut down on her sodium intake but she doesn't really like the taste of food without salt, so sometimes she doesn't bother to eat. Her niece shops for her once every two weeks to pick up food to supplement her home-delivered meals, and her neighbor stops by now and then when she is going to the store to see if Mrs. J needs anything. However, if it is nearing the end of the month and Mrs. J has no money remaining from her Social Security check, she tells her neighbor that she doesn't need anything, even if her food supply is low.

1. What are factors relating to Mrs. J's health and living situation that will influence her nutrient intake? What might you suspect regarding Mrs. J's nutritional status?

2. What types of food is Mrs. J likely to be eating less frequently than she should? What nutrients are likely to be low in Mrs. J's diet?

3. Plan a menu for one week for Mrs. J that incudes all food items that will not be included in the home-delivered meals. Use a computer program to verify that your menus will met 67% of the RDA and provide all additional food portions needed to meet the recommendations of the Food Guide Pyramid. You can assume that each of the food portions listed in the Title III Meal Pattern in Table 14-1 will be contained in all meals delivered, including the two cold weekend meals, and that all will contain 33% of the RDA. Be sure to keep in mind Mrs. J's mobility and vision problems that limit her ability to prepare meals as well as her limited financial resources.

4. Develop a shopping list that includes all items to be purchased by Mrs. J's niece when she shops for her every two weeks. Include foods that will have a shelf life of at least one week or indicate items that Mrs. J's neighbor may be able to bring her in between her niece's visits.

The largest provider of nutrition services for people age 60 and older is the Elderly Nutrition Program (ENP) funded under the Older Americans Act. When the ENP began in 1972, it was intended to provide both a nourishing meal and social interaction in a congregate setting for older people who, because of low income, disability, loneliness and depression, or lack of meal preparation skills, were unable to provide adequate meals for themselves. Since that time the home-delivered meals program was established with separate funding to provide for those individuals who because of physical disability or health problems cannot leave their home. The nutrition standards of the ENP require that each meal provide at least one-third of the Recommended Dietary Allowances and meet the Dietary Guidelines for Americans. A recent national evaluation indicated that the average meal contains well above 33% of the RDA for many micronutrients. Also, these meals are the major source of the nutrients consumed by the participants, providing almost half of their total daily intake. Overall, congregate meal participants have higher nutrient intakes than home-delivered meal participants, and both congregate and home-delivered meal participants have higher intakes than nonparticipants who are similar in age and socioeconomic status. The growing demand for meals, especially home-delivered meals, has not resulted in a commensurate increase in the resources available. This has led to tension within the ENP as administrators are faced with increasing waiting lists for home-delivered meals and difficult decisions as to the relative importance of congregate versus home-delivered meals. Congregate meals supply nutrients that help to prevent the downhill spiral that results in functional disability in frail older people. Home-delivered meals play a role in community-based long-term care and prevent or delay institutionalization. Thus, both programs are important. Seeking innovative ways of providing home-delivered meals at lower cost, such as delivering frozen meals on a weekly basis, must be an important objective.

Recent federal legislation has established standards for nursing facilities that emphasize the importance of nutritional care and the rehabilitation of elderly residents to the highest possible level of function, including self-feeding. Making food attractive and palatable and improving the dining environment encourages food intake.

Older people are receptive to nutrition education but value information that is of immediate use to them. Focus groups are an effective way to obtain ideas from older people about preferred topics and format for nutrition education programs. Encouraging older people to emphasize food as their major source of nutrients rather than numerous and costly supplements should be a central theme of nutrition education to preserve for older people the best possible quality of life.

REVIEW QUESTIONS

1. What does long-term care mean? Discuss the issues surrounding the shift in emphasis from institutionalization to community-based long-term care. Distinguish between formal and informal services. List the types of formal services that are currently available and give an example of each. What is the role of the case manager in community-based long-term care?

2. What is the Elderly Nutrition Program (ENP) and how is it funded? What are the nutrition standards for the ENP? Discuss problems and strategies for home-delivered meal programs relating to food safety, food packaging, and participants' need for social contact.

3. What was the target population for the ENP as described in the original version of the Older Americans Act? Is that target population currently being served? How has the philosophy of the ENP regarding congregate versus home-delivered meals changed in recent years, and why has it changed? Are home-delivered meal recipients more in need of meals than congregate recipients? Defend your answer.

4. What does the ENP contribute to the nutrient intake of participants? What are the limitations of the current amount of food provided? What recommendations would you make for food and nutrition services in the future?

5. What legislation has established standards for nutritional care in nursing facilities, and what are those standards? What factors influence nutrient intake in nursing home residents? Is the food and nutrient intake of nursing home residents better or worse than that of older people living at home?

6. What are common sources of nutrition information used by older people? What are characteristics of the older learner that are important for nutrition educators? What are some successful ways of identifying nutrition education needs and formats for older people?

SUGGESTED LEARNING ACTIVITIES

1. Call the dietitian or food service director at a nursing facility near your home and ask if you can visit the dining room at lunch or dinner. Note the amount of plate waste. Are the residents consuming all of their meal, most of their meal, or a small amount of their meal? What food items are they most likely to eat, and what food items are they most likely not to eat? Are there particular characteristics of the food eaten or not eaten (e.g., easy or difficult to chew, served in a container that is difficult to open, or needing to be cut in pieces)? Record your observations about the ambiance of the dining room, the interaction of the staff and the residents, and the interaction of the residents with each other. Summarize what you have observed about the food intake and dining environment.

2. Accompany a person who delivers home-delivered meals for one week and observe the functional ability of the recipients. Note what type of packaging is used for the meals and what type of delivery case is used in transport. How long was the holding time between when the food was packaged and loaded in the car and when the last meal was delivered? Does the delivery person have much time to visit with the clients when the meal is delivered? Summarize what you have observed about the program and the meal recipients. Work with a student who visited a nursing facility and in a report to the class, compare the general functional ability of these recipients and the residents in the nursing facility.

3. Visit a Title III or Title VI congregate meal site in your area. Note the type of food service used and how long the food was held before being

served. Are the meals preportioned or served cafeteria style? Are there options for modified meals or a choice of dessert for those with diet restrictions? Note the amount of plate waste, and if the participants are consuming all of the meal, most of the meal, or a small amount of the meal. What food items are they most likely to eat and what food items are they most likely not to eat? Record your observations about the ambiance of the dining area and the interaction of the participants with each other. Summarize what you have observed about the program, the functional ability of the participants, and their food intake. Work with a student who visited a nursing facility and in a report to the class, compare the functional ability of the congregate meal participants and the nursing home residents, the amount of food and type of food most likely to be eaten or left by each group, and the interaction at the table of each group.

4. Interview 10 to 15 older people at a senior center or congregate meal site about their possible interest in a nutrition education class. What topics would they like to learn more about, and what type of class would they like to have? Based on their suggestions, develop a nutrition class using the article by Kicklighter[28] as a resource in preparing visuals and developing activities that will be easily read and of use to the older learner.

REFERENCES

1. Abbasi, A.A., and Rudman, D.: Undernutrition in the nursing home: prevalence, consequences, causes, and prevention, Nutr. Rev. 52(4):113, 1994.

2. American Dietetic Association: ADA's testimony on reauthorization of the Older Americans Act, J. Am. Diet. Assoc. 91:849, 1991.

3. American Dietetic Association: Position of the American Dietetic Association: nutrition, aging, and the continuum of care, J. Am. Diet. Assoc. 96:1048, 1996.

4. Asp, E.H., and Darling, M.E.: Home-delivered meals: food quality, nutrient content, and characteristics of recipients, J. Am. Diet. Assoc. 88:55, 1988.

5. Balsam, A.L., and Carlin, J.M.: Frozen meals for the homebound elderly, Catering and Health 1:253, 1990.

6. Balsam, A., and Rogers, B.L.: Service innovations in the elderly nutrition program: strategies for meeting unmet needs, Medford, MA, July 1988, Tufts University School of Nutrition.

7. Bonnel, W.B.: The nursing home group dining room: managing the work of eating, J. Nutr. Elderly 13(1):1, 1993.

8. Buckler, D.A., Kelber, S.T., and Goodwin, J.S.: The use of dietary restrictions in malnourished nursing home patients, J. Am. Geriatr. Soc. 42:1100, 1994.

9. Chapman, K.M., and others: Applying behavioral models to dietary education of elderly diabetic patients, J. Nutr. Ed. 27:75, 1995.

10. Coulston, A.M.: Nutrition management in nursing homes. In: Morley, J.E., Glick, Z., and Rubenstein, L.Z., editors: Geriatric nutrition. A comprehensive review, ed. 2, New York, 1995, Raven Press.

11. Crockett, S.J., and others: Mailed-home nutrition education for rural seniors: a pilot study, J. Nutr. Ed. 24:312, 1992.

12. Dollahite, J., Franklin, D., and McNew, R.: Problems encountered in meeting the Recommended Dietary Allowances for menus designed according to the Dietary Guidelines for Americans, J. Am. Diet. Assoc. 95:341, 1995.

13. Ellis, L., and Roe, D.A.: Home-delivered meals programs for the elderly: distribution of services in New York State, Am. J. Public Health 83:1034, 1993.

14. Elmstahl, S., and others: Hospital nutrition in geriatric long-term care medicine. 1. Effects of a changed meal environment, Compr. Gerontol. A1:29, 1987.

15. Fogler-Levitt, E., and others: Utilization of home-delivered meals by recipients 75 years of age or older, J. Am. Diet. Assoc. 95:552, 1995.

16. Gallagher, A.: Elegance adds appeal to nursing home food service, J. Am. Diet. Assoc. 90:1663, 1990.

17. Gallagher-Allred, C.R.: OBRA: A challenge and an opportunity for nutrition care, Columbus, OH, December 1992, Ross Professional Development Series, Ross Laboratories.

18. Glassman, M.H.: Housing for the elderly. In: Reichel, W., editor: Care of the elderly. Clinical aspects of aging, ed. 4, Baltimore, 1995, Williams and Wilkins.

19. Goldberg, J.P., Gershoff, S.N., and McGandy, R.B.: Appropriate topics for nutrition education for the elderly, J. Nutr. Ed. 22:303, 1990.

20. Greene, J.: Coordination of Older Americans Act programs, J. Am. Diet. Assoc. 78:617, 1981.

21. Gregoire, M.B., Nyland, N., and Morcos, S.: Use of frozen meals by and food preferences of various age groups of adults, J. Nutr. Elderly 13(2):23, 1993.

22. Haynes, J., and Kendrick, O.W.: Plate waste and perception of quality of food prepared in conventional vs commissary systems in the Nutrition Program for the Elderly, J. Am. Diet. Assoc. 95:586, 1995.

23. Iszler, J., and others: Formative evaluation for planning a nutrition intervention: results from focus groups, J. Nutr. Ed. 27:127, 1995.

24. Johnson, R.K., Tonore, M.F., and Gallagher, F.A.: Medical nutrition therapy and health-care reform: strategies of the American Dietetic Association, Persp. Appl. Nutr. 2(1):1994.

25. Johnson, R.M., and others: Nutrient intake of nursing home residents receiving pureed foods or a regular diet, J. Am. Geriatr. Soc. 43:344:1995.

26. Keeney, D.B., and others: Nutrition evaluation of a grocery delivery program for rural homebound elderly, Fed. Proc. 48:829, 1983.

27. Kicklighter, J.R.: Characteristics of older adult learners: a guide for dietetic practitioners, J. Am. Diet. Assoc. 91:1418, 1991.

28. Koren, M.J.: Care in nursing homes and other long-term care facilities. In: Abrams, W.B., Beers, M.H., and Berkow, R., editors: Merck manual of geriatrics, ed. 2, Whitehouse Station, NJ, 1995, Merck Research Laboratories.

29. Koren, M.J.: Home health care. In: Abrams, W.B., Beers, M.H., and Berkow, R., editors: Merck manual of geriatrics, ed. 2, Whitehouse Station, NJ, 1995, Merck Research Laboratories.

30. Krinke, V.B.: Nutrition information topic and format preferences of older adults, J. Nutr. Ed. 22:292, 1990.

31. Kumanyika, S., and others: Picture-sort method for administering a food frequency questionnaire to older adults, J. Am. Diet. Assoc. 96:137, 1996.

32. Kupka-Schutt, L., and Mitchell, M.E.: Positive effect of a nutrition instruction model on the dietary behavior of a selected group of elderly, J. Nutr. Elderly 12(2):29, 1992.

33. Medeiros, L., Russell, W., and Shipp, R.: Nutrition knowledge as influenced by source of nutrition information, Nutr. Research 11:979, 1991.

34. McCool, A.C., and Posner, B.M.: Nutrition services for older Americans: food service systems and technologies. Program management strategies, Chicago, 1982, American Dietetic Association.

35. Militello, J., Coleman, L.J., and Haran, E.: Food management for the aging population, J. Nutr. Elderly 15(2):15, 1995.

36. National Council on the Aging: Home-delivered meals for the ill, handicapped, and elderly, Am. J. Public Health 55(suppl.):1, 1965.

37. Neyman, M.R., Zidenberg-Cherr, S., and McDonald, R.B.: Effect of participation in congregate-site meal programs on nutritional status of the healthy elderly, J. Am. Diet. Assoc. 96:475, 1996.

38. Nutrition Strategic Study Committee: Nutrition strategic study. A report to the director of the Ohio Department of Aging, Columbus, OH, 1989, Ohio Dept. of Aging.

39. Oakland, M.J., and Thomsen, P.A.: Beliefs about and usage of vitamin/mineral supplements by elderly participants of rural congregate meal programs in central Iowa, J. Am. Diet. Assoc. 90:715, 1990.

40. OBRA '87 update, J. Am. Diet. Assoc. 91(11):1381, 1991.

41. Ponza, M., and others: Serving elders at risk. The Older Americans Act Nutrition Programs: National Evaluation of the Elderly Nutrition Program 1993–1995, Vol. I, Title III Evaluation Findings, Princeton, NJ, June 1996, Mathematica Policy Research. Available on the web site of the National Policy and Resource Center on Nutrition and Aging, Florida State University; access at http://www.aoa.dhhs.gov/aoa/pages/nutreval.html.

42. Ponza, M., Ohls, J.C., and Millen, B.E.: Serving elders at risk. The Older Americans Act Nutrition Programs. National Evaluation of the Elderly Nutrition Program, 1993–1995, Executive Summary, Princeton, NJ, June 1996, Mathematica Policy Research.

43. Probart, C.K., and others: Factors that influence the elderly to use traditional or nontraditional nutrition information sources, J. Am. Diet. Assoc. 89:1758, 1989.

44. Rabin, D.L., and Barry, P.P.: Community options for elderly patients. In: Reichel, W., editor: Care of the elderly. Clinical aspects of aging, ed. 4, Baltimore, 1995, Williams and Wilkins.

45. Ranno, B.S., Wardlaw, G.M., and Geiger, C.J.: What characterizes elderly women who overuse vitamin and mineral supplements, J. Am. Diet. Assoc. 88:347, 1988.

46. Rhodes, S.S., editor: Effective menu planning for the elderly nutrition program, Chicago, 1991, American Dietetic Association.

47. Sahyoun, N.: Nutrient intake by the NSS elderly population. In: Hartz, S.C., Russell, R.M., and Rosenberg, I.H., editors: Nutrition in the elderly. The Boston Nutritional Status Survey, London, 1992, Smith Gordon and Company.

48. Sanders, H.N., Hoffman, S.B., and Lund, C.A.: Feeding strategy for dependent eaters, J. Am. Diet. Assoc. 92(11):1389, 1992.

49. Sempos, C.T., and others: A dietary survey of 14 Wisconsin nursing homes, J. Am. Diet. Assoc. 81:35, 1982.

50. Short, P., and Leon, J.: Use of home and community services by persons ages 65 and older with functional difficulties, National Medical Expenditure Survey Research Findings 5, DHHS Publication No. (PHS) 90-3466, Rockville, MD, 1990, U.S. Dept. of Health and Human Services.

51. Stevens, D.A., Grivetti, L.E., and McDonald, R.B.: Nutrient intake of urban and rural elderly receiving home delivered meals, J. Am. Diet. Assoc. 92:714, 1992.

52. Taeuber, C.: Sixty-five plus in America, Curr. Pop. Rep., Special Studies P23-178, Washington, DC, August 1992, U.S. Bureau of the Census.

53. Tak, J., Gregoire, M.B., and Morcos, S.H.: Commercial frozen meals: a cost-effective alternative for home delivery in feeding programs for the elderly?, J. Nutr. Elderly 12(3):15, 1993.

54. Thole, C., and Gregoire, M.B.: Time-temperature relationships during freezing of packaged meals in feeding programs for the elderly, J. Am. Diet. Assoc. 92:350, 1992.

55. Torres-Gil, F.M., Lloyd, J.L., and Carlin, J.: Role of elderly nutrition in home and community-based care, Persp. Appl. Nutr. 2(4):9, 1995.

56. Turner, J., and Glew, G.: Home-delivered meals for the elderly, Food Technol. 36:46, 1982.

57. U.S. Department of Health and Human Services: Healthy People 2000. National health promotion and disease prevention objectives, DHHS Publication No. (PHS) 91-50212, Washington, DC, 1991, U.S. Government Printing Office.

58. U.S. Department of Health and Human Services: Long-term care for the functionally dependent elderly, Vital and Health Statistics Series 13, No. 104, Washington, DC, 1990, U.S. Government Printing Office.

59. U.S. Senate Special Committee on Aging: Home care at the crossroads. An information paper, Serial No. 100-H, Washington, DC, 1988, U.S. Government Printing Office.

60. Van der Wielen, R.P., and others: Dietary intake of energy and water-soluble vitamins in different categories of aging, J. Gerontol. 51A(1):B100, 1996.

61. Wetle, T.: Social issues. In: Abrams, W.B., Beers, M.H., and Berkow, R., editors: Merck manual of geriatrics, ed. 2, Whitehouse Station, NJ, 1995, Merck Research Laboratories.

62. Williams, P.G.: Vitamin retention in cook/chill and cook/hot-hold hospital food services, J. Am. Diet. Assoc. 92(11):1389, 1992.

63. Wilson, S., and Barry, J.: Serve Our Seniors, Inc. A demonstration program for proposed California menu guidelines for senior nutrition, J. Nutr. Elderly 13(1):37, 1993.

A
Recommended Dietary Allowances

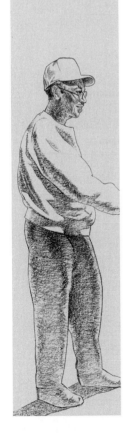

TABLE A-1 Recommended Dietary Allowances for Persons Ages 51 and Over (Revised 1989)

	Males	Females
Weight*		
(kg)	77	65
(lb)	170	143
Height*		
(cm)	173	160
(in)	68	63
Protein (g)	63	50
Vitamin A (µg RE)†	1,000	800
Vitamin D (µg) ‡	5	5
Vitamin E (mg α-TE)§	10	8
Vitamin K (µg)	80	65
Vitamin C (mg)	60	60
Thiamin (mg)	1.2	1.0
Riboflavin (mg)	1.4	1.2
Niacin (mg NE)‖	15	13
Vitamin B-6 (mg)	2.0	1.6
Folate (µg)	200	180
Vitamin B-12 (µg)	2.0	2.0
Calcium (mg)	800	800
Phosphorus (mg)	800	800
Magnesium (mg)	350	280
Iron (mg)	10	10
Zinc (mg)	15	12
Iodine (µg)	150	150
Selenium (µg)	70	55

*Weights and heights given are actual median values for the U.S. population ages 51 and over as reported by NHANES II. These height-to-weight ratios may not be ideal.

†Retinol equivalents: 1 retinol equivalent = 1 µg retinol or 6 µg β-carotene.

‡As cholecalciferol: 10 µg cholecalciferol = 400 IU of vitamin D.

§α-Tocopherol equivalents: 1 mg d-α tocopherol = 1α-TE.

‖1 NE (niacin equivalent) = 1 mg niacin or 60 mg dietary tryptophan.

TABLE A-2 Estimated Safe and Adequate Daily Dietary Intakes of Selected Vitamins and Minerals for Adults

Vitamin/Mineral	Intake*
Biotin	30–100 µg
Pantothenic acid	4.0–7.0 mg
Copper	1.5–3.0 mg†
Manganese	2.0–5.0 mg†
Fluoride	1.5–4.0 mg†
Chromium	50–200 µg†
Molybdenum	75–250 µg†

*Because there is less information on which to base allowances, these figures are provided in the form of ranges of recommended intakes.

†Because the toxic levels for many trace minerals may be only several times usual intakes, the upper levels given in this table should not be habitually exceeded.

TABLE A-3 Estimated Sodium, Chloride, and Potassium Minimum Requirements of Healthy Adults

Mineral	Intake
Sodium*	500 mg
Chloride*	750 mg
Potassium†	2,000 mg

*No allowance has been included for large, prolonged losses from the skin through sweat. No evidence suggests that higher intakes confer any health benefit.

†Desirable intake may considerably exceed this value (about 3,500 mg for adults).

Adapted from Food and Nutrition Board: Recommended dietary allowances, ed. 10, Washington, DC, 1989, National Academy Press.

B

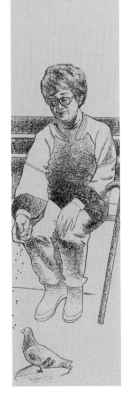

Government Agencies and Professional and Voluntary Organizations Providing Information and Assistance to Older People

AGENCIES–U.S. GOVERNMENT

ACTION
  1100 Vermont Ave., N.W.
  Washington, DC 20525
  (Administers programs serving the aged,
    including RSVP and Foster Grandparents
    Program)
Administration on Aging
  Wilbur J. Cohen Bldg., Room 4646
  330 Independence Ave., S.W.
  Washington, DC 20201
Arthritis and Musculoskeletal Interagency
  Coordinating Committee
  National Institutes of Health
  Bldg. 31, Room 4C32
  Bethesda, MD 20892
Department of Agriculture
  Human Nutrition Information Service
  6505 Belcrest Rd., Room 360
  Hyattsville, MD 20782
Gerontology Research Center, National
  Institute on Aging
  Baltimore City Hospitals
  4940 Eastern Ave.
  Baltimore, MD 21224
National Institute on Aging
  Public Information Office
  Bldg. 31, Room 5C27
  9000 Rockville Pike
  Bethesda, MD 20892
Office of Disease Prevention and Health
  Promotion
  National Health Information Center
  P.O. Box 1133
  Washington, DC 20013-1133
  800-336-4797
  (Provides information regarding health
    organizations and support groups)
Social Security Administration
  6401 Security Blvd.
  Baltimore, MD 21235
U.S. Department of Education
  National Institute on Disability and
    Rehabilitation Research
  330 C St., S.W., Room 3060
  Washington, DC 20202-2572

U.S. Department of Education
  Clearinghouse on Disability Information
  Switzer Bldg., Room 3132
  Washington, DC 20202-2524
U.S. Senate
  Special Committee on Aging
  Dirkson Senate Office Bldg.
  Room G-31
  Washington, DC 20510-6400
U.S. House of Representatives
  Select Committee on Aging
  H1-A712 O'Neil House Office Bldg.
  Washington, DC 20515-6361
Veterans Administration
  810 Vermont Ave., N.W.
  Washington, DC 20420

PROFESSIONAL AND VOLUNTARY ORGANIZATIONS
General Aspects of Aging

Aging in America
  1500 Pelham Parkway, S.
  Bronx, NY 10461
American Aging Association
  c/o Denham Harman, M.D.
  College of Medicine
  University of Nebraska
  Omaha, NE 68105
American Bar Association
  Commission on Legal Problems of the Elderly
  1800 M Street, N.W.
  Washington, DC 20036
American Society on Aging
  833 Market Street
  Suite 512
  San Francisco, CA 94103
Asian and Pacific Coalition on Aging
  1102 Crenshaw Blvd.
  Room 43
  Los Angeles, CA 90019
Association for Adult Development and Aging
  c/o American Association for Counseling
    and Development
  5999 Stevenson Ave.
  Alexandria, VA 22304

Association for Gerontology in Higher Education
600 Maryland Ave., S.W.
West Wing 204
Washington, DC 20024
Gerontological Society of America
1275 K Street, N.W.
Suite 350
Washington, DC 20005-4006
International Federation on Aging
1909 K Street, N.W.
Washington, DC 20049
Legal Services for the Elderly
132 W. 43rd Street, Third Floor
New York, NY 10036
Little Brothers–Friends of the Elderly
1658 W. Belmont Ave.
Chicago, IL 60657
National Association of Counties
Aging Program
440 First Street, N.W.
Washington, DC 20001
National Association of Foster Grandparents
Program Directors
195 East San Fernando Street
San Jose, CA 95112
National Caucus and Center on Black Aged
1424 K Street, N.W.
Suite 500
Washington, DC 20005
National Committee for Senior Americans
P.O. Box 9009
Valley Forge, PA 19485
National Council on the Aging
409 Third St., S.W., Second Floor
Washington, DC 20024
National Hispanic Council on Aging
2713 Ontario Rd., N.W.
Suite 200
Washington, DC 20009
National Indian Council on Aging
P.O. Box 2088
Albuquerque, NM 87103
National Interfaith Coalition on Aging
P.O. Box 1924
Athens, GA 30605
National Pacific/Asian Resource Center on
Aging
2033 6th Ave.
Suite 410
Seattle, WA 98121

National Retired Teachers Association (NRTA)
1909 K Street, N.W.
Washington, DC 20049
National Senior Citizens Law Center
2025 M Street, N.W.
Suite 400
Washington, DC 20036
Service Corps of Retired Executives Association
1825 Connecticut Ave., N.W.
Suite 503
Washington, DC 20009
U.S. Conference on Mayors
Task Force on Aging
1620 I Street, N.W.
Washington, DC 20006

Long-Term Care Facilities and Services

American Association of Homes for the Aging
1129 20th Street, N.W.
Suite 400
Washington, DC 20036
American College of Health Care
Administrators (Nursing Homes)
325 S. Patrick Street
Alexandria, VA 22314
American Health Care Association
1201 L Street, N.W.
Washington, DC 20005
Council of Home Health Agencies
and Community Health Services
National League for Nursing
10 Columbus Circle
New York, NY 10019
Health Insurance Association of America
1025 Connecticut Ave., N.W.
Suite 1200
Washington, DC 20036
National Association for Families Caring for
Their Elders
1141 Loxford Terrace
Silver Spring, MD 20901
National Association for Home Care
519 C Street, N.E.
Washington, DC 20002
National Citizens' Coalition for Nursing Home
Reform
1424 16th Street, N.W.
Suite L2
Washington, DC 20036

National Hospice Organization
    1901 N. Moore Street
    Suite 901
    Arlington, VA 22209
National Institute on Adult Daycare
    c/o National Council on the Aging
    409 Third St., S.W., Second Floor
    Washington, DC 20024

Physical and Mental Health

Alzheimer's Association
    919 N. Michigan Ave., Suite 1000
    Chicago, IL 60611-1676
Alzheimer's Disease Education and Referral
    Center
    P.O. Box 8250-JML
    Silver Spring, MD 20907-8250
American Cancer Society
    1599 Clifton Road, N.E.
    Atlanta, GA 30329-4251
American Diabetes Association
    National Service Center
    P.O. Box 25757
    1660 Duke Street
    Alexandria, VA 22314
American Geriatrics Society
    770 Lexington Ave.
    Suite 300
    New York, NY 10021
American Heart Association
    7320 Greenville Ave.
    Dallas, TX 75231-4599
American Lung Association
    1740 Broadway
    New York, NY 10019
American Medical Association
    Committee on Aging
    515 N. State Street
    Chicago, IL 60610
American Nurses' Association
    Council of Nursing Home Nurses
    Division on Gerontological Nursing Practice
    2420 Pershing Rd.
    Kansas City, MO 64108
American Parkinson's Disease Association
    60 Bay St., Suite 401
    Staten Island, NY 10301
American Psychiatric Association
    Council on Aging
    1400 K Street, N.W.
    Washington, DC 20005

American Psychological Association
    Division of Adult Development and Aging
    750 First St., N.E.
    Washington, DC 20036
American Public Health Association
    Section of Gerontological Health
    1015 15th Street, N.W.
    Washington, DC 20005
American Society for Geriatric Dentistry
    211 E. Chicago Ave.
    Suite 1616
    Chicago, IL 60611
Arthritis Foundation
    P.O. Box 19000
    Atlanta, GA 30326
National Center for Health Promotion
    and Aging
    c/o National Council on the Aging
    409 Third St., S.W., Second Floor
    Washington, DC 20024
National Osteoporosis Foundation
    2100 M St., N.W., Suite 602
    Washington, DC 20037
National Safety Council
    444 North Michigan Ave.
    Chicago, IL 60611
National Voluntary Organizations
    for Independent Living for the Aging
    c/o National Council on the Aging
    409 Third St., S.W., Second Floor
    Washington, DC 20024
North American Association of Jewish Homes
    and Housing
    2525 Centerville Road
    Dallas, TX 75228
Special Constituency Section on Aging and
    Long-Term Care Services
    c/o American Hospital Association
    840 N. Lake Shore Drive
    Chicago, IL 60611

Physical Rehabilitation Services

American Dance Therapy Association
    2000 Century Plaza
    Suite 108
    Columbia, MD 21044
American Foundation for the Blind
    15 W. 16th Street
    New York, NY 10011

American Occupational Therapy Association
  1383 Piccard Drive, Box 1725
  Rockville, MD 20850
American Physical Therapy Association
  1111 N. Fairfax
  Alexandria, VA 22314
American Self-Help Clearinghouse
  St. Clare's Riverside Medical Center
  Pocono Road
  Denville, NJ 07834
American Speech-Language-Hearing Association
  10801 Rockville Pike
  Rockville, MD 20852
IBM National Support Center for Persons with
  Disabilities
  P.O. Box 2150-H06R1
  Atlanta, GA 30301
Lighthouse National Center for Vision
  and Aging
  800 Second Ave.
  New York, NY 10017
National Hearing Aid Society
  20361 Middlebelt Road
  Livonia, MI 48152
National Information Center for Deafness
  Gallaudet University
  800 Florida Ave., N.E.
  Washington, DC 20002-3625
National Library Service for the Blind and
  Physically Handicapped
  1291 Taylor St., N.W.
  Washington, DC 20542
National Rehabilitation Association
  633 S. Washington Street
  Alexandria, VA 22314
National Rehabilitation Information Center
  8455 Colesville Rd., Suite 935
  Silver Spring, MD 20910
National Self-Help Clearinghouse
  Graduate School and University Center of
    the City University of New York
  25 W. 43rd St., Room 620
  New York, NY 10036
National Society to Prevent Blindness
  500 E. Remington Road
  Schaumburg, IL 60173
National Stroke Association
  300 E. Hampden Ave., Suite 240
  Englewood, CO 80110-2654

Nutrition Information and Research

American Dietetic Association
  216 W. Jackson Blvd.
  Suite 800
  Chicago, IL 60606
American Association for Nutritional Sciences
  9650 Rockville Pike
  Bethesda, MD 20814
American Society for Clinical Nutrition
  9650 Rockville Pike
  Bethesda, MD 20814
Society for Nutrition Education
  1700 Broadway
  Suite 300
  Oakland, CA 94612

Nutrition and Social Services

Catholic Golden Age
  1012 14th Street, N.W.
  Suite 1003
  Washington, DC 20005
Jewish Association for Services for the Aged
  40 W. 68th Street
  New York, NY 10023
National Association of Area Agencies
  on Aging
  1112 16th St., Suite 100
  Washington, DC 20036
National Association of Meals Programs
  204 E Street, N.E.
  Washington. DC 20002
National Association of Nutrition and Aging
  Services Programs
  2675 44th Street, S.W.
  Suite 305
  Grand Rapids, MI 49509
National Association of Older American
  Volunteer Program Directors
  1148 Bingham Terrace
  Reston, VA 22091
National Association of RSVP Directors
  RSVP of El Paso
  Two Civic Center Plaza
  El Paso, TX 79999
National Association of Senior Companion
  Project Directors
  Street Landry Parish Community Action
    Agency
  P.O. Box 1510
  Opelousas, LA 70570

National Association of State Units on Aging
  2033 K Street, N.W.
  Suite 304
  Washington, DC 20006
National Institute of Senior Centers
  National Council on the Aging
  409 Third St., S.W., Second Floor
  Washington, DC 20024

Research on Aging

American Federation for Aging Research
  725 Park Ave.
  New York, NY 10021
Center for Study of Aging and Human
    Development
  Duke University Medical Center
  Box 3003
  Durham, NC 27710
U.S. Dept. of Agriculture
  Human Nutrition Research Center
    on Aging
  Tufts University
  711 Washington Street
  Boston, MA 02111

ADVOCACY GROUPS–GENERAL MEMBERSHIP

American Association of Retired Persons
  601 E. St., N.W.
  Washington, DC 20049
Gray Panthers Project Fund
  1424 16th St., N.W., Suite 602
  Washington, DC 20036
International Senior Citizens Association
  1102 S. Crenshaw Blvd.
  Los Angeles, CA 90019
National Alliance of Senior Citizens
  2525 Wilson Blvd.
  Arlington, VA 22201
National Council of Senior Citizens
  1331 F St., N.W.
  Washington, DC 20004-1171
Villers Advocacy Associates
  1334 G Street, N.W.
  Washington, DC 20005

C

Mini Nutritional Assessment Form (MNA)

Reprinted with permission of the Nestlé Research Center/Clintec Nutrition Company

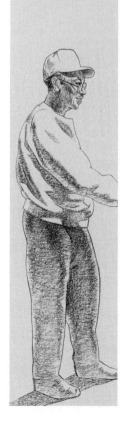

MINI NUTRITIONAL ASSESSMENT
MNA®

ID# _____

Last Name: _____ First Name: _____ M.I. _____ Sex: _____ Date: _____

Age: _____   Weight, kg: _____   Height, cm: _____   Knee Height, cm: _____

Complete the form by writing the numbers in the boxes. Add the numbers in the boxes and compare the total assessment to the Malnutrition Indicator Score.

ANTHROPOMETRIC ASSESSMENT

	Points
1. Body Mass Index (BMI) (weight in kg) / (height in m)^2 a. BMI < 19 = 0 points b. BMI 19 to < 21 = 1 point c. BMI 21 to < 23 = 2 points d. BMI ≥ 23 = 3 points	☐
2. Mid-arm circumference (MAC) in cm a. MAC < 21 = 0.0 points b. MAC 21 ≤ 22 = 0.5 points c. MAC > 22 = 1.0 points	☐.☐
3. Calf circumference (CC) in cm a. CC < 31 = 0 points b. CC ≥ 31 = 1 point	☐
4. Weight loss during last 3 months a. weight loss greater than 3kg (6.6 lbs) = 0 points b. does not know = 1 point c. weight loss between 1 and 3 kg (2.2 and 6.6 lbs) = 2 points d. no weight loss = 3 points	☐

GENERAL ASSESSMENT

	Points
5. Lives independently (not in a nursing home or hospital) a. no = 0 points b. yes = 1 point	☐
6. Takes more than 3 prescription drugs per day a. yes = 0 points b. no = 1 point	☐
7. Has suffered psychological stress or acute disease in the past 3 months a. yes = 0 points b. no = 2 points	☐
8. Mobility a. bed or chair bound = 0 points b. able to get out of bed/chair but does not go out = 1 point c. goes out = 2 points	☐
9. Neuropsychological problems a. severe dementia or depression = 0 points b. mild dementia = 1 point c. no psychological problems = 2 points	☐
10. Pressure sores or skin ulcers a. yes = 0 points b. no = 1 point	☐

DIETARY ASSESSMENT

	Points
11. How many full meals does the patient eat daily? a. 1 meal = 0 points b. 2 meals = 1 point c. 3 meals = 2 points	☐

	Points
12. Selected consumption markers for protein intake • At least one serving of dairy products (milk, cheese, yogurt) per day? yes ☐ no ☐ • Two or more servings of legumes or eggs per week? yes ☐ no ☐ • Meat, fish or poultry every day? yes ☐ no ☐ a. if 0 or 1 yes = 0.0 points b. if 2 yes = 0.5 points c. if 3 yes = 1.0 points	☐.☐
13. Consumes two or more servings of fruits or vegetables per day? a. no = 0 points b. yes = 1 point	☐
14. Has food intake declined over the past three months due to loss of appetite, digestive problems, chewing or swallowing difficulties? a. severe loss of appetite = 0 points b. moderate loss of appetite = 1 point c. no loss of appetite = 2 points	☐
15. How much fluid (water, juice, coffee, tea, milk,...) is consumed per day? (1 cup = 8 oz.) a. less than 3 cups = 0.0 points b. 3 to 5 cups = 0.5 points c. more than 5 cups = 1.0 points	☐.☐
16. Mode of feeding a. Unable to eat without assistance = 0 points b. self-fed with some difficulty = 1 point c. self-fed without any problem = 2 points	☐

SELF ASSESSMENT

	Points
17. Do they view themselves as having nutritional problems? a. major malnutrition = 0 points b. does not know or moderate malnutrition = 1 point c. no nutritional problem = 2 points	☐
18. In comparison with other people of the same age, how do they consider their health status? a. not as good = 0.0 points b. does not know = 0.5 points c. as good = 1.0 points d. better = 2.0 points	☐.☐

ASSESSMENT TOTAL (max. 30 points): ☐☐.☐

MALNUTRITION INDICATOR SCORE

≥ 24 points	well-nourished	☐
17 to 23.5 points	at risk of malnutrition	☐
< 17 points	malnourished	☐

Ref.: Guigoz Y, Vellas B and Garry PJ. 1994. Mini Nutritional Assessment: A practical assessment tool for grading the nutritional state of elderly patients. *Facts and Research in Gerontology*. Supplement #2: 15-59.

©1994 Nestec Ltd (Nestlé Research Center)/Nestlé Clinical Nutrition

APPENDIX

D

Selected Resources

SELECTED RESOURCES FOR PROFESSIONAL USE
Nutrition Education and Health Promotion

American Association of Retired Persons:
  Activities with Impact: Innovative Program Ideas for Adult Housing Residences, 1987
  Minority Affairs Information Packet—Materials include:
  Celebrating Diversity: A Learning Tool for Working with People of Different Cultures
  Health Risks and Preventive Care Among Older Blacks
  Health Risks and Preventive Care Among Older Pacific/Asian Americans
  Health Risks and Preventive Care Among Older American Indians and Alaska Natives
  Health Risks and Preventive Care Among Older Hispanics (also available in Spanish), 1992
  AARP Health Promotion Publications List
  Perspectives in Health Promotion and Aging (bimonthly newsletter)
  Available from Health Advocacy Services, AARP, 601 E Street, N.W., Washington, DC 20049.
American Dietetic Association:
  Ethnic and Regional Food Practice Series:
  Soul and Traditional Southern Food Practices, Customs, and Holidays, 1995
  Navajo Food Practices, Customs, and Holidays, 1991
  Alaska Native Food Practices, Customs, and Holidays, 1993
  Hmong American Food Practices, Customs, and Holidays, 1992
  Mexican American Food Practices, Customs, and Holidays, 1989
  Filipino American Food Practices, Customs, and Holidays, 1994
  Chinese American Food Practices, Customs, and Holidays, 1990
  Jewish Food Practices, Customs, and Holidays, 1989
  Indian and Pakistani Food Practices, Customs, and Holidays, 1996

Cajun and Creole Food Practices, Customs, and Holidays, 1996
  Available from American Dietetic Association, 216 W. Jackson Blvd., Suite 800, Chicago, IL 60606-6995.
Corbin, D.E., and Metal-Corbin, J.: Reach for It! A Handbook of Exercise and Dance Activities for Older Adults, 1983. Available from Eddie Bowers Publishing Co., 2600 Jackson St., Dubuque, IA 52001.
Donavin, D.P.: Aging with Style and Savvy: Books and Films on Challenges Facing Adults of All Ages, 1990. Available from American Library Association, ALA Books, 50 East Huron St., Chicago, IL 60611-2795.
Food and Drug Administration: Current Issues in Women's Health, ed. 2 (Articles previously published in FDA Consumer cover a broad scope of health issues, including cancer, osteoporosis, and menopause). Available from Superintendent of Documents, P.O. Box 371954, Pittsburgh, PA 15250-7954.
Food and Drug Administration:
  Using the New Food Label to Choose Healthier Foods, 1994
  How the New Food Label Can Help You Plan a Healthy Diet, 1994
  Available from Food and Drug Administration, Office of Public Affairs, Room 15A-19, 5600 Fishers Lane, HFI-40, Rockville, MD 20857
Food-Medication Interactions, ed. 8, available from Box 6590, Pottstown, PA 19464.
Franklin, B.A., and others: On the Ball: Innovative Activities for Adult Fitness and Cardiac Rehabilitation Programs, 1990. Available from Brown and Benchmark, 25 Kessel Court, Madison, WI 53711.
Gonzalez, V.M., Gonzalez, J.T., Freeman, V., and Howard-Pitney, B.: Health Promotion in Diverse Cultural Communities, Stanford Health Promotion Resource Center, 1991, Palo Alto, CA.
Helgeson, E.M., and Willis, S.C.: Handbook of Group Activities for Impaired Older Adults, New York, 1987, Haworth Press.
Holmes, L., Bernstein, P., Rodriques-Trias, H., and Ruzek, S.B.: Enhancing Cultural

Awareness and Communication Skills: A Training Program for Health Care Providers and Educators, Memphis, TN, 1989, Memphis State University, Center for Research on Women (one manual, one videotape).

Horn, B.J.: Facilitating Self Care Practices in the Elderly, New York, 1990, Haworth Press.

Hurley, O.: Safe Therapeutic Exercise for the Frail Elderly: Introduction, ed. 2, Center for the Study of Aging of Albany, 1996, Suite 8, 706 Madison Ave., Albany, NY 12208.

Kobriger, A.M.: Prevention of Weight Loss in the Elderly, 1995. Available from Kobriger Presents, Box 55, Chilton, WI 53014-0123.

Massachusetts Office of Elder Affairs: Nutrition and Health Education for Older Adults at Home. Available from Executive Office of Elder Affairs, 38 Chauncy St., Boston, MA 02111.

Medicine Is No Mystery (program kit for group session on medication management), 1991. Available from National Council on the Aging, 409 Third St., S.W., Second Floor, Washington, DC 20024.

National Agricultural Library: Nutrition and the Elderly: Resource Listing. Available from U.S. Dept. of Agriculture Food and Nutrition Information Center, Room 111, Beltsville, MD 20705.

National Arthritis and Musculoskeletal and Skin Diseases Information Clearinghouse: Osteoporosis Patient Education Materials: An Annotated Bibliography. Available from NAMSIC, Box AMS, 9000 Rockville Pike, Bethesda, MD 20892.

National Cholesterol Education Program: There's No Wrong Way to Eat, As Long As You Eat Right, Stock No. 55-685 (poster of people of different ages and races eating different types of food), NHLBI, Box 30105, Bethesda, MD 20824-0105.

National Council on the Aging, National Institute on Aging, President's Council on Physical Fitness, and Food Marketing Institute:

To Your Health: Food and Activity Tips for Older Adults (package includes two

brochures, Eat Well and Stay Active, and six newsletters)

Supermarket Health Campaign for Older Shoppers (package contains brochures and promotional materials)

Available from Food Marketing Institute, 800 Connecticut Ave., N.W., Washington, DC 20006-2701.

National Food Processors Association: Label Facts for Healthful Eating. Educator's Resource Guide, 1995. Available from Label Facts, Box 964, Bensalem, PA 19020.

National Heart, Lung, and Blood Institute: Stay Young at Heart Kit (contains 50 heart healthy recipes for quantity food service and companion recipes for use at home; camera-ready handouts included), NIH Publication No. 94-3648. Available from NHLBI Information Center, P.O. Box 30105, Bethesda, MD 20824-0105.

North Dakota State University: Harvest Health at Home—Eating for the Second Fifty Years (series of newsletters and implementation guide), Fargo, ND, 1990, North Dakota State University Extension Service.

Pynoos, J., and Cohen, E.: Home Safety Guide for Older People: Check It Out, Fix It Up, 1990. Available from Serif Press, 1331 H St., N.W., Suite 110LL, Washington, DC 20005.

Smiley, J.: Creative Recreation and Socialization for Senior Citizen Centers, 1988. Available from Community Nutrition Institute, 2001 S St., N.W., Suite 530, Washington, DC 20009.

Womack, P.: The Dysphagia Challenge. Techniques for the Individual, 1993. Available from P. Womack, 13320 S.E. 43rd Place, Bellevue, WA 98006.

Long-Term Care Facilities

Alta Bates-Herrick Rehabilitation Center: Dysphagia Dining (handbook for people with swallowing disorders). Available from Alta Bates-Herrick Rehabilitation Center, Dept. of Nutrition and Food Services, 2001 Dwight Way, Berkeley, CA 94704.

American Dietetic Association Consulting Dietitians in Health Care Facilities: Dining

Skills: Practical Interventions for the Caregivers of Eating-Disabled Older Adults, Chicago, 1992. Available from CD-HCF, P.O. Box 2067, Pensacola, FL 32513.

Dietary Policy and Procedure Manual (for nursing home or group home dietary managers). Available from Nutrition Consulting Services, 843 N. Cleveland-Massillon Rd., Bldg. 9, Akron, OH 44333-2174.

Dietary Training Manual (modular inservice training manual for long-term care facilities), Hillhaven Corporation, Printing Services, Box 2264, Tacoma, WA 98401-2264.

Gallagher-Allred, C.R.: OBRA: A Challenge and an Opportunity for Nutrition Care, Ross Professional Development Series, Columbus, OH, 1992, Ross Laboratories.

Gerwick, C.L.: Nutrition Care in Nursing Facilities, revised 1992, American Dietetic Association, 216 W. Jackson Blvd., Chicago, IL 60606-6995.

Kansas Dietetic Association: Best Ideas in Gracious Dining (ideas for the dining room in long term care facilities. Available from KDA, Box 8704, Wichita, KS 67208.

National Kidney Foundation: Nutritional Care for Renal Patients in Extended Care Facilities. Available from NKF/NCA, 5335 Wisconsin Ave., N.W., Suite 830, Washington, DC 20015.

Puree Pizzazz (kitchen-tested puree recipes for multiple servings). Available from Nutrition Consulting Services, 843 N. Cleveland-Massillon Rd., Bldg. 9, Akron, OH 44333-2174.

Womack, P.: The Puree Challenge. A Recipe Book for Health Care, 1991. Available from P. Womack, 13320 S.E. 43rd Place, Bellevue, WA 98006.

Nutrition Program Planning, Implementation, and Management

ACTION and University of Maryland Center on Aging: A Guide to Volunteering for Older Americans. Available from Consumer Information Center, Dept. 82, Pueblo, CO 81009.

American Dietetic Association
Chef's Handbook: Low-Fat Quantity Food Preparation (developed through Project Lean, Low-Fat Eating for America Now), 1993
Project LEAN Resource Kit: Tips, Tools, and Techniques for Promoting Low-Fat Lifestyles, 1995
Available from ADA, 216 W. Jackson Blvd., Chicago, IL 60606-6995.

California Department of Aging: Title III Nutrition Program Manual (provides guidelines on menu planning, home-delivered meals, and participant assessment). Available from California Dept. of Aging, Nutrition Unit, 1600 K St., Sacramento, CA 95814.

Central Texas Dietetic Association: Martha's Kitchen Cookbook (recipes, menus, and kitchen procedures for a homeless shelter/soup kitchen), 1992. Available from CTDA, P.O. Box 2585, Temple, TX 76504.

Jones, L.M., and Fischer, B.R.: Simplified Recipes for Adult Care Centers, Florence, KY, 1990, Van Nostrand Reinhold.

LifeCare Alliance, Central Ohio Area Agency on Aging, Ohio Dept. of Aging: Cookbook for Change. Homebound Meals for the 1990s (notebook of comprehensive material for operation of a home-delivered meals program), 1992. Available from LifeCare Alliance, 1699 West Mound St., Columbus, OH 43223.

National Association of Nutrition and Aging Services Programs (NANASP): Many Hats (newsletter for congregate meal site managers). Available from NANASP, 2675 44th St., S.W., Suite 305, Wyoming, MN 49509.

National Association of State Units on Aging:
Preparing the Nutrition Program for the '90s (comprehensive material for operation of a congregate meals program), 1992
Collection of Innovative Models (comprehensive material describing innovative community meals programs for older people), 1992
Available from National Association of State Units on Aging, 2033 K. St., N.W., Washington, DC 20006.

Pettit, J., and Weinstein, J.: Programs to Help Older People Eat Better, 1989. Available from Community Nutrition Institute, 2001 S St., N.W., Suite 530, Washington, DC 20036.

Puerto Rican Dietetic Association: Recipe Manual. Available from Regional Nutrition Specialist, Administration on Aging, Region II Office, 26 Federal Plaza, Room 4149, New York, NY 10278.

Rhodes, S.S.: Effective Menu Planning for the Elderly Nutrition Program, 1991. Available from American Dietetic Association, 216 W. Jackson Blvd., Chicago, IL 60606-6995.

Shugart, G.S., Molt, M.K., and Wilson, M.E.: Food for Fifty, ed. 9, New York, 1993, MacMillan Company.

Turner, S., and Aronowitz, V.: Healthwise Quantity Cookbook, Washington, DC, 1990, Center for Science in the Public Interest.

U.S. Department of Agriculture:
Child and Adult Care Food Program. Adult Day Care Handbook (discusses food service and meal reimbursement), 1993
Quick and Easy Commodity Recipes for the Food Distribution Program on Indian Reservations (70 traditional and nontraditional recipes for Native Americans)
Available from Food and Nutrition Service, Nutrition Science and Education Branch, 3101 Park Center Drive, Room 607, Alexandria, VA 22302.

Wood, M., and Harris, K.: Quantity Recipes, New York College of Human Ecology, Ithaca, NY, Cornell University.

Nutrition Screening Initiative

Screening Older Americans' Nutritional Health: Current Practices and Future Possibilities, Full Report, 1991
Nutrition Screening Manual for Professionals Caring for Older Americans, 1991
Nutrition Interventions Manual for Professionals Caring for Older Americans, 1992
Implementing Nutrition Screening and Intervention Strategies, 1993

Strong and Healthy: Your Guide for Better Nutritional Health (brochure for older people)
Available from Nutrition Screening Initiative, 4407 Wheeler Ave., Alexandria, VA 22304.

FOR THE LAY PUBLIC
Nutrition Education and Health

Alzheimer's Caregiver's Support Kit. Available from The Alzheimer's Project, 1360 Beverly Rd., Suite 305, McLean, VA 22101.

American Association of Retired Persons:
Action for a Healthier Life: A Guide for Mid-Life and Older Women
Healthy Eating for A Healthy Life
How Does Your Nutrition Measure Up
Pep Up Your Life: A Fitness Book for Seniors
Stay Strong: For Men Over 50
Using the New Food Label to Choose Healthier Foods (large type)
Available from AARP, 601 E St., N.W., Washington, DC 20049.
Coping and Caring: Living with Alzheimer's
Nursing Home Life: A Guide for Residents and Families
Available from AARP Fulfillment (EE0636), Box 22796, Long Beach, CA 90801-5796.

American Dietetic Association:
Lactose Intolerance
Meal Planning with Mexican American Foods, 1989
Osteoporosis
Planificacion De Comidas Con Alimentos Mexicanoamericanos, 1990
Safe Cooking for Safe Eating: Tips on Proper Food Preparation
Safe Keeping for Safe Eating: Tips on Proper Food Storage
Vitamins, Minerals, and Food Supplements
Staying Healthy—A Guide for Elder Americans (revised)
Available from ADA, 216 W. Jackson Blvd., Suite 800, Chicago, IL 60606-6995.

American Foundation for the Blind:
Environmental Modifications for the
Visually Impaired: A Handbook
Low Vision Questions and Answers:
Definitions, Devices, Services
Available from American Foundation for the
Blind, 15 W. 16th St., New York, NY
10011.
American Geriatrics Society: Complete Guide
to Aging and Health, Washington, DC,
1995, American Geriatrics Society.
American Heart Association: Low-Fat, Low-
Cholesterol Cookbook, New York, 1989,
Random House.
American Institute for Cancer Research:
Healthy Meals on Hand
Cooking Solo—Healthful Eating for One
or Two
Be Your Best: Nutrition After Fifty
Available from AICR, 1759 R St., N.W.,
Washington, DC 20060.
California Dietetic Association, Los Angeles
District: La Dieta Diabetica (English-
Spanish booklet of exchange lists for meal
planning). Available from CDA–Los Angeles
District, P.O. Box 3506, Santa Monica, CA
90403.
Campbell Soup Company: Yes You Can
(brochure describing eating choices for
diabetics). Available from Yes You
Can/JDF, Box 48K, Campbell Place,
Camden, NJ 08103-1799.
Healthy Habits for the Best of Your Life (large
print brochure). Available from the Egg
Nutrition Center, 1819 H St., N.W., Suite
250, Washington, DC 20006.
Hachfeld, L., and Eykyn, B.: Cooking a'la
Heart. Delicious Heart Healthy Recipes to
Reduce the Risk of Heart Disease and
Stroke, ed. 2, 1992. Appletree Press, 151
Good Counsel Drive, Mankato, MN 56001.
Harris, S., and Hurley, O.: Who? Me? Exercise?
Safe Exercise for People Over 50. Center for
the Study of Aging of Albany, 1995, Suite
8, 706 Madison Ave., Albany, NY 12208.
Healthwise for Life: Medical Self-Care for
Healthy Aging (large print book covering
common health problems of older people),
1995. Available from Healthwise, Box 1989,
Boise, ID 83901.

Langholz, E., and others:
The Nutrition Game. The Right Moves If
You're Over 50, 1990
Over 50 and Still Cooking: Recipes for
Good Health and Long Life, 1990
Available from Bristol Publishing
Enterprises, Inc., P.O. Box 1737, San
Leandro, CA 94577.
Maryland Office on Aging and Maryland
Cooperative Extension Service: Check It
Out, series of leaflets on food groups and
diet concerns. Available from Maryland
Cooperative Extension, Room 0109,
Symons Hall, University of Maryland,
College Park, MD 20742.
National Dairy Council:
Calcium: You Never Outgrow Your Need
for It
For Mature Eaters Only: Guidelines for
Good Nutrition
Getting Along with Milk: for People with
Lactose Intolerance
Health Dividends: A Plan for Balancing
Your Fat Budget
Osteoporosis: Are You at Risk (also available
in Spanish)
Available from National Dairy Council,
6300 North River Road, Rosemont, IL
60018-4233.
National Institute on Aging:
Age Page (series of fact sheets covering a
variety of health topics including food
shopping, nutrition, drugs, and alcohol)
Directory of available resources
Single copies available free from NIA
Information Center, P.O. Box 8057,
Gaithersburg, MD 20898-8057.
National Meals on Wheels Foundation: Set of
10 camera-ready brochures with diet tips
and recipes to accompany the Nutrition
Screening Initiative Determine Your
Nutritional Health Checklist. Available from
National Meals on Wheels Foundation,
2675 44th St., S.W., Suite 305, Grand
Rapids, MI 49509.
National Osteoporosis Foundation:
Bone Basics for Men of All Ages
Bone Basics for Older Women and Men
Menopause and Osteoporosis: Choices for a
Healthy Future

Osteoporosis and Medications
Osteoporosis: A Woman's Guide
The Older Person's Guide to Osteoporosis
Booklets available from NOF, 1150 17th
St., N.W., Suite 500, Washington, DC
20036.
Ponichtera, B.: Quick and Healthy, Vol. II,
1995 (contains low-fat, easy to prepare
recipes with menus and grocery lists).
Available from Scale Down, 1519 Hermits
Way, The Dallas, OR 97058.
Rippe, J.M., and Ward, A.: Complete Book of
Fitness Walking, New York, 1989, Prentice
Hall.
Ross Laboratories: Eating to Make the Most of
Maturity, 1991. Available from Ross
Laboratories, Columbus, OH 43216.
U.S. Department of Agriculture:
Dietary Guidelines and Your Diet: Eating
Better When Eating Out, HG 232-11,
1989
Dietary Guidelines and Your Diet: Making
Bag Lunches, Snacks, and Desserts, HG
232-9, 1989
Dietary Guidelines and Your Diet: Preparing
Foods and Planning Menus, HG 232-8,
1989
Dietary Guidelines and Your Diet: Shopping
for Food and Making Meals in Minutes,
HG 232-10, 1989
Food Facts for Older Adults. Information on
How to Use the Dietary Guidelines,
Home and Garden Bulletin No. 251, 1993
Food Guide Pyramid, Home and Garden
Bulletin No. 252, 1992
Making Healthy Food Choices, Home and
Garden Bulletin No. 250
Using Less Sugar, Fat, and Salt, Program
Aid No. 1388, 1986
Available from U.S. Department of
Agriculture Human Nutrition
Information Service, 6505 Belcest Road,
Hyattsville, MD 20782.
U.S. Department of Agriculture and U.S.
Department of Health and Human Services:
Nutrition and Your Health: Dietary
Guidelines for Americans, Home and
Garden Bulletin No. 232, ed. 4,
Washington, DC, 1995, U.S. Government
Printing Office.

Wheat Foods Council:
How to Get Enough (ways to reach 6 to 11
servings from the grain group each day)
Bread: Enjoy Today's Low-Fat Choices
Available from Wheat Foods Council, 5500
S. Quebec, Suite 111, Englewood, CO
80111.

Resources for Helping the Functionally Impaired

Anonymous: Making Life a Little Easier: Self-
Help Tools for the Home (slide/tape or
video and brochure). Available from AARP
A/V Programs, Program Resources Dept.,
601 E St., N.W., Washington, DC 20049.
Arthritis Center and the Department of
Nutrition Sciences, University of Alabama at
Birmingham:
Arthritis Cookbook: Kitchen Basics for People
With Arthritis, Fibromyalgia, and Other
Pain and Fatigue. Available from Appletree
Press, 151 Good Counsel Drive, Suite 125,
Mankato, MN 56001
Catalogue of Resources for Persons with
Disabilities. Available from the Disability
Bookshop, Twin Peaks Press, P.O. Box 129,
Vancouver, WA 98666-0129
Klinger, J.L., and the Institute of
Rehabilitation Medicine, New York
University Medical Center: Mealtime
Manual for People with Disabilities and the
Aging, ed. 2, Camden, NJ, 1978, Campbell
Soup Company.
Sargent, J.V.: An Easier Way: Handbook for
the Elderly and Handicapped, Ames, IA,
1981, Iowa State University Press.

AUDIOVISUAL RESOURCES
Nutrition Education and Health Promotion

Anonymous: Put Away Your Frying Pan (10-
minute videotape on healthy cooking
techniques for Black Americans). Available
from Health Promotion Council of
Southeastern Pennsylvania, 311 S. Juniper
St., Philadelphia, PA 19197-5803.
Food and Drug Administration: The Food
Label and You: Check It Out (7-minute

video on using the food label). Available from Duplication Dept. of Interface Video Systems (telephone: 202-861-0500).

Los Angeles Project LEAN: Heart Healthy: Healthy Food Choices or Escasa La Grasa, Salud En Su Casa (25-minute videotape directed toward the Latino diet). Available from the LA Latino Project LEAN, P.O. Box 802864, Santa Clarita, CA 91380-2864.

National Dairy Council: Spice of Life (15-minute videotape giving practical suggestions for healthy eating for older adults). Available from National Dairy Council, 6300 North River Road, Rosemont, IL 60018-4233.

National Livestock and Meat Board and American Dietetic Association:
  Lean 'n Easy: Preparing Meat with Less Fat and More Taste (25-minute videotape with leader's guide, activity sheets, and take home handouts; developed for Project LEAN, Low-Fat Eating for America Now)
  MVE-TV: The Channel for Moderation, Variety, and Exercise (25-minute video with leader's guide and camera-ready activity sheets)
  Available from National Livestock and Meat Board, 444 North Michigan Ave., Chicago, IL 60611.

Pawtucket Heart Health Program: After Fifty (30-minute videotape in the Controlling Cholesterol series). Available from Pawtucket Heart Health Program, Memorial Hospital of Rhode Island, 111 Brewster St., Pawtucket, RI 02860.

Texas Agricultural Extension Service:
  Fanny (an educational kit including video and user guide focusing on late onset diabetes for black elderly), 1990
  Reverend Jones (an educational kit including video and user guide focusing on high blood pressure for black elderly), 1990
  Available from Minority Peer Education Project, Texas A&M University, College Station, TX.

Turner Educational Services (CNN):
  Eating Healthy for Life (20-minute video)

Eating Healthy for Heart Health (20-minute video)
Eating Healthy When Dining Out (20-minute video)
Eating Healthy for Weight Control (20-minute video)
User guide and videos available from Turner Broadcasting, 1 CNN Center, P.O. Box 105366, Atlanta, GA 30348.

Wisconsin Cooperative Extension and Ross Laboratories: Medication and Your Nutritional Health (9-minute videotape directed to older people). Available from Ross Laboratories, Columbus, OH 43216.

Nutrition Program Development

American Association of Retired Persons: Healthy Aging: Model Health Promotion Programs for Minority Elders (45-minute video and companion booklet). Available from National Resource Center on Health Promotion and Aging, AARP, 601 E St., N.W., Washington, DC 20049.

Beverly Foundation: Geriatric Nutrition, Patient Assessment, and Care Planning Reconsidered (51-minute video). Available from Beverly Foundation, 70 South Lake Ave., Suite 750, Pasadena, CA 91101.

Consultant Dietitians in Health Care Facilities, American Dietetic Association: Dining Skills: Restoring Pleasure to Mealtime: Techniques for Helping the Older Adult (video for training; manual also available). Available from ADA/CD-HCF, Box 2067, Pensacola, FL 32513.

San Francisco Commission on Aging: Getting It Right (45-minute video developed for in-service training of congregate meals site staff and volunteers); series available in Chinese, English, Japanese, Spanish, and Tagalog. Available from Spot 52 Productions, P.O. Box 460903, San Francisco, CA 94146-0903.

U.S. Department of Agriculture: Food Safety Is No Mystery (34-minute training video in English or Spanish). Available from Modern Talking Picture Service, 5000 Park St., N., St. Petersburg, FL 33709.

This resource list is provided for reader information and does not imply endorsement by the author.

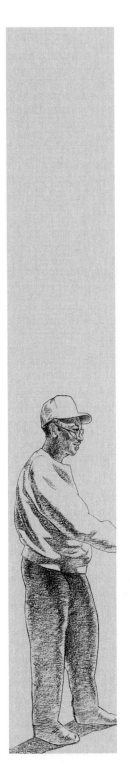

Glossary

abdominal fat fat located around the waist or abdominal area; fat deposits in this area are associated with hyperinsulinemia and hyperlipidemia.

accommodation the process by which the body decreases nutrient reserves, the amount of a particular tissue, or the level of function in response to a reduced or inadequate supply of nutrients.

acetaminophen drug used to relieve pain and reduce fever.

acetylcholine a neurotransmitter; acts as a vasodilator and depresses cardiac function.

achlorhydria absence of hydrochloric acid in the gastric juice.

acidosis an above-normal concentration of hydrogen ions in the body because of abnormal retention of acid or abnormal loss of base; occurs in poorly controlled diabetes when ketones accumulate or when the kidney is unable to excrete hydrogen ions or reabsorb bicarbonate ions.

Activities of Daily Living (ADLs) list of activities used to measure the ability of an individual to handle self-care; includes eating, dressing, bathing, transfer from bed to chair, walking, and toileting.

acute phase response first response of the body to infection or inflammation, with synthesis of cells and proteins of the immune system and other body defense systems.

acute sharp or intense; disease or illness that begins suddenly, reaches a peak rapidly, and then subsides after a short period.

ad-libitum fed allowed to eat as much as desired.

adenosine triphosphate molecule that stores energy in the cell.

adiposity relative amount of body fat.

adrenergic inhibitor drug that blocks the effects of the sympathetic nervous system that are mediated by norepinephrine.

adrenergic relating to the neurotransmitter epinephrine and activity of the sympathetic nervous system.

adult day care center facility that provides personal assistance and physical and social activities to frail or physically or mentally impaired older people who live in the community but require care throughout the day.

adverse drug reaction (ADR) a harmful unintended effect of a drug.

aerobic capacity the maximum amount of air that can be moved in and out of the lungs in a given amount of time.

aerobic exercise exercise that increases oxygen uptake and improves cardiovascular fitness, such as jogging, brisk walking, or cycling.

age-appropriate patterns of behavior considered by the general public to be appropriate for or associated with older people.

aged old; having lived a long time.

agitation restlessness, emotionally tense.

albumin a protein in the blood which serves as an indicator of protein status; contributes to maintenance of appropriate osmotic pressure and fluid balance between extracellular and intracellular fluids.

aldosterone a hormone produced in the adrenal cortex that acts on the kidney to cause sodium reabsorption and, in turn, water reabsorption.

alkalosis a situation in which the pH of extracellular fluids rises above 7.44; can be caused by an excess of bicarbonate ions or an abnormally low level of hydrogen ions.

alpha islets groups of cells in the pancreas that synthesize and release glucagon.

alpha tocopherol the form of vitamin E having the highest biological activity.

aluminum hydroxide a compound in many antacids that binds phosphates and prevents their absorption.

alveoli small air sacs in the lungs where gases are exchanged.

ambulatory able to walk.

American Heart Association Step I Diet diet recommended to lower serum triglycerides and LDL cholesterol; total fat is restricted to 30%, saturated fat to less than 10%, and polyunsaturated fat to no more than 10% of total energy.

American Hospital Formulary reference book on drugs published by the American Association of Hospital Pharmacists.

amitriptyline hydrochloride drug used to treat depression.

amylase enzyme that breaks down starch to dextrins and maltose.

analgesic drug that relieves pain.

anemia of chronic disease an anemia resulting from the effects of inflammation, liver disease, heart disease, or kidney disease on erythropoiesis and not from a lack of dietary iron.

anemia a decrease in the number or hemoglobin content of red blood cells.

angiotensin converting enzyme (ACE) inhibitor drug used to treat high blood pressure; it interferes with the production of angiotensin and reduces vasoconstriction.

angiotensin polypeptide in the blood that causes the release of aldosterone from the adrenal cortex.

anorexia nervosa a psychologic disorder in which the individual is obsessed with thinness and refuses to eat; leads to emaciation and possibly death.

anorexia lack of appetite.

anosmia loss or impaired sense of smell.

antacid drug that neutralizes the acid in the stomach.

antagonist a drug or agent that exerts an opposite action to that of another or competes for the same receptor site.

anthropometric measurement a body measurement such as height, weight, skinfold thickness, or body circumference used to estimate body composition.

anthropometric see anthropometric measurement.

antiarrhythmic drug prevents or alleviates abnormal heart rhythm.

antibiotic drug that destroys microorganisms; used to treat infections.

anticholinergic agent blocks the effects of the parasympathetic nervous system that are mediated by acetylcholine.

anticoagulant prevents or delays blood clotting.

antidiabetic agent drug used to control diabetes; lowers blood glucose levels.

antidiuretic hormone (ADH) hormone formed in the hypothalamus and released from the posterior pituitary; increases the reabsorption of water by the renal tubule and decreases the formation of urine.

antigen a foreign protein that causes the immune system to produce antibodies against it.

antigenic causing the production of antibodies.

antihypertensive agent reduces high blood pressure.

antineoplastic agent controls the proliferation of or kills cancer cells.

antioxidant a chemical substance that prevents or retards the oxidation of the double bonds in unsaturated fatty acids; this reaction occurs in the body and in foods containing fats and oils.

antipsychotic agent diminishes psychotic symptoms associated with mental disorders.

antipyretic reduces fever.

antirheumatic agent reduces or prevents the chronic inflammation of a joint, ligament, or muscle.

antivitamin activity the ability of a substance to prevent a vitamin from carrying out its biological function.

antivitamin a substance that inactivates a vitamin.

apathy lack of motivation.

apolipoprotein A-1 activates the enzyme necessary to release cholesterol from the peripheral tissues and allow its removal by high density lipoproteins.

apraxia a psychomotor disorder in which the ability to program muscle movements and control voluntary motions necessary to carry out tasks is impaired.

arachidonic acid an omega-6 fatty acid composed of 20 carbons and 4 double bonds that can be synthesized from linoleic acid.

area agency on aging local agency established by a state government to administer and implement social and nutrition services to older adults in a given geographic area.

aromatic amino acid decarboxylase enzyme required for the synthesis of norepinephrine and serotonin (neurotransmitters).

arterial pressure the stress exerted on the arterial walls by the circulating blood.

arthritis see osteoarthritis.

ascorbic acid a water-soluble vitamin required for formation of collagen; acts as an antioxidant.

aspartate aminotransferase apoenzyme the enzyme without its vitamin B-6 cofactor; in this form the enzyme is inactive.

aspartate aminotransferase an enzyme required for the transfer of an amino group for the formation of glutamic acid; serum levels increase following myocardial infarction or liver damage.

aspiration pneumonia pneumonia caused by the inhalation of food or fluid into the lungs; can be caused by swallowing disorders or feeding an older person who is lying down.

assisted-living housing facility for resident care of functionally impaired older people that provides meals, supervision, and assistance with personal care as needed.

atherosclerosis see atherosclerotic plaque.

atherosclerotic see atherosclerotic plaque.

atherosclerotic lesion see atherosclerotic plaque.

atherosclerotic plaque yellow lipid deposits on the inner walls of the large arteries that over time become calcified and covered with connective tissue; sometimes called "hardening of the arteries."

atrial fibrillation rapid random contractions of the atrial compartments of the heart.

atrial natriuretic peptide hormone that increases the excretion of sodium and water.

atrial tachycardia rapid heart beat of over 100 beats per minute originating in the atrium; begins suddenly and can end abruptly.

atrophic gastritis chronic inflammation of the stomach lining with loss of mucosal cells and reduced secretion of HCl.

atrophy wasting away of body tissue.

autoimmune reaction developing antibodies to one's own tissues.

avidin a substance in raw egg white that binds with biotin and prevents its absorption.

B-cells cells of the immune system that produce antibodies (immunoglobulins) that defend against virus and bacteria.

baby boom generation the large number of babies born following World War II, between 1946 and 1964; this generation will be responsible for the rapid rise in the number of older people beginning about 2005.

bacterial overgrowth extensive proliferation of bacteria in the upper duodenum as a result of low acid secretion in the stomach; bacteria can bind with vitamins and prevent their absorption and break down bile salts.

bactericidal able to destroy bacteria.

balance method method used to determine the requirement for protein or a mineral; the requirement is the level of intake at which equilibrium is reached (intake equals losses in urine, feces, and sweat).

Baltimore Longitudinal Study of Aging (BLSA) a longitudinal study of men and women ranging in age from young adults to age 100 and over conducted by the National Institute on Aging; participants' nutrient intake and physiologic and psychologic function are evaluated every two years.

baroreceptor nerve endings in the major blood vessels that are sensitive to changes in blood pressure.

basal metabolism the amount of energy required to maintain essential body processes when an individual is awake, at rest, and has not eaten for at least 14 hours.

benzodiazepine psychotropic drug used to reduce anxiety and as a sedative.

beta carotene a precursor of vitamin A found in plant foods, especially dark green and deep yellow vegetables and fruits.

beta islets groups of cells in the pancreas that synthesize and release insulin.

beta tocopherol a form of vitamin E with reduced biological activity.

bicarbonate an ion (HCO_3-) resulting from the dissociation of carbonic acid; acts in the acid-base buffering system.

bile acid sequestrant substance that binds with bile acids in the intestine and prevents their reabsorption.

bile salts emulsifiers synthesized by the liver and released by the gallbladder to aid in the digestion of fat.

biliary colic pain resulting from the passage of a stone through the bile duct.

bioavailability ability to be absorbed.

bioelectrical impedance analysis (BIA) a method of determining body fat content based on the electrical resistance of particular tissues.

biopsy the removal of a small piece of tissue from a body part for microscopic examination.

biphosphate a group of compounds that inhibit activity of the osteoclasts and bone resorption.

board and care facility facility for resident care that provides meals and supervision and may assist with personal care.

body cell mass (BCM) the body compartment that includes the metabolically active cells in muscle, visceral organs, blood and brain; cells in connective tissue that have slow turnover rates are not included.

body mass index (BMI) Quetelet index; body weight divided by body height squared (kg/m^2).

bone marrow soft tissue found in the center of the long bones where hematopoiesis takes place.

Boston Nutritional Status Survey a survey of 686 community-living and 266 institutionalized economically advantaged people age 60 and over living in metropolitan Boston; available data include dietary records, anthropometric measurements, socioeconomic and health characteristics, dental status, and clinical and nutritional blood parameters.

bradykinesia a condition in which all voluntary movements and speech are slowed.

branched-chain amino acids leucine, isoleucine, and valine; these amino acids have an important role in muscle protein metabolism.

breath hydrogen expired hydrogen used to measure the completeness of digestion of disaccharides, particularly lactose.

bronchiole small airway within the lungs that transports inspired air and waste gases.

bronchodilation increase in the diameter of the bronchioles to increase the flow of air in and out of the lungs; brought about by a drug or action of the sympathetic nervous system.

bronchodilator drug that relaxes the smooth muscle lining the bronchioles, allowing them to expand in diameter.

c-reactive protein a protein that appears in the serum as part of the acute phase response and acts on the immune system.

cachexia general wasting and emaciation associated with serious disease such as cancer.

calcitonin a hormone that opposes the action of parathyroid hormone in regulating blood calcium levels.

calcitriol term used for 1,25-dihydroxycholecalciferol, the active metabolite of vitamin D.

calcium carbonate a form of calcium used as a calcium supplement.

calcium channel blockers drugs that inhibit the flow of calcium ions across muscle membranes, thereby relaxing muscle tone and reducing muscle spasms.

calcium-citrate-malate compound a form of calcium added to orange juice as a calcium supplement.

calcium-dependent ATPase adenosine triphosphatase enzyme splits adenosine triphosphate into adenosine diphosphate and inorganic phosphate and energy; action is necessary for muscle contraction; calcium is a necessary cofactor.

calcium a mineral required by the body; most body calcium is found in the bone although it also is required for nerve impulse transmission and muscle contraction; serum levels are regulated by parathyroid hormone and calcitonin.

calculi small stones formed by the precipitation of mineral salts; can block the bile duct or urinary tract.

cancellous bone porous, spongy bone with a lattice-like structure.

carbamazepine drug used to relieve pain and prevent convulsions.

carcinogenesis the initiation and promotion of a cancer.

cardiac arrhythmia an abnormal rate or rhythm of contraction of the heart muscle.

cardiac cachexia a condition characterized by lack of appetite, malnutrition, and weight loss associated with serious heart disease; often related to use of digoxin which causes anorexia and nausea.

cardiac glycosides drugs that increase the force of the contraction of the cardiac muscle and decrease the heart rate.

cardiac output quantity of blood pumped per minute (average value is approximately 5 liters).

cardiovascular disease condition involving dysfunction of the heart vessels; atherosclerosis, systemic hypertension, and cardiac failure are types of cardiovascular disease.

carotenoids type of yellow, red, and orange pigments found in plant foods; some are precursors of vitamin A, and some appear to protect against cancer.

case management process by which a health professional or social worker assesses an older person's need for health and social services, arranges for the services required, and conducts ongoing supervision and reassessment.

cataract (senile) degenerative change in the lens of the eye resulting in a loss of transparency and, if untreated, loss of vision.

catharsis purging or violent emptying of the bowel.

cathartic a type of laxative that brings about an emptying of the bowel by stimulating peristalsis.

celiac disease see gluten-sensitive enteropathy.

cell-mediated immune function immune responses involving T cells rather than antibodies; provides resistance to infectious disease, certain immune diseases, and possibly cancer.

centenarian a person age 100 years or over.

cerebral hemorrhage rupture of a blood vessel in the brain.

cerebrovascular accident stroke; interruption of blood flow to an area of the brain because of blockage or breakage of the blood vessel supplying blood to that region.

cerebrovascular disease pathologic changes in the blood vessels in the brain.

ceruloplasmin a plasma transport protein for copper.

chelating agent a substance that combines with a mineral ion in a ring-like structure.

chemotherapy the use of chemicals to destroy cancer cells.

chief cells cells in the lining of the stomach that secrete pepsinogen and intrinsic factor.

chloride the chloride ion (Cl^-) or a compound containing the chloride ion such as sodium chloride; chloride ions are found in the extracellular fluid and help to regulate acid-base balance.

chlorpromazine drug used to control psychotic symptoms and vomiting.

cholecalciferol vitamin D-3.

cholecystectomy removal of the gallbladder.

cholecystokinin a hormone produced by the upper intestinal mucosa that stimulates contraction of the gallbladder and secretion of pancreatic digestive enzymes.

cholesterol a complex lipid molecule with a sterol structure found in animal fat and egg yolk; it is synthesized by the liver and found in many body tissues; inappropriate serum cholesterol levels are associated with atherosclerosis and increased cardiovascular risk.

cholestyramine drug used to lower blood cholesterol or lipid levels.

cholinesterase enzyme that breaks down acetylcholine to choline and acetate.

chromium a trace mineral required for normal carbohydrate and lipid metabolism; appears to help insulin bind to the cell membrane.

chronic obstructive pulmonary disease (COPD) a progressive and irreversible lung disease in which the airways are decreased in size and the passage of air is reduced.

chronic prolonged; a disease that develops slowly and persists for a long time, possibly for the remaining years of life.

chronologic age a person's age in years.

chylomicron remnant the cell fragment remaining after the free fatty acids have been taken up by muscle and adipose cells; the remnant particles are removed from the blood and metabolized by the liver.

chymotrypsin an enzyme produced in the pancreas that flows into the small intestine and breaks down protein.

cimetidine drug that inhibits the production and secretion of acid in the stomach.

cinchonism condition of headache, deafness, and ringing in the ears caused by excessive intake of quinine.

circumference measurement measurement of the outer boundary of specific locations on the arm, waist, hip, or leg used in standardized equations to estimate body composition.

citric acid cycle the sequence of metabolic reactions by which carbohydrates, fatty acids, and amino acids can be broken down to form water, carbon dioxide, and ATP.

clinical trial a research study designed to test a medical treatment or nutritional intervention.

clofibrate drug used to lower high blood cholesterol or triglyceride levels.

cobalamin the cobalt-containing portion of the vitamin B-12 molecule.

cofactor a metal ion or small molecule that is required for the action of a larger molecule such as an enzyme; an example is the heme component within the hemoglobin molecule.

cognitive status a person's level of intellectual function relating to reasoning, thinking, or remembering.

cognitive related to the mental processes of acquiring knowledge, judgment, reasoning, and memory.

cohort study a group of individuals in a scientific study who share a common characteristic such as age, sex, or health status.

colchicine drug used to treat gout.

colestipol drug used to lower high blood cholesterol levels.

collagen a protein consisting of small bundles of fibers found in tendons, ligaments, and bone matrix.

community-based long-term care an integrated system of health and social services designed to maintain the chronically ill or functionally impaired individual in his or her home and delay or prevent institutionalization.

computed tomography an x-ray technique used to determine body composition.

congestive heart failure condition caused by the inability of the heart to pump all the blood returned to it; associated with retention of sodium and water by the kidney and development of edema.

congregate housing apartment complexes for older people that often provide some social services or referral.

congregate meal program program funded under the Older Americans Act that provides a hot meal at noon Monday through Friday in a social setting for people age 60 and over.

constipation difficulty in passing stools.

Consumer Price Index index that reports the average percent rise in prices of goods and services over the previous year.

continuing-care retirement community a retirement community designed to provide a range of housing options and services to support independent living for healthy older people and provide

skilled nursing care for those who come to require more specialized care.

Continuing Survey of Food Intakes by Individuals (CSFII) a dietary survey conducted by the U.S. Department of Agriculture of all age groups in the 48 coterminous states; data collected included three-day dietary records, food eaten away from home, and times of meals and snacks.

continuum of care the range of health, support, and nutrition services that will allow an individual to maintain the highest level of independence and personal well-being possible.

copper a trace element required by the body which acts as a cofactor for many enzymes and assists in the absorption and metabolism of iron and production of normal red blood cells.

core foods foods eaten daily; staple foods in the dietary pattern.

coronary artery disease development of atherosclerotic plaques that reduce the diameter of the artery and the blood flow carrying oxygen and nutrients to the heart.

coronary heart disease see coronary artery disease.

cortical bone compact, dense bone found in the shafts of the long bones.

coumarin a drug that prevents blood clotting.

creatinine clearance the amount of creatinine removed from the blood by the kidneys, expressed on the basis of the volume of blood filtered per unit of time; used to evaluate the glomerular filtration rate.

creatinine a product of muscle metabolism; urinary creatinine excretion can be used to estimate body muscle mass.

cross-sectional study a comparison of data from two or more groups of people evaluated at the same time.

cyanocobalamin vitamin B-12.

cytochrome C oxidase a copper-containing enzyme within the respiratory chain necessary for electron transport.

cytokinin a hormone-like protein that regulates the duration and intensity of an immune response.

D-xylose a pentose used to measure the completeness of carbohydrate absorption; substance is not metabolized so the total amount absorbed will be excreted in the urine

dehydration abnormally low body fluid volume resulting from inadequate fluid intake or high fluid loss.

7-dehydrocholesterol compound in the skin that on exposure to sunlight is synthesized into vitamin D.

delta-6-desaturase the regulatory enzyme that controls the first step in the conversion of linoleic acid and alpha linolenic acid to arachidonic acid and other nonessential fatty acids.

dementia a progressive loss of mental function caused by physiologic changes or disease.

demographic relating to the size, geographic distribution, and general characteristics of human populations, including age, sex, income, race, or health.

dendrite a tree-like branch of a nerve cell that conducts impulses toward the nerve cell body.

dental caries tooth decay.

depression feeling sad, worthless, hopeless about the future.

desolates term applied to older people living alone who are discontented and long for their spouses or other family members who have died or moved away.

desquamated cells cells lost from the surface of a tissue through normal erosion such as from the skin or gastrointestinal tract.

desquamation the shedding of the outer layer of cells.

diabetes mellitus a disorder of carbohydrate, fat, and protein metabolism resulting from a lack of insulin secretion by the pancreas.

diabetic neuropathy damage to the peripheral nerves caused by high blood glucose levels in poorly controlled diabetes.

diagnosis related groups (DRGs) classifications of patients based on primary and secondary diagnoses and procedures; used to determine the level and extent of care eligible for Medicare reimbursement.

diarrhea the passage of loose, watery stools.

diastolic blood pressure the blood pressure when the heart muscle is relaxed and blood is entering the heart chambers.

diazepam a drug used as a sedative, tranquilizer, and anticonvulsant.

diazoxide a drug used to lower blood pressure.

dietary recall a method of collecting food intake information in which a person is asked to remember the food eaten recently, usually for the last 24 hours.

dietary status the relative adequacy of the diet as compared to the Recommended Dietary Allowances for an individual of that age, sex, or condition.

digitalis cachexia loss of weight and general malnutrition resulting from loss of appetite and nausea associated with use of digitalis.

digitalis glycoside chemical name for digitalis noting its structure as a carbohydrate with a sugar and a nonsugar component.

digitalis intoxication excessive intake of digitalis leading to drug poisoning.

digoxin a drug that increases the strength of the contraction of the cardiac muscle and slows the heart rate.

1,25-dihydroxyvitamin D the active form of vitamin D; also called calcitriol.

disability loss or impairment of physical or mental fitness.

disordered taste perception changes in the degree of recognition of the basic tastes, or changes in taste (e.g., bitter taste with many foods; unpleasant taste with sweet items).

diuretic a drug that decreases the reabsorption of water in the renal tubule and increases urine output.

diurnal variation a change in level or secretion of a substance over a 24-hour period.

divalent cation an atom with a positive valence of 2.

diversity representing many different varieties or types.

diverticulitis inflammation and infection of the pouch-like projections (diverticuli) found in the colon in advanced age.

diverticulosis pouchlike projections in the colon common among older people; may be related to low fiber intake.

dizygous twins developing from two fertilized ova; fraternal twins.

DNA (deoxyribonucleic acid) the molecules of nucleic acids that form the genetic material in the chromosomes.

docosahexaenoic acid an omega-3 fatty acid found in fish; has 22 carbon atoms and 6 double bonds.

dolomite a naturally occurring mineral containing calcium that is unsuitable as a calcium supplement as it may contain toxic minerals such as lead or mercury.

dopamine a neurotransmitter and precursor of norepinephrine.

dual-energy x-ray absorptiometry (DEXA) an x-ray technique used to determine body composition.

dyspepsia discomfort in the abdominal region following eating.

dysphagia difficulty in swallowing.

eating-dependent requires help with eating, cannot feed himself or herself.

edentulous without teeth.

eicosapentaenoic acid an omega-3 fatty acid found in fish; has 20 carbon atoms and 5 double bonds.

elastin protein found in elastic tissues such as the blood vessels that are capable of vasoconstriction and vasodilation.

Elderly Nutrition Program (ENP) a program funded by the Older Americans Act that provides congregate or home-delivered meals to people age 60 and over.

electrolyte an element or compound that forms ions when placed in water (e.g., potassium, sodium chloride).

elixir a mixture of sugar, alcohol, and water used as a vehicle for drugs; also, a potion believed to have powers for curing disease or restoring youth.

emollient substance that softens the skin or mucous membranes.

endometrial relating to the inner lining of the uterus.

endothelial surface the cells making up the inner surface of the heart, blood vessels, and body cavities.

envelope measurements circumference measurements of the waist or hip.

epidemiology study of the factors or conditions associated with the incidence, prevalence, or control of a particular disease.

epinephrine neurotransmitter in the sympathetic nervous system.

error catastrophe theory that a change in DNA caused by an environmental insult, such as polluted air or water, leads to synthesis of defective proteins and aging.

erythrocyte aspartate transaminase enzyme requiring vitamin B-6 as a coenzyme; enzyme activity used as an indicator of vitamin B-6 status.

erythrocyte glutathione reductase enzyme requiring riboflavin as a coenzyme; enzyme activity used as an indicator of riboflavin status.

erythrocyte protoporphyrin a component necessary for the formation of the hemoglobin molecule; used as an indicator of iron status and a developing anemia.

erythrocyte sedimentation rate the rate at which red blood cells settle to the bottom of the tube when unclotted blood is allowed to stand; used to establish if inflammation is present.

erythrocyte transketolase enzyme requiring thiamin as a coenzyme; enzyme activity used as an indicator of thiamin status.

erythrocyte a red blood cell.

erythropoiesis production of red blood cells.

erythropoietin hormone secreted by the kidney that stimulates the production of red blood cells.

estrogen replacement therapy (ERT) giving estrogen to postmenopausal women to prevent or alleviate bone mineral loss or reduce cardiovascular risk.

estrogen female sex hormone produced by the ovaries.

ethacrynic acid a diuretic.

ethnic pertaining to a particular national, racial, or cultural group.

etidronate biphosphate compound used in treatment of osteoporosis.

extended family several generations of a family or adult brothers and sisters and their children living together.

factorial method method to determine the requirement for protein by adding all routes of obligatory nitrogen loss and calculating the level of dietary protein required to replace those losses.

failure to thrive syndrome in older people who lose physical, social, and cognitive function with no immediately apparent cause.

fasting refraining from eating for a specific period of time.

fat-free mass (FFM) the body mass with all fat removed including the fatty acids found in cell membranes and essential structures.

fat-soluble vitamin a vitamin that dissolves in a lipid or oil; vitamins A, D, E, and K are fat-soluble.

fecal fat undigested fat appearing in the feces.

ferric iron trivalent form of iron that occurs naturally in foods but cannot be absorbed.

ferritin a protein-iron complex that serves as a storage form of iron; serum ferritin is highly correlated with liver iron stores.

ferrous iron divalent form of iron; form in which iron is absorbed.

ferrous sulfate form of iron found in supplements given to treat iron-deficiency anemia.

fibrin protein formed in blood clotting; helps to form the clot.

Five A Day health promotion program of the National Institutes of Health to encourage people to eat five servings of fruits and vegetables every day.

flavor enhancer concentrated flavors added to foods to strengthen the natural flavor.

fluorapatite a bone mineral crystal composed of calcium, phosphate, hydroxyl, and fluoride ions that is highly resistant to bone resorption.

fluoride the fluoride ion (Fl^-) or a compound such as sodium fluoride that is added to the water supply in small amounts to prevent tooth decay; fluoride supports the development of a less soluble mineral crystal in bones and teeth.

focus group method involving small discussion groups for obtaining information from older people regarding their preferences or satisfaction regarding services or programs.

folate a form of folic acid; required by the body as a coenzyme in reactions involving transfer of one carbon units.

food aspiration the accidental inhalation of food into the lungs.

food assistance programs government-supported programs that provide food or meals or increased income to purchase food; includes congregate or home-delivered meals programs, commodity food distribution programs, and food stamps.

food idiosyncrasy a food habit or pattern that is unique to a particular individual.

food insecurity the limited availability or uncertainty of adequate food as related to income, inability to shop for groceries, no one to assist with food preparation, or limited ability to feed oneself.

food intake regulation ability of the body to monitor food intake and regulate appetite and satiety to maintain a constant weight.

food intolerance an adverse reaction to a particular food resulting in discomfort or physical symptoms; may relate to a problem in digestion or absorption or metabolism of a nutrient.

food sensitivity reaction to a food or a particular substance in a food brought about by an immunologic response.

food stamps plan by which low-income people can receive stamps for food purchases that will raise their food money to meet the lowest cost food plan set by the U.S. Dept. of Agriculture.

frail physically weak; requiring assistance with heavy household chores or when going outside the home.

Framingham Heart Study a long-term prospective epidemiologic study being carried on in the community of Framingham, Mass., to evaluate risk factors associated with cardiovascular and other chronic diseases.

free radical an unstable high-energy compound with an unpaired electron that causes oxidation reactions in unsaturated fatty acids.

functional disability the inability or difficulty in carrying out Activities of Daily Living, such as bathing, eating, or toileting, or the Instrumental Activities of Daily Living, such as shopping or meal preparation.

functional related to the special work or acuity of an organ or body part.

furosemide a diuretic drug.

gallstone a small stone formed by the accumulation of bile salts that can block the bile duct.

gastrectomy removal of all or part of the stomach.

gastric emptying time amount of time required for a test meal to completely pass out of the stomach and into the duodenum.

gastric emptying the movement of food from the stomach into the duodenum (small intestine).

gastric motility the spontaneous peristaltic movements in the stomach that mix food and gastric secretions and move food through the stomach and into the duodenum.

gastric mucosa the layer of cells lining the stomach.

gastric phytobezoar a solid mass of vegetable fiber or seeds forming in the stomach; a food ball.

gastrin a hormone secreted by the stomach that stimulates the flow of gastric juice and acts to stimulate the secretion of bile and digestive enzymes by the pancreas.

gastroesophageal reflux the backflow of stomach contents into the esophagus as a result of poor function of the lower esophageal sphincter.

gastrointestinal bleeding bleeding from any location in the gastrointestinal tract including the esophagus, stomach, small intestine, or colon; usually is related to an ulcer, diverticulitis, ulcerative colitis, or cancer.

genetic code information carried by the DNA molecule and used for the synthesis of identical proteins.

Georgia Centenarian Study an ongoing longitudinal study of community living people age 100 and over in Georgia.

geriatrics the branch of medicine dealing with changes in physiologic function, diseases, and care of older people.

gerontologic nurse practitioner (GNP) a nurse who has completed specialized training and certification in the health needs and health care of older people.

gerontology the scientific study of the aging process including biologic, sociologic, psychologic, and clinical aspects.

gingivitis red, swollen, or bleeding gums.

glomerular filtrate the fluid portion of the blood that is filtered by the kidney.

glomerular filtration rate (GFR) the amount of blood plasma that can be filtered in a given amount of time (GFR of a young adult is about 125 ml per minute).

glossitis inflammation of the tongue.

glucagon a hormone produced by the alpha islets of the pancreas that stimulates the conversion of glycogen to glucose and gluconeogenesis in the liver to bring about a rise in plasma glucose levels.

glucocorticoid hormone steroid hormone secreted by the adrenal cortex that promotes the release of amino acids from muscle for gluconeogenesis and exerts an anti-inflammatory effect.

gluconeogenesis the formation of glucose from other compounds, usually amino acids, from which the amino group has been removed.

glucose intolerance reduced ability to metabolize glucose, resulting in elevated serum glucose following a test dose of glucose or a meal.

glucose tolerance factor a chromium amino acid complex that facilitates the binding of insulin to its cell receptor.

glucose tolerance the ability of the body to metabolize a load of glucose; is measured by administering a standard dose of glucose by mouth and measuring blood glucose levels for two to three hours thereafter.

glutamine a nonessential amino acid that serves as an amino group donor in synthetic reactions.

glutathione peroxidase enzyme that participates in antioxidant reactions and protects tissues against damage from free radicals.

glutathione reductase enzyme that catalyzes the oxidation-reduction reactions necessary for the antioxidant activity of glutathione disulfide.

glutathione component of enzymes that act as antioxidants; prevents hemolysis of red blood cells.

gluteal relating to the buttocks.

gluten-sensitive enteropathy a condition resulting from an immunologic response to the gliadin fraction in gluten, a protein in wheat and some other grains; results in diarrhea, steatorrhea, and general malabsorption unless gluten is eliminated from the diet; also referred to as celiac disease.

gluten a protein found in wheat and some other grains.

glyburide an oral antidiabetic drug.

glycation chemical reaction in which a sugar joins with an amino group on a protein.

glycemic control an effort to control blood glucose levels in people with diabetes mellitus through defined treatment involving diet, injection of insulin, or use of other drugs.

glycogen storage form of glucose found in the liver and muscle.

glyconeogenesis forming glycogen from a noncarbohydrate such as protein by converting it first to glucose and then to glycogen.

glycosuria an abnormally high level of glucose in the urine occurring in diabetes mellitus.

glycosylated hemoglobin compound formed by the combining of glucose with the end amino group of a hemoglobin chain; used to monitor blood glucose control in diabetes mellitus.

glycyrrhizic acid a substance found in licorice root that mimics the action of aldosterone.

grazing food pattern in which an individual eats many small meals or snacks throughout the day rather than several large meals.

growth hormone a hormone secreted by the anterior pituitary that promotes protein synthesis, increases fat mobilization and use of fatty acids for energy, and increases breakdown of glycogen and gluconeogenesis to raise blood glucose levels.

gynecomastia abnormal enlargement of the breasts in men.

H$_2$-receptor antagonist drug that prevents the secretion of acid in the stomach.

half-life the time required for a substance to lose half of its activity or for half to be metabolized or excreted.

health maintenance organization (HMO) a type of managed health care in which group members pay a fixed fee and then receive all diagnostic, preventive, and medical treatment covered by the plan; such groups emphasize preventive care.

Healthy Eating Index a method of rating the adequacy and appropriateness of daily food intake based on the number of servings from the milk, meat, fruit, vegetable, and grain groups, and percentage of kilocalories coming from fat.

Healthy People 2000 National Health Promotion and Disease Prevention Objectives: a national strategy to promote health and prevent unnecessary disease and disability in Americans of all ages by the year 2000.

heartburn a burning pain in the esophagus caused by the backflow of gastric contents and acid.

helicobacter pylori the pathogenic microorganism associated with the development of gastric ulcers.

hematocrit the packed cell volume of the red blood cells as a percentage of the total blood volume.

hematopoiesis the formation of blood cells in the bone marrow.

hematopoietic see hematopoiesis.

heme iron iron complexed in the hemoglobin molecule; found in animal tissues.

heme the iron-containing complex of the hemoglobin molecule.

hemochromatosis condition involving excess deposition of iron in the tissues as a result of inappropriately high iron absorption; may have a genetic basis.

hemodialysis process by which a patient's blood is shunted through a dialysis machine which removes urea and other waste products and then returns the blood to the body; extends the life of people with chronic renal failure.

hemoglobin the protein-iron complex in erythrocytes that binds and transports oxygen to the tissues and removes carbon dioxide.

hemorrhagic stroke when a blood vessel in the brain bursts and blood drains into surrounding tissue; brain cells deprived of their blood supply die.

hemorrhoids swollen veins around the anus; can be caused or aggravated by straining to pass hard stools.

hepatic retinyl ester hydrolase enzyme in the liver that breaks down retinyl esters and releases retinol for transport to body tissues.

hepatotoxicity the situation in which drug or alcohol is harmful to the liver.

heterogeneous dissimilar; not uniform throughout.

heterogenicity being dissimilar or different.

hiatus hernia a protrusion of the stomach upward toward the diaphragm which can result in backflow of stomach acid into the esophagus.

high density lipoprotein (HDL) a plasma lipoprotein complex relatively high in protein and low in cholesterol and believed to slow the development of atherosclerosis by assisting in the transport of cholesterol to the liver where it is excreted in the bile.

Hispanic Health and Nutrition Examination Survey (HHANES) a survey conducted by the U.S. government to determine the nutritional status and chronic disease risk of the Hispanic population.

histamine a compound formed by the breakdown of histidine that stimulates gastric secretion, acts as a vasodilator on arteries and capillaries, and constricts bronchial passageways.

home care a combination of health, medical, personal, and home management services that maintain the frail or physically disabled person at home.

home-delivered meals meals prepared and delivered by a government or community agency to homebound older people.

home health agency an agency that provides and supervises health-related services in the home, ranging from personal care and homemaking services to skilled nursing care.

home health aide provides personal care services, such as help with bathing or dressing, to functionally disabled individuals in their home.

home study providing nutrition education materials to older people to study at home.

homebound unable to leave home because of illness or physical disability.

homemaker services home management services, such as food shopping and meal preparation, provided to older people with functional disability under the supervision of a nurse or home health agency.

homeostasis maintaining the internal environment of the body within the conditions required for living cells including parameters such as temperature, pH, and oxygen supply.

homocysteine an intermediate compound in the synthesis of cysteine which accumulates in the blood when folate or vitamin B-12 is lacking.

hydralazine drug used to lower blood pressure.

hydrochloric acid HCl; secreted in the stomach by the parietal cells as a part of gastric juice.

hydrolysis a chemical reaction which occurs with the addition of water, resulting in a compound splitting into two parts.

25-hydroxy vitamin D metabolite of vitamin D formed in the liver.

hydroxyapatite the major mineral crystal found in bone; contains calcium, phosphate, and hydroxyl ions.

1-α-hydroxylase see renal 1-α-hydroxylase.

hypercalcemia abnormally high blood calcium level.

hypercalciuria abnormally high level of calcium in the urine.

hypercapnia abnormally high level of carbon dioxide in the blood.

hyperfiltration situation in which the kidney increases the amount of blood plasma filtered in response to a high flow of blood to the kidney.

hyperglycemia abnormally high blood glucose level.

hyperinsulinemia excessively high blood insulin level.

hyperkalemia abnormally high level of potassium in the blood.

hyperkeratosis overgrowth of the dry, cornified layer of the epidermis.

hypermagnesemia abnormally high level of magnesium in the blood.

hypernatremia abnormally high level of sodium in the blood.

hyperparathyroidism excessive secretion of parathyroid hormone.

hyperperfusion situation in which an abnormally large quantity of blood is delivered to the kidney for filtration.

hyperphagic to overeat, excessive appetite.

hypertension blood pressure that is above normal; often defined as systolic pressure ≥ 140 mm Hg and diastolic pressure > 90 mm Hg.

hypertensive see hypertension.

hyperthyroidism above normal secretion of thyroid hormones.

hypertrophy an increase in the size of an organ, such as the heart, brought about by an increase in cell size.

hypervitaminosis A condition resulting from excessive intakes of preformed vitamin A over an extended period; leads to liver damage.

hypnotic agent substance with a calming effect; reduces anxiety.

hypoalbuminemia abnormally low blood albumin level.

hypoalbuminemic malnutrition protein-energy malnutrition identified by a serum albumin of less than 30 g/l.

hypochlorhydria a lower than normal level of hydrochloric acid in the gastric juice.

hypoglycemic agent a drug that lowers blood glucose levels used in the treatment of diabetes mellitus.

hypokalemia abnormally low level of potassium in the blood.

hyponatremia abnormally low level of sodium in the blood.

hypophagic poor appetite, anorexia.

hypoprothrombinemia abnormally low level of prothrombin in the blood resulting from vitamin K deficiency.

hypoprothrombinemic effect a decrease in the amount of prothrombin in the blood resulting in less efficient clot formation; can result from a vitamin K deficiency or use of an anticoagulant drug.

hypothalamic-neurohypophyseal axis relating to the hormonal pathway existing between the hypothalamus and the posterior lobe of the pituitary gland (neurohypophysis); controls release of antidiuretic hormone.

hypothalamus part of the brain that controls the endocrine system, appetite, the autonomic nervous system, and possibly mood and motivation.

hypothyroidism below normal secretion of thyroid hormones.

hypoxia lack of sufficient oxygen for the tissues.

iatrogenic disorder caused by a drug, treatment procedure, or diagnostic procedure.

ibuprofen a nonsteroidal anti-inflammatory drug (NSAID) used for mild pain relief and treatment of rheumatoid arthritis and osteoarthritis.

imipramine drug used to treat depression.

immunoglobulin group of humoral antibodies that defend against microorganisms or environmental toxins.

incontinence loss of ability to control urination or defecation.

inflammatory bowel disease chronic inflammation and infection of the colon and rectum resulting in watery diarrhea containing blood and pus.

initiation the first step in the development of cancer; a carcinogen acts on a cell to produce an irreversible genetic mutation.

insensible water loss unnoticed loss of fluid from the body through expired air, feces, and continual loss from the skin.

insoluble fiber indigestible cellulose, hemicellulose, and lignin found in cereal grains and vegetables that increase fecal bulk.

insoluble will not dissolve in water or other solvent.

Instrumental Activities of Daily Living (IADLs) a list of activities used to determine an individual's ability to live independently; activities include shopping, preparing meals, managing money, using the telephone, doing housework, and going outside unassisted.

insulin-dependent diabetes mellitus (IDDM) form of diabetes mellitus in which the beta cells are incapable of producing any insulin; patient is prone to ketoacidosis.

insulin-like growth factor a peptide synthesized in the liver that acts on peripheral tissues to bring about the anabolic effects associated with growth hormone; sometimes referred to as somatomedin C.

insulin a hormone secreted by the beta cells of the pancreas in response to increased blood glucose levels; promotes the movement of glucose into fat and muscle cells and the use of glucose for energy or glycogen synthesis and lowers blood glucose levels; promotes protein and fatty acid synthesis.

interleukin-1-b a protein that activates the inflammatory response and activates the immune system to respond to infection.

intestinal motility the rhythmic contractions of the intestinal muscle layer that move the intestinal contents along the passageway.

intrinsic factor substance secreted by the gastric mucosa that is necessary for the normal absorption of vitamin B-12.

iron depletion loss of iron from the body resulting in low or no iron stores; usually caused by chronic blood loss.

iron-deficiency anemia anemia resulting from inadequate iron intake or excessive iron (blood) loss; red blood cells are small in size with a below-normal level of hemoglobin.

iron-deficient erythropoiesis disruption in the normal production of red blood cells because of a lack of available iron for heme synthesis; may be caused by inadequate iron intake, excessive iron (blood) loss, or failure of the body to release iron to the bone marrow as a result of infection or inflammation.

iron trace mineral found in the heme molecule; also acts as a cofactor for enzymes in the respiratory chain.

irritable bowel syndrome abnormally increased motility in the small and large intestines resulting in diarrhea and pain; appears to be caused by emotional stress and not disease.

ischemic heart disease damage to the heart from a decreased blood supply and insufficient oxygen.

isolates term used to describe older people who live alone and lead fairly solitary lives but are content with their level of social interaction.

isoniazid drug used to treat tuberculosis.

isotope a form of a chemical element that differs in molecular weight from the standard and can be used to track metabolic processes in the body.

isotopic applied to the surface of the skin.

jaundice yellowing of the skin caused by abnormally high levels of bilirubin in the blood; may indicate liver disease or obstruction of the bile duct.

jejunum the middle section of the small intestine located between the duodenum and the ileum.

ketoacidosis complication of diabetes mellitus in which ketones accumulate in the blood, resulting in acidosis, mental confusion, dyspnea, and, if untreated, coma.

ketones products arising from incomplete oxidation of fatty acids which accumulate in the blood and urine in uncontrolled diabetes mellitus (e.g., beta-hydroxy-butyric acid, acetoacetic acid, and acetone).

Kupffer cells specialized liver cells that remove bacteria from the blood delivered to the liver from the gastrointestinal tract through the portal vein.

kyphosis abnormal curvature of the spine resulting in a hunchback appearance; caused by osteoporosis in the vertebrae; also known as dowager's hump.

labeled amino acid an amino acid containing a radioactive atom; used to study amino acid and protein metabolism.

labeled trace mineral a trace mineral with a radioactive marker attached; used to study mineral absorption, metabolism, and excretion.

lactase enzyme that breaks down lactose into glucose and galactose.

lactobacillus a nonpathogenic bacteria normally found in the intestine that ferments lactose to lactic acid.

lactose intolerance inability to break down lactose because of a deficiency of the enzyme lactase.

laxative drug causing emptying of the bowel.

lean body mass (LBM) compartment of the body that includes all tissues (e.g., muscle, bone, water, visceral organs) except the fat contained in the adipose tissue; lean body mass does include the "essential fat," which refers to the fatty acids in membranes and other structural tissues.

leanness having a low amount of body fat but an appropriate amount of lean body tissue.

leukocyte a white blood cell that defends against bacteria and toxic substances.

leukopenia a below normal level of white blood cells.

leukotrienes compounds found in white blood cells that produce allergic and inflammatory reactions and are associated with development of rheumatoid arthritis.

levodopa drug used to treat Parkinson's disease.

life expectancy the number of years a person of a given age, sex, and race can be expected to live.

lingual lipase lipase secreted by the serous glands in the mouth.

linoleic acid an omega-6 fatty acid with 18 carbon atoms and 2 double bonds which cannot be synthesized by the body; the essential fatty acid.

linolenic acid an omega-3 fatty acid with 18 carbon atoms and 3 double bonds that is a substrate for the synthesis of eicosapentaenoic and docosahexaenoic acids.

lipase enzyme that breaks down triglycerides into fatty acids and glycerol.

lipoprotein lipase enzyme located on the inner surface of the blood vessels that hydrolyzes triglycerides in the chylomicrons and very low density lipoproteins and allows the fatty acids to enter the cells.

lipoprotein a molecule composed of protein and lipid; the form in which lipids are transported in the plasma.

long-term care facility a personal care home, boarding home, or nursing home that provides ongoing residential care for older people based on their personal or medical needs.

long-term care services or facilities that will maintain an older individual for a period of months or years.

longevity a long life (beyond that normally expected for a particular species).

longitudinal study a scientific study of changes occurring within the same individuals over time.

lordosis an increased curvature of the back; individual appears to be bent over.

low density lipoprotein (LDL) a plasma lipoprotein complex high in cholesterol content and believed to contribute to the development of atherosclerosis.

lutein a yellow-red carotenoid found in fruits, vegetables, and egg yolk.

lymph the clear fluid similar to plasma that is collected from body tissues and carried by the lymphatic vessels back to the venous circulation.

lymphocyte a type of white blood cell; includes the B cells and T cells.

macrocytic anemia blood disorder with impaired production of normal red blood cells and the presence of abnormally large red blood cells; usually related to vitamin B-12 or folate deficiency.

macromineral a mineral present in the body in substantial amounts (e.g., calcium, phosphorus).

macronutrient a nutrient required by the body in relatively large amounts; often used to refer to carbohydrate, protein, and fat.

macular degeneration damage to the macula, located in the center of the retina of the eye; results in a blurred area in the center of the visual image.

magnesium hydroxide the active ingredient in Milk of Magnesia, an over-the-counter drug used as a laxative and antacid.

magnesium a mineral required by the body that is found in bone mineral and is a necessary cofactor for many enzyme reactions, nerve transmission, and muscle contraction.

magnetic resonance imaging (MRI) an x-ray method used to determine body composition.

Maillard reaction chemical reaction between a carbohydrate and protein that denatures the protein.

malabsorption impaired absorption of one or more nutrients as a result of incomplete digestion, changes in the cells of the mucosa, pattern of nutrient intake, or disease.

mandible the lower jaw bone.

manganese a trace mineral required by the body that is a necessary cofactor for many enzyme reactions.

mastication chewing food; food also is mixed with saliva.

maximum oxygen consumption the greatest amount of oxygen that the cardiovascular system can transport from the lungs to the exercising muscles at any given time.

mean corpuscular volume (MCV) the average size of the red blood cells; used to diagnose anemia.

median the middle value in a distribution, with half of the values falling above and half below.

Medicaid program funded by state and federal dollars that provides medical assistance to low-income elderly; pays for doctor's fees and, in some states, other health services.

Medicare federal health insurance program for people age 65 and older who are eligible for Social Security; pays for hospitalization and doctor's fees.

metabolic alkalosis abnormal condition in which blood pH rises above 7.45; caused by an abnormal loss of acid or an increased level of bicarbonate or other basic compound.

metabolic efficiency relative gain in weight per unit of energy intake.

metabolic rate oxygen consumption per unit of body weight in a given period of time.

metalloenzyme enzyme with a mineral element as part of its structure.

metastasize the spread of cancer cells from one organ to another.

methionine an essential amino acid that contains sulfur.

methotrexate drug used to treat cancer.

3-methylhistidine an amino acid synthesized in the muscle; urinary 3-methylhistidine excretion is used to estimate total muscle mass.

methylmalonic acid a metabolite that accumulates in blood and urine in vitamin B-12 deficiency.

methylmalonyl coenzyme A an intermediary metabolite that is elevated in vitamin B-12 deficiency.

metoclopramide drug used to treat nausea and vomiting.

micelle a particle containing lipids and bile salts that moves fatty acids from the intestinal lumen to the intestinal mucosa for absorption.

microcytic hypochromic anemia anemia in which cells are small in size and contain below normal levels of hemoglobin.

micronutrient a nutrient such as a vitamin or trace mineral that is needed by the body in very small amounts.

microvascular relating to the capillaries.

mid-arm circumference the circumference of the arm taken halfway between the acromion and olecranon processes; used in the calculation of arm muscle circumference.

mid-arm muscle circumference used to assess protein and energy status; low muscle circumference indicates protein-energy malnutrition; mid-arm muscle area can be calculated using the mid-arm circumference and the triceps skinfold measurement.

milk-alkali syndrome a condition of alkalosis brought about by very excessive consumption of milk, calcium-containing antacids, or other alkaline substances; most likely to occur in older people with peptic ulcer.

Mini Nutritional Assessment Form a scoring system for evaluating nutritional risk in older adults based on food intake, anthropometric measurements, cognitive status, functional status, and prescription drug use.

mitogenic response a response to infectious bacteria or other foreign substance that involves increased cell division and activation of T cells.

modified diet diet developed for the alleviation or treatment of a physiological or medical problem that requires or restricts certain foods.

monoamine oxidase (MAO) inhibitor drug used to treat depression and anxiety; has a potentially dangerous interaction with foods high in tyramine (e.g., red wine, aged cheeses).

monoamine oxidase enzyme that oxidizes amines such as tyramine found in cheeses and red wine; these foods can cause headache and heart palpitations in people on monoamine oxidase inhibitor drugs.

monounsaturated fatty acid a fatty acid containing only one double bond (e.g., oleic acid).

monozygous identical twins coming from a single fertilized ovum.

morbidity illness or disease.

mortality rate the number of deaths per unit of population for a specific region, age group, or disease; usually expressed as deaths per 1,000, 10,000, or 100,000.

mortality ratio the total number of deaths among persons of a given sex or condition divided by the total number of individuals in the population.

mucin a mucopolysaccharide found in mucus that acts as a lubricant and protects the surface of the gastrointestinal tract.

mucopolysaccharide a compound comprised of protein and carbohydrate found in connective tissue, collagen, and bone matrix.

mucosa layer of epithelial cells that secrete mucus and line cavities of the body that open to the outside such as the mouth and digestive tract.

multi-infarct dementia loss of cognitive function because of damage to the brain by a cerebrovascular accident.

myasthenia gravis a nerve condition resulting in chronic fatigue and weakness of the muscles of the face and throat.

myelin a lipid-containing substance that forms a covering for the major nerves.

myocardial contractility the degree of strength of the heart contraction.

myocardial infarction heart attack; condition resulting from the occlusion of a coronary artery and interruption of the blood supply to cardiac tissue.

myocardial stimulation action of epinephrine or similar hormone or drug that increases the rate or strength of contraction of the heart muscle.

myocardium the muscle layer of the heart.

myoglobin the iron-protein molecule in the muscle that stores oxygen.

n-3 fatty acid see omega-3 fatty acid.

naproxen sodium a nonsteroidal anti-inflammatory drug (NSAID) now available without prescription.

narcotic drug that acts on the central nervous system to relieve pain and induce sleep.

National Aging Services Network network of area agencies on aging receiving funds under the Older Americans Act to provide nutrition, social, and support services to community-living older people.

National Center for Health Statistics Longitudinal Study of Aging a continuing follow-up study of older people who participated in the National Health Interview Survey.

National Cholesterol Education Program (NCEP) a program developed and implemented by the U.S. government to develop public awareness of the cardiovascular disease risk associated with elevated blood cholesterol levels and to implement intervention strategies

National Food Consumption Survey (NFCS) A survey conducted by the U.S. Department of Agriculture to determine the types and quantities of foods consumed and the nutrient intakes of the general population.

National Health and Nutrition Examination Survey (NHANES) a survey conducted by the U.S. government at regular intervals to determine the nutritional status and chronic disease risk of the general population.

National Health Interview Survey an ongoing survey conducted by the U.S. government to determine the health habits, utilization of health and medical services and facilities, extent of chronic and acute illnesses, prevalence of disability, and unmet needs for health care in the general population.

National Institutes of Health (NIH) a government agency made up of several divisions, including the National Cancer Institute, the National Heart, Lung and Blood Institute, and the National Institute on Aging, which all sponsor research and health promotion activities.

National Long-Term Care Survey a national study carried out by the U.S. government that provides information on nursing homes, the number of people cared for in nursing homes, their social, functional, and medical characteristics, and their length of care.

National Medical Expenditure Survey an ongoing survey conducted by the U.S. government to determine out-of-pocket expenses for health care and public and private insurance reimbursement for physicians' visits, hospital services, drugs, and related expenses.

negative nitrogen balance situation in which the amount of nitrogen consumed is less than the amount of nitrogen lost through all excretory routes, resulting in a net loss of body nitrogen.

neomycin drug used to treat infection.

neoplastic disease abnormal growth of cells forming tumors; cancer.

nephritis kidney disease resulting in some loss of function.

nephron the functional unit of the kidney that filters the blood plasma.

neuroendocrine relating to the functional interaction between the nervous system and the endocrine glands.

neuroleptic agent a drug that leads to an altered degree of consciousness with reduced anxiety and motor activity and indifference to surroundings.

neurologic relating to nerve function.

neuromuscular relating to nerves controlling muscle function.

neuropathy degenerative changes in the peripheral nerves often associated with diabetes mellitus.

neurotransmitter a chemical such as acetylcholine and norepinephrine that is released at the synapse of nerve cells and causes the transmission of nerve impulses.

neutron activation analysis an irradiation technique to determine body composition based on body content of particular mineral elements.

neutrophil a type of white blood cell that engulfs and destroys bacteria.

NHANES Epidemiologic Follow-Up Study (NHEFS) a study conducted by the U.S. government to reinterview NHANES participants and determine any changes in their nutrient intake, health status, and chronic disease risk factors.

niacin a water-soluble vitamin of the B complex that participates as a coenzyme in the breakdown and metabolism of carbohydrate, fat, and protein and the production of energy.

nicotinamide adenine dinucleotide phosphate (NADP) a coenzyme containing niacin that is required for energy metabolism; serves as an electron and hydrogen donor and receptor in the electron transport chain.

nicotinamide form of niacin.

nicotinic acid a form of niacin.

nitrogen retention positive nitrogen balance with a net increase in total body nitrogen.

nonambulatory unable to walk.

nonheme iron iron found in plant foods and in animal tissues other than hemoglobin or myoglobin.

non-insulin-dependent diabetes mellitus (NIDDM) type of diabetes mellitus resulting from a reduced output of insulin by the beta islets of the pancreas and the reduced effectiveness of insulin in moving glucose into muscle and adipose cells.

nonsteroidal anti-inflammatory drug (NSAID) type of drug used to treat osteoarthritis and rheumatoid arthritis; available over-the-counter as ibuprofen.

nonulcer dyspepsia discomfort in the abdomen after eating, caused by unknown factors, not an ulcer.

nootropic drug drug that improves cognitive function used to treat senile dementia of the Alzheimer type.

norepinephrine hormone produced by the adrenal medulla that increases blood pressure by constricting the blood vessels.

normotensive having normal blood pressure.

nursing facility a facility providing health and personal care under the supervision of a physician to residents with medical problems who require a high level of skilled nursing care.

nutrient dense foods foods that contain protein, vitamins, or minerals in a percentage of the RDA equal to or above the percentage of kilocalories provided.

nutrient density see nutrient dense foods.

nutrition education providing individuals or groups with practical information to assist in meal planning and food selection for optimum nutrition.

nutrition survey collecting nutrition information such as food intake, anthropometric data, or biochemical data from particular population groups to determine their nutritional status.

nutritional anemia anemia caused by a lack of a particular nutrient such as iron, vitamin B-12, or folate.

nutritional risk having a high probability of poor nutritional status or inadequate nutrient intake.

nutritional status the nutritional health of an individual as determined by past and present intakes of protein, fat, carbohydrate, vitamins, and minerals, and related health and physiological factors; evaluation must be based on dietary, clinical, biochemical, and anthropometric measurements.

obesity having an excessive amount of body fat.

obligatory nitrogen loss the lowest level of nitrogen excretion that can be reached by an individual on a protein-free diet.

occult blood concealed or hidden; not easily observed; often refers to blood in the stool.

occupational therapist a certified professional who plans activities to assist the impaired individual (who may have experienced illness or injury) in regaining self-feeding, food preparation, or other motor skills.

Older Americans Act the major piece of federal legislation providing nutrition and social services for noninstitutionalized people age 60 and over.

oldest-old people age 85 and older.

oleic acid a monounsaturated fatty acid having one double bond.

olfactory function sharpness of the sense of smell.

omega-3 fatty acid a polyunsaturated fatty acid that has its first double bond after the sixth carbon from the methyl end; is found in fish and is believed to prevent blood platelet aggregation and retard the progression of vascular disease.

omega-6 fatty acid a polyunsaturated fatty acid that has its first double bond after the third carbon from the methyl end; includes linoleic acid, alpha linolenic acid, and arachidonic acid.

Omnibus Budget Reconciliation Act of 1987 (OBRA) law that set standards for rights of nursing home residents and requirements for optimum nutrition and efforts toward rehabilitation, including self-feeding.

omnivore an individual who consumes both plant and animal foods.

oophorectomy surgical removal of the ovaries.

oral antidiabetic agent a drug taken by mouth for treatment of non-insulin-dependent diabetes mellitus; these drugs stimulate pancreatic secretion of insulin.

oral glucose tolerance test test to evaluate the body's ability to metabolize carbohydrate and diagnose the presence of diabetes mellitus; a standard amount of glucose is given by mouth and blood glucose levels are measured for two to three hours following.

oral consumed by mouth.

organic brain disease brain disorder related to a physiologic change or injury in brain cells

organic brain syndrome change in behavior or cognitive function caused by a physiological alteration such as loss of brain cells, cerebral arteriosclerosis, or decreased synthesis of neurotransmitters.

orthostatic hypotension abnormally low blood pressure that occurs when a person stands up.

osmolality the osmotic pressure exerted by a solution expressed on the basis of the number of ions or particles per kg of water or solvent.

osmoreceptor nerve cell in the hypothalamus sensitive to the concentration of electrolytes or molecules in the blood.

osmotic cathartic cathartic that induces bowel emptying by drawing water into the large intestine and diluting intestinal contents; magnesium hydroxide acts this way.

osmotic diarrhea a diarrhea resulting from an accumulation of a nonabsorbable sugar such as mannitol that causes large amounts of water to move into the large intestine.

osmotic diuresis increased excretion of water resulting from a substance present in the renal tubule at a level that is too high to be effectively reabsorbed (e.g., glucose or urea).

osmotic pressure the pressure that must be exerted to prevent particles or solute from drawing fluid across a semipermeable membrane.

osteoarthritis localized degenerative changes in the joints resulting in pain, swelling, and often some degree of disability.

osteoblast a cell that synthesizes bone matrix and assists in the deposit of mineral to form new bone.

osteoclast a cell that dissolves bone mineral and removes remaining matrix in the resorption of bone.

osteomalacia adult rickets; bone disorder in which mineral but not matrix is lost from the bone.

osteopenia bone mass falling between 1 and 2.5 standard deviations below the mean value for young adults.

osteoporosis a bone disorder occurring in older individuals leading to loss of bone mineral and matrix, loss of bone strength, and increased risk of bone fracture.

osteoporotic bone disease see osteoporosis.

out-of-pocket having to pay the costs of medical or health services from personal funds.

over-the-counter (OTC) drug available without a prescription.

oxalate compounds found in spinach and various other vegetables that bind divalent cations, such as calcium and iron, and prevent their absorption.

pancreas organ in the abdominal cavity that secretes glucagon (alpha islets), insulin (beta islets), and digestive enzymes.

pancreatic insufficiency inadequate secretion of pancreatic hormones or enzymes as a result of physiologic deterioration or disease.

pancreatic lipase enzyme contained in the pancreatic juice that breaks down dietary fats to glycerol and fatty acids; flow stimulated by the presence of food in the duodenum.

para-aminohippuric acid substance actively secreted into the urine by the kidney; used to measure total plasma flow through the kidney.

para-aminosalicylic acid drug used to treat tuberculosis.

paralysis loss of muscle function.

parathyroid hormone (PTH) controls the calcium level in the blood.

parenteral feeding providing nutrients by a route other than through the gastrointestinal tract; usually refers to intravenous delivery of glucose, amino acids, vitamins, and minerals.

parietal cell cells lining the stomach that produce hydrochloric acid.

Parkinson's disease a neurologic disorder occurring in people above age 60 characterized by tremors, muscle weakness and rigidity, and a shuffling gait.

parotid glands the largest pair of the salivary glands.

passive absorption/reabsorption absorption occurring by diffusion; not energy-requiring.

penicillamine drug that binds with and removes minerals from the blood; acts as an anti-inflammatory agent and is used to treat rheumatoid arthritis.

pepsinogen protein secreted by the chief cells in the gastric mucosa that is converted to pepsin in the presence of gastric acid.

peptic ulcer a loss of the protective mucous membrane in an area of the stomach or duodenum as a result of excessive acid production, stress, or certain drugs.

perceived health benefit an individual's impression of the value of a particular behavior in developing or maintaining good health.

periodontal disease inflammation of tissues around the teeth; can result in loosening and loss of teeth and damage to the jaw bone.

peripheral neuropathy a functional disorder affecting the motor or sensory nerves outside of the brain and spinal cord; can be a complication of diabetes or a particular vitamin deficiency.

peripheral relating to the areas of the body outside of the viscera.

pernicious anemia an anemia characterized by immature macrocytic red blood cells and accompanied by the deterioration of neural tissues; caused by a lack of intrinsic factor necessary for normal absorption of vitamin B-12.

peroxidation the addition of an oxygen atom at a double bond in an unsaturated fatty acid; can occur in the body or in a foodstuff.

personal care home a facility that provides room, board, and supervision for older people but no medical or health services.

pH a measure of the concentration of hydrogen ions in a solution; 7.0 is neutral, a value above 7.0 is alkaline, and a value below 7.0 is acid.

phagocyte a cell that can surround and digest bacteria or dead cells.

phagocytosis process by which cells of the immune system surround, enclose, and digest microorganisms, cell debris, or foreign matter.

pharmacodynamics the study of how drugs act in a living person and the relationship between drug dosage and the observed response.

pharmacokinetics the study of the absorption, metabolism, and excretion of drugs and the duration of activity.

pharynx the throat.

phenobarbitol a drug that acts as a sedative and anticonvulsant by depressing the activity of the central nervous system.

phenolphthalein a laxative that increases the motor activity of the lower intestinal tract.

phenothiazine drugs a family of drugs used to control psychotic behavior.

phenytoin drug used to prevent seizures or convulsions.

phosphorus a mineral required by the body which along with calcium makes up bone mineral; is essential for glycolysis and the metabolism of carbohydrate and formation of high energy molecules (adenosine triphosphate).

phylloquinone vitamin K.

Physician's Desk Reference (P.D.R.) a reference book published annually containing information supplied by manufacturers regarding drugs used in the United States.

phytate phosphoric acid compounds found in grains that bind iron, magnesium, and other divalent cations and prevent their absorption.

picture-sort method using pictures of food portions to assist older people in providing information about their food intake patterns.

plasma amino acid response curve a method for determining the requirement for a specific amino acid.

plasma pyridoxal phosphate the blood level of plasma pyridoxal phosphate is sometimes used as a measure of vitamin B-6 status.

plasma the fluid portion of the blood.

plasminogen activator a molecule that can promote the formation of small blood clots by acting on fibrinogen to form fibrin.

platelet aggregation the joining together of blood platelets in response to an injury in the blood vessel; the first step in forming a blood clot.

pneumonia infectious disease of the lungs in which the airways and alveoli fill with fluid, making breathing and gas exchange difficult.

polydipsia excessive thirst; classic sign of diabetes mellitus.

polypharmacy use of a number of drugs at one time.

polyphenols a group of substances that occur in tea and interfere with the absorption of iron and possibly other minerals.

polyunsaturated fatty acid fatty acid with more than one double bond.

polyuria excessive amounts of urine; classic sign of diabetes mellitus.

positive nitrogen balance situation in which the amount of dietary nitrogen consumed exceeds the amount of nitrogen excreted by all routes leading to a net gain in body nitrogen.

postmenopausal osteoporosis (Type 1) osteoporosis resulting from loss of bone mass that occurs after menopause and estrogen withdrawal.

postmenopausal after menopause.

postprandial plasma glucose plasma glucose level after a meal; a two-hour postprandial plasma glucose is used in diagnosis of impaired glucose tolerance or diabetes mellitus.

postprandial after eating.

potassium salts potassium chloride is used as a substitute for table salt (sodium chloride) by those wishing to reduce their sodium intake; is also used as a potassium supplement.

potassium sparing diuretic type of diuretic that does not increase loss of body potassium.

poverty income ratio a measure of the income status of an individual or family relative to the minimum income needed to meet basic needs as determined by the federal government; a value of < I indicates poverty status.

poverty level the minimum income required to provide the basic necessities of food, clothing, and shelter as determined by the federal government.

prealbumin a plasma transport protein with a short half-life used as an indicator of protein status.

preformed vitamin A form of vitamin A present in animal foods.

premature menopause menopause occurring at a young age because of removal of the ovaries or other medical reason.

premenopausal prior to menopause.

presbyesophagus loss of elasticity of the esophagus interfering with the movement of food down the passageway.

prescribed diet see modified diet.

pressure ulcer ulcer occurring over a bony prominence from continued pressure on the tissue covering the bone; occurs in people confined to chair or bed who change position infrequently; also called decubitus ulcer.

preventive health efforts to reduce chronic disease and disability through appropriate lifestyle practices, optimum nutrition, and regular physical examinations and treatment.

pro re nata (PRN) Latin term used in prescription writing that means "as the occasion arises."

probability sample determined by a multistaged selection method designed to achieve the target number of sample persons by age, sex, race, and ethnicity and used in the National Health and Nutrition Examination Survey and the Continuing Survey on Food Intakes by Individuals.

progression process in which a cell undergoes more than one mutation to become a cancer cell.

proliferative capacity the ability of cells to multiply.

promotion the second step in the development of cancer; a carcinogen or chemical agent acts on a genetically altered cell to stimulate uncontrolled growth.

propranolol drug used to lower blood pressure and control cardiac arrhythmias.

prospective payment system payment system based on the diagnostic related groups (DRGs) in which hospitals are reimbursed by Medicare according to the procedures and days of care considered to be necessary for the treatment of a particular condition.

prospective a study designed to examine the relationship between a particular illness or disease and a specific habit or environmental factor, such as diet or smoking; healthy subjects are recruited for study and observed over time to determine the rate at which the disease develops.

prostaglandin substance found in many tissues that acts on smooth muscle and causes vasoconstriction, vasodilation, and increased muscle contraction in the intestinal tract.

protease enzyme that breaks peptide bonds.

protein turnover the continuous process of protein breakdown and synthesis occurring in the body.

protein-energy malnutrition (PEM) a condition resulting from a deficiency in both kilocalories and protein.

psychotherapeutic drugs drugs used to treat personality or mental disorders such as anxiety, depression, or paranoia.

psychotropic agents drugs that affect behavior or mental activity.

psyllium natural seed fiber used in bulk-forming laxative preparations and in treating constipation.

pteroylglutamic acid folic acid.

pteroylpolyglutamate hydrolase enzyme the enzyme that breaks down pteroylpolyglutamic acid

to pteroylmonoglutamic acid so it can be absorbed; these are forms of folate.

pteroylpolyglutamic acid the form of folate that occurs naturally in food.

pulmonary embolism blockage of an artery in the lung by air, a blood clot, or an atherosclerotic particle.

pureed food food blended to the consistency of a smooth thick liquid.

pyridoxal kinase enzyme that transfers a phosphate group to the pyridoxine molecule to form pyridoxal phosphate.

pyridoxal phosphate (PLP) a coenzyme containing vitamin B-6 that is necessary for transamination reactions; plasma PLP levels are used as an indicator of vitamin B-6 status.

quality assurance an evaluation of nutrition and health services provided and the results achieved as compared to accepted standards.

quinidine drug used to prevent fibrillation of the atria and rapid heart beat.

receptor sensitivity the ability of a receptor to respond to a stimulus or recognize a substance such as a hormone or antigen that must bind to it.

receptor site a chemical structure on the cell membrane where a hormone or antigen binds.

Recommended Dietary Allowances (RDAs) the level of intake of an essential nutrient considered to be adequate to meet the daily needs of practically all healthy people of a particular age, sex, or condition.

red cell folate is highly correlated with liver folate stores and used as an indicator of folate status.

redox agent a molecule that can accept or donate electrons and acts as an antioxidant.

refined grains grain foods from which the bran has been removed with loss of fiber and micronutrients.

reflux backward flow of stomach contents into the esophagus.

regression analysis a method of statistical analysis that considers the value of one variable in relation to the value of other variables related to it.

relative weight the body weight of an individual divided by the average or desirable body weight of people of the same height, sex, and age.

renal 1-α-hydroxylase enzyme in the kidney that converts 25-hydroxyvitamin D to 1,25-dihydroxyvitamin D, the active form of vitamin D.

renal insufficiency inability of the kidney to excrete waste materials and conserve water, electrolytes, and other important molecules to the extent needed.

renal tubular reabsorption the reabsorption by the kidney of water, glucose, vitamins, and electrolytes from the glomerular filtrate.

renal tubular secretion the energy-requiring elimination of ions or molecules by the kidney (e.g., H$^+$, drug metabolites).

renin-angiotensin-aldosterone system enzyme-hormonal feedback system that controls blood pressure through the reabsorption and excretion of water and sodium.

renin an enzyme produced in the kidney in response to low blood pressure; it causes the formation of angiotensin.

reserve capacity the ability of an organ system to adjust to an increased need that may rise from physiologic stress or disease.

residual lung volume air remaining in the lungs after the individual has exhaled.

resorption (bone) the loss of bone matrix and mineral.

respondent-assessed health respondents are asked to rate their health as excellent, good, fair, or poor; physical examinations or assessment by a health professional do not occur.

resting cardiac output amount of blood pumped per minute when the individual is resting quietly.

resting energy expenditure (REE) the amount of energy required to maintain essential body processes when the individual is at rest and neither perspiring nor shivering; differs from basal metabolism in that the individual has not fasted and the measurement may include the thermic effect of food.

restricted diets diets used in the treatment of chronic diseases that limit energy, fat, sodium, or carbohydrate intake.

reticuloendothelial cells cells lining the blood vessels that attack virus and bacteria and produce antibodies against foreign molecules.

retinol equivalent unit of measure of vitamin A; 1 retinol equivalent equals 1 μg of retinol or 6 μg of beta carotene.

retinol-binding protein a protein that transports retinol in the plasma and is sometimes used as an indicator of protein status.

retinol the form of vitamin A with the highest biological activity.

retinyl ester form in which vitamin A is stored in the liver.

rheumatoid arthritis a chronic, systemic, inflammatory disease resulting in swelling of the joints, destruction of the cartilage, and muscle atrophy.

rickets a bone disorder occurring in growing children in which bone matrix is not mineralized because of a lack of vitamin D and failure to absorb calcium.

roughage older term for foods high in fiber.

salicylic acid precursor for a family of drugs used to relieve pain, reduce fever, and control inflammation.

sarcopenia abnormally low amount of muscle mass.

SCALES a scoring system to identify older people at nutritional risk; criteria are sadness, serum cholesterol, serum albumin, loss of weight, and problems with eating and shopping.

sebaceous glands glands in the skin that secrete oil that prevents drying of the skin.

Second National Health and Nutrition Examination Survey (NHANES II) a survey conducted between 1976 and 1980 by the U.S. government to determine the nutritional status and chronic disease risk of the general population.

secondary not the major or usual cause of a disorder but the result of an associated factor or disorder.

secretin a hormone secreted by the upper small intestine in response to foods containing fatty acids; it stimulates the secretion of pancreatic enzymes and bile.

secular changes changes related to the passage of time.

sedative drug used to induce sleep or reduce anxiety.

selenium a trace mineral required by the body that is a cofactor for glutathione reductase, an enzyme that acts as an antioxidant to prevent the formation of free radicals.

senescence the process of growing old.

senile dementia of the Alzheimer type (SDAT) degenerative brain disease occurring beyond middle age and resulting in loss of memory, cognitive function, and speech and changes in behavior.

senile dementia loss of mental and cognitive function occurring in extreme old age; believed to result from atrophy and changes in cells in the brain.

senile osteoporosis (Type 2) osteoporosis resulting from aging changes in the ability to convert vitamin D to its active form, resulting in lower calcium absorption.

senna extract a type of cathartic that increases motor activity in the lower intestine.

serotonin reuptake inhibitor drug used to treat depression.

serotonin a neurotransmitter derived from tryptophan.

serum albumin used as a measure of protein status and visceral protein stores; levels below 35 g/l are less than optimum.

serum aspartate aminotransferase enzyme the blood level of this enzyme increases after a myocardial infarction; increased levels also indicate liver damage or dysfunction.

serum osmolality the osmotic pressure of the serum which is based on the number of molecules or ions it contains.

serum triglycerides blood fats; elevated serum triglycerides are associated with increased risk of cardiovascular disease.

sickle cell disease a genetic disorder causing synthesis of an abnormal hemoglobin and production of crescent-shaped and fragile red blood cells.

single room occupancy older people living in inner city hotels that provide a small sleeping area but no other services or supervision.

skinfold calipers an instrument used to measure the thickness of a skinfold as an indicator of the level of body fat.

skinfold compressibility the degree to which the skinfold is pressed together when grasped with the skinfold caliper; an increase in connective tissue will decrease compressibility.

skinfold thickness the width of a skinfold as measured with a skinfold caliper.

Social Security a federal government insurance system that provides income payments to retired people age 65 and over based on their income while still employed; a major source of income for retired people in the U.S.

socially impaired individuals with behavioral or psychological problems relating to alcoholism, mental illness, organic brain disease, or the mental and emotional stress related to homelessness.

sodium-induced hypertension sensitivity of some individuals to develop hypertension as a result of excessive sodium intakes.

sodium a mineral required by the body; it is the principal cation in the extracellular fluid and is involved in body fluid regulation, acid-base balance, nerve transmission, and muscle contraction; excessive dietary sodium is related to high blood pressure in sensitive people.

soft diet diet soft in texture that requires only limited chewing; includes custards, ground meat, well-cooked vegetables and fruits that are not fibrous or stringy.

soluble fiber components of pectins and gums found in fruits, oats, and legumes that reduce the rate of gastric emptying, have water holding properties, increase fecal bulk, and contribute to the lowering of serum cholesterol levels.

somatic mutation a change in the genetic material of a body cell leading to synthesis of defective proteins; theory of how aging occurs.

somatomedin C see insulin-like growth factor.

somatostatin a hormone produced in the hypothalamus that inhibits the release of somatotropin (growth hormone releasing hormone) from the anterior pituitary and the release of adrenocorticotrophic hormone, glucagon, insulin, cholecystokinin, secretin, and gastrin.

spastic colon increased or uncontrolled contractions of the colon; irritable bowel syndrome.

special diet see modified diet.

speech-language pathologist person with training in speech and language disorders and organs involved with speech; can assess and assist with swallowing problems.

splanchnic blood flow see splanchnic blood perfusion.

splanchnic blood perfusion blood flow to the visceral organs, including the liver, heart, lungs, kidneys, and digestive organs.

staple foods foods that are consumed regularly and provide a major portion of an individual's nutrient intake on a daily basis.

stearic acid saturated fatty acid found in many animal fats.

stem cell an immature cell that has the potential to develop into one of several different mature cells.

sterol large molecule with a ring structure and carbon side chain; cholesterol and cholecalciferol are sterols.

stimulant laxative substance that induces emptying of the bowel by irritating the intestinal mucosa which increases peristalsis; phenolphthalein acts this way.

stomatitis inflammation or soreness of the mouth.

streptococci bacteria causing infections such as pneumonia or urinary infections.

stroke volume the amount of blood ejected from the heart with each contraction.

stroke loss of blood supply to a part of the brain caused by a blockage or rupture of a blood vessel.

Strong Heart Dietary Survey a dietary survey conducted by the Indian Health Service on American Indian adults, ages 45 to 74, living in South Dakota, Arizona, and Oklahoma; 24-hour recalls and food frequency questionnaires were obtained.

subcutaneous fat fat located directly under the skin.

successful aging the prevention or amelioration of physiologic aging through positive health practices such as an appropriate diet, regular physical exercise, avoidance of cigarette smoking, and no or limited use of alcohol.

succinyl coenzyme A an intermediate compound in the citric acid cycle.

sulfonylurea an oral antidiabetic agent that stimulates production of insulin by the pancreas.

superoxide dimutase an enzyme that acts as an antioxidant in destroying free radicals.

supine lying on the back.

support services medical, health, personal, or home management services provided to older people in their homes to delay or prevent institutionalization.

surfactant lipoproteins that reduce the surface tension of the fluid in the lungs and promote gas exchange.

swivel spoon a spoon with a link in the middle of the handle that allows the bowl of the spoon to move from side to side.

sympathetic nervous system component of the autonomic nervous system that increases the heart rate, constricts the blood vessels, and raises blood pressure.

synapse the area between two nerve cells.

systemic circulation movement of the blood throughout the arteries and veins of the entire body and back to the heart.

systolic blood pressure the blood pressure when the heart muscle contracts and blood is being ejected from the heart; systolic pressure is usually higher than diastolic pressure.

T-cells activated white blood cells that attack fungi, viruses, and tumors; responsible for cell mediated immunity.

tachycardia rapid heart beat (over 100 beats per minute).

taste acuity the sharpness of perception of the basic tastes: sweet, salty, bitter, sour.

taste threshold the lowest concentration of a flavor or taste that can be detected.

testosterone the male sex hormone secreted by the testes.

tetracycline drug used to treat infections.

theophylline (xanthine derivative bronchodilator) increases the diameter of the bronchi; used in the treatment of asthma and emphysema.

therapeutic index the difference between the minimum therapeutic dose and the minimum toxic dose of a drug.

thermal buffer physiologic mechanism to avoid fluctuations in body temperature (e.g., body fluids can absorb or give off heat).

thermic effect of food (TEF) energy expended in the digestion, absorption, and metabolism of ingested food.

thiamin pyrophosphate (TPP) a coenzyme containing thiamin that is necessary for decarboxylation reactions and the transketolase pathway forming five carbon sugars.

thiamin a water-soluble vitamin of the B complex; a necessary cofactor for the breakdown of carbohydrates and for normal cardiovascular and nerve function; alcohol interferes with absorption of thiamin.

thiazide diuretic type of diuretic associated with urinary loss of potassium and sodium and urinary conservation of calcium.

thioridazine hydrochloride used to treat mental disorders and depression in the elderly.

Third National Health and Nutrition Examination Survey (NHANES III) a survey conducted between 1988 and 1991 by the U.S. government to determine the nutritional status and chronic disease risk of the general population.

thrombocytopenia an abnormally low level of blood platelets needed for normal blood clotting.

thrombosis a blood clot attached to the wall of a blood vessel that may occlude the flow of blood.

thyroid hormone hormone secreted by the thyroid gland that controls the rate of metabolism in the cell and influences cardiac function, mental function, and muscle tone.

thyroid stimulating hormone (TSH) a substance released by the anterior lobe of the pituitary that causes the thyroid gland to release thyroid hormone.

thyroxin (T_4) hormone produced by the thyroid gland that controls the metabolic rate of body cells.

tinnitus ringing in the ears.

Title III nutrition program the program funded by the Older Americans Act that provides for the implementation of congregate and home-delivered meals for people age 60 and over.

Title III section of the Older Americans Act that provides funds for congregate and home-delivered meals for the general population age 60 and older.

Title VI section of the Older Americans Act that provides funds for congregate and home-delivered meals for Alaskans, Hawaiians, and Native Americans age 60 and older.

tocopherol equivalent basis for expressing the vitamin E activity of compounds as compared to the activity of 1 mg of alpha tocopherol.

tolazamide an oral antidiabetic drug.

tolbutamide an oral antidiabetic agent used in management of non-insulin-dependent diabetes mellitus.

total body water (TBW) includes all the water in the intracellular and extracellular body compartments.

total energy expenditure (TEE) total energy cost for an individual including energy required for basal metabolism, the thermic effect of food, and physical activity.

total lymphocyte count (TLC) used as an indicator of protein and energy status and immune function.

total meal cost the total cost of providing a congregate or home-delivered meal, including food, packaging, labor, delivery, and administrative costs.

toxicity degree to which a substance is harmful or poisonous; a substance such as a drug or vitamin may have a positive effect at low levels but be poisonous at high levels.

trabecular bone spongy bone with a lattice-like structure found in the ends of the long bones and the vertebrae.

trace elements minerals present in the body in very small amounts.

transaminase enzyme that transfers amino groups and requires vitamin B-6 as a coenzyme.

transferrin receptor location on the transferrin molecule that binds iron.

transferrin saturation the relative proportion of transferrin in the blood that is combined with an iron molecule.

transferrin the transport protein for iron.

transketolase activity red blood cell transketolase activity is used as a measure of thiamin status.

transketolase an enzyme essential in carbohydrate metabolism that requires thiamin as a coenzyme.

transthyretin a transport protein for thyroxin; below-normal levels may indicate protein-energy malnutrition.

tricyclic antidepressant drug such as imipramine or amitriptyline that has a three ring structure; used to treat depression.

triglyceride the primary form of fat found in food and the storage form of fat in the body; it is made up of three fatty acids joined to one molecule of glycerol.

triiodothyronine (T_3) a form of thyroid hormone; arises from the metabolism of thyroxine (T_4) in the tissues.

tryptophan load test test used to evaluate vitamin B-6 status.

tryptophan an essential amino acid; is used in the synthesis of serotonin.

tuberculosis chronic infection of the lungs with accumulation of cell masses and connective tissue that interfere with air passage and gas exchange.

type 1 muscle fiber (slow twitch fiber) muscle fibers that perform extended repetitive motions and are slow to fatigue; endurance runners have a high proportion of slow twitch muscle fibers.

type 2 muscle fiber (fast twitch fibers) muscle fibers that perform short, rapid motions and become fatigued rapidly; sprinting, jumping, and weight-lifting are activities that use fast twitch fibers.

tyramine an amino acid that can be synthesized in the body from tyrosine that stimulates the release of epinephrine and norepinephrine; also found in various food products, including aged cheeses and red wine.

tyrosine hydroxylase enzyme necessary for the synthesis of epinephrine and serotonin.

tyrosine an amino acid used to synthesize epinephrine.

U.S. Recommended Daily Allowance (USRDA) standards for daily nutrient intake that were developed by the Food and Drug Administration for use on nutrition labels but are no longer used.

undernutrition condition characterized by an insufficient level of kilocalories and/or protein, vitamins, and minerals.

unintentional weight loss loss of weight occurring without a deliberate dietary or exercise modification; unwanted weight loss.

U.S. Pharmacopeia Dispensing Information (U.S.P.D.I.) a reference recognized officially by the Food and Drug Administration that contains descriptions, uses, strengths, and standards of purity for selected drugs.

unsaturated fatty acids this reaction occurs in the body and in foods containing fats and oils.

urinary creatinine the amount of creatinine excreted in the urine is related to body muscle mass; a 24-hour urinary creatinine measurement can be used to estimate total muscle mass and body composition.

usual aging the normal physiologic and biologic changes occurring as a result of aging but uncomplicated by chronic disease.

vasoconstrictor agent that causes the blood vessels to decrease in diameter.

vasodilator agent that causes blood vessels to increase in diameter.

vasopressin less common name for antidiuretic hormone (ADH).

vegan an individual who consumes no food of animal origin.

very low calorie diet diet used for weight loss that contains only 400 to 800 kcal; should be used only under strict medical supervision.

very low carbohydrate diet popular but dangerous diet for weight loss that leads to high losses of body fluids, protein, and electrolytes; contains little (less than 50 g) or no carbohydrate.

very low density lipoprotein (VLDL) a plasma lipoprotein with a high content of triglycerides.

visceral fat see abdominal fat.

visceral organs organs found in the abdominal cavity (e.g., heart, liver, kidney, spleen, digestive organs).

visceral proteins the proteins synthesized in the liver, including albumin, transferrin, and retinol-binding proteins.

vitamin B-12 water-soluble vitamin required for maintenance and function of the nerves and maturation of the red blood cells; deficiency results in pernicious anemia.

vitamin D a fat-soluble vitamin necessary for the absorption of calcium and development of normal bone; it can be synthesized in the skin when directly exposed to sunlight.

waist-to-hip ratio waist circumference divided by the hip circumference; a higher ratio is associated with greater abdominal fat (male pattern) and higher risk of chronic disease; a lower ratio is associated with greater fat in the hip region (female pattern) and lower disease risk.

warfarin drug that prevents blood clotting.

wasting disease a disease or syndrome that leads to weight loss, loss of appetite, and lack of energy for physical activity; examples are cancer and cardiac cachexia.

water miscible substance that can be mixed with water.

whole grains grain foods from which the bran has not been removed.

x-ray absorptiometry method used to evaluate bone density.

xanthurenic acid a metabolite of tryptophan that is present at high levels in the urine of vitamin B-6 deficient people.

xerostomia dry mouth; abnormally low secretion of salivary fluids.

young-old people between the ages of 65 and 74.

zeaxanthin a yellow carotenoid found in corn, fruits, and egg yolk.

zinc a trace mineral required by the body that is a cofactor for many important enzymes and participates in protein and DNA metabolism, wound-healing, immune function, and taste.

Index